The Healing Hand
Man and Wound in the Ancient World

Harvard University Press
Cambridge, Massachusetts
London, England

Guido Majno

The Healing Hand

Man and Wound in

the Ancient World

Copyright © 1975 by the President and Fellows of Harvard College
All rights reserved
Printed in the United States of America
10 9 8 7 6 5 4

First Harvard University Press paperback edition, 1991

Library of Congress Catalog Card Number 74-80730
ISBN 0-674-38330-3 (cloth)
ISBN 0-674-38331-1 (paper)

To my generous wife
who for ten years
never quite knew
whether I was there
or somewhere
around 400 B.C.

Preface

Ten years ago, my wife and I went to an afternoon party in a lovely garden near Boston. As the crowd gathered, our host came searching for me. "You know," he said, "since you are planning to write a history of the wound, you really ought to come and talk to Dr. Churchill." I knew Dr. Churchill, one of Boston's prominent surgeons in the Grand Old Tradition. So I told him about my project. He took one step back, raised his glass, and said, after an ominous pause: "Young man"—I was forty-three— "I have been trying that for thirty years. It can't be done."

He was probably right. A complete history of the wound would be difficult to write and impossible to read. It would have to cover all of surgery, much about wars and warfare, and the history of mankind altogether.

This book is far less ambitious. It is not even, strictly speaking, a medical book; I tried to write it plainly enough for anyone who would care to read it. In fact, I wrote it by accident. It was going to be the preface to a monograph on inflammation, which is more properly my field, and the preface took over.

The jump from inflammation to wounds, and from biology to history, was short. Most inflammations are the result of infection, and infection has always been a central issue in wound care. Ultimately, Lister's great crusade against bacteria was fought around wounds.

There are other reasons for being fascinated by the history of wounds. In ancient texts, diseases in general are difficult or impossible to recognize. What is, for instance, the *aaa* disease mentioned in the Egyptian papyri? Perhaps schistosomiasis, but nobody really knows. Wounds, instead, are always wounds: they speak right out of the page. The problems of the patients, as of those who attend them, are obvious.

And then, long before the birth of anything that could be called experimental medicine, wounds also functioned as natural experiments, multiplied millions of times. They were treated with dressings, and in the long run the better dressings stood out. In this permanent battle between man and bacteria, it is thrilling to watch the birth of the first antiseptics, coupled with the history of wine, copper, honey, myrrh, and many other plant drugs and resins. In this sense, the wound was the first medical laboratory.

Besides infection, wounds have raised a series of problems, biological as well as human. Why do they bleed? Is there anything good about the bleeding? Does it have anything to do with pus, and how can one stop it? Can wounds be used as windows, to study live organs inside? What is the flesh made of? And for the historian, if a patient in any given place and time sought help from a physician, what were his chances of actually being helped? What did the physician do, why did he do it, and could it possibly work?

Because I am primarily interested in sick people, I have paid a great deal of attention to this last problem: trying to find out whether the patients were made better, or worse, by the treatment. In this respect, the medical writer can help the lay reader as well as the classical scholar, for the answers are usually buried in obscure drug names and cryptic medical explanations.

I have tried to find answers within the perspective of the time. This could not be done without a broad historical framework. The syringe, for instance, was invented in Alexandria, and its first medical use seems to have been on wounds. But to understand why this happened just in Alexandria required an excursion beyond the field of medicine.

My "patients," those whom you will meet in these pages, come from all parts of the ancient world, including China. In a recent treatise on the history of medicine, China was not even mentioned—silence was preferred to misinformation. But today, Joseph Needham's *Science and Civilisation in China* provides that guide to Chinese literature which had earlier been missing. So, with the courage of the amateur, I have dealt also with China.

This is my first experience with history, and I found it, from the point of view of the scientist, thoroughly exciting, yet often frustrating. Scientists like to run experiments and modify nature. Here all the experiments had been done, the records had not been well kept, and practically all the authors had died. To make up for the uncertainties, I chose some problems that could be tested in the laboratory and actually attempted some "experimental history," mainly with antibacterial drugs. These were most rewarding efforts.

I must also mention here a happy coincidence. As the last chapters were being completed, we happened to discover in our laboratory one of the basic mechanisms in healing a wound: the mechanism that draws one lip of the wound toward the other and closes the gap. I hope it is a good omen.

A history of the wound is necessarily born of untold human suffering. May this book be a drop in the sea of human understanding.

Acknowledgments

This book is the gift of hundreds of people. During the past eight years I have knocked at so many doors, and sent out so many calls for help, that I could not possibly acknowledge all my debts. The following list includes my major benefactors; others will be mentioned in the text and notes; to all, including my friends, colleagues, correspondents not mentioned here by name, I wish to express my perennial gratitude.

Financial support. It was Dr. George P. Berry, former Dean of Harvard Medical School, who made me realize that I would never succeed without substantial bibliographic help. This was made possible through a generous grant from the Commonwealth Fund of New York; my former chief, Dr. Arthur T. Hertig, Dean Berry, and Dean Robert H. Ebert, assisted me in obtaining it. When this grant ran out, the Société Académique de Genève came to my rescue. The experimental work was supported incidentally by research grants that I held while at Harvard Medical School (mainly from the National Institutes of Health) and in Switzerland (from the Fonds National Suisse pour la Recherche Scientifique and from Zyma S. A., Nyon); the Honey Industry Council of America, and Hood and Sons, Inc., Boston, supported specific projects.

Bibliographic assistants. Mrs. Ann M. Barry was the pioneer, courageous enough to get me under way when the book was merely a gleam in the eye. Mrs. Marie-Louise Bowditch was a jewel of insight and competence. Mrs. Martine Reed helped me wade through Chinese literature; Mrs. Pamela

Seldon, Miss Mary Perry, and Mr. Bert Collins carried the torch at various times. In Geneva, the intricacies of bibliographic work were handled with infinite care and precision by Miss Jeannine Merlo, whose finds figure in most of the following pages. Mrs. Meredith Frapier was my invaluable aide in Paris, always ready to tackle the most difficult subjects with the thoroughness and devotion of a true collaborator. After having shared so much research, anguish, and satisfaction, it seems absurd to acknowledge my debt in just a few words.

Libraries. The staff of the Francis A. Countway Library of Harvard Medical School, particularly Mr. Richard Wolfe and Miss C. L. Binderup, turned into pleasure for me what could have been a nerve-racking experience, extending their help even across the ocean. In Paris, I am greatly indebted to the Bibliothèque de la Faculté de Médecine (especially to Miss Germaine Le Noir and Mrs. Germaine Verhague); and in Geneva, to the Bibliothèque Publique et Universitaire (especially to Mr. Marc-A. Borgeaud).

Artists. Of the nearly four hundred pictures in this book, one hundred were drawn especially for it by the following artists—all of whom were delightful collaborators:

Mr. Joshua B. Clark, Framingham, Massachusetts: Plates 3.8, 4.1, 4.2; Figures 1.2, 1.6, 4.17, 4.26, 4.35, 4.36, 6.1, 6.4, 9.15, 9.33, 9.44, and all the chapter symbols.

Mr. Pierre Duvernay, Geneva, Switzerland: Plate 4.3; Figures 1.3, 1.17, 1.19, 2.3, 2.5, 2.8, 2.9, 2.13, 2.14, 2.17, 2.21, 2.24, 2.25, 2.27, 2.28, 3.1, 3.3, 3.11, 4.1, 4.3, 4.12, 5.4, 6.16, 7.2, 7.7, 7.8, 7.12, 7.13, 7.17, 7.21, 7.22, 7.23, 7.25, 7.28, 8.21, 9.12, 9.31, 9.32, 9.39, 10.6, 10.7, 10.13, 10.20.

Mr. Gilbert Sesenna, Geneva, Switzerland: Figures 1.5, 3.24, 4.8, 4.13, 4.14, 4.16, 4.23, 4.34, 5.12, 8.1, 8.15, 8.16, 8.17, 8.18, 8.19, 8.20, 9.6, 9.34.

Mr. Michel Czech and Mr. André Ruffieux, Geneva, Switzerland: Figures 2.1, 3.9, 3.16, 3.29, 4.33, 5.2, 6.4, 6.7, 6.20, 9.28, 9.34, 9.36, 10.18.

Mr. Axel Ernst, Geneva, Switzerland: Figures 4.15, 7.27, 8.9, 10.5.

Miss Judith D. Love of the Rhode Island School of Design: Figure 10.15.

Mr. Charles Ryser and his staff, Geneva, Switzerland: Figures 3.27, 3.28, 4.37, 6.5. The ability of Mr. Michel Czech in retouching photographs was always a pleasure to behold.

Secretaries. The trying business of typing and retyping corrected versions of the same text was gallantly faced by several young ladies, who were also generous with advice (and not only in matters of English). In chronological order, I wish to thank Mrs. Henrietta Bins, Miss Mary Viveiros, Mrs. Del Ryan, Mrs. Annemarie Lardelli, and Mrs. Karen E. Melia. To Miss Lise Piguet, who carried for five years the major responsibility of this enterprise—all the correspondence in four languages (usually not in her own), almost all the typing, some of the literature, the filing of some five thousand photographs, all the administration, and the endless series of loose ends that at times seemed to form a hopeless forest—I will never be able to repay my debt; her criticisms, penciled in the margin of the drafts, invariably led to an improvement in the manuscript. Her sure sense of aesthetics is reflected in many of the illustrations. And how could I thank her for keeping her smile, even when work was not yet finished on Sunday afternoon?

Laboratory experiments. Mrs. Jean Thurston planned and carried out a number of experiments on the effect of honey-salve on wounds; Mrs. Elisabeth Bouchardy was responsible for similar experiments on the effect of the *barbarum* ointment of Celsus; to both, and to Miss Geneviève Leyvraz, I am also indebted for beautiful histological slides. Experiments on the bactericidal power of wine and ancient drugs were carried out in Geneva by Dr. Daniel Kekessy, and more extensively by Dr. Elisabeth Schorer and Mrs. Sylvie Dersi. The experiments on the bactericidal power of the honey-butter salve were carried out by Dr. H. L. Wildasin of H. P. Hood & Sons, Boston, and his collaborators. For several other projects of "experimental history" I enjoyed the help of Dr. Isabelle Joris, whose work is always flawless as well as aesthetic.

Photographers. Almost all the pictures in this book were taken, modified, or rephotographed by Jean-Claude Rumbeli, photographer of the Institute of Pathology of Geneva. Mr. Rumbeli rose to many a challenge and improved many a subject. I never resented the comment of a colleague—that my book was a series of legends to Rumbeli's photographs. The remaining pictures were taken at Harvard Medical School by Mr. Eduardo Garriga, in Geneva by Mr. Etienne Denkinger, and in Worcester by Mr. Peter W. Healey.

Help on specific chapters. Ch. 1 (Prehistory) was read and criticized by Prof. A. Leroi-Gourhan of the Collège de France, and by Dr. J. Dastugue of the Faculté de Médecine of Caen (France). To both go my warmest thanks, also for their patience with views that could not be their own. For advice in matters of ancient bones I am much indebted to Dr. Ronald Singer of the University of Chicago, Mr. Gilbert Stucker of the American Museum of Natural History in New York, and Dr. Léon Pales of the Musée de l'Homme in Paris.

Ch. 2 (Mesopotamia) would never have been without the help of the late Prof. René Labat and Pablo Herrero of the Collège de France, who also read and corrected the manuscript. I often resorted to the generous advice of Mrs. Françoise Brüschweiler of Geneva and Dr. Miguel Civil of the Oriental Institute, Chicago.

Ch. 3 (Egypt) was read and criticized by Prof. Charles Maystre, Head of the Department of Egyptology of the University of Geneva. For the interpretation of *wḥdw* I enjoyed the advice of Dr. Robert O. Steuer in Paris, and for topics of Egyptian technology I was greatly helped by correspondence with Dr. John R. Harris of the Institute of Egyptology, Copenhagen.

Ch. 4 (Greece) was read by my friend Prof. Jean Starobinski, who was always on call—and always ready with treasures of knowledge.

Ch. 6 (China) would have been a disaster without the help of Professor Joseph Needham of Cambridge, whose precious letters I came to regard as blood transfusions. Prof. Needham and Dr. Lu Gwei-Djen also took the trouble of combing through the chapter, helping me remove the major flaws (any left are strictly my own), and suggesting important additions (a forthcoming volume of Prof. Needham's *Science and Civilisation in China* will give the reader a much closer view of chinese medicine). In Geneva I was greatly helped by Prof. Jean-François Billeter.

For Ch. 7 (India) I obtained invaluable advice from Prof. Jean Filliozat, Director of the Ecole Française de l'Extrême-Orient in Paris; Prof. Henri Frei of Geneva; Miss Jeannine Auboyer, Conservateur en Chef, Musée Guimet, Paris; and Gopal Sukhu of Boston—who first introduced me to Sanskrit, with occasional lapses into Chinese, and delightful intermezzi on his classical guitar.

Ch. 9 (Rome) was weeded—of the major weeds—by Prof. R. W. Davies of the Sunderland College of Education. Prof. Davies was also generous with references and advice, as was Prof. Paul Collart of Geneva.

Dr. Graeme B. Ryan was kind enough to comb through several chapters, with a keen eye for flaws and contradictions; Miss Rindy Northrop took the trouble of doing the same with the entire manuscript; and so did Dr. Isabelle Joris, who also identified and numbered every single Egyptian hieroglyph, and helped correct all the galley proofs. A few words of thanks, for a job of this magnitude, are again an absurdity.

Other debts. The Latin and Greek texts I checked with the help of Mrs. Martine Vodoz, who also solved for me a host of disparate, historic, and philologic problems.

In matters surgical I enjoyed the advice of my old friend Dr. John P. Remensnyder of the Massachusetts General Hospital and Dr. Denys Montandon of Geneva.

Also in Geneva, I spent many enriching hours with Jacques Vicari, discussing matters of ancient architecture, Assyriology, hospital structure, philology, and humanity altogether.

Dr. Luigi Belloni, now Professor of the History of Medicine in Milan and long ago my teacher of pathology in Geneva, promptly rose to help on many occasions. So did Prof. Erwin Ackerknecht of Zürich, whose critical, "no-nonsense" way of dealing with medical history has been a guiding light. I owe him much advice and encouragement, and dearly hope that this book will live up to it.

I also enjoyed a vast amount of negative help. There were times, especially in Geneva, when the members of my department would have liked to see me in the autopsy room or before a microscope—while I was before my typewriter or buried in some ancient text. Hence, this book is also the product of their patience, and to all of them goes my unending gratitude. I wish to thank them personally: Drs. Anne-Marie Schindler, Isabelle Joris, Jocelyne Grobéty, Pierre Vassalli, Guilio Gabbiani, Yusuf Kapanci, François Chatelanat, René Lagier, SvenWidgren, Jeremiah Cox, Chadli Bouzakoura, and Bernard Portmann.

The memory of Andrew Turnbull, a much lamented friend and one-time neighbor, lingers throughout these pages. Long ago, while he was finishing his masterpiece, *Scott Fitzgerald*, Andrew came over to check some medical facts in my library. To my amazement, he was genuinely pained, not at the contents, but at the poor style of what he read. So real was his shock that he tried his best to prevent me from doing the same; he rewrote the introduction to one of my own scientific papers, and then took the trouble of explaining to me, patiently, some of the tricks of writing in English, like replacing nouns with verbs—not *reaching a conclusion* but just *concluding*. I must have thought of that lesson thousands of times since. Though English is not my language, it came closer to being so thanks to Andrew Turnbull.

My friends at Harvard University Press left their masterly touch in every part of this book: Arthur Rosenthal in the title and first chapter, William Bennett in every chapter, Virginia LaPlante in every paragraph, and Gretchen Wang in the design.

To thank my family in just a few words is another impossible task. The text is mine, but the time was largely theirs—hence the authorship should read, more precisely, "Guido and Fritzi Majno, with the assistance of Corinne, Lorenzo, and Luca."

Contents

Illustrations

Illustrations

Illustrations

Illustrations

Illustrations

Illustrations

Color Plates
Following page 294

Illustrations

The Healing Hand

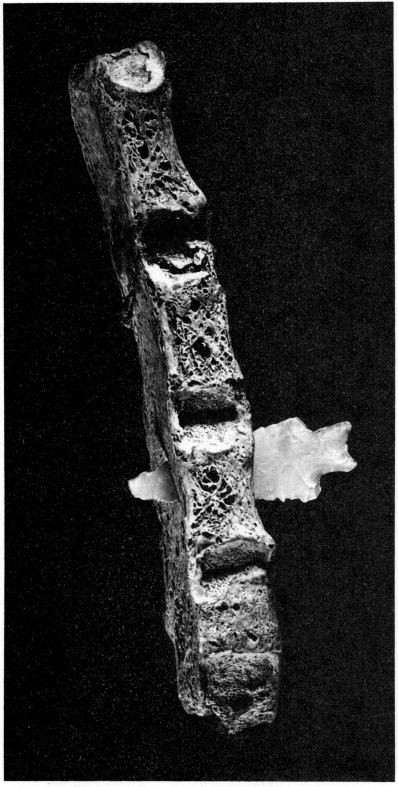

1.1 A flint arrowhead in a human sternum. It struck the bone from the front (right to left on the photograph) and penetrated into the chest deep enough to reach the heart: a deadly wound.

1   Prelude

Sample of prehistoric life from Patagonia: an arrowhead in a human bone (Fig. 1.1). This timeless opposition of stone and flesh will recur like an echo to the end of this book: life is fragile, to be hurt is part of the game.

There are many ways to be hurt, of course, and it can happen without arrowheads. Yet physical trauma has always fared high on the list of man's problems. Prehistoric man left pictures of himself pierced by arrows. Thousands of years later, trauma is just as inevitable: coping with this reality is one of our chores. Mexican children begin to adjust while playing with one-legged dolls, or nibbling at candy coffins.

But then, injury has also helped to shape life itself, by eliminating the unfit.[1] It has left its imprint in our tissues, even in our cells, in the form of built-in, life-saving reactions, ready to be triggered at an instant's notice. And myriads of wounds have become stepping stones to one of man's greatest creations—the art of healing.

A Five-Minute Lecture on Wounds

In classical Greece, every cultured layman was supposed to know the basic principles of medicine.[2] These first few pages are dedicated to my nonmedical readers, in that same spirit, for I do believe that everyone should know the beautiful deeds of which his or her tissues are capable.[3]

The first point to grasp is that a wounded salamander does much better than man. It can afford to lose a whole limb, because it will grow a new one, skeleton and all. In scientific terms, it has a great capacity to regenerate. In mammals, only a few tissues, like the epidermis, regenerate really well; severed muscles never grow back, and even as modest an item as a hair root is too complicated to rebuild. So man's wounds heal mainly by a patching-up process called "repair." The loss is made good not with the original tissue but with a material that is biologically simple, cheap, and handy: connective tissue. This is a soft but tough kind of tissue, specialized for mechanical functions, primarily that of holding us together; it fills the spaces in and around all other tissues. Under the microscope both its softness and its toughness are explained, for it is constructed of a loose, three-dimensional network of fibers—some inextensible, others rubbery—bathed in a jellylike fill (the technical names of these three components are collagen fibers, elastic fibers, and mucopolysaccharides). Scattered throughout this system are several types of cells, including the ones that built it. In normal life these slender cells, called fibroblasts ("fiber-makers"), lie peacefully in their self-made jungle (Fig. 1.2A).

Now imagine a wound in this system. It disturbs millions of fibroblasts, which promptly set about the task of repair. But at the same time the wound has created a dreadful mess of spilled blood, dead cells, foreign material, and some bacteria. To cope with the debris, nature has devised an automatic mopping-up operation, called acute inflammation. As the first step in this sequence of events, blood flow around the injured area increases, helping to meet the emergency by bringing in extra "manpower" in the form of white blood cells, as well as supplies of antibacterial proteins and other chemicals. This rush of supplies is speeded up by another emergency device: the finest vessels, especially the venules, develop temporary leaks, so that fluid, without cells, actually pours out (hence the local swelling). The white blood cells, however, crawl out of the blood vessels by their own means and set about their different jobs. Some, specialized to fight bacteria, concentrate on swallowing and killing the intruders; these cells are called polymorpho-nuclear granulocytes, or polys for short (Fig. 1.2B). White cells of another kind, called macrophages (literally "big eaters"), consume and destroy the other debris left lying around. All these events are triggered by chemicals released from the damaged tissue. Note the elegant coordination: the tissue injury itself sets off the mechanisms for cleaning up the effects of that injury.

The two operations, clean-up and rebuilding, go on side by side. But just as a burning house cannot be rebuilt while the fire is raging, healing cannot be effective if bacteria keep on destroying tissues. So the wound can take, schematically, two different courses, depending on the presence or absence of infection (Fig. 1.2). If infection is absent—or minimal—the white blood cells undertake their routine clean-up, and in the meantime the fibroblasts bring about repair undisturbed. Slowly they multiply and fill up the gap with new fibers and the jellylike substance; blood vessels also grow into the region of repair, to support the building operations. The result is a new mass of connective tissue, called *granulation tissue* because—to the eye of the surgeon—its fleshy red surface looks bumpy or "granular." This type of

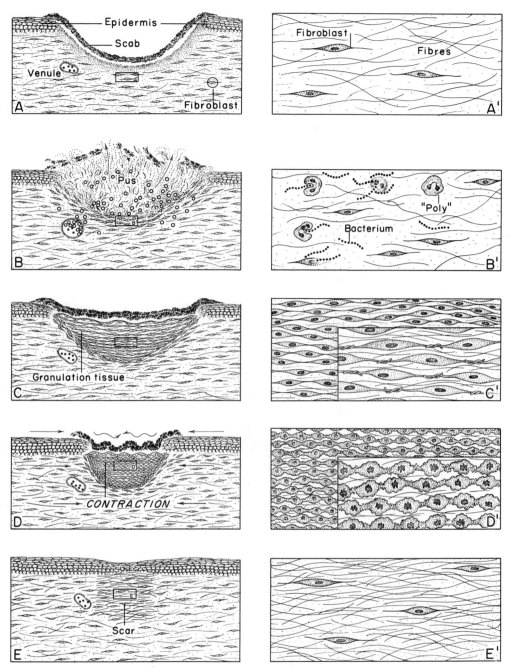

1.2 Stages in the healing of a wound, as seen through the microscope. The column at right shows details of the figures at left.

wound healing, in which bacteria do not interfere, goes under the ancient and venerable name of "healing by first intention" (Fig. 1.2 omitting phase B).

Things are very different when infection flares up. Bacteria delay healing in two main ways. First, they destroy live cells and tissues, so that the repair work of the fibroblasts is continually frustrated. Second, many types of bacteria raise havoc by starting a battle: they cause defending polys to flood the scene in such numbers as to form a thick cream, called pus. As the polys die within the pus, they let loose chemicals that were not used up in digesting bacteria. This is both good and bad: good because it helps to digest away dead tissue, where bacteria lurk; bad because the same wave of breakdown interferes with the constructive efforts of the fibroblasts (Fig. 1.2B). Healing can really get under way only after the infection has been beaten back. This course of events is called, in traditional terms, "healing by second intention."

Pus is therefore a noble substance: it is made of brave cells that never sneak back into the blood vessels to escape; they all die in the line of duty. Note also the double meaning of suppuration: it indicates that there is an infection, but also that the body is fighting it well. The outcome of the battle can be predicted, to some extent, from the aspect of the pus, as was observed even in ancient times. The whitish, creamy kind (and therefore rich in polys) is "preferable," because it indicates that an infection is being fought effectively. Hence its ancient Latin name of *pus bonum et laudabile*, "good and laudable pus." Thin or malodorous pus suggests a poor defense or especially vicious bacteria.

Either mode of wound healing—by first or second intention—leads to the same result: a gap filled or lined with granulation tissue, and covered by a scab of dried-up blood. The wound is now ready for the final step in the healing process (Fig. 1.2C). At this stage, although man lags behind the salamander, he is at least ahead of the tree. In an injured tree-trunk, new tissue simply grows in from the sides of the wound, very, very slowly. There is no other option. Human granulation tissue goes one step further: as it fills the gap, it also pulls the margins together—a process called wound contraction. As the wound closes, new epidermis creeps in beneath the scab and seals off the raw area. Deep down, more fibers are formed, while most of the cells die and disappear. The end result is a dense mass of fibers with few living cells: a scar.

Several things can go wrong with the process of wound healing. Most of the mishaps are caused by bacteria; and their visible effect depends on the kind of bacteria as well as on the response of the tissue (Fig. 1.3). The most common accident is suppuration, which brings about healing by second intention. Suppuration, incidentally, is caused by bacteria that have the property of attracting many white blood cells (a truly suicidal trait). A spreading, superficial infection forms a red halo, for which the Greeks coined the term *erysipelas*. An infection spreading into the depths of the tissue and causing blood vessels to leak extensively produces much swelling (*tumor* in ancient Latin terminology). Sometimes, unaccountably, an excess of soft red granulation tissue mushrooms out of the wound, a complication once known

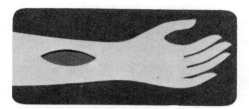

Fresh, uncomplicated wound

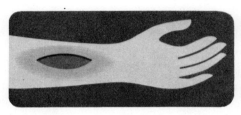

Reddening caused by superficial inflammation ("erysipelas")

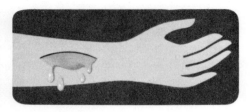

Suppuration

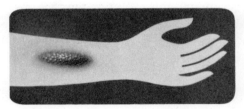

Swelling caused by deep inflammation

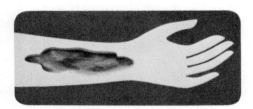

Spreading ulcer

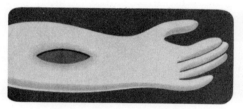

Excess of granulation tissue ("proud flesh")

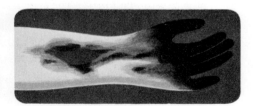

Gangrene

1.3 Six major "wound diseases": complications that can occur to a wound. The cause of "proud flesh" is not understood; all the others are due to bacteria.

as proud flesh. If the bacteria gain ground on the defenses, spread, and kill more and more tissue, the wound becomes a spreading ulcer, called also serpiginous or phagedenic. A massive death of tissue goes under the name of gangrene; the Greeks also called it "blackening" (*melasmós*). A hard, bulging, overgrown scar is called a keloid. Its cause still unknown, the keloid is the curse of plastic surgery. These various clinical problems of healing wounds can be so distinctive that the ancients thought each kind represented a special disease, requiring its own special treatment: a view that was not totally wrong, for some of the clinical peculiarities do correspond to differences in the invading bacteria.

The mechanism that makes an open wound contract, as if an invisible force were drawing its margins together, was an ancient puzzle. Clinical and experimental observations suggested that the source of the pull was in the granulation tissue, but neither the fibroblasts nor the various kinds of fibers seemed to have the qualifications of a pulling machine. The answer is extraordinary. When a wound must close by contraction, the versatile fibroblasts perform two feats that allow them to behave like a pulling machine: they join end to end, and they develop internal bundles of contractile fibers, similar in all respects to the contractile component of muscle (Fig. 1.2C,D). Thus transformed, they respond to the same substances that cause involuntary, or "smooth," muscle to contract. In the laboratory, a little strip of granulation tissue, taken from the floor of a wound and maintained in a warm bath, can be made to contract or relax like a muscle when certain drugs or chemicals are added to the bath.[4]

Still unknown is how the fibroblasts are induced to join together and pull, but the fact is that they do. I suspect that during evolution they became programmed to respond in this manner because of the great advantages to wound healing. If there is any truth to this suggestion, it follows that injury has shaped the behavior of human cells.

A Glance at the Fossil Evidence

Wounds involving bones or shells left traces in fossils long before man or mammals appeared on the scene. The healing process of wounds in ammonites, about 200 million years ago, left imperfections in their lovely spirals.[5]

Moving up to about five million years ago, we meet the man-ape who seems to be our likeliest ancestor:[6] *Australopithecus africanus*, "the South African ape,"[7] whose remains perhaps bear witness to the "first wound." It all began when Raymond Dart, examining the skulls of his newly-found australopithecines and of baboons lying with them, noticed peculiar double depressions shaped like a squat 8 (Fig. 1.4).[8] Encouraged by a professor of forensic medicine, who saw the marks as evidence of attack with a weapon, he searched the fossil-bearing limestone for objects that could have been used as a club, and found remains of antelope bones that could have served the purpose: the best candidate was the lower end of the humerus, which had

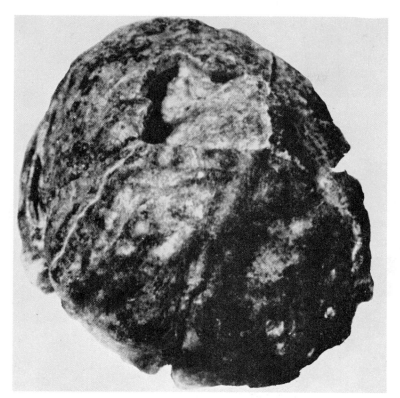

1.4 The skull of an australopithecine who, according to Dart, was clubbed to death by another australopithecine—the double depression reflecting the shape of the bone club. If Dart's interpretation is right, this accurate, vertical blow was delivered, perhaps from the rear, as much as three or four million years ago.

two knuckles that fitted neatly into the double depression.[9] The overall conclusion was such bad news that it could not fail to make headlines: the australopithecines, having discovered the principle of bashing skulls with clubs, placed such demands on their primitive nervous system to develop this skill in weaponry that the evolution of their brain was accelerated; hence, violence created man.[10]

Recent developments are more optimistic. Flaked stones found among the fossils show that the australopithecines were already exploring the possibilities of handicraft, and fashioning simple tools from pebbles, as early as 2.6 million years ago.[11] Now here is a more constructive occupation to have given our ancestor's brain a push in the right direction. In the wake of this discovery, the double depressions in the skull have been almost forgotten.[12] Although it turns out that chimpanzees in the wild use clubs to attack leopards,[13] and even hurl stones at baboons,[14] nobody has tried to find out, experimentally, whether an antelope bone could really produce an acceptable double depression in a baboon skull.

To sum up the story of the "first wound," we are left with the portrait of a stone-chipping artisan painted over a somewhat faded image of Cain. Perhaps both are authentic. In any event, after having been told that bloodshed is inevitably our lot, because we are the product of violence, we

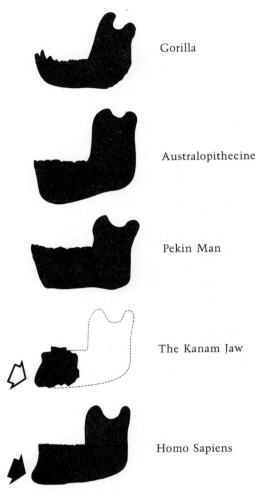

Gorilla

Australopithecine

Pekin Man

The Kanam Jaw

Homo Sapiens

1.5 The chin that caused most trouble: the Kanam fragment.

should find it welcome news that work may be our lot, because we descend from a craftsman.[15]

Among the fossils that stirred up controversy was a small piece of jaw from Kanam, Kenya, dating roughly from the time of the australopithecines—an impossible jaw, because it had a chin (Fig. 1.5).[16] Nobody but man has a chin. Even Pliny said so: *mentum nulli praeter hominem*.[17] It is true no one knows exactly when man appeared (we were definitely here 30-35,000 years ago, perhaps as early as 100,000 years ago, side by side with the Neanderthals), but surely we did not live at the time of our australopithecine ancestors. The jaw remained a puzzle until P. V. Tobias decided to cut the Gordian knot. In fact, he cut the jaw and looked at it with the microscope. The chin was a lump of callus over a nasty infected fracture; so its owner was just a miserable hominid who had been hit in the face.[18]

The Neanderthals are a mysterious lot. They lived from approximately 150 to 40,000 years ago, had clothes and fire, and spoke some sort of Neanderthalese.[19] Their brains were at least as large as ours, and they looked very much like us. *Homo sapiens* and *Homo neanderthalensis* may even have intermarried.[20] Then, unaccountably, the Neanderthals vanished. Yet one of them must be remembered here because he has been described as the first known case of surgical amputation (whereas the story itself, I fear, should be amputated). The facts are as follows.

Some 46,000 years ago there lived in a cave of northern Iraq a sorry specimen of Neanderthal.[21] Early in life something went wrong with his arm, which remained stunted. Years later he lost half of the same arm.[22] He carried on by gripping things with his jaw, so he wore down his teeth quite badly.[23] Then he lost two front teeth.[24] A blow received on the top of his head healed well, but another one that smashed the left side of his face probably left him blind in that eye. In the meantime, he reached the ripe old age of forty (equivalent to about eighty in our day) and developed a bad case of arthritis. Finally the roof caved in, and he was killed near his hearth.

His discoverers grew rather fond of him. They called him Nandy[25] and composed over his bones a bit of romance.[26] Perhaps his amputation was an example of "very early surgery" (although there were surely more lions than surgeons in the immediate neighborhood). And perhaps Nandy's remains were themselves mute evidence of "man's humanity to man."[27] Nandy could have been making himself useful around the place; his comrades, though cannibals, were human enough to recognize his virtues and allowed him to live on; when he died, they even took the trouble of piling rocks over his remains.[28]

Maybe it is true that Nandy represents fossilized compassion, to the extent that a cripple was allowed to live on rather than being reutilized as food (a level of human decency that is current among animals). But asking Nandy to play the role of surgical patient is too much; it assumes that Neanderthal surgery had gone beyond the level even of Hippocrates, who did not know how to amputate. The real lesson of Nandy, I believe, is that nature alone is able to staunch the bleeding and stamp out the infection, even after such major accidental wounds as those of amputation.

Stepping into the era of *Homo sapiens*, among Stone Age fossils we find scores of arrowheads embedded in bones, especially in lumbar vertebrae, possibly because shields protected the upper part of the body.[29] In many cases it is obvious that the wounded must have died immediately (Fig. 1.1); others lived long enough to produce an intense bony reaction (Fig. 1.6). For the medical historian there is not much to learn from these fossils, except that killing technology had advanced a great deal since the primordial clubs.

A Role for Pleasure

Sometime, somewhere, the striking hand must have also learned to accomplish a healing, soothing gesture. It is difficult to discuss prehistoric therapy without running into Calvin Wells' veto: "imaginative insight must stop well short of delirium."[30] But we can try to look back and see when the footsteps of medicine began to emerge from the night of time.

Certain gestures, like scratching, have defied time and evolution as

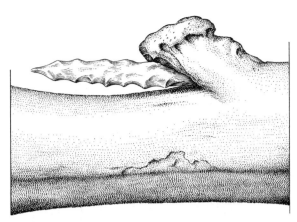

1.6 In prehistoric France, a grazing shot landed this flint arrowhead against a human tibia. The subject survived, and the arrowhead, presumably helped by bacterial infection, caused the formation of a peculiar bony lump (top right). This development must have taken months, possibly years.

effectively as fossils.[31] As to medical gestures, nobody knows how long they may have survived. However, professional historians in search of man's earliest medicine do not refrain from looking into the habits of primitive tribes.[32] Not being a professional historian, I feel even less inhibited: how about inquiring into our relatives the apes?[33]

Nobody alive could testify more competently than Jane van Lawick-Goodall, who actually shared the forest with wild chimpanzees.[34] Here is the status of wound care among wild chimpanzees, as I learned it directly from Dr. Goodall.[35] A wounded chimpanzee takes care of himself to some extent: "a chimpanzee will pick leaves, dab at a fresh bloody wound, lick the blood off the leaves, and then dab again. A sore on the back, or side, or head will often be pressed with the fingers, which are then licked, then pressed again to the wound." Care of a wounded companion, however, is somewhat disappointing. Dr. Goodall has seen, "on one or two occasions, one chimpanzee lick the wound of another. On the other hand, when one female had a really bad puncture wound in her shoulder, which she repeatedly presented for grooming to an adult male, he appeared fearful, whimpered, and hurried away from her . . . We have seen chimps, especially youngsters, staring intently at a wound of another chimp, putting their faces close to it, but not doing anything else; even in the case of a mother carrying a badly wounded infant."

The same species in captivity seems to have done better. First aid among captive chimpanzees was actually recorded in a unique photographic sequence (Fig. 1.7).[36] Pan and Wendy, a pair in their early thirties, had been sharing a Florida enclosure for twenty-nine years. One morning in February 1954, Dr. Walter Miles happened to be standing nearby, armed with a camera. Pan was engaged in his usual noisy, belligerent display. Suddenly,

. . . in the midst of Pan's excited behavior, Wendy came up behind him whimpering. Pan suddenly turned, looked, and approached her. She sat down on the ground; he immediately crouched in front of her and with his two forefingers began manipulating her left eyelid . . . The first photograph taken shows Pan crouching in

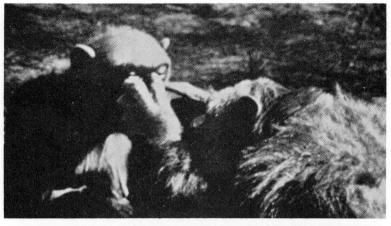

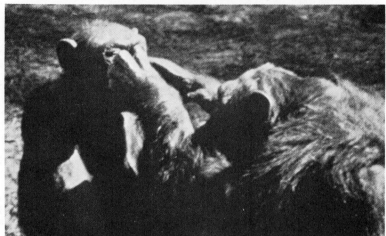

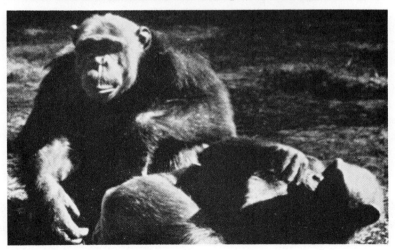

1.7 Medical aid among chimpanzees. *Top:* Wendy, at left, has just
signaled that something is in her left eye. Pan crouches before her and
pulls down her lower eyelid. *Center:* The search goes on. Wendy has
pulled back her head a little, as most patients would. Pan seems to
stabilize it with his left hand (note the little thumb of his right hand).
Bottom: Just after success, both chimps relax. They have switched
places. Wendy lies down; Pan, who moments before had been romping
wildly, is now in a pensive mood.

front of Wendy and very near, as he views her left eye. He is using both his hands for the task of searching. With his left hand he appears to stabilize Wendy's head. With his right forefinger he has drawn down the lower eyelid exposing the pink mucous membrane. Wendy's head is tipped toward Pan, who is viewing her eye from a distance that we estimate as 5 to 6 inches . . . The moment when Pan withdrew his fingers from Wendy's face, signalling success of his attempt, occurred with such suddenness it was not captured by a photograph. As Wendy experienced relief, there was a quick change in her posture from sitting to lying down. Pan turned so that he could again see his two human observers. He glanced briefly at Wendy's genital area and then assumed the relaxed sitting posture immediately behind Wendy . . . He seemed to look at his human observers with a much altered perceptual attitude . . . He sat quietly . . . for about five minutes.

The motives behind ape first aid—as seen by a human primate—have been explored by W. Koehler:

Monkeys of many kinds have a custom of mutual personal "inspection," and skin treatment. But we are at present in the dark as to the reasons for the popularity of this investigation of skin, hair, and hind quarters, which is carried out with the greatest eagerness and attention—and is a pleasure shared equally by the active and passive parties in the process . . . As a branch of the same activity, the chimpanzee likes to pay attention to wounds or injuries received by his fellows; but hardly urged thereto by motives of "mutual aid." *To handle such things gives him pleasure* [italics mine] and there is sometimes a helpful and beneficial result. Once an enormous abscess had appeared on the lower jaw of one of our chimpanzees. When it became noticeable through the extent of the inflamed surface and secretion of pus, another of the apes would not stir from the patient's side, but pressed and kneaded the injured jaw, until the pus was removed, revealing a raw, gaping wound. The animal thus treated made no objections. As apes like using diverse objects in all eager manipulations, the operator worked with a large piece of old rag in his hand. Yet, wonderful to relate, the wound—itself probably originally caused by skin treatment with filthy hands—healed rapidly and completely. Chimpanzees also like very much to remove splinters from each other's hands or feet, by the method in use among the ordinary human laity. Two fingernails are pressed down on either side and the splinter levered upwards, to be caught and removed by the teeth. At the risk of infection, I went up to a chimpanzee on one occasion when I had run a splinter into one of my fingers and pointed it out to him. Immediately his mien and expression assumed the eager intensity proper to "skin treatment"; he examined the wound, siezed my hand and forced out the splinter by two very skillful, but somewhat painful, squeezes with his finger-nails; he then examined my hand again, very closely, and let it fall, satisfied with his work.[37]

In summary, nature does most of the job, while the chimps perform a few helpful gestures. And some of these gestures are derived from grooming, *in the pursuit of pleasure.* No barber-surgeons are left to testify on the basic interrelations of pleasure, grooming, and surgery.[38] But to turn to my surgical colleagues: would anyone deny that cleaning up an untidy wound still is, deep down, a pleasure?

News of more chimpanzee medicine came recently from the Delta Regional Primate Center in Louisiana, where seven young chimps, seven to eleven years old, had been living together for three and a half years.[39] Their

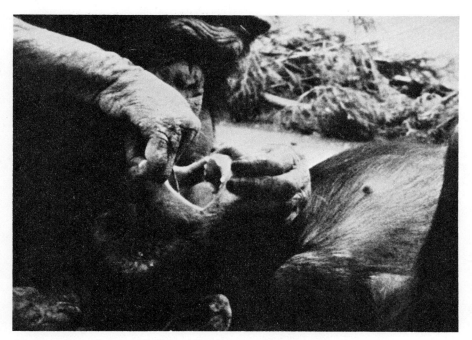

1.8 Dental care between Belle and Bandit, two chimpanzees.

home was a one-acre outdoor enclosure, with an overhead deck from which
Dr. William McGrew and Caroline Tutin could study their behavior. The
greatest surprise came from Belle, a female, who had developed a definite bent
for dental grooming. In six weeks of observation she was seen performing this
service forty-five times, especially on a young male, Bandit, who seemed to be
the perfect patient because he was both losing his baby teeth and enjoying the
attention. "Her usual procedure was to begin normal social grooming directed
to the hair of Bandit's torso, limbs or head. She then concentrated on his face
and, finally, opened his mouth . . . Belle adopted a variety of postures while
working: sitting, bipedal standing, crouching, reclining. The patient usually
lay supine, but Belle maneuvered him through other postures."[40] On four
occasions she found it necessary to pick up a stick to use as a tool (Fig. 1.8);
once it was a twig of red cedar, which she stripped of leaves before using it.
Her major feat was the removal of a deciduous molar with the help of a pine
twig (Fig. 1.9).

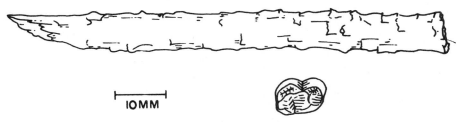

IOMM

1.9 A unique surgical specimen: Bandit's lower left deciduous second premolar, and
the pine twig used by Belle in removing it.

Why Belle developed this specialty is not explained. There is no reason to believe that she was copying human behavior, such as tooth picking; and no encouragement was offered. I submitted the problem to Dr. Goodall, who replied that chimpanzees in captivity "typically *do* more things—they have more leisure time." Belle is now dead and she took her secret with her: perhaps a blend of pleasure, leisure time, and skill.

The Wound As a Problem

A million years ago, as now, a wound implied three major medical problems: mechanical disruption, bleeding, and infection. Nature is prepared to cope with all three; but man can help, even with simple means.

On the question of mechanical damage, nature's contribution to repair needs no advertising. In a survey of 118 wild gibbons, 42 had fractures (up to four apiece) and all healed, even in the humerus and femur,[41] with just enough exceptions to show that gibbons can be human.[42] Whatever apes do or do not do, it works. As to wounds, apes make no active attempt to help, such as holding the margins together; but man too has been very slow at that, perhaps because nature proved so fast. Stitching of wounds among primitive people is exceptional.[43] Sometimes the wound is really sewn with fibers or shreds of tendon; sometimes the lips of a wound are pinned together by a thorn or spike used like a skewer, and its protruding ends are wound around with fiber (Fig. 1.10)—a technique that is not wholly obsolete. But we cannot be certain that any of the few examples observed nowadays is truly native or had a prehistoric equivalent.

Yet the act of sewing is probably older than *Homo sapiens*, since Neanderthal man wore some sort of clothing.[44] So why the delay? Was it lack of imagination? I doubt it. Perhaps stitching was tried off and on, but without enough success. In wounds contaminated with bacteria, sutures are a mixed blessing: they favor infection and may actually prevent the wound from healing. We teach today that dirty wounds are better off unsewn. Besides, there are three good ways to hold a wound closed even without thread and needle: a simple bandage, adhesive tape, and clips. Bandages must be as old as clothing; the oldest known were found in Egypt and represent an advanced state of the art, since they were applied with splints.[45] Adhesive tape has a shockingly modern ring, but the notion may well be four thousand years old and possibly older than sutures, for "stickiness" is a very early and basic concern, bound to the use of resin, that all-purpose material.[46] As to clips, insect mandibles are used to this end by primitive people today. Their use in prehistoric times cannot be documented, however, and they first appear in history with ancient Hindu medicine.

For clearcut evidence of stitches in live flesh (which the Egyptians may have tried) we have to wait for the classical writings of India and Greece. But the overall priority for stitching goes to the ants. They had the idea long before man, perhaps millions of years ago. *Oecophylla smaragdina*, as we shall see, discovered a way to sew leaves with a triple combination of clamping, stitching, and gluing.[47]

The problem of hemorrhage was mastered even later than stitching. Mankind had great difficulty in grasping the main facts about bleeding and how to stop it. Minor hemorrhages are checked by the simple act of bandaging, and a few among the infinity of materials that have been stuffed into wounds may actually help blood clotting. The most effective means developed by primitive people to stop bleeding is the cautery,[48] which might possibly have been used as far back as 3000 B.C.;[49] but wounds to any major vessel meant bleeding to death until well into historical times. Even the Greeks had very vague notions about hemostasis; if Hippocrates ever tied a spurting vessel, he never said so. By the time the tourniquet was a well-recognized procedure, people were shooting guns.

How could it take so long to understand something so simple—in concept—as turning off a faucet? Although it did take a long time, in retrospect the problem was not so simple. First, there is no closing of a faucet for people who have never seen a faucet. Then in many cases, such as a major blow on the head, the wound itself is the lethal event; bleeding is incidental. In other cases it does not help at all to stop the outward loss of blood, because bleeding continues inside. This holds for all penetrating wounds of the chest and abdomen. Besides, the ligature itself is a hazard. Consider the case of a Neanderthal man who has his femoral artery torn open in fighting off a cave bear. His neighbor is a genius and ties off the thigh with a strip of hide. The bloody fountain dries up. But then what? The magic gesture has simply traded hemorrhage for gangrene: the great first-aid principle of the tourniquet fails unless the torn vessel itself is tied and the tourniquet is released within a very few hours. Finally, to the unprepared mind, the blood lost is only that which was contained in the wounded part, which deprives the event of some of its urgency. To take an optimistic view of this prolonged human failure, let us say that death by hemorrhage was given an extended chance to work for natural selection.

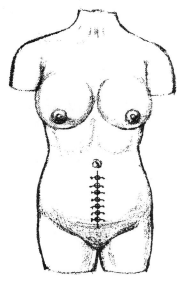

1.10 Primitive wound closure with iron spikes, wound around with thread. A successful Caesarean section, under anesthesia with banana wine, from Uganda, 1879.

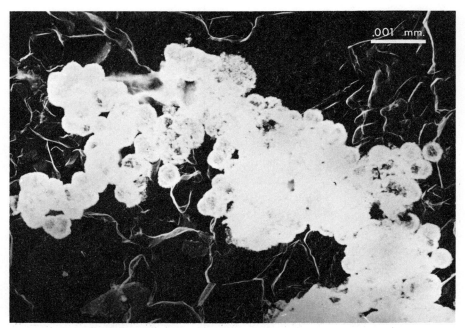

1.11 Fossil bacteria two billion years old. From gunflint chert, a Precambrian sediment in southern Ontario. Enlarged about 15,000x.

As for the problem of infection, bacteria should have been old hands at causing trouble by the time that man came around. Clostridia in particular should have been rampant, for they are able to survive in inanimate nature and also happen to cause two of the deadliest wound infections, tetanus and gas gangrene.[50] For those who like concrete evidence I will submit a picture of fossilized bacteria 2 billion years old (Fig. 1.11) (primates began to appear only about 65 million years ago).[51] These fossils were embedded in rocks that could be dated—some as far back as 3200 million years.[52] From their shape, their arrangement in little chains, and their remains of organic content, there can be little doubt that they represent fossil bacteria.[53]

Bone disease caused by infection (osteomyelitis), if long standing, usually causes the bone to swell and become riddled with channels (sinuses) through which the pus drains. The first acceptable evidence of osteomyelitis is far older than man: it concerns a Permian reptile, whose gnarled bony spine suggests that the basic changes of osteomyelitis have not changed much in the last 200 million years (Fig. 1.12).[54] Osteomyelitis has been described in many other fossils, animal and human.[55]

To me as a pathologist, the diagnosis of "infected bone" in most of the fossils thus labeled seems acceptable, although nobody can guarantee that these infections were caused by bacteria rather than by other agents, such as protozoa or fungi.[56] However, we do know that tooth cavities are the work of bacteria, and of bacteria alone. Thus, unless the biology of caries has changed a lot in the last 3 to 4 million years, the teeth of *Australopithecus* have preserved the oldest known evidence of bacterial infection, albeit of a special variety (Figs. 1.13–1.14).[57]

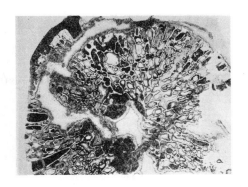

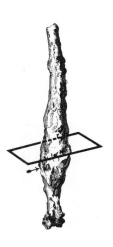

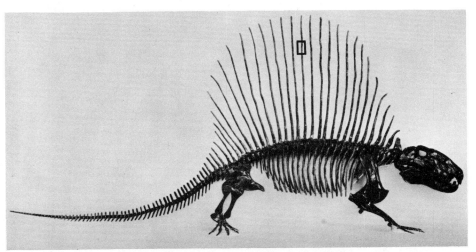

1.12 Oldest known trace of an infected wound. About 200 million years ago, in Texas, a Permian reptile broke one of its dorsal spines: it was a *Dimetrodon*, like this nine-foot specimen (bottom). The bone healed but remained swollen (center), as if it had become infected through a break in the skin (arrow: site of fracture). A microscopic section across the spine (top) shows a honeycombed structure, which Moodie interpreted as infected bone riddled by sinuses full of pus. Unfortunately he gave no picture of a normal spine.

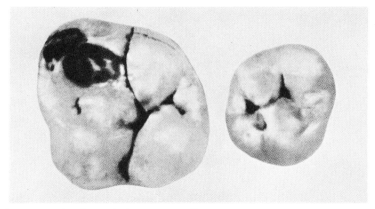

1.13 *Left:* Bacterial infection about two million years ago—two cavities in an upper molar of an australopithecine. *Right:* A comparable human molar.

1.14 Caries in a modern human tooth, photographed through the electron microscope, to show that caries is a bacterial infection. A swarm of bacteria (B) are burrowing into the enamel. The small black segments (C) are enamel crystals; they are being dissolved by lactic acid produced by the bacteria. Enlarged about 21,000x.

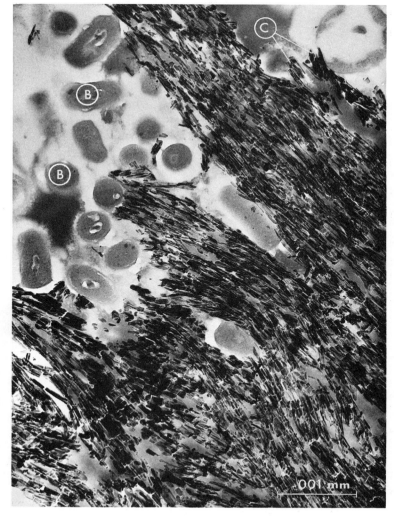

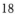

Franz Weidenreich suggested, on rather slim grounds, that primitive man may have been generally more resistant to infection. His argument was based on the jaws of Pekin man, which remained perfectly healthy despite the teeth, which had been heavily worn down by a gritty diet.[58] Yet there are jaws of Neanderthal men with retreating gums and related problems,[59] and the full-blown picture of dental infection is painfully clear in a famous skull of Rhodesian man, 30 to 40,000 years old. Its teeth, worn or decayed, allowed bacteria to penetrate into the bone, which is honeycombed with abscesses.[60] These isolated cases are clearly not enough to decide whether our ancestors were better off than us in their daily fight against bacteria.

Messages from Primitive Art

Not long after the disappearance of Neanderthal man, *Homo sapiens* invented art; that was about 35,000 B.C.[61] From then on the wound was potentially available as a subject of artistic expression. But astonishingly, our ancestors did not seem to think so, for the drawings they left are infinitely milder than those of historical times. In the caves of France and Spain, the catalog of prehistoric art runs to 2260 figures:[62] only a fraction of these portray wounds or scenes of violence (Fig. 1.15). The most common victim is the bison, and even his casualty rate is less than 2.5 percent.[63] I can offer no explanation.

A prehistoric message that may or may not concern medicine is painted all over the Gargas cave in southern France.[64] Something very strange went on there, perhaps 25,000 years ago. Men of the Aurignacian culture left "signatures" on the walls of the cave, as negative imprints made by smearing or

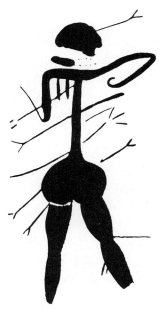

1.15 This wretched little man, surrounded by archers, is painted on a rock in eastern Spain. Is he trying to pull out one of the arrows?

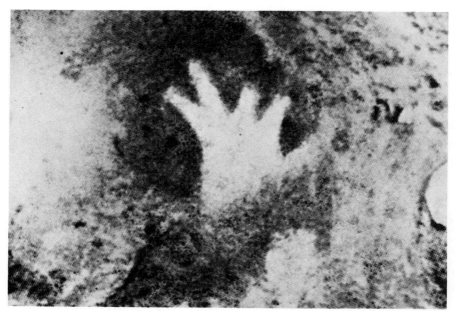

1.16 Negative imprint left on a wall of the Gargas cave in southern France about 25,000 years ago, when a human being smeared red color around a hand. Four fingers are too short. Of over one hundred hand imprints in the cave, most are "incomplete." Ritual amputation? Disease? Sign language?

blowing black or red color around the hand laid on the rock (Fig. 1.16). Many of these hands lack one or more fingers; the thumb seems to be spared.[65] One possible explanation is that the whole group suffered from Raynaud's disease, a familial condition that could have led to gangrene of the fingers in a cold land where the mammoth still roamed.[66] But similar hands turned up in the Maltravieso cave in central Spain, where the climate was milder.[67] Could it have been ritual amputation?

For once, the truth may not be as gruesome as it seemed. A. Leroi-Gourhan noticed recently that the commonest types of "abnormalities" correspond to fingers that are most easily bent down, alone or in combination (Fig. 1.17). Thus, the hands could have been laid backward against the rock, while the fingers were making a conventional hunting sign. Some of the hands also seem to show that a finger was retouched off, as one would retouch an *E* to make it look like an *F* (Fig. 1.18). The prevailing combination, "thumb only, all fingers down," could have been the sign for the prevailing bison.[68] Bushmen still use such a code (Fig. 1.19).[69]

But the Bushmen also do something else that casts new light on the problem. Like other primitive peoples, they have been known to chop off fingers as a form of sacrifice (Fig. 1.20).[70] Several Indian tribes of northwestern Canada do the same thing "when death is too assiduous in his visits to a family: the survivors . . . place the little finger on the edge of the coffin and sacrifice the first joint, in order, as they say, *to cut off the deaths*."[71] Robert Gardner recently filmed a similar rite in New Guinea among the Dugum Dani tribe.[72] The occasion was the death in combat of a tribesman, and the sacrificial victims were, as usual, little girls, selected for a certain consanguinity (Fig. 1.21). That particular sacrifice was a way of expressing the solidarity of the kin group and the grief of the family; it also served to placate the ghost of the dead relative.[73] Almost all Dani girls lose several fingers yet maintain a high degree of manual skill (Fig. 1.22).[74]

From the medical point of view, the overall conclusion—once again—is that mutilated fingers can heal quite predictably, without much danger of infection. At least in the forest.

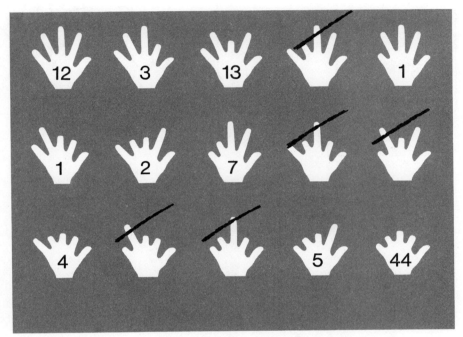

1.17 Finger formulas of the Gargas cave. The figures indicate their frequency, in a total of 92 that were readable (slashed formulas are not found). Conclusion: the commonest configurations are also among the easiest to mimic by bending fingers.

1.18 Occasional fingers of the Gargas hands seem to have been retouched off: another blow to the amputation hypothesis.

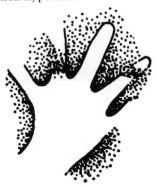

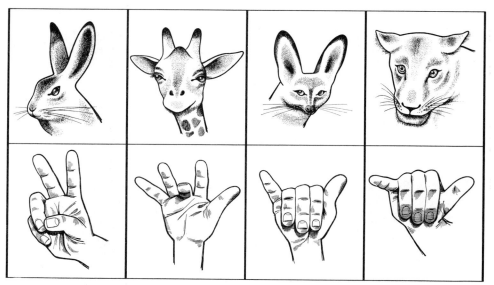

1.19 Four highly suggestive "hand-words" used by hunting Bushmen: "scrub hare," "giraffe," "bat-eared fox," "lion." This sign language may be a clue to the "amputated" fingers of the Gargas cave.

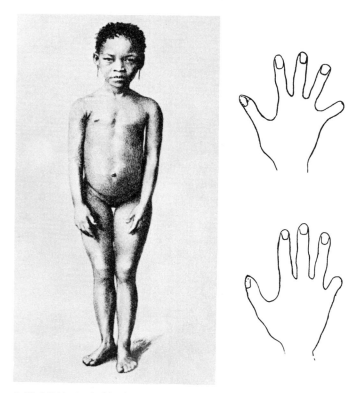

1.20 N'Aissi, child of a Bushman family that was exhibited in Berlin in 1886. In four of the six members of the family, one or more fingers were stunted, as shown on right. "In every sickness of what kind soever it is usual with them to take off extreme joints of the fingers, beginning with the little finger of the left hand."

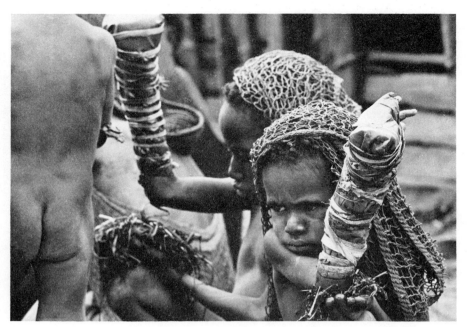

1.21 New Guinea, 1961: these little Dani girls just lost one or two fingers under a stone adze, as a sacrifice, with no more anesthesia than a hard rap on the elbow. The wounds were dressed in ashes and clay, then the remaining fingers were bent into a fist and wrapped in leaves. Blood ran for several hours; the brave little creatures soaked it up in a handful of grass held under the elbow. They knew they would heal, and that it might happen again.

1.22 Grown-up Dani women, like this one, fondle their children "with hands that are mostly thumbs." Their fingers went to placate the ghosts, together with pigs and shell goods. Infection must have taken place, but it does not seem to have caused much trouble. (Now that the Dani have been civilized, they have traded ritual amputation for cigarettes.)

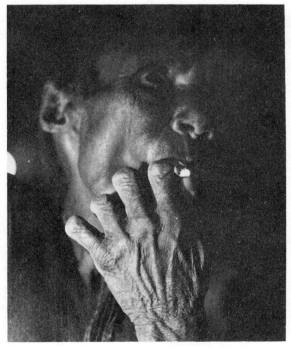

The Birth of Surgery

And when did *Homo sapiens* discover the peaceful use of wounds that we call surgery? The priority is usually assigned to the man who had the idea of making a hole in the head. But before giving him credit, I would like to place on record another possible claim, for the unsung genius who castrated a bull and thereby invented the ox. His case must ultimately hinge on discovery of the proper fossil. Although the bones of an ox are not quite the same as those of a bull (Fig. 1.23), the difference, unfortunately, is relatively small, and the distinction is even more difficult in the presence of female bones. To sort out the three kinds of skeletons would thus be a matter of statistics and would require a large heap of bones.[75] To date, prehistoric sites have not been so generous. However, it is not impossible that archeologists will some day come up with the homely discovery that the first gesture of surgery to leave its mark was castration.[76] The domestication of animals could have started in the neighborhood of 8000 B.C.,[77] but so far it has been impossible to decide just when man discovered that castration was more efficient than persuasion.[78]

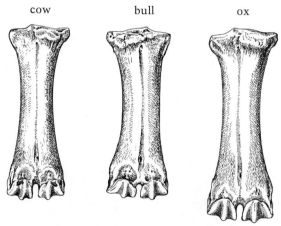

cow   bull   ox

1.23 Marks of castration that could defy millennia: metacarpal bones of a cow, bull, and ox. Contemporary.

As for trepanation of the skull, an operation to remove a portion of the bone, it may have been performed as far back as 10,000 B.C.[79] Examples have been found all over the world, and they never cease to astonish: the several thousand papers on the subject probably exceed the number of specimens. Some of the perforated skulls have nothing to do with surgery: a few may have represented birth defects; many more were worn through by tumors or infections; others were gnawed by rats and mice, or even sanded down by the wind.[80] But those that bear the marks of carving instruments must be the work of man. As far as I know, these are the oldest traces of a surgical act, and of a bold one too, if not a logical one by today's standards.

When the patient died soon after the operation, which was by no means the rule, the marks of the instrument are often so clear that it has been possible to reconstruct the four basic techniques (Fig. 1.24). In a number of skulls the hole is over or near a recent crack, so that the plan of the operator was probably to "relieve" the effect of a fracture. This is certainly true for many, perhaps most, of the skulls from Peru,[81] where the ancient Incas were masters in the art of trepanning (Figs. 1.25–1.26). As the Incas fought with

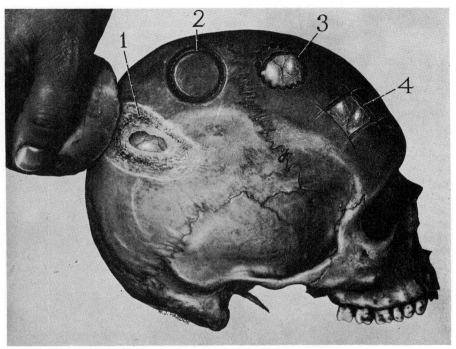

1.24 Different methods of trepanation: (1) scraping, (2) grooving, (3) boring and cutting, (4) rectangular intersecting incisions. From Lisowski 1967; courtesy of Charles C Thomas, Publisher, Springfield, Illinois.

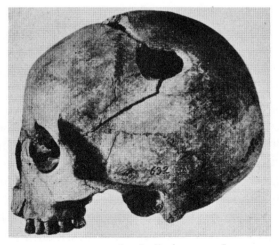

1.25 Traces of violence and mercy on the skull of a young Inca woman. This is one case in which trepanation was performed for a recognizable purpose: relieving the effect of trauma. The two surgical openings are clearly placed along a crack. Marks of the instrument are visible on the specimen. Incas were all-time masters at trepanation, but this patient must have died of her fracture.

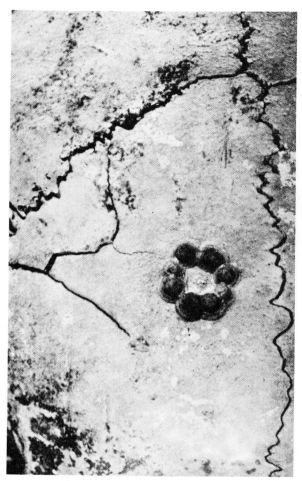

1.26 Frontal bone of another prehistoric Inca woman. Between two recent cracks, trepanation was accomplished by the rare method of drilling. The operator was probably planning to remove the central disk of bone, but left it in place for unknown reasons. The smooth edges of the drill holes suggest some survival. Patients with bad fractures like this one were doomed from the start.

great clubs and sling stones,[82] most of the injuries and trepanations are found on the left side of the skull.[83] In one collection of 273 skulls from Peru, 47 had been trepanned one to five times.[84]

Another specimen comes from prehistoric Sardinia. Its four operations must have been performed about one thousand years before Hippocrates. Three openings have smooth edges indicative of bone healing; the fourth and largest (Fig. 1.27) seems freshly cut and may have been fatal, unless death was related to the fracture that is visible.

When a prehistoric skull shows a man-made hole but no crack, rather than speculating about the reasons that made the patient ask for (or stand for) a vent in his head, we can go into the brush and ask. Trepanning is an ongoing practice among primitive and not-so-primitive tribes. A British anthropologist who worked in the mountains of Algeria between 1913 and 1921 gave the following account:

The scar of the trepan is very frequently to be found upon the living natives . . . The removal of bone from the skull is, certainly, the most important operation which the Shawiya surgeon attempts, and is the one in which he glories above all others; he therefore, performs it with remarkable frequency. The operation, though believed to require care, is certainly not regarded . . . as critical or even dangerous, indeed . . . Shawiya women . . . have been known to undergo trepanation in order to support fictitious charges of assault against husbands from whom they were seeking grounds for a divorce . . . The native surgeons . . . are unanimous in declaring that injuries resulting from a blow are the sole cause of the favourite operation . . . all . . . agreed that on no account must the *dura mater* be disturbed, as death will inevitably result should this be done, and that the sutures, which are believed to be the patient's destiny written by the hand of Allah [*they are indeed very wiggly*] must be left untouched.[85]

In modern Algeria, then, skulls were trepanned only after local injuries. Historically, magic certainly played a role. In the words of Dr. Margetts, a Canadian psychiatrist who interviewed both operators and operated in East Central Africa, the reasons for operating could be "practically everything relating to the head."[86]

The rate of survival from primitive trepanning, indicated by healing processes at the edges of the bone, is astonishing in practically all the series that have been studied: it can come close to 100 percent. One modern operator interviewed by Dr. Margetts boasted of over one hundred operations with no casualties. One of his patients had given up thirty square inches of skull in a series of sittings, with no complications except a very soft head. Doubtless men who undertook these operations with stone or bronze tools

1.27 Traces of prehistoric surgery in a skull from Nuraxi Figu in southwest Sardinia, 2000–1500 B.C. At that time southern France was a major center for trepanation. This subject was operated on in four places (two on the opposite side). The crack (center) is probably a fracture caused by a blow just before death; the last, large trepanation (right) may have been a treatment for this blow.

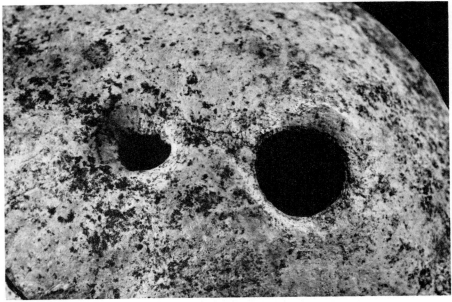

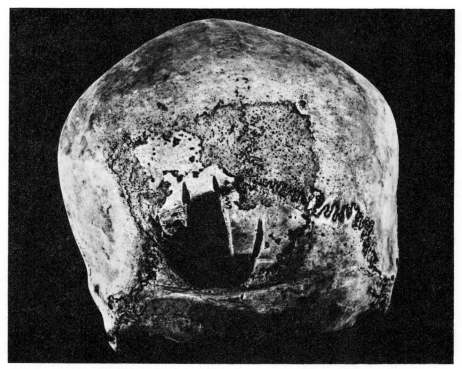

1.28 Not all prehistoric surgeons got away without infection, even in Peru. The abnormal surface around this trepanation hole betrays osteomyelitis; its angular outline probably corresponds to the extent of the surgical scalping. The surgical technique is uncommonly rough, which may well have had something to do with the poor result.

were encouraged by previous "success." This is not to say that prehistoric patients were never plagued by infection; but in most cases the outer surface of the skull around the operated site is smooth, indicating that bacteria caused no major complication. In only a few cases did osteomyelitis leave its marks (Fig. 1.28).[87]

On the whole, therefore, skull trepanning in the brush has always been, and still is, a substantially safe procedure. So we have here the paradox of primitive cultures obtaining a survival rate approaching 100 percent for the same operation that in highly differentiated cultures—during the first half of the 1800s—caused a mortality rate approaching 100 percent. By then, trepanation was so dangerous that the first requirement for the operation, wrote one authority, was "dass der Wundarzt selbst auf den Kopf gefallen sein müsse"—"that the wound surgeon himself must have fallen on his head."[88]

And here lies a partial answer, short of delirium, to the question of early man's resistance to infection. Stone Age man—whatever other worries he may have had—was safer from wound infection than many of his successors on three counts at least: there were no attending physicians to carry embattled staphylococci from one patient to the next; crowding in cities and hospitals had not yet led to the breeding of virulent strains; and man-made complications, which will occupy a large part of this book, were at a minimum.

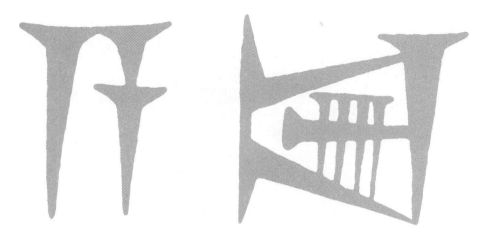

2   The Asu

Homo sapiens threw another switch, and History was turned on. That was the invention of writing.

Where did it happen? Most likely in southern Mesopotamia, now Iraq, where the Sumerians were writing around 3100 B.C.[1] Hence, the Sumerians deserve to come next on the stage, after the fossils.

Mesopotamia: A Tale of Mud

A miraculous combination took place in Mesopotamia: rivers carrying the right kind of mud, and people knowing exactly what to do with it. Of course, the Sumerians were not alone in doing great deeds in the Bronze Age world; other great civilizations were being nourished by the Nile, the Hindus, the Yellow River (Fig. 2.1). But when the days of Mesopotamia were over, after more than three millennia, it could be said that nowhere else had men and mud done more for each other.

Surely it was not an easy land to live on. Its scorching winds, its torrential rains were unknown in Egypt. Two rivers, the Tigris and the Euphrates, gave it life, but theirs were unruly waters (Fig. 2.2), prone to rise fitfully,[2] and quite unlike those of the majestic and predictable Nile. They had to be tamed by a precarious system of canals that was a constant worry, and they carried silt at such a rate that the Sumerian beaches on the Persian gulf are now perhaps one hundred miles inland (Fig. 2.3).[3] Marshes offered plenty of reeds—called in Akkadian *qanū*, related to the English *cane*[4]—but timber and stone were scarce.

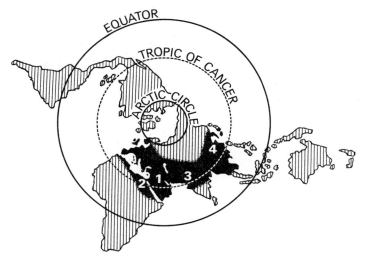

2.1 The four main river-valley civilizations of the ancient world: (1) Mesopotamian, (2) Egyptian, (3) Indian, (4) Chinese. Areas where bronze was used are shown in black.

The houses were built of sun-dried bricks, hidden behind an extra layer of mud.[5] When a house became obsolete, its walls were pushed over and a new one was built over the fill, a foot or two higher. Slowly the cities became perched on mounds of clay. The clay, of course, was also shaped into pottery; then the pottery was turned on wheels; and later the wheels were applied to carts, a step that the Egyptians were unable to make on their own.[6]

Wheel and clay were also combined to produce legal documents. Strung around their neck, worthy citizens carried a little cylinder of stone or other hard material, engraved all around. Whenever they were called upon to sign their name on legal documents, which must have been often in that highly bureaucratic society, they rolled their cylinder over the wet clay tablet (Fig. 2.4). And finally, not long after the invention of the wheel—perhaps only a few centuries later—the men of the lowlands turned mud and reeds into writing materials.

The first Sumerian writings were not cuneiform at all: they were drawings of objects (pictograms), traced in clay, probably with a pointed reed. Later the continuous line-drawing was replaced with many bits of short, wedge-shaped ("cuneiform") lines, obtained by pressing the tip of the reed, held sideways, into the clay. Thus, the Sumerians put together a set of about 350 signs, mostly ideograms, well suited to their monosyllabic language (Fig. 2.5).

Around 2600 B.C. these inventive people were overrun by the Akkadians, who spoke an entirely different, Semitic language. The newcomers borrowed the Sumerian written signs (somewhat as the Japanese borrowed Chinese signs), while Sumerian itself survived as Mesopotamia's classical language, just as Greek and Latin survive today. In fact, the single continuous thread that runs through all of Mesopotamia's turbulent history, apart from the mud, is its Sumerian heritage.

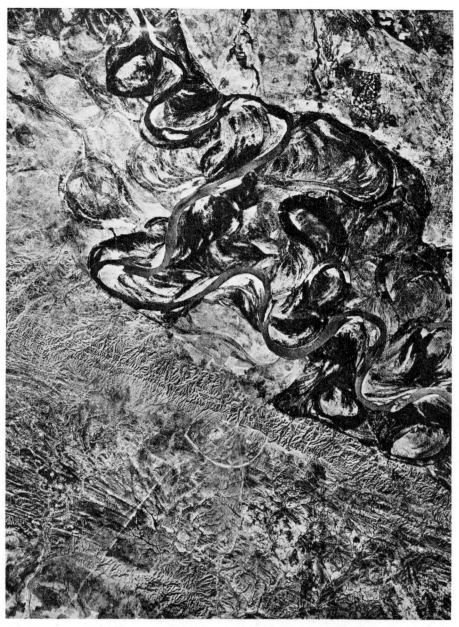

2.2 Rivers, floods, and silt were at the heart of Mesopotamian life. The sacred city of Dur-Untash (bottom center) was built around 1250 B.C. with clay carried from the banks of the treacherous river above. Aerial view.

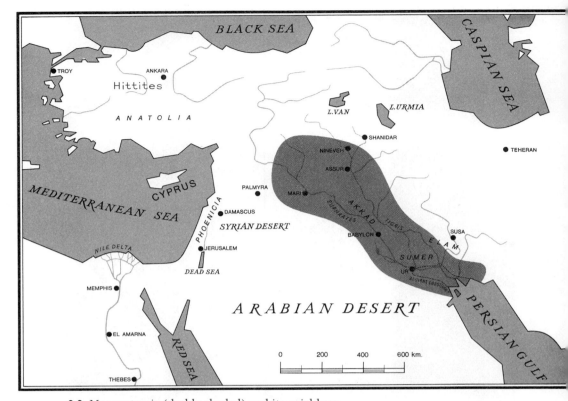

2.3 Mesopotamia (darkly shaded) and its neighbors.

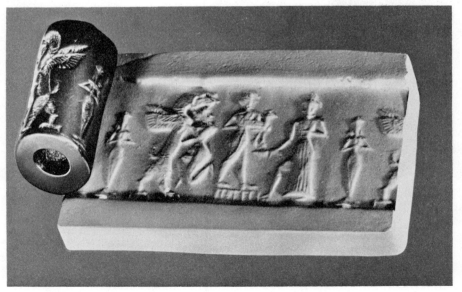

2.4 Cylinder seal in action: a winged dragon trying to bite off a man's head; the offering of a goat to Shamash, the sun-god; and Ishtar, goddess of both love and war. The scene might possibly tell the gratitude of a patient after a narrow escape. Circa 1700 B.C.; almost twice actual size.

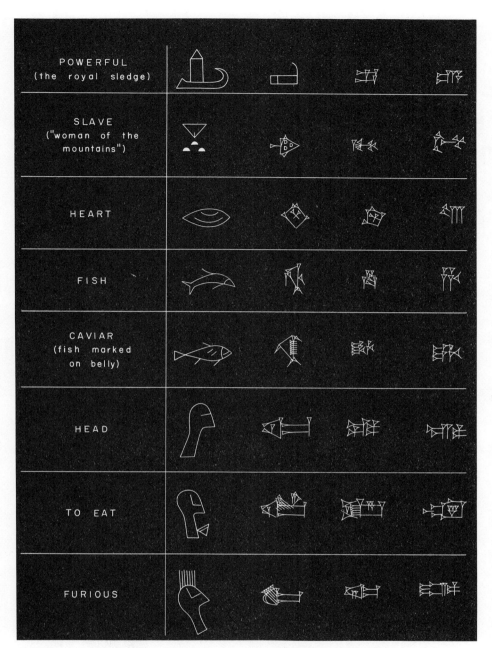

2.5 The development of writing from Sumerian pictograms (first column) to late Assyrian and Babylonian cuneiform (fourth column). At an early stage (second column) the symbols were turned 90 degrees counterclockwise (probably for convenience, as the clay tablet was held in the left hand) and drawn with cuneiform signs; then the drawings were progressively simplified. The Sumerian signs have a charm of their own, but lack the beauty of Egyptian hieroglyphs; for example, compare the symbol for *heart* with the corresponding Egyptian sign (Fig. 3.6).

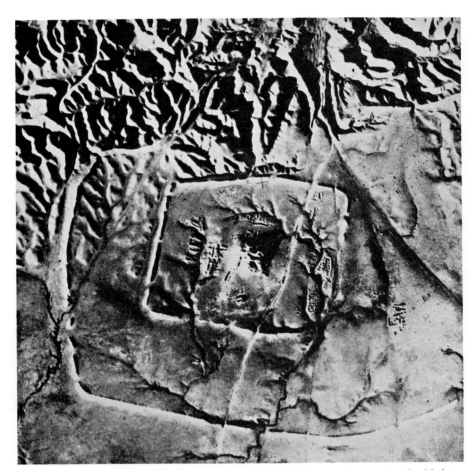

2.6 Closer view of Dur-Untash, silted up and scarred by rainwater, as time had left it. The temple-tower or *Ziggurat* (center) is barely distinguishable from any other hill. Ziggurats were made of large, sun-dried clay bricks, covered with a thin shell of baked brick. When this facing was gone, the whole tower was exposed to erosion.

As kingdoms came and went, and Akkadian dialects took shape— Assyrian, Babylonian, Chaldean—the number of cuneiform signs grew tremendously and then settled to about 600, a number that only an elite of scribes could master. The man in the street continued to sign the clay with his cylinder seal or, if he had none, with the hem of his garment, or even with his fingernails.[7] This cumbersome way of writing in clay lasted more than three thousand years and spread over much of western Asia, while the civilization that had produced it reached its peak around 1600 B.C., then began to decline. It was already dying in 547 B.C. when Cyrus the Persian conquered Babylon.[8] Cuneiform writing lingered on, despite wave after wave of new invaders and competition from the far simpler alphabetic systems, until finally it flickered out around 75 A.D.[9] As the writing sank into oblivion, it carried with it most of its messages. All the rest vanished too: the cities melted back into the ground (Fig. 2.6); silt erased the network of canals; the huge temple-towers of biblical fame—one was the Tower of Babel[10]— crumbled into mounds to match those of the countryside. Time did its job so

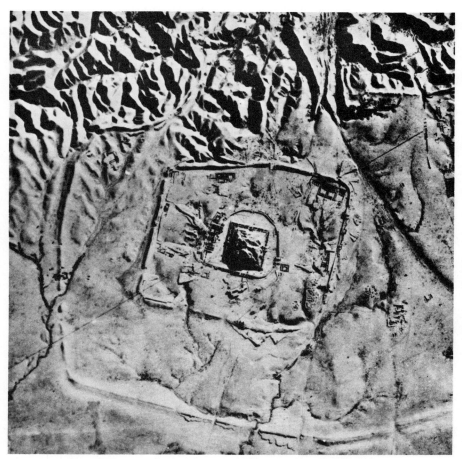

2.7 Dur-Untash begins to reappear. The three walls enclosed the clergy (inner square), the king and nobles (middle ring), and the people (outer square).

thoroughly that in the year 1800 anyone interested in Mesopotamian history would have to rely, primarily, on a few paragraphs in the Bible.

The resurrection began in 1802, when the first few words of cuneiform script were deciphered.[11] Today, Assyriology—the study of all the Mesopotamian civilizations—is a world of its own, so sophisticated that the translations of cuneiform tablets include, quite routinely, a list of scribal errors. The mounds that were Mesopotamian cities, gigantic crystals laid down by dozens of generations of busy people, are now the archeologist's dream. A typical mound contained fourteen periods layered within one hundred feet[12] (Fig. 2.7).

The Sumerians, whose name had been lost, were rediscovered less than a century ago.[13] It turned out that their civilization had never died at all: some of their myths were echoed in the Bible. Even the Biblical Deluge was a reality of Sumerian history.[14] Babylonians listed their kings as "before the Deluge" and after. They even had a Noah, complete with ark and dove, whose name was Ut-Napishtim in Sumerian, Atra-ḫasīs in Akkadian.[15]

Mesopotamian Medicine: The Sources

Cuneiform writing is practically the only source of information about Mesopotamian medicine. No instruments, no artistic representations are known, and skeletal remains are minimal.[16] The literature of neighboring countries is almost silent; the Greeks could have little to tell us about it anyway, since the greatest period of Mesopotamian civilization, the centuries around 1600 B.C., came long before Homer.

The texts of medical interest amount to no more than a thousand tablets or fragments. Consider that we are exploring a period that ranges—roughly— from 3000 B.C. all the way to the beginning of the Christian era. All along this path the "medical" tablets are sprinkled sparingly, a couple here, a fragment there, with huge time gaps in between. The great bulk occurs very near the end and derives from one single treasure-trove: the library of Assurbanipal, the last great king of Assyria.[17] This collection was buried with the palace when Nineveh was destroyed in 612 B.C., and it reappeared in 1853 as a ditch full of tablets: about 20,000 in a layer five feet deep. The king had been so systematic that his archives are a near-complete fossil of the literature in his day.[18] It was already late, of course; but not too late, because the scribes were in the habit of copying and recopying ancient tablets, so that many of the texts are actually much older than Assurbanipal's reign, perhaps by as much as a millennium[19].

Out of this mass of material, Campbell Thompson of Oxford collected 660 tablets of a medical nature.[20] The vast majority contain prescriptions. Real medical books with flowing text do not exist; however, certain series of tablets with similar entries are often referred to as treatises,[21] such as the "Treatise on Prescriptions for Diseases of the Head."[22]

The largest collection of this kind is the "Treatise of Medical Diagnoses and Prognoses,"[23] a group of three thousand entries on forty tablets, whereby the future of patients could be foretold, depending on certain signs, bodily, natural, or other. Here, too, most of the tablets were actually written a millennium or more after the peak of Akkadian civilization. The patience and knowledge required to reassemble these forty tablets is hard to conceive. Labat inherited the problem as a transcendental puzzle in cuneiform, with bits of different editions that had been written centuries apart in various parts of Mesopotamia, and are now scattered among the museums of two continents. The text is both interesting and entertaining despite the large number of incomplete lines. It is a list of diseases arranged from head to foot. In fact, many are not true diseases but "situations" of prognostic significance, like the number of openings on the nipple of an expectant mother (5 and 6 are bad, 7 to 10 are good). The actual prognostic significance of the work, in the modern sense, is about nil. Its value is more general, for many of the symptoms described are real (like *amurriqânu*, "jaundice"), and some relationships, like venereal infection, are correctly observed. However, the treatise is essentially a handbook of the sorcerer,[24] not a manual of medicine.

The remaining sources are marginal: allusions in laws, letters, and literary texts. Not much, if you wish; but how dangerous. The non-Assyriologist who tries to explore this material is bound to make a fool of himself unless an expert leads him step by step. Translations and books with all the outward appearance of classics are painfully outdated and misleading; recent reviews of the medical material are almost nonexistent;[25] whole volumes of new material are being "published," but in cuneiform;[26] much else is still in the form of tablets.[27] As if this were not enough, one also has to contend with a shattering truth, so obvious to every Assyriologist that it is not spelled out anywhere: Akkadian does not handle like Greek or Latin. The translation of many words still carries a *probability tag*, which is well known to the professional and may or may not keep changing with time, so that the printed translation has no absolute value. This is a fact of life; nothing much can be done to help the outsider. It follows that no text can be quoted, let alone interpreted in medical terms, without consulting first an Assyriologist. Roses may have become mustard; cress may have become a bush with thorns.[28] A beautiful charm that begins "The Sieve, the Sieve, the Red Sieve"[29] read in an earlier translation "O Willow, Willow, dark Willow."[30]

Without the help and understanding of some of the world's leading Assyriologists, this chapter would have been a comedy of errors.

Searching for Mesopotamian Wounds

Since the wound came before the surgeon, we shall begin by searching the cuneiform texts for the word *wound*. Please note that this is much more significant than looking up an entry in a dictionary: until that time, the wound had been a fact in the flesh; from then on it was also a concept inscribed in clay.

Surprisingly, there seems to have been no single, precise Akkadian equivalent for our term *wound*. I was looking forward to some telling Sumerian pictogram, but none with this meaning has come down to us. In most cases the text has the rather loose word *mursu* (Fig. 2.8), which meant "disease" as well as "diseased part," so that the idea of wound must be guessed from the context, as in the following examples:

> pān   mursi   takappar...
> the surface   of the sick part   you shall clean ...
>
> pān   mursi   himēta   tapasshash...
> the surface   of the sick part   with butter   you shall anoint ...
>
> ana   libbi   mursi   tashakkan.
> into   the inside   of the sick part [wound?]   you shall put [it].[31]

Other words come closer to *wound* but have a special connotation: *niksu*, "cut"; *liptu*, "blow"; *shimittu*, "bruise"; and *dikshu* (Fig. 2.9), "piercing pain" or "wound caused by piercing," but a German dictionary translates it as "swelling."[32] A host of words are tentatively translated as "abscess," "pustule," "eczema," and other kinds of skin lesions. If the Assyriolo-

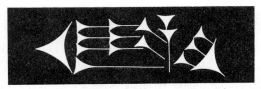

2.8 An Akkadian ideogram: *murṣu*, "the sick place"—sometimes a wound.

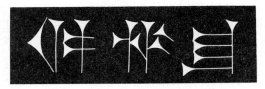

2.9 Another Akkadian ideogram: *dikshu*, written here *di-ik-shu*, as it might have appeared around 1000 B.C.; meaning either "piercing wound" or "piercing pain".

gist called to become a diagnostician is sometimes puzzled, the layman is outright bewildered to find that holes and bumps are thrown together, since the *Reallexikon der Assyriologie* registers a single entry for *Geschwulst* and *Geschwür*, "tumor" and "ulcer."[33] Perhaps each Akkadian term had a reasonably precise clinical equivalent in its day; but now, I suspect that most could be translated just as well by "sore."

With medical art at such a primitive stage, we cannot expect to find much evidence of a correlation between wounds and symptoms. However, it would be unfair not to recall two bas-reliefs which are almost textbook evidence of anatomo-clinical correlations: the famous lioness wounded in the spinal cord, showing the expected paralysis of the rear end (Fig. 2.10), and a lion wounded in the chest, demonstrating that torn lungs cause bleeding by the mouth (Fig. 2.11).

Two Ways To Treat

Given this ample supply of *liptu* and *dikshu*, it remains to be seen what a citizen could do about them. The tablets offer a choice of remedies, which seem to fall into two broad categories: primitive first aid and outright sorcery. The choice was real, for it is well established that injuries, in the days of Babylon, could be treated in two different but complementary ways, like any other disease.[34] Here is one method:

> *Incantation.* If a man has a blow on the cheek, practical prescription for this: Bray [*a plant*] in water from the well of Marduk, collect therein dust from four crossroads . . . Seven and seven times cleanse his mouth.[35]

Here is the other method, prescribed for the same injury:

> If a man is sick with a blow on the cheek: pound together fir-turpentine, pine-turpentine, tamarisk, daisy, flour of *Inninnu*. Strain; mix in milk and beer in a small copper pan; spread on skin, bind on him, and he shall recover.[36]

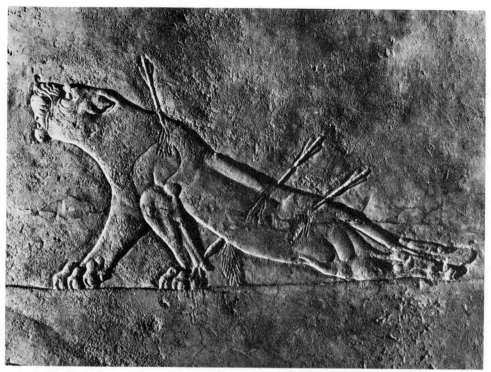

2.10 Clinical observation in art: an injury to the spinal cord (top arrow) paralyzes the rear end.

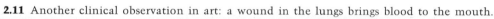

2.11 Another clinical observation in art: a wound in the lungs brings blood to the mouth.

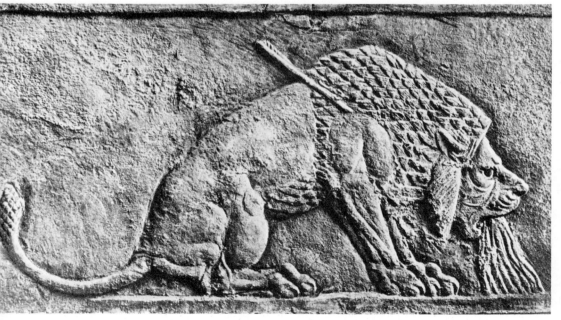

The first remedy is from the *áshipu* or "sorcerer," the second from the *asu* or "physician" (pronounced *ah'zoo*).[37] In the mind of the scribes these two forms of therapy must have had similar value, because they were recorded pell-mell on the same tablets.[38] Kings certainly used both; their correspondence with royal physicians is preserved in several court archives, together with whole volumes of general advice from sorcerers.[39] The two types of healers were probably collaborators rather than competitors: the sorcerer used drugs, and occasionally the asu used charms.[40]

With time, as the Akkadian world declined, the asu ceased to be mentioned and the sorcerer took over; a retreat of physic before magic that we shall find in another ultraconservative society, the Egyptian.[41] It is therefore not surprising that the only medical event recorded by art, as far as is known, was treatment by magic: several amulets show the patient lying on a bed, arms raised, between masked sorcerers who are chasing away Lamashtu, a fierce, lion-headed goddess who specialized in persecuting pregnant women (Fig. 2.12).[42]

How the sick Akkadians chose between the asu and áshipu we do not know. One factor may have been that the sorcerer was a member of the clergy.[43] Today we equate drugs and magic with good and bad, respectively. Given the drugs of the time, we might well have preferred magic. But whatever the choice, one point is clear: both men filled a need; *both practiced medicine.*

The name of the asu has survived in the Biblical name of King Asa, which was probably short for Asa-El, "God-Heals" (another way to say God-Heals was Rapha-El, which gave the name Raphael).[44] There was no particular term for surgeon, probably because the asu himself took to the knife when necessary. This he definitely did. The word for knife was the same as for "barber's razor," *naglabu.*[45] Two of the signs used to write it derive from the Sumerian pictograms for dagger and hand (Figs. 2.13–2.14). In the Royal Library at Nineveh the medical tablets bear an official stamp, in which King Assurbanipal boasts of having registered on tablets the three ways to health: "the art of healing with drugs" (*bultítu*), "the way of operating with the brass knife" (*šipir bêl imti*), and "the prescriptions of the sorcerers" (*urti mashmashē*).[46] Perhaps he did, but somehow the brass knife has left few written traces, as we shall see.[47] And not a single tablet describes what was done about war wounds on the battlefield.

Tꟻ ⌸

This scarcity of surgical literature might be, of course, a matter of chance. Labat suggests a different explanation.[48] The scribes did not try to record all existing knowledge. They concentrated only on those traditions that required an *aide-mémoire*, a written guide, leaving the rest to oral transmission. So they never bothered to describe the daily tasks of most artisans. They did make an exception for the perfume makers and the glass makers; apparently these craftsmen thought enough of their work, or thought that there was enough theory about it, to have it explained in writing.[49] But the simple ways of Mesopotamian surgery may not have been worth explaining in the clay.

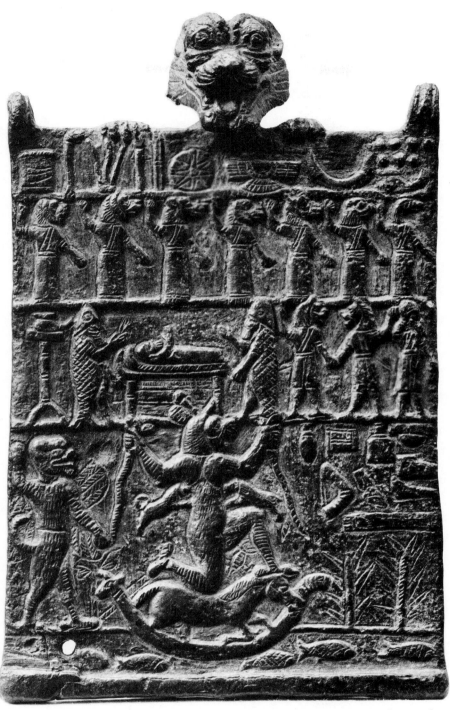

2.12 Amulet depicting the "other way" of treating disease: two sorcerers disguised as fish try to induce Lamashtu (the lion-headed goddess) to retreat from the patient, cross the Bitter River, and go back to the world below. Slightly enlarged.

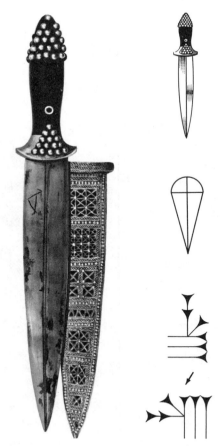

2.13 Sumerian dagger of solid gold, c.2500 B.C. From daggers such as this came the Sumerian pictogram (middle right), and finally the cuneiform ideogram (bottom right), for the surgeon's knife, *naglabu*. In this figure and in following ones, the oblique arrow indicates the 90-degree turn incurred by the cuneiform symbols.

2.14 The connection between barbers and surgeons goes a long way back. The Assyrian word for the surgeon's knife, *naglabu*, could also be written with three signs that originally meant "knife [of] barber." In the original Sumerian pictograms (bottom) the barber's hand is quite obvious (the meaning of the last sign is not clear).

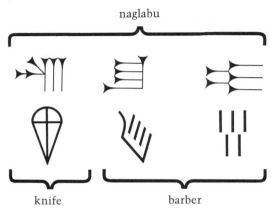

Surgery As Seen by the Law

The proudest document of Akkadian surgery, and one of the oldest, is not a tablet but a huge black stone; a block of polished diorite, eight feet high, engraved with the 282 laws of King Hammurabi's Code, about 1700 B.C. It was found—broken—in 1901–1902 by a French expedition, reassembled, photographed, translated, and published in a superb volume, all within eleven months.[50] As one of the outstanding documents of humanity, this stone deserved the haste. It is now at the Louvre (Fig. 2.15).

The stone will speak for itself; but notice, to begin, that the laws concerning the surgeon follow those that deal with assault and battery:

204: If a commoner has struck the cheek of a[nother] commoner, he shall pay ten shekels of silver. . .

206: If a seignior has struck a[nother] seignior in a brawl and has inflicted an injury on him, that seignior shall swear "I did not strike him deliberately," and he shall also pay for the physician . . .

215: If a physician performed a major operation on a seignior with a bronze lancet and has saved the seignior's life, or he opened the eye-socket [nakkaptu] of a seignior with a bronze lancet and has saved the seignior's eye, he shall receive ten shekels of silver.

216: If it was a member of the commonalty, he shall receive five shekels.

217: If it was a seignior's slave, the owner of the slave shall give two shekels of silver to the physician.

218: If a physician performed a major operation on a seignior with a bronze lancet and has caused the seignior's death, or he opened the eye-socket [nakkaptu] of a seignior and has destroyed the seignior's eye, they shall cut off his hand.

219: If a physician performed a major operation on a commoner's slave with a bronze lancet and caused [his] death, he shall make good slave for slave.

220: If he opened up his eye-socket [nakkaptu] with a bronze lancet and has destroyed his eye, he shall pay one-half his value in silver.

221: If a physician has set a seignior's broken bone, or has healed a sprained tendon, the patient [lit. "the owner of the injury"] shall give five shekels of silver to the physician.

222: If it was a member of the commonalty, he shall give three shekels of silver.

223: If it was a seignior's slave, the owner of the slave shall give two shekels of silver to the physician. . .

226: If a brander cut off the slave-mark of a slave not his own without the consent of the owner of the slave, they shall cut off the hand of that brander.[51]

These entries are all that may be considered to have any reference to medical practice: which means that *the Code did not hold the physician responsible unless he used his knife*, as in law 215. Other translations of that particular law are actually phrased, "If a physician . . . operates a man of a severe wound"[52] or "makes a deep incision."[53] Any other condition, treated by nonsurgical means, was not subject to the penalty of malpractice. This was in keeping with the Akkadian concept of disease: if someone became ill, it was either his own fault for having committed a sin, or he had become the victim of outside agents, such as an evil spirit, a god, cold, dust, or a bad smell.[54] The physician could not be held responsible for any of these causes.

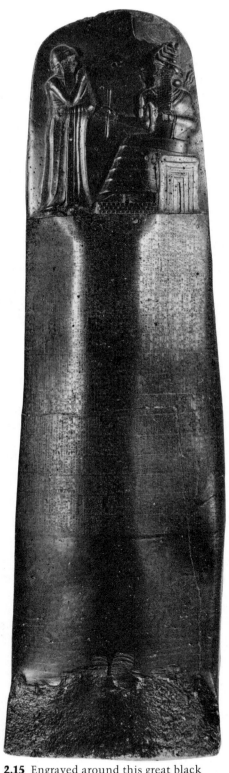

2.15 Engraved around this great black stone, nearly eight feet tall, are the laws of Hammurabi, c. 1700 B.C. At the top is the king himself, receiving the word from Shamash, the Sun-god.

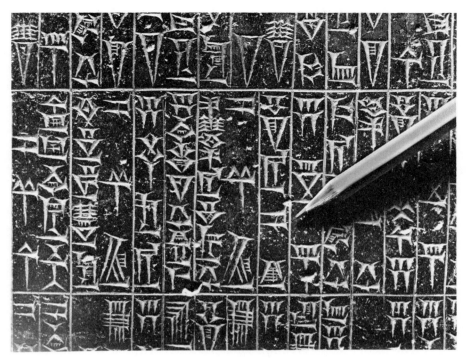

2.16 Hammurabi's law 215, which refers to the surgeon's knife. The pencil, shown for scale, points to the letter ⬦ *A* of *asu*, "physician."

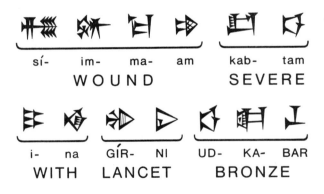

sí- im- ma- am kab- tam
WOUND **SEVERE**

i- na GÍR- NI UD- KA- BAR
WITH **LANCET** **BRONZE**

2.17 Locating the *wound* and the *lancet* in the text of Fig. 2.16, tipped to the left so that the lines read horizontally. (In the transcription, as customary, small letters correspond to Akkadian words, capitals to Sumerian.)

In contrast, a wound wilfully caused by a man, physician or not, had to be the responsibility of that man (Figs. 2.16–2.17).

The cutting of the *nakkaptu* has given rise to half a dozen translations, mostly centered on the notion that the asu was operating for a cataract, as was surely done in ancient India. A close look at the word itself rather suggests some operation around the eye.[55] Even less is known about the nature of the other surgical operations, except that the surgeon's fees appear to have been as stiff as the punishments mentioned in the Code. The fee for a "deep incision on a seignior" was ten shekels of silver: enough to cover the labor for a substantial house or to pay a carpenter for 450 working days (that was when the Code was written; now, 85 grams of silver are worth just 9 dollars[56]).

However, it is not at all sure that the asu really made a fortune on his surgery, or that he staked both his hands at it, because ancient codes did not necessarily correspond to real life. Judges did not feel bound by the written law. Of the legal documents that have been found, none refers to a law of Hammurabi's Code.[57]

Two laws in the Code mention the *asu alpim u lu imērim*, "physician of an ox or an ass":

224: If a veterinary surgeon [*lit. "a physician of an ox or an ass"*] performed a major operation on either an ox or an ass and has saved [*its*] life, the owner of the ox or ass shall give to the surgeon one-sixth [*shekel*] of silver as his fee.
225: If he performed a major operation on an ox or an ass and has caused [*its*] death, he shall give to the owner of the ox or ass one-fourth its value.

Of this veterinary surgery there are no other records, but it certainly included castration, at least of animals. And if the asu alpim did not practice castration on people, somebody else certainly did,[58] because it was a form of punishment[59] and possibly a form of "domestication." Court employees were distinguished as either "bearded" or "eunuchs."[60]

To sum up, if it were not for Hammurabi's Code of Laws, all memory of surgical deeds in Babylon around 1700 B.C. would have been lost. Note that surgery as a craft was barely worth mentioning in clay; but *when it became an object of the law, it was engraved in stone.* Such was the scale of values in the Land Between the Rivers. The Sumerians alone left us at least 150,000 legal and administrative documents,[61] but only two medical tablets.[62] I take this to mean that—in those days at least—wrong was considered worse than disease.

Three Healing Gestures

In the treatment of wounds, there are three gestures that must be practically as old as writing: washing (which is surprisingly not mentioned in Egyptian medicine), making plasters, and bandaging. This we know for sure, because all three appear in the world's oldest medical manuscript: a small clay tablet carefully written in Sumerian around 2100 B.C. (Fig. 2.18). In a sense this precious document is disappointing, because it carries only prescriptions with no mention of diseases. However, of the fifteen prescriptions, twelve are for external use, and eight of these are plasters, which suggests that they may have been intended for local diseases or injuries.

The text is difficult; it was tackled several times,[63] and the translation may have to be retouched in years to come, but the unknown author's selection of drugs comes through quite clearly. There is no real difference between his pharmacy and that of much later texts.[64] For example, one prescription reads:

Pound together: dried wine dregs, juniper and prunes; pour beer on the mixture. Then rub [*the diseased part*] with oil, and bind on [*as a plaster*].[65]

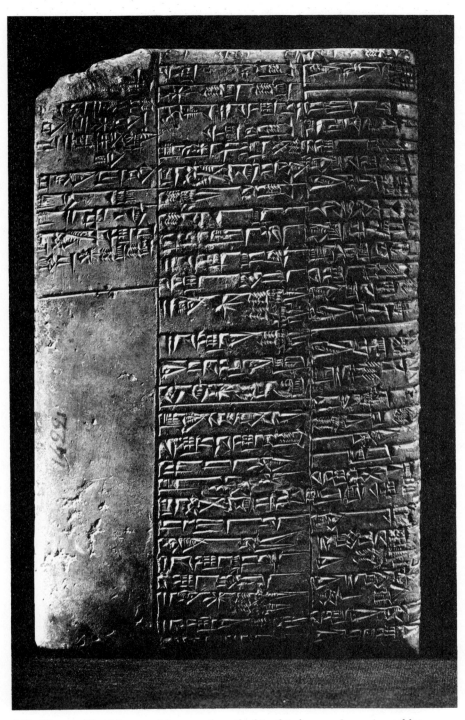

2.18 The world's oldest poultices are described in this famous Sumerian tablet, which is also the world's oldest medical text. The style of writing dates it from the Third Dynasty of Ur, c.2158–2008 B.C. or a little earlier. The oldest Egyptian papyrus, the Kahun papyrus, was written around 1850 B.C.

The Sumerians were great beer lovers: they brewed at least nineteen brands—there is a whole book on the subject.[66] The alcoholic content of beer is much too low to have any significance as an antiseptic. However, as the antiseptic properties of wine depend on components other than alcohol, it is possible that beer too contains such antibacterial substances. As to juniper, under the name of *burashu* it later became the most used ingredient of Akkadian pharmacy.

The following prescription is more ambitious:

> Pass through a sieve and then knead together: turtle shell, naga-si plant, salt and mustard. Then wash the diseased part with beer of good quality and hot water, and rub with the mixture. Then friction and rub again with oil, and put on [*a plaster of?*] pounded pine." [67]

Note that the diseased part is first washed with beer and hot water. A Sumerian could scarcely have chosen a better wound-wash, though a kind of liquid soap was also already available.[68] The first rubbing, with a mixture including salt and mustard, may have been intended to cause stinging; perhaps by then the patient already felt that if the medicine stings, it really works. Another prescription reads:

> Take some river sediment, pound it, knead it with water; then rub the diseased part with mineral oil, and bind on as a plaster.[69]

There goes the mud again. If it was meant for an aching joint, the main difference with twentieth century medicine is that our mud plasters are hot. If it was meant for a wound, the practice is still current in the same land: an archeologist returning from Iraq told me that his native diggers treated their wounds with clay (sometimes also with eggwhite and chicken feathers).

So much for Sumerian plasters. If we now skip fifteen centuries and roam through the archives of Assurbanipal in search of more attractive stuff to put on wounds, we will find one such item—sesame oil—though drowned among so many other Sumerian-sounding drugs that the overall impression is scarcely one of progress.

The asu, alas, never knew very much. His knowledge of anatomy remained at the level of butchery. His physiology was about nil: the heart was the site of intelligence; liver harbored anger; strength was in the kidneys, and the brain was more or less forgotten.[70] Of sutures, of ligatures of bleeding vessels, apparently also of cauteries, he had no inkling. The crux of his art, *bultîtu*, lay in concocting for each case just the right kind of *bultu*: a sort of mush made of herbs and other ingredients, usually pounded, cooked, and strained.[71] You would swallow your bultu or apply it externally, take it as an enema or even inhale it.[72] Two bultu would probably never be the same, because the amounts were not stated and probably not measured, and the choice of ingredients was large—including such imaginative items as dung of lizard and marrow of long bone.[73] In the remains of a drugstore of the first millennium, tablets were found listing all the drugs on the shelves, about 230 in all (Fig. 2.19).[74]

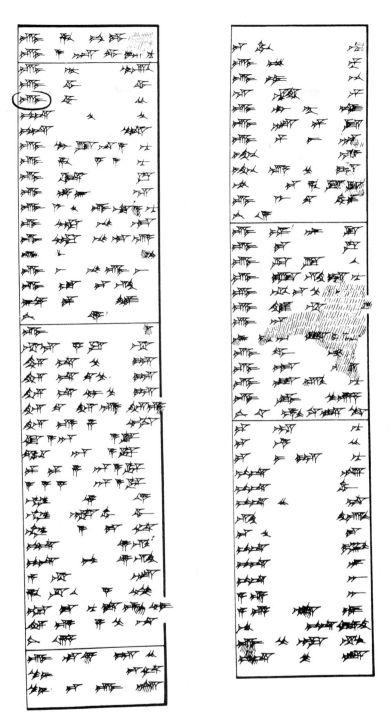

2.19 Part of the inventory of an Assyrian pharmacy. The
repeated sign along the left margin (see circle) reads *shammu*,
literally "herb" (also "drug"). Listed were some 230 items,
almost the entire Assyrian pharmacopoeia. First half of the first
millennium B.C.

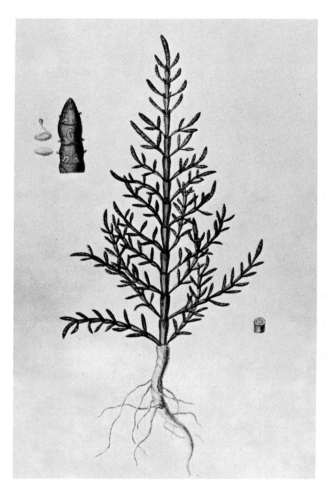

2.20 *Salicornia herbacea* L., a kind of glasswort common in Mesopotamia. Glasswort was the general name for plants that gave ashes rich in alkali, later used for glass making (*kâlati,* "burned," gave the Arabic *al-quali,* "the [plant] ash," hence *alkali*).

However, the asu seems to have known two procedures that qualify—for his time—as advanced technology. Some of the plasters required the heating of resin or fat with alkali, which yields soap. The alkali was obtained by burning certain plants, like *Salicornia* (Fig. 2.20). Coniferous resins contain abietic acids, which also form excellent soaps with alkali; many modern soaps are prepared from a mixture of fats with resins. Perhaps these prescriptions aimed at a detergent effect, although the resulting soap is never mentioned.[75]

Then, a "wrapping for the head" includes pine, spruce, myrrh, gum of aleppo pine, honey, fat from the kidney of a male sheep (so far a standard mixture), but also "essence" of cedar.[76] Thus, the asu must have had at his service the process of distillation, once thought to be a much later invention.[77] Suitable pots have actually been found (Fig. 2.21).

Both procedures, the "soap" and the "essence," were already hinted at in the famous Sumerian medical tablet discussed above.[78] We are free to choose how to conclude: either progress was very slow, or the starting level was relatively high . . .

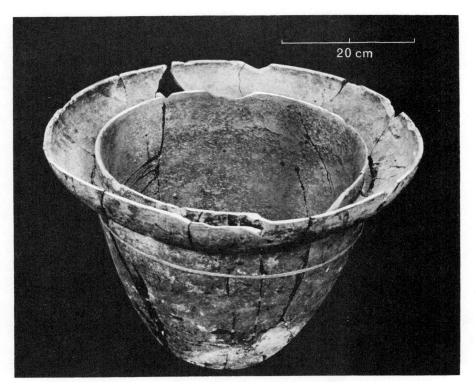

2.21 Akkadian drugs included distillates, which could have been prepared with vessels like this one (above), about 5500 years old. According to a chemist-Assyriologist, it would be possible to obtain a distillate with the pot, as shown below: the raw material is placed on the bottom and heated gently; vapors, such as volatile oils, condense against the cooler lid and trickle into the rim, where they are wiped up with a rag.

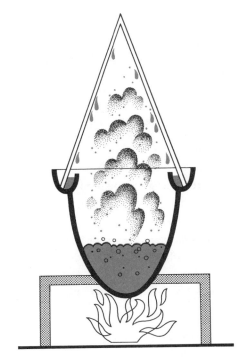

Three Surgical Wounds

Definite, bona fide wounds are mentioned in relation to the bronze knife, which makes, by the latest count, four appearances in the clay tablets—thanks to the archives of Assurbanipal. Each one of these is an exercise in frustration: "You shall take the knife . . ." and the rest is broken off.[79] In one tablet, although the text is damaged, these intriguing words stand out: "three ribs . . . fourth rib cut open . . . fluid . . ." a strong suggestion that the asu was cutting his way into the chest.[80] In principle this operation would not be anything extraordinary: a collection of pus in the pleura, or even in the liver (where amoebae are able to carve out large abscesses), can bulge under the skin and open out spontaneously, so that the knife would just help the natural process. But in either case the cut would need to be much lower than the third rib.

To rescue the sense, Labat proposed that the Akkadians may have counted the ribs backward, that is, upward, which is actually more natural.[81] In this way the cut would fall just where it should. In fact, I was elated to find that Labat's idea is borne out by ancient Greek medicine. The Hippocratic treatise *On Internal Diseases* describes the incision of the chest for pleural empyema as follows: "Having established this, incise over the third rib, beginning from the last."[82]

The two remaining operations referred to are in the collection of "Prescriptions for Diseases of the Head."[83] In one case the knife goes as far as scraping the skull, which was to become a favorite occupation of Greek medicine.[84] This patient seems to suffer from an abscess under the scalp.

If the ailment mentioned above [*the text above is lost*] is painless, and the very surface of the flesh is intact; if, when you open, [pus squirts out and] keeps flowing: the name of this disease is "little she-fly" [*meaning unclear*]. If the wind has blown onto the patient, it is a case of Pabil-sag [the god]: you can operate it [*lit. "you can make a prescription."* In other cases the physician is advised not to intervene[85]]. To remove it, attack this disease with the point [of the knife. After cutting it open] grind: boiled plaster, salt of ammonia and powder of . . . [*a mineral, possibly belemnite*]. Apply all this onto the diseased surface and make a dressing of it. If the disease [has reached] into the bone, cut all around, scrape and remove [*that is, scrape off and remove the sick bone[86]*].

The other fragment preserves in some detail the postoperative care of the wound. If the top of this tablet had been broken off, it would have been impossible to appreciate its treasure, because the wound of the scalp is referred to literally as "the sick place." Here it is, the best of three surgical dressings to represent one hundred generations of Mesopotamian practice:

Wash a fine linen in water, soak it in oil, and put it on the wound.
Bray powder of acacia and ammonia salt, and put it on the wound; let the dressing stand for three days. When [*you remove it*] wash a fine linen in water, soak it in oil, put it on the wound, and knot a bandage over it.
Leave the dressing three more days . . .
Thus continue the dressing until healing ensues.[87]

This is essentially a dressing with oil. Now it may seem delirious to discuss this single dressing, one of millions that were lost; but no statistician could argue that where there is a leaf, there was at least a tree. And then we can check this lone tablet against one other source on Mesopotamia, the Bible:

> O sinful nation, people loaded with iniquity . . .
> from head to foot there is not a sound spot in you—
> nothing but bruises and weals and raw wounds
>   which have not felt compress or bandage
>   or soothing oil.[88]

So this *was* a common dressing; presumably with sesame oil in Mesopotamia, olive oil in Palestine. Oil and grease cannot do much harm on raw flesh, and they also serve the useful purpose of preventing the bandage from sticking to the wound, like today's first-aid creams. Bacteria do not grow in oil. In fact, we tested the survival of staphylococci in sesame oil and found that they were rapidly killed.[89] Beyond these practical facts, oil had very special connotations. To us it means salad dressing and lubrication; in the ancient Near East it was a basic need of life; it was the main source of light, a ritual offering, a measure of wealth, and a spiritual symbol in the many anointing ceremonies.[90] When the asu applied it to a wound, he certainly felt that he was doing something basically good, and so did his patient.

Traces of Medical Theory

While the tablets are fairly explicit about what the physician did, they do not explain why he did it. This we have to read between the lines. The single exception is a startling letter in which Arad-Nana, the *rab asi* or "chief physician" to King Esharaddon (680–669 B.C.), explains a mechanism—not for the sake of science, but to straighten out an ignorant colleague before the king.[91] This is also the one and only reference to a treatment for bleeding:

To the King my lord, your servant Arad-Nana. May it be surpassingly well with the King my lord. May Ninurta and Gula grant health of mind and body to the King my lord.

It is exceedingly well with the son of the King. The treatment that we had planned for him, we gave it for five-sixths of a double hour [*100 minutes*]. He has walked, he has felt better and regained strength. However, he has not yet gone out . . .

In regard to the patient who had a hemorrhage from the nose, the Rab-Mugi [*a high official charged with the care of horses and chariots, possibly the Rabmag of Jeremiah 39:3*[92]] reported to me: "Yesterday toward evening much blood ran." That is because the dressings [*that I had*] prescribed are applied without knowledge. They are placed over the nostrils, [*so that*] they [*only*] obstruct the breathing [*but*] come off when there is hemorrhage. They should be placed within the nostril: [*then*] they will stop the breath and hold back the blood. If it is agreeable to the King, I will go tomorrow and give instructions. Now [*meantime*] let me hear of his condition.

Arad-Nana was absolutely right: dressings placed over the nose are of little help; they must be stuffed inside. Except for the Rab-Mugi, this letter could have been written yesterday. (Arad-Nana sounds less cocky in another letter, after the king had rebuffed him for being unable to diagnose and cure a royal disease.[93])

Let us now shift to that colorful text, the "Treatise of Prognoses."[94] Your eye will be caught by statements such as these, the first two being for *ambiance:*

> If [*the sorcerer*] sees pigs which keep lifting up their tails, [*as to*] that sick man, anxiety will not come near him.
>
> If a snake falls on the sick man's bed, that sick man will get well.
>
> If blood flows out of his penis, it is the hand of Shamash [*the Sun-god*]; sign of Land-of-no-Return [*The Underworld*].
>
> If his penis and his testicles are inflamed, the hand of the goddess Dilbat [*equivalent to Venus*] has reached him in his bed.
>
> If his testicles are inflamed, if his penis is covered with sores, he has gone in to the High Priestess of his god.[95]

Disregard the comment on the high priestess: she was only a short step beyond the line of duty (ritual prostitution was the lot of the *Qadishtu*, other women of the temple community).[96] What is most remarkable here is the use of the word *inflammation*, one of the key terms and key concepts of modern medicine.

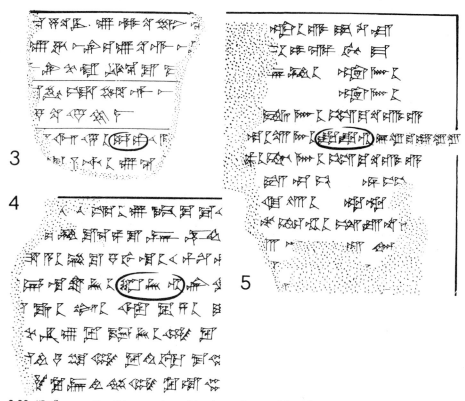

2.22 "Inflammation" is mentioned in these three tablets from Assurbanipal's library. They read: (3) "If a man, his right eye is inflamed . . ."; (4–5) ". . . his guts are inflamed . . ." The word *inflamed* (in circles) is written differently in each case.

Dans le n° 3 : [cuneiform signs]

náp - hât : "est enflammée" (œil est féminin)

le mot (forme verbale) est écrit phonétiquement ; c-à-d. que les deux
signes ont une valeur syllabique (celle du son prononcé)

Dans le n° 4 : [cuneiform signs] : innappahu "sont enflammées"
(sujet : "ses entrailles")

le mot (3ᵉ pers. pl. présent du verbe napāhu) est ici écrit
idéographiquement (c'est à dire que le signe exprime, non plus
un son, mais une idée).

Ce signe est [cuneiform] (en sumérien : MÚ) : il est suivi d'un
déterminatif ([cuneiform]) qui indique le pluriel, et d'un complément
phonétique ([cuneiform] : hu), qui précise la prononciation de la syllabe
finale du mot (innappahu).

Dans le n° 5 :

nous retrouvons la même expression que dans le n° 4 :
" ses entrailles sont enflammées " irrē-šu innappahu

Pour innappahu, il s'agit du même signe, mais, ici, dans
l'écriture assyrienne ([cuneiform]) et non plus dans l'écriture babylonienne ([cuneiform]).

D'autre part, l'idée du pluriel est marquée, non par l'emploi
d'un déterminatif spécifique ([cuneiform]), mais par le redoublement
de l'idéogramme ([cuneiform] [cuneiform]).

Suit, enfin, le même complément phonétique (hu : [cuneiform])
précisant la prononciation de la syllabe finale du mot.

2.23 Part of a letter from Prof. René Labat, explaining how it can be that the three different sets of signs in the preceding figure may all read "inflamed."

The appearance of this term is indeed a great event, worth exploring in detail. My first reaction was to find out if it was true. The word *inflammation* comes up also in Campbell Thompson's translations. I compared these with the cuneiform originals, sign by sign (Fig. 2.22). No set of signs seemed to recur. Perhaps the scholar of Merton College had been taking liberties? The first Assyriologist I consulted threw up his arms in despair, and advised me to have faith in Campbell Thompson. The second was too busy (there are far too many tablets around for the number of Assyriologists available), but would I please not rely on Campbell Thompson's translations, notoriously outdated. I wound up at the Collège de France, knocking at the door of René Labat. It was like turning on the light. In the first place, there are several words that can be rendered as "inflammation." Second, even if the same word were repeated, it might take on very different looks by being spelled either ideographically or phonetically (just like 5 or *five*, + or *plus*) and with either Assyrian or Babylonian signs (Fig. 2.23). Third, in this instance Thompson had been right. The commonest expression for "burning," "inflamed," is *nappaḫu;* and oddly enough it comes from a verb, *napāḫu*, which means "to blow." To us, accustomed as we are to matches, blowing is connected rather with extinguishing. We blow our fires *off.* It was quite otherwise for people who had to start their fires by friction: they blew their fires *on* and must have puffed a lot to kindle them. In fact, the Akkadian way of saying "to light a fire" was "to blow a fire." The blacksmith was called *nappâḫu,* and if the accent is removed, the word becomes his bellows.[97] So, when the asu said "inflammation," to his patient it must have sounded like something between "the burning thing" and "the blown thing."[98]

There is also a term for the "hot thing," *ummu.* More often it causes all the body to burn, in which case it must be fever; but when the burning is local, the most likely equivalent is inflammation. Take the following example:

Shumma	amīlu	ina	sili´tishu	ummu	ina	libbi
If	a man	during	his disease	inflammation	into	the inside

uznēshu	ippushma . . .
of his ears	spreads . . .[99]

The word *ummu* can be written phonetically, *um* + *mu*, or with an ideogram (Fig. 2.24). And when the ideogram is traced back to the original Sumerian pictogram, perhaps two thousand years older, one ends up with a flaming brazier[100] (Fig. 2.25).

The next step in my investigation of *ummu* failed. I tried to find a real Sumerian brazier, to make sure that it looked like the pictogram, but none seems to exist. Contenau pointed out a flaming brazier in the reproduction of a Sumerian bas-relief; I had to drop it when I discovered that in an earlier work he called it a flowerpot[101] (Fig. 2.26).

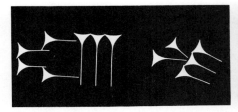 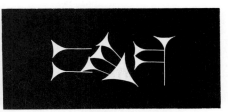

2.24 *Ummu*, one of the Akkadian words meaning "fever" and "inflammation," here written phonetically, with two syllables: *um + mu*.

The same word, *ummu*, written with a single ideogram. For the origin of this sign, which to a layman does not appear to suggest anything hot, see next figure.

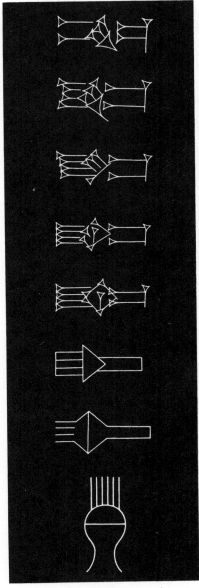

2.25 *Top:* the final writing of *ummu*, c.500 B.C. *Below:* progressively earlier forms, until the earliest one (bottom) turns out to be a Sumerian pictogram for *brazier* (rotated 90 degrees).

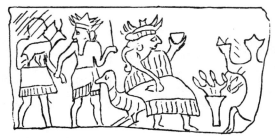

2.26 Dilemmas of interpretation: the flowerpot that became a brazier.

Anyway, it would be unreasonable to doubt the translations of "fever" and "inflammation." And surely none of my readers could afford a shadow of doubt after having shared my last bit of evidence (which is also evidence of phenomenal ingenuity on the part of the Assyriologists). At the top of Fig. 2.27 is a Sumerian word representing a nonclinical type of inflammation; the symbol for inflammation or fever, *ummu*, appears inside a sort of frame. Trace this cuneiform word back to the Sumerian pictogram: it turns out to be the same old brazier, but inside a thorax. "Inflammation inside the chest": what else but *love?*

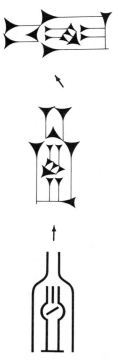

2.27 A timeless Sumerian word, too obvious to require explanation . . .

As to the treatment of inflammation (or infection), I must disregard all plasters except to say that they qualify as either horrible, indifferent, or incomprehensible. But buried among them is one procedure that belongs to modern medicine. It is mentioned once only, in the last and longest surgical

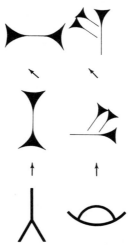

2.28 Akkadian word for "pus," *sharku* (top). Its two signs derive from Sumerian pictograms (bottom) meaning "blood" (a branching vein?) and "white" (a sunrise). This is not a prophetic reference to white blood cells, but rather has the general meaning of "white sap."

fragment.[102] The patient seems to suffer from a boil or abscess of the scalp; he is the same one whose wound was being dressed with oil:

> If a man, his skull contains some fluid, with your thumb press several times at the place where the fluid is found. If the swelling gives way [*under your finger*], and [*pus*] is squeezed out of the skull, you shall incise, scrape the bone and [*remove*] its fluid . . .
>
> If [*instead*] when you press [*the diseased part*], the swelling does not give way [*under the finger*], you will make all around his head an application of hot stones [*lit. "a fire of stones"*].

I read the line of thought as follows: "If you can feel a collection of pus, then cut: if the abscess is not yet ripe, bring it out with heat." The asu seems to have realized the helpful effect of heat in speeding up the formation of an abscess. The process, empirically referred to as maturation, is not an old wives' tale but a fairly precise biological fact. It is the last stage in a sequence of events whereby a focus of infection is first surrounded by white blood cells (pus), then walled off, cut off, and finally digested by the enzymes contained in the pus; at this stage it is "ripe" and ready to be let out. Heat tends to speed up this process by increasing the flow of blood, hence the supply of white blood cells. The word for pus, incidentally, was *sharku*, "white sap" (Fig. 2.28).

What was thought about the cause of inflammation? When the wounds of his operated patients became all red and hot and began to throw pus, it could not dawn upon the asu that it might be his own fault. Note that he did work out one basic mechanism of man-made infection, venereal disease: but then, he could hardly be expected to realize that the high priestess and an inflamed penis stood in the same relationship as a dirty surgical knife and a wound. If inflammation was not his fault (as in many cases it certainly was not), there were two other possibilities: the gods, and the patient himself.

Inflammation was blamed on gods and ghosts quite freely:

> If there is a red swelling on the man's body . . . it is the Hand of Sin [*the Moon god*] . . .
> If there is a white swelling on the man's body, it is the Hand of Shamash . . .[103]
> If a sick man, his face, his guts, his hands, his feet are inflamed. . . Hand of Shamash.
> If his guts are severely inflamed: Hand of Kubû[104] [*a demon arising from the stillborn fetus, which could turn into a wicked ghost, like the dead left without burial*[105]].

This "hand" is very Mesopotamian. Diagnoses were often expressed with the pat formula: if a man shows such and such a symptom, "Hand of Shamash" or "hand" of some other entity, the oddest being the "Hand-of-the-power-of-an-oath." The wording recurs with such automatism, that one comes to wonder whether it had any real medical significance; that is, whether it literally meant that the god was the sole cause of the disease.[106] In some cases a natural cause was mentioned at the same time, as in the following: "If a baby, his bowels are stopped, and his body is yellow, he has been seized by the bad smell; Hand of Gula."[107] Perhaps this "hand" was more like a ritual statement, such as one might expect from a people who did not make a clearcut distinction between the natural and the supernatural.[108]

But the patient also had to look for causes within himself: he might have committed a sin. Perhaps in such cases the cure was confession to a priest, since confession[109] was an established part of Akkadian religion. In one extremely interesting letter Nabu-nasir blames the king's *ṣarāḫu* "on his teeth." *Ṣarāḫu* is another word for "burning," so we can picture old King Esharaddon with a bad case of caries and high fever. Here is one translation:

> [*To the King my lord, your servant Nabu-nasir*] . . . Regarding that which the King my lord has written, saying "According to your [*usual*] integrity, send" I have spoken the truth with the King my lord. The burning of his head, his hands, his feet wherewith he burns is because of his teeth. His teeth should be drawn, his residence should be sprinkled. He has been brought low. Now he will be well exceedingly.[110]

Another translation reads that "the King's teeth are coming out [*to come out*]: that is why he burns."[111]

Whichever reading is right, the fact remains that Nabu-nasir connected tooth problems with fever, which is a perfectly sound idea. I doubt that he had in mind to pull good teeth for stamping out the fever; but even if he had, he was again anticipating a twentieth century practice. In certain febrile diseases one suspects a hidden focus of infection, and physicians take a close look at the teeth. This is the theory of *focal infection*. In my student days it was carried to extremes, especially in Great Britain, where if the blame could not be pinned on a visibly carious tooth, all the teeth were pulled out, good or bad!

By the way, notice that Nabu-nasir saw fit to blame the king's aches and pains on his teeth, not on the gods. Disease was not always a matter of sins, gods, or devils.[112] In fact, religion had little impact on the daily life of the Akkadian. The religious attitudes of Akkadians in general have been greatly overemphasized, probably reflecting the bias of historians who, consciously or unconsciously, felt that they were writing about the land of the Bible.[113]

These are the few specks of pathology that I could gather from the clay tablets. Now for the pharmacology.

The Problem of Ancient Drugs

Did any of those dubious plasters help, or was it all nonsense? The question holds for all of antiquity; and the answer must be gleaned in two stages. First the philologist must tell us exactly what he reads in the text.

The identity of some drugs, like milk, beer, or honey, poses no problem; Akkadian botany is quite another matter. Until recently the authority on drug identifications was the late R. Campbell Thompson, who spent years assembling all possible data on the present and ancient flora of Mesopotamia and on its minerals, including the distance in miles from Nineveh, the frequency with which the names occurred, the conceivable affinities in Arabic, Syrian, and Hebrew, not to mention Latin and Greek. The result was a labor of love but an impossible challenge for any printer: the *Assyrian Herbal*[114] has an index in nine languages and seven alphabets, and each page is a mosaic of these (Fig. 2.29); the front page is printed, but Thompson wrote all the rest in longhand and mimeographed it himself. Today's scholars, alas, have chilled Thompson's enthusiasts. The comparison between languages is dangerous (just recall that the Spanish *aceite* means "oil," the Italian *aceto* is "vinegar," yet both are Latin languages) and even literal translation of Akkadian has its traps: *lion's fat*, for instance, probably means opium, *human sperm* is a kind of gum, and *human excrements* is a plant.[115] What the Germans call *Dreckapotheke*, "filth-drugstore," is not as rich as it looks. As matters now stand: for plants, no identification is absolutely certain. Some are likely; some are possible (*perhaps* the sleep-plant was poppy); *burashu*, on August 1, 1972, was juniper.

Next comes the physician, who looks over the list of identifiable drugs and wonders why they were used and what were their effects, real or expected. It is now certain that some herbs were used, and not only in Meso-potamia, for reasons purely linguistic: that is, because their name punned with a given disease. This is, of course *our* view. At that time, "the name of an object was part of the essence of the object. What we regard as a *play* on the name . . . was . . . an indication of what the thing itself is."[116] For example, a tablet of the Maklû series lists a number of incantations, expressing the wish that the witch (to be taken as the agent of disease) be pierced, bound, lacerated, etc., by different plants. In each case the name of the plant puns with the verb:

On the other hand Assyrian appears to have borrowed certain words: *budulḫu*, bdellium; *ladiru* (attar of roses?), *liaru* (Juniperus Oxycedrus, L.), *lardu* (nard)

A study of the plant-names shews numerous variations from the equivalents in other languages, when the liquids *l, m, n, r*, are components: e.g., *lardu* (nard), *şilurtu* (ليو), *kuniphu* (ܟܘܢܦܬ ?)[1], *anameru* (حمور ?)[1], *liaru* (Ar. 'ar'ar)[1] *zabalum* (Ar. *lizzâb*)[1] *ilṭakku* (ܟ ...)[1], *nushu* (زو ?)[1], *arzallu* (azarolus?)[1], *šalluru* (سرور)[1] *kurkanû* (curcuma), *bişru* (ܒܨܪ), *ḥasarratu* (خريب)[1], *nurmû* (רמון)[1], *sarmadu* (ܐܪܡܕܐ)[1] *labiše* (لبسا)[1] *saqilatu* (שקדל)[1] *ussurâli* (عصفر ?)[1], *kullaru* (ܟܠܠ)[1], *baluḫḫu* (*galbanum*)[1], *urkarinnu* (ערבון), *muştu* (שקמים ?)[1], *ḫalluru* (חרדל), *kudimeru* (κάρδαμον ?)[1], *pillû* (Ar. *luffah*)[1], NAM.TAR.IRA (μανδράγορα)[1], *musukkanu* (συκάμινος)[1].

št is curious: *ḫašḫuru*, long known as ܚܙܘܪ, would lead us to identify *nushu* with زو, and *antaḫšum* with الخشم, even if there were no other reason.

Sex in plants was recognized, but apparently only in the date-palm properly. But the term "male" is applied to *ašlu* (cyperus), NAMTAR (mandrake), and "male" and

[1] These are new identifications and will be found under their respective sections.

2.29 A sample of the effort and knowledge that went into Campbell Thompson's *Assyrian Herbal* (1924).

> Like the *shiklu* plant [*a thorny plant*]
>   may her enchantment *likshulu* her [*pierce her*] . . .
> Like the *sammu* plant
>   may her enchantment *lisammu* her [*blind her*] . . .
> Like the *sammu* plant
>   may her enchantment *liruru* her [*curse her*] . . .[117]

In most cases the reasons that prompted the choice of one drug or another (if there were any) are entirely lost to us; and even guessing is difficult. Read this, for instance, in the typical Akkadian construction:

> If a man, his head is full of sores: dissolve boiled dung in hot water, shave . . . cleanse until blood issues.[118]

Now I am not going to support the surgical use of dung, boiled or not. However, I do wish to make it clear that even a plaster like this one—dung on sores—cannot be branded as "irrational" because our point of view is so terribly different. People who depended on dung for several daily needs would have a much friendlier disposition toward it. To us it means outdoors, manure, and pollution; Akkadians spread rubble as fertilizer, of all things,[119] and brought their dung indoors as fuel. After burning it, they probably extracted ammonium salt from its soot.[120] Another important use of dung was strictly chemical, as an infusion for the bating of hides prior to tanning (perhaps the reason that the tanners were made to live apart).[121] In the bating process "as we now know it today, proteolytic enzymes act upon a hide or skin to reduce its swollen state."[122] *To reduce the swelling:* it is quite possible that the asu had this in mind when he chose this particular plaster.

Thoughts on Mesopotamian Wound Drugs

Luckily for the asu and for mankind, it is not easy to prevent a wound from healing, except by infecting it. In the normal process a wound heals under a layer of dead material, the scab. Injurious chemicals might kill an extra layer of superficial cells, but granulation tissue will push up anyway from beneath it. This being said, for most Akkadian plasters it is impossible to guess whether they were good, bad, or indifferent because one or more drugs are not identified; it is more feasible to judge some of the ingredients. Fats are fairly safe and mechanically soothing; for the patients this may be good enough. Inorganic salts in high concentrations make life uncomfortable for bacteria (and also for tissues).[123] Their antiseptic effect was known in antiquity, but Akkadian formulae preferred vegetable drugs. Here is a typical example from Campbell Thompson's *Assyrian Prescriptions for Bruises and Swellings;* it illustrates well his botanical acrobatics:

> [*If*] . . . his flesh has poison and lassitude, and shrinking of the flesh . . . *Artemisia*, *balsam, *sagapenum, sumach . . . hellebore, cedar, cypress, juniper, *Acorus calamus, cypress of the cemeteries . . . box (?), fir-turpentine, pine-turpentine,

oleander(?), myrtle, tamarisk . . . *Conium maculatum*, shredded[2] daisy, date-palm, juice(tops) of *lemon, juice(tops) of plane . . . juice(tops) of fig, juice(tops) of apple, juice(tops) of medlar, juice(tops) of *TIL.LA karani*,[3] juice(tops) of fir . . . [pist]achio(?), all orchard-fruit, all plant-drugs, all aromatics . . . thou shalt put, boil in a small copper pan, wash him therewith.[124]

As in this formula, most Akkadian drug ingredients fall into two groups: plant extracts, and resins and spices (Thompson's turpentine really means resin). As to plant extracts and decoctions, nothing is known of their possible effects on wounds, with one interesting exception. Many higher plants, perhaps all, contain antibacterial substances, and under the proper circumstances these might play a role in a wound plaster. A large-scale screening of green plants for antibacterial activity was undertaken for the first time in Oxford in 1943, about the time that penicillin was being born. It turned out that 2300 species, belonging to 166 families, gave a positive result. Plants of 28 families were active against *Staphylococcus aureus, E. coli,* or both.[125] This study also brought out several facts that complicate the interpretation of ancient plasters. In some cases the plant begins to lose its inhibitory power within two days of being picked, and loses it altogether when dried; in other cases, even drying for a year will not affect it. Moreover, the inhibitory substance may be distributed throughout the plant or restricted to one part only. In the continuing quest for new antibiotics, many more species have since been studied. In 1959, a review of 2222 plants reported some antibiotic activity in 1362, none in 860.[126] As to the meaning of this antibiotic effect, plants seem to use it for their own protection. Antifungal agents may well explain the resistance to decay of certain trees, like cedar.[127] Insects appear to take advantage of plant antibiotics to protect themselves against their own bacterial enemies.[128] We have not yet seen them on the market because those tested were found to be too toxic. Raphanine, for instance, the potent antibiotic of radish seeds, kills mice in the dose of 7–10 mg given intravenously.[129] But the fact is that they are there. They might surprise us some day.

Resins and spices, the other main category of Akkadian drugs, were part of a cultural passion that started in prehistoric days and still runs strong. Resins of pine, fir, and cedar were common ingredients in Akkadian medicine; and if we can believe the translations, so were cassia, frankincense, myrrh (*murru*), and even turpentine—of course not the distillate now understood by that name, but the resin of *Pistacia terebinthus* (Fig. 2.30), one of the most persistent drugs in history.[130] *Some* of these fragrant substances have *some* antiseptic value; they made the patient's malodorous sores smell better; and their toxicity was practically nil. In this respect, it was safer to have one's wound dressed by the asu than by a sophisticated Greek physician, whose multicolored salves were loaded with arsenic, mercury, and lead.

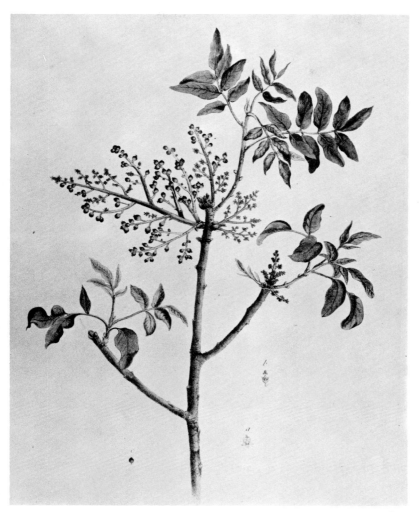

2.30 *Pistacia terebinthus,* the original source of turpentine (resin), a tree or shrub common on the islands and shores of the Mediterranean and in the Near East.

Aquim-Addu and Itûr-Asdu

Nobody alive can guess whether the asu's dressings worked. But somewhere in the dust that blows over Iraq are the remains of two men who knew. Chance preserved two letters that the king of Mari on the Euphrates received around 1800 B.C. and kept in his archives. Here is one:

> To my Lord say this: thus speaks I Aquim-Addu, thy servant. A child who is with me is ill. From beneath his ear, an abscess is discharging. Two physicians of mine are tending him but his disease does not change. Would my Lord, now, dispatch his physician to me . . . or an expert physician, that he may examine the disease of the child, and treat him . . .[131]

So there was still hope in *asûtu,* the medical art, even where two physicians had already failed. In this particular case, however, no royal asu could have lived up to the call: the disease was either tuberculosis of the

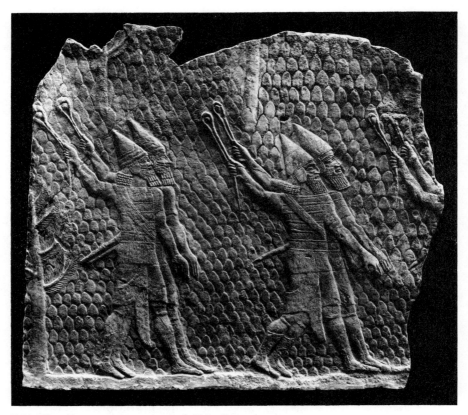

2.31 The sling-stone was a typical Akkadian weapon.

lymph glands or a middle ear infection that had spread to the bone, the dreaded mastoiditis.

The other letter is a touching tribute to the asu as a healer of wounds. It came from a remote military outpost. Sling-stones were flying (Fig. 2.31), ramparts were crumbling.[132] A message went out to the king:

> To my Lord say this:
> thus speaks Itûr-Asdu, thy servant.
> There is no physician, no mason.
> The wall is crumbling,
> and there is no one to rebuild it.
> And if a sling-stone . . .
> wounds a man,
> there is not
> a single physician.
> If it please my lord,
> may my lord send me
> a physician and a mason . . .[133]

My portrait of the Mesopotamian healing art will have to end here, because we have run out of documents. More will surely appear, but those at hand tell us that the asu practiced a humble folk medicine,[134] a step or two below that of his Egyptian colleagues. His flashes of insight were not enough to outshine the competition and discourage the sorcerer. Even that clean, logical, effective treatment with "a fire of hot stones" is offered in competition with another approach, for just below it is a charm designed to help the same patient: a marvellous opportunity to compare once again the procedures of the asu with those of the sorcerer, who could be filthy at times, but also had a touch of the poet:

CHARM.

The sieve, the sieve
The red sieve hath come
   And masked the red cloud
The red rain hath come
   And deluged·the red wastes
The red flood hath come
   And filled the red river
The red gardener hath come
   And brought spade and *tupsikku*-board
   That he may dam back the red waters
Red door forsooth, red bolt forsooth
   Their gateway is shut [?]
But that which shall open you
[*Is*] planting and watering,
   Planting and watering.

End of the charm.[135]

It is obvious, says Campbell Thompson, that this is a sympathetic charm, describing the disease of the head in the previous section, and that the pus is symbolized in the "red rain," "red wastes," "red flood," and so on: "As usual, the charm begins with the beginning of things, in this case the rain-clouds which bring the flood ultimately to be dammed back by the Red Gardener."[136]

I am not aware that pus ever rose to higher poetry.

Assurbanipal, the maniac collector of texts, came just in time. The great culture of his land was already on its way to break up into collector's items. A couple of centuries later a foreigner—Herodotos, the Father of History—seems to have found nothing left of the asu. His remark about Babylonian medicine, whether true or not, must be understood as reflecting only the situation of his day, for he himself was as remote from the Sumerian physicians as we are from Julius Caesar: "They bring out the sick to the market place; for they do not use physicians. People who walk by, and have suffered the same ill as the sick man's, or seen others in like case, come near and advise him about his disease and comfort him, telling him by what means they have themselves recovered of it, or seen others to recover. None may pass by the sick man without speaking and asking what is his sickness."[137]

So the asu faded away. Whether or not he paved the way for Greek medicine, or laid down a few cobblestones—the evidence is meager[138]—it is a fact that commoners and kings begged for his help. Should he appear before us today half-naked, his hair shaved off, carrying a bag of herbs, a libation jar, a censer with coals ablaze,[139] and a barber's knife, he would scarcely qualify as a physician. We would have to remember that what makes a physician is not only what he knows, or what he does, or even how he does it—much of the time, *just that he does it.*

> Babylon falls suddenly and is broken.
> Howl over her,
> fetch balm for her wound;
> perhaps she will be healed.[140]

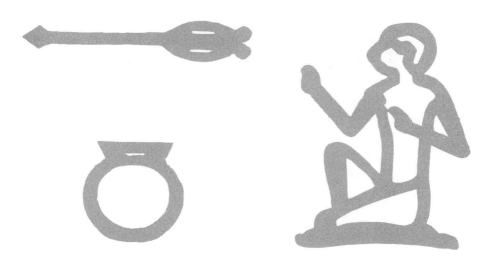

3   The Swnw

Soo-noo, perhaps; we may never know. Egyptian words came down to us mummified: consonants only, with a few shreds of vowels attached.

The *swnw* was the physician in the land of the pyramids.

The Setting

From Babylon to the Nile we have come only a thousand miles as the crow flies (Fig. 2.3), but we are in a different, separate world: so separate that we can discuss Egyptian medicine almost without referring to Mesopotamia. The fact is that Egypt is, really, nobody's neighbor; Egypt was and still is a peculiar sort of island, a greenhouse in the desert (Fig. 3.1).

The live part of the country amounts essentially to the Nile Valley, the Nile Delta, and a few oases. The Nile Valley itself is no more than "a gorge  between the cliffs forming the escarpment, on the one side of the Arabian, on the other of the Libyan, desert. This valley is quite narrow; its maximum breadth is about fourteen miles, but in Middle Egypt the average width is more like nine miles, and in Upper Egypt it shrinks to a mile or two, in some places to no more than a narrow strip of cultivation on one bank only of the river. Egypt is in shape like a tadpole with a very long tail. The length of this tail, from Cairo . . . to Aswan, where for long periods . . . ancient Egypt really ended, is rather less than 550 miles."[1] The habitable surface is only 3.5 percent, about the size of Switzerland,[2] and surrounded by formidable

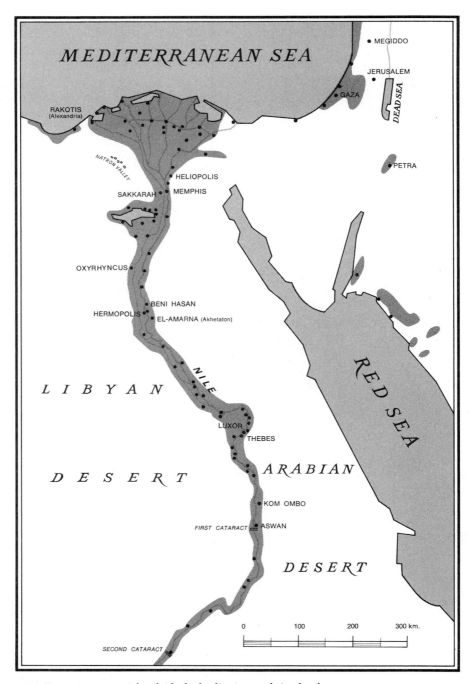

3.1 Egypt is a green island (dark shading), a gash in the desert.

deserts. In this rainless, self-contained, symmetric world, the Egyptians depended for survival on the Nile that rose and fell once a year like clockwork; they could hardly afford to look beyond the desert. Their name for the land of Egypt was *earth*, their word for north was *downstream*, their hieroglyph for foreign country was *desert* ᴗᴗ and the word *people* meant "Egyptians"; foreigners were nonpeople (Fig. 3.2).[3]

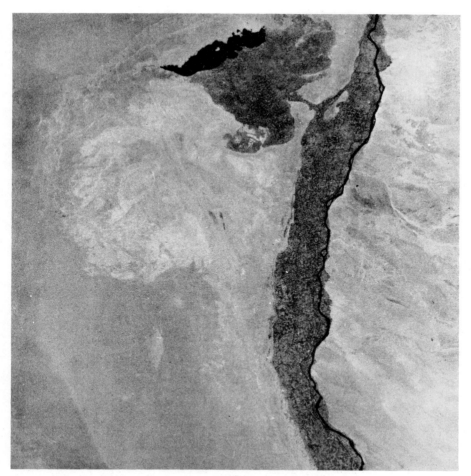

3.2 The geography of the Nile Valley and the precise timing of the floods left their special mark on Egyptian civilization. Compare this view, taken from a satellite, with the aerial view of untidy Mesopotamian rivers (Fig. 2.2).

Somehow this environment favored the cult of medicine. Whatever contacts it may have had with Mesopotamia,[4] the Egyptian art of healing flourished as a national glory, acquiring fame throughout antiquity and beyond. It outlasted the Pharaohs and merged with Greek medicine. Herodotos, who seems to have found nothing left of the asu, wrote about Egypt that "physicians are all over the place."[5]

Egyptian Medicine: The Sources

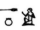

A museum exhibit of Akkadian medicine would have little more to show than cuneiform writings. Egyptian soil has been more generous: with the writings it preserved some of the patients and several artistic works related to medicine (Fig. 3.3). The first samples of writing appeared a little later than in Mesopotamia, around 2900 B.C., when the hieroglyphs seem to have sprung up readymade;[6] papyri from this time—medical or otherwise— have not been found.

The first known practitioner of the medical art survives as a stately profile:

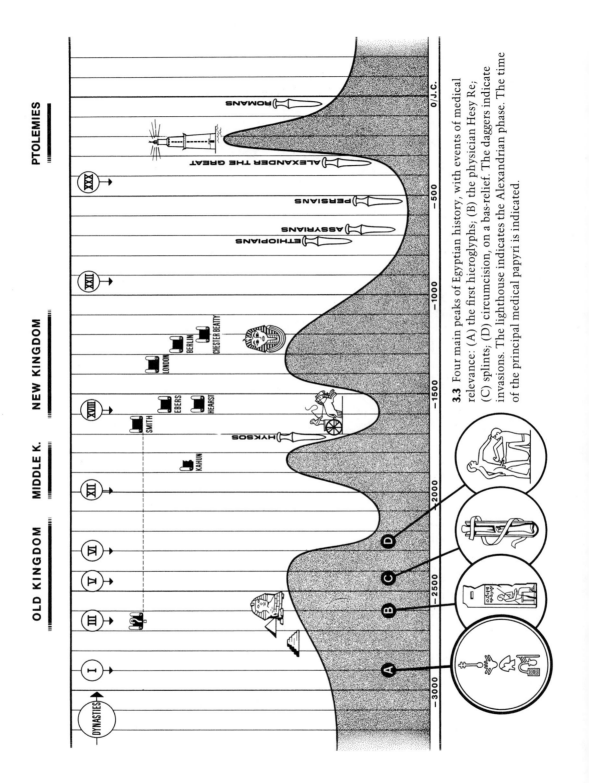

3.3 Four main peaks of Egyptian history, with events of medical relevance: (A) the first hieroglyphs; (B) the physician Hesy Re; (C) splints; (D) circumcision, on a bas-relief. The daggers indicate invasions. The lighthouse indicates the Alexandrian phase. The time of the principal medical papyri is indicated.

Hesy Re, Chief of Dentists and Physicians to the pyramid builders of the Third Dynasty around 2600 B.C.[7] (Fig. 3.4). What he did for royal toothaches the inscription does not tell. Surely he did not drill teeth, but some say that he may have drilled bones to drain dental abscesses. The evidence is a much photographed Old Kingdom mandible, with bad teeth, an abscess, and two little holes draining it.[8] The truth is probably the reverse (or 𓏎, "upside down," as Hesy Re might have written): the holes are better interpreted as sinuses dug by the pus itself, which had to find its own way out,[9] because the dentists of the time had not discovered the simple device of pulling a bad tooth in order to drain the abscess around its root.[10]

Foolproof signs of surgical activity from this period were found on two bodies from tombs of the Fifth Dynasty: fractured limbs set by means of splints and bandages, with the world's oldest bloodstains (Fig. 3.5).[11]

The first known medical text, the battered Kahun papyrus, appears in the Middle Kingdom around 1900 B.C.; it is followed by half a dozen others. Egyptian history is so long that on a chart the medical papyri appear to be clustered together, but actually they are spread out over 800 years or so (Fig. 3.3). Translated and printed, they would amount to less than 200 pages. Their text, reminiscent of the Akkadian tablets, consists of short paragraphs that are either prescriptions, spells against a given disease, or diagnoses, that is, short descriptions of a disease. There are roughly 1200 such paragraphs, of which 900 are prescriptions[12]—which amounts to saying that the Egyptian papyri read on the whole like catalogs.

There is one major exception. Anyone in search of a treat should procure and read the Smith papyrus in its magnificent Breasted edition of 1930; it is especially satisfying to the uninitiated, because the translation of each word is explained and critically analyzed in such a way that even a layman can grasp the essentials. As to the Ebers papyrus (the longest: over twenty meters), its English version could be fun to read if one did not feel at the mercy of an over-enthusiastic translator—B. Ebbell, a Norwegian county medical officer—without the benefit of critical comments.[13] In general, a comparison of the oldest papyri with the more recent ones reveals a trend for magic spells to replace down-to-earth medicine; hence, the number of papyri defined as medical varies from five to ten, according to the writer's indulgence toward witchcraft.

To the outsider, this literature is far more available and less treacherous than the cuneiform medical texts. Egyptology is an older science than Assyriology and more stabilized; in fact, its progress is now much slower. As for the language itself, Sir Alan Gardiner's *Egyptian Grammar*, which unveils the mystery of the hieroglyphs, is probably the world's only fascinating grammar.

For those who can trade hieroglyphs for German, all Egyptian medicine comes incredibly packaged in the ten volumes of a German *Handbuch*, Grapow's *Grundriss der Medizin der alten Ägypter*, in which every single word is spelled out, catalogued, analyzed, and cross-filed in every possible way as the philologist sees it. This magnificent opus is, in a sense, the gravestone of Egyptian medicine: it implies that the sources are drying up.

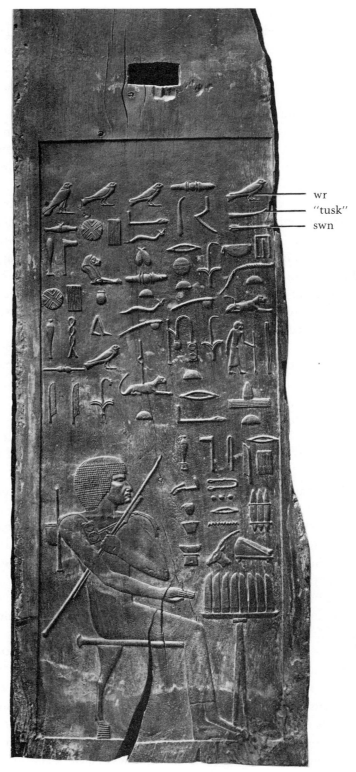

wr
"tusk"
swn

3.4 Hesy Re; the first known Egyptian physician, about 2600 B.C. The three signs 🐦 〰 ◦→ (swallow, tusk, arrow) read *wr*, *ibkh*, *swn*—the most concise possible way to write "chief," "tooth," "physician." A learned man, Hesy Re wore the scribe's palette and reed holder.

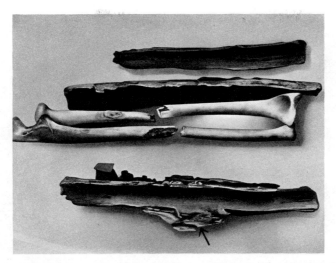

3.5 Fracture of the forearm set with bark splints, c.2450 B.C. The blood-stained lint (arrow), perhaps made of palm fiber, may be the *ftt* mentioned in the Smith papyrus.

How To Write "Swnw"

To understand Egyptian views on wounds, it is essential to grasp the principles of hieroglyphic writing. The total number of hieroglyphs is of the order of 1000, but the standard list used by modern scholars, which includes only the commonest, comes to 743.[14] Quite unlike the cuneiform signs, which gradually changed shape and lost all resemblance to the original pictograms, the commonest hieroglyphs acquired their shape very early and then retained it with astonishingly little change for about 3500 years (Fig. 3.6).[15]

The first thing to know about Egyptian hieroglyphs is that they represent consonants, or groups of consonants. Signs for vowels did not exist, but four guttural sounds come close to them and are known as semivowels or weak consonants (Fig. 3.7, first five hieroglyphs). This means that from the writing itself we have no clue as to the actual sound of the words. Luckily, the vowels of some Egyptian words left traces in other languages, mainly Coptic. Thus, it is possible to make informed guesses as to their position and quantity; their actual quality is much more difficult to ascertain.[16]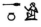

Coptic (probably a corruption of the Greek *Aigyptos*, "Egypt") was the language of the Christian descendants of the Egyptians, in whose churches it is read, though not understood, to the present day. To some extent it is a semiartificial literary language elaborated by native Christian monks about the third century A.D. The vocabulary is part Greek, part Egyptian, and the letters are Greek supplemented by signs derived ultimately from the hieroglyphs.[17] Unfortunately, Coptic came so late that it can throw but a dim light on ancient Egyptian; vowels and even consonants had ample time to change

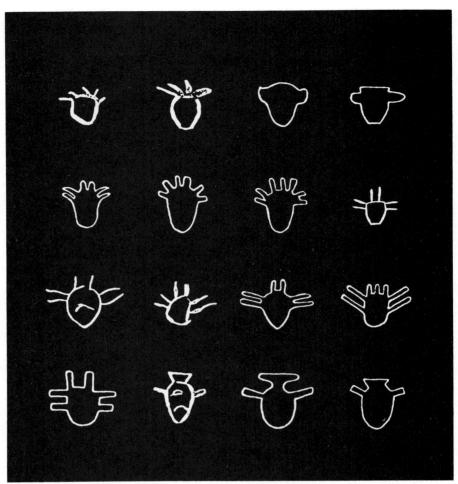

3.6 Many hieroglyphs acquired their final shape very early. These are the earliest forms of the sign for "heart," from the first two dynasties, about 2900–2700 B.C.; they differ but little from the final form (lower right).

in many words. (The Coptic for "physician," for instance, obviously a derivative of *swnw*, is *saein*.[18] The reading swnw seems to prevail, though some prefer *sinw*.[19])

The next most important fact about hieroglyphs is that they can be used in two ways. Sometimes the little figure means just what it shows; that is, it has the function of a pictogram. For instance, if it is written of a drug:

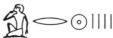

the entire sequence can be guessed: "take in—by mouth—day[s]—four (you are also required to guess that "one sun" means one day).[20]

More often the same sign is used phonetically: it stands not for the object itself, but for its name, which is being used to make up a part of another word. For instance, the "sandal strap" ⸙ called *ankh* (ʿnḫ), may stand for the letter-group *ankh*, so it can be used to write part of the name

76

3.7 The Egyptian alphabet. These are also the commonest signs in hieroglyphic writing, though they represent a fraction of the signs available: 26 of about 1000. From A. Gardiner's *Egyptian Grammar.*

Sign	Trans-Literation	Object Depicted	Approximate Sound-Value
𓄿	*ꜣ*	Egyptian vulture	glottal stop heard at the commencement of German words beginning with a vowel, ex. *der Adler*
𓇋	*i*	flowering reed	usually consonantal *y*; at the beginning of words sometimes identical with *ꜣ*
(1) 𓇌 (2) 𓏭	*y*	(1) two reed-flowers (2) oblique strokes	*y*
𓂝	*ꜥ*	forearm	guttural sound unknown to English
𓅱	*w*	quail chick	*w*
𓃀	*b*	foot	*b*
𓊪	*p*	stool	*p*
𓆑	*f*	horned viper	*f*
𓅓	*m*	owl	*m*
𓈖	*n*	water	*n*
𓂋	*r*	mouth	*r*
𓉔	*h*	reed shelter in fields	*h* as in English
𓎛	*ḥ*	wick of twisted flax	emphatic *h*
𓐍	*ḫ*	placenta (?)	like *ch* in Scotch *loch*
𓄡	*ẖ*	animal's belly with teats	perhaps like *ch* in German *ich*
(1) 𓊃 (2) 𓋴	*s*	(1) bolt (2) folded cloth	*s*
𓈙	*š*	pool	*sh*
𓈎	*ḳ*	hill slope	backward *k*, rather like *q* in *queen*
𓎡	*k*	basket with handle	*k*
𓎼	*g*	stand for jar	hard *g*
𓏏	*t*	loaf	*t*
𓍿	*ṯ*	tethering rope	originally *tsh* (*č* or *tj*)
𓂧	*d*	hand	*d*
𓆓	*ḏ*	snake	originally *dj*; also a dull emphatic *s* (Hebrew צ)

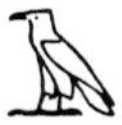

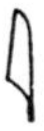

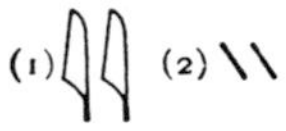

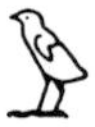

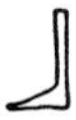

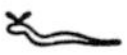

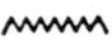

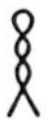

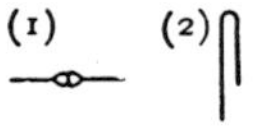

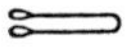

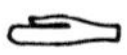

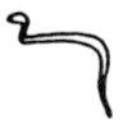

Tutankhamun.[21] When the hieroglyphs are used phonetically, they represent either one, two, or three consonants:

⌓ a loaf of bread = t

⌷ a house = pr

♀ a windpipe attached to the heart = nfr

It follows that Egyptian words, read in their unvoweled state, feel like a mouthful of bones:

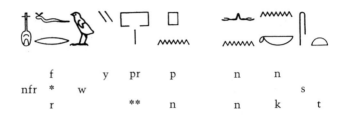

nfr	f	y	pr	p	n	n	
	*	w					s
	r		**	n	n	k	t

* The repetition nfr+f+r will be explained further.

** The vertical stroke below ⌷ means: "the preceding sign (in this case 'a house') stands for exactly what it looks like; it is not part of a rebus." One must therefore read the word as "house," which is pronounced pr.

Read consecutively, this passage comes to: "nfr.wy pr pn   nn n.k st," which stands for: "How beautiful this house! It does not belong to thee."[22]

To make the words more readable, it has been agreed to refill them with as many vowels as necessary, usually e's. This is how the beautiful Queen Nefertiti came about. All anyone knows for sure is Nfr-t-yy-t-y ("beautiful-she-has-arrived"):

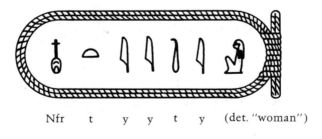

Nfr　　t　　y　　y　　t　　y　　(det. "woman")

A major drawback to writing without vowels is that a number of unrelated words look alike. Consider the problem that would arise if we were to write just rt for the English words art, rat, rite, riot, rot, rut, and root. To guide the reader, the Egyptian scribe used a device known also in Mesopotamia: that of adding after the word a *determinative* (abbreviated in our examples as "det."). This symbol was not to be pronounced; its only function was to suggest the general idea or classification of the preceding word.

Something to do with air or wind would be determined with ⊥ "a sail"—
even the word for shortness of breath, *y-t-tm-m-w* or *ytmw*:[23]

(hieroglyphs)

    y   m   w   (det.)
         t
       tm

The sign *(hieroglyph)* suggests "garden"; *(hieroglyph)* "lifting, carrying"; *(hieroglyph)* "high, rejoice,
support"; *(hieroglyph)* "weary, weak"; and so on. Thus, it no longer mattered that the
letters *ḥrt* ⊂⊃ (a head, a mouth, a loaf of bread) could mean "sky" as well
as "road" or "tomb"; in each case the meaning was decided by an appropriate
determinative: the ideogram for "sky" *(hieroglyph)* (when used as a determinative)
conveyed the notion "high, above"; a little segment of road bordered by
shrubs *(hieroglyph)* suggested "road, distance"; and the dunes of the desert *(hieroglyph)*
indicated "foreign land," including the Great Yonder, as required to give the
idea of "tomb." Hence, each of the three words acquired its own identity:[24]

(hieroglyphs)

   "sky"   "road"   "tomb"

Or if a patient suffered from *ḥaty*, whatever that may have been—

(hieroglyphs)

                t
       ḥ   a   (det.) (det.)
             y

it was likely that *water was raining* from his *eye.*

Sometimes two and even three determinatives were tagged onto a single
word. About one hundred determinatives were in common use, and they
have been of great help in deciphering texts. Often the name of a drug is not
understood, but the determinative retains the principal notion: ₀ ₀ ₀ suggests
"grains" or "mineral," *(hieroglyph)* "plant," and *(hieroglyph)* "weed."

Another basic notion about hieroglyphs is that the same word could be
written in several ways, because the list of signs offered a vast number of
alternatives. One way was to break the word into bits and choose signs to
represent the necessary consonants, singly or in groups. According to this
principle, which is the same as a rebus, one can write CATERPILLAR by

suggesting either CATER + PILLAR, or CAT + TAR + PILLAR, or CATER + PILL + R, plus one feature of hieroglyphs that in modern rebuses would be considered unfair: suggesting the same sound twice in a row (for safety, as it were), but meaning it only once. To keep the example of CATERPILLAR, we might get something like C + CAT + TAR + R + PILL + PILLAR.

Take a deep breath, you are not through. There was the added possibility of *drawing* a caterpillar.

And of spelling it out letter by letter.[26] Yes, letter by letter: this is one of the most puzzling features of Egyptian writing. Sprinkled among the hieroglyphs is a respectable alphabet of twenty-four letters at least. Why did the scribes continue to use signs for combined letters, when the alphabet would have been so much simpler? Why were they so pig-headed about using ⦶ for *nfr*, or even wild spellings like ⦶⟷ *nfr f r*, or ⟿ ⦶⟷ *n nfr f r*,[27] instead of writing alphabetically ⟿ *n*, ⟍ *f*, ⟷ *r*, and throwing out the ⦶ *nfr* with hundreds and thousands of other signs? Could it be that, like Molière's character who wrote prose without even realizing it, they invented the alphabet but never noticed it? It seems likely that they knew what they had, but for a number of reasons (religion, aesthetics, secrecy) the more involved system suited them better.[28] I might add that the difficulties I listed here may not be as great as they sound. A professional Egyptologist reminded me at this point that learning 𓅓 and ⟝ is no worse than learning *a* and *A*; and it is certainly easier to teach *r* to a pupil when one can also say "*r* is drawn ⟷ like your mouth *ra*."

These few indications should make clear that reading an Egyptian text is similar to deciphering a puzzle. Does each particular sign, in each particular instance, stand for the object it represents, or does it stand for a part of a word, as in a rebus? Or does it happen to function as a determinative? And where does each sentence, each word, begin or end? This last detail did not seem to matter in any ancient language; nor did it worry the Egyptian scribes, whose only concern was to space the signs aesthetically in imaginary squares or rectangles, so as not to leave unsightly gaps. No matter to them if two words had to flow together.[29] As if these difficulties were not enough, when the scribes wrote on papyrus, they did not use the classical hieroglyphs but simplified versions known as *hieratic* writing, so that the Egyptologist has to work by stages:[30] first he transcribes the cursive signs into hieroglyphs, then he proceeds to decipher these (Fig. 3.8).

Despite the forbidding sound of the word *hieroglyphs*, decoding a few words requires no magic. To begin, look at the animals: they will tell you which way to read, which can be right or left. The rule of thumb is to read head to tail (or front to back for the people). And if, within one line, two hieroglyphs are written one above the other, read the top one first.

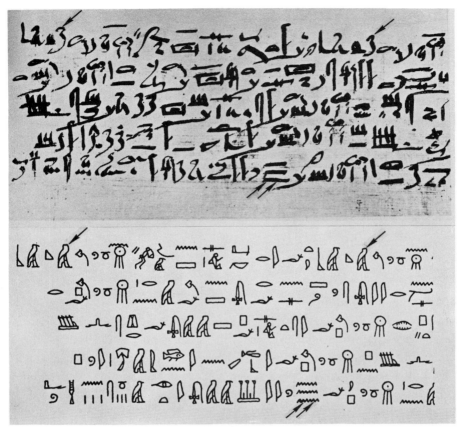

3.8 Hieratic writing (top) is made of simplified hieroglyphs: a passage of the Smith papyrus, with Breasted's hieroglyphic transcription below. Equivalent signs are marked: "water," the letter *n* (double arrow); the owl, which stands for *m* (single arrow). The simplified version of the owl looks intriguingly similar to the Phoenician *m* and to our *m*.

Now for the *swnw*. The ordinary spelling was the first one in the following series; the others are some of the variants:[31]

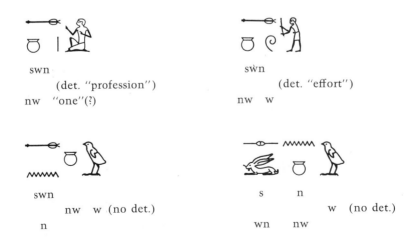

The determinative of swnw is ordinarily the sitting man  as it is for male occupations in general. In a few cases the scribe chose instead the sign for "abstraction" (the papyrus scroll tied up with a knot ⟱); in others, a man or just a forearm striking with a stick ⟶ which means "force, effort." I had hoped that the latter symbols might carry the connotations, respectively, of "scholarship" and "struggle with disease," but I doubt that the scribe intended to convey these flattering concepts, because he used the same determinatives for the word *barber* (something like *ẖaḳu*):[32]

   ẖ   ḳ   (det.)
         (det.)
   a   w   (det.)

Note, in fact, the simultaneous use of three determinatives (the first is a razor).

The determinative "man with a stick" is rather deceptive, because it is also used when the expenditure of energy is quite small, as in the case of a haircut. This leaves us in the dark as to the expenditure of energy involved in teaching, for the verb *sba*, "to teach," was also determined with ⟰.[33] May the reader decide for himself, taking into account that the Egyptians used the stick rather freely, and that among the fragments preserved on papyrus are the following: "The young man has a back, he listens to him who strikes," and "The ear of the young man is on his back."[34]

Some royal physicians attached to their title the drawing of a tired-looking man leaning on a cane ⟰. This is taken to be the hieroglyphic equivalent of "dean," *semsu* (*śmśw*).[35] In two cases the name of the swnw is contaminated by a "loaf of bread" ⌒ or t, which seems to make no sense; Jonckheere listed it with the scribal errors.[36] However, the ending t, probably vocalized as -*at*,[37] also indicates the feminine gender. Since one of these aberrant t's appears on the stele of Peseshet, Chief Woman Physician (Fig. 3.9) *swnw-t* must have been the feminine version of swnw.[38]

3.9 One of the eminent ladies of antiquity: "Peseshet (*P-s-sh-t*), overseer (*mr*) woman-doctor (*swn-nw-t*)."

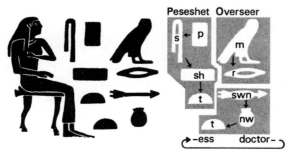

If this spelling is unusual, it is even more unusual to find an ancient woman in this profession, and in so eminent a position. Yet the social status of women in Egypt was quite powerful even before Cleopatra.[39] A subtle sign of this power is the possessive, almost protective attitude of women in many Egyptian sculptures of couples, in which the wife holds the husband with both hands (Fig. 3.10).[40]

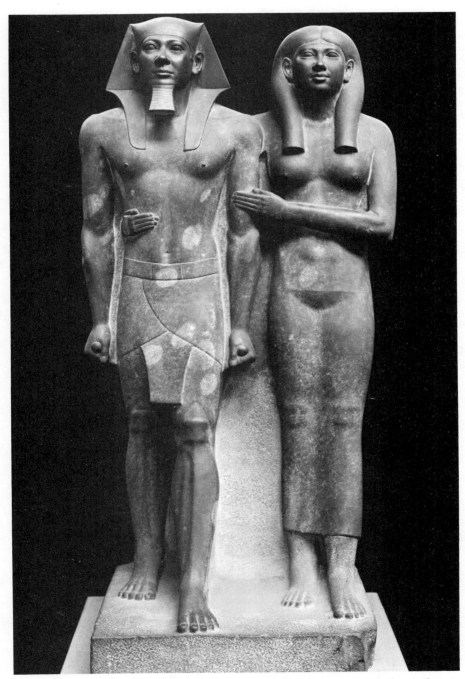

3.10 This lady's protective gesture tells a lot about women's role in her day, in her country. Pharaoh Mn-ka-re and his queen, Fourth Dynasty.

It was lucky for Peseshet that she was born in Egypt. The combined records of ancient Mesopotamia, Greece, and Rome preserved the names of perhaps ten women physicians, and none was a "Chief." And trust the male-oriented Greeks: the word for physician, *iatrós*, was masculine; it could be twisted into a feminine form, like *iatráina*, but probably lost breadth in the process and came to mean "midwife."[41]

Wounds Without Surgeons

Despite the splendid isolation of Egypt, its citizens were not immune from the trauma of warfare. War injuries are dramatically shown in a mass grave of about 2000 B.C., in which the bodies of sixty soldiers are preserved well enough to show mace injuries, gaping wounds, and arrows still infixed.[42] The lot of the soldier is well described in this fragment written around 1200 B.C.: "I will instruct thee concerning the condition of the soldier . . . He is taken to be a soldier as a child of a reed's length . . . He rises in the morning only to receive castigation, and will be wounded with bloody wounds. He is accoutred with weapons in his hand, and stands on the battle-field every day. A lacerating blow is dealt his body, a double blow descends on his skull. A blow that knocks him head over heels is dealt his eyes, and a shattering blow falls on his nose . . . He leaves off work beaten like a papyrus and battered with castigations."[43] To be "beaten like a papyrus" was the equivalent of being "beaten to a pulp" (Fig. 3.11).

The scribes were better off. A favorite theme of Egyptian literature is to extoll their comfortable way of life: "Be a scribe. It will save thee from taxation, and will protect thee from all labours . . . It stoppeth thee from hardships . . . Be a scribe, that thy limbs may be sleek, and thy hands become soft."[44]

In a survey of 6000 skeletons it was found that one of every 32 individuals had suffered a fracture;[45] today we break many more bones than that, at least in skiing countries. The Swiss National Accident Insurance informed me that in the period 1966–1968 there were about 2.6 fractures per 100 insured persons *per year* (if the data on the ancient skeletons are reliable, only 3 percent of the Egyptians broke a bone in their whole lives). In contrast, today we have fewer encounters with angry jaws. The Egyptians had enough mishaps of this kind to fill a whole *Book of Bites*.[46] This book is now lost, but many prescriptions of the time refer to human bites (the most common kind), hippopotamus bites, and lion bites, the latter perhaps from the tame lions (a Ptolemaic queen, Berenice, had her face licked by a lion to improve her complexion[47]). And crocodile bites. The effect of a crocodile on an army officer is described in a letter: "He jumps into a thorny bush; his legs are chewed by the reptile, his heel is pierced."[48]

Other accidents were recorded by the foremen who kept track of the absentees on the pharaoh's building sites. These efficient bureaucrats kept records on slabs of stone, including date, name of absentee, and justification.

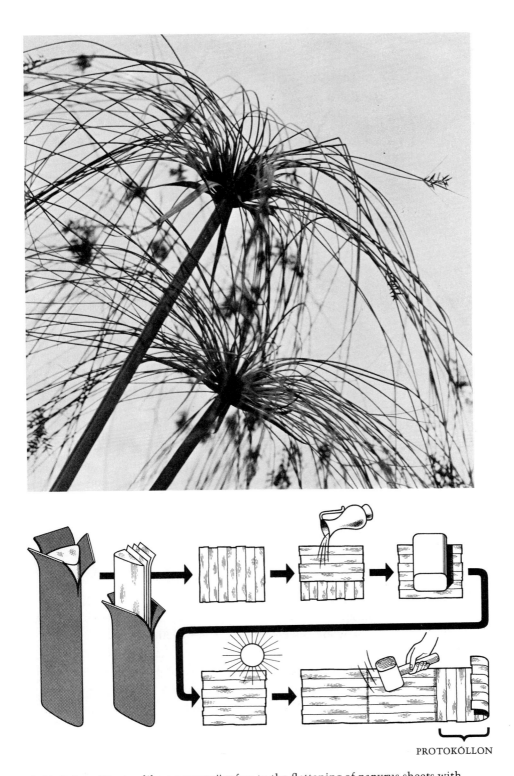

3.11 *Below:* "Beaten like a papyrus" refers to the flattening of papyrus sheets with mallets, the last step in making a papyrus scroll. Here is the whole process, beginning with the papyrus stems (left). *Protokóllon* is the name given by the Greeks to the special end-sheet or *kóllema,* bearing the official authentication of the scroll (hence our *protocol*). Its outer strips ran lengthwise, to avoid fraying. *Above:* The flowering tops of two papyrus reeds, about eight feet high.

One example: "Fourth month of the flood day 27 Nbnfr was ill was stung by the scorpion."[49]

Life had other dangers too in that matriarcal society:

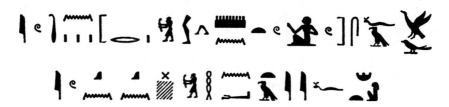

First month of winter day 21 Tlmntw was absent had a fight with his wife[50]

Poor Tlmntw must have been in bad shape. His predicament is described with the word *knkn* (or), which was also used for "grinding up" a drug in a mortar.[51] Note, incidentally, the *l* in Tlmntw: it is written by combining *n* + *r* and other signs, and indicates a foreign name.

Who took care of all these wounds? In a country of specialists like Egypt it would have been reasonable to expect a guild of wound surgeons. There were doctors for the eyes, the teeth, the belly, the "hidden diseases."[52] The narrowest field, but certainly one in great demand, was that of the famous Shepherd of the Anus[53] (a title that should perhaps be toned down to Custodian of the Bottom). Yet there seem to have been no specialized surgeons. Wounds were probably treated by general practitioners, that is, by the lay swnw and the priests of the goddess Sekhmet.[54] It may be that surgeons were unnecessary because the operations performed were few and not too complex: the primary concern of surgery was the dressing of accidental wounds, as described in the great Smith surgical papyrus.

When Blades Fell from Heaven

In the Smith surgical papyrus, odd as it may seem, the surgical knife is never mentioned; the wounds were already made. Seeing those lovely pages neatly written in black and red, it is hard to imagine that they are so old that some of the injuries were caused by flint weapons and probably none by iron. There is a bas-relief with a scene of circumcision about 2250 B.C., in which  the blade is probably of stone (Fig. 3.3). Bronze and iron, like the wheel, came to Egypt from the East and relatively late: bronze, definitely an Asiatic discovery, had to trickle in through Mesopotamia, so that the Egyptian Bronze Age did not begin until the Middle Kingdom, sometime after 2000 B.C. Although the beginning of the Iron Age in Egypt is a classical subject of dispute, iron knives could scarcely have been used at the time of the two great papyri, Smith and Ebers (1650 and 1550 B.C).[55]

The beginnings of Egyptian iron make for a story literally out of this world. In 1911, G. A. Wainwright found two groups of iron beads in pre-

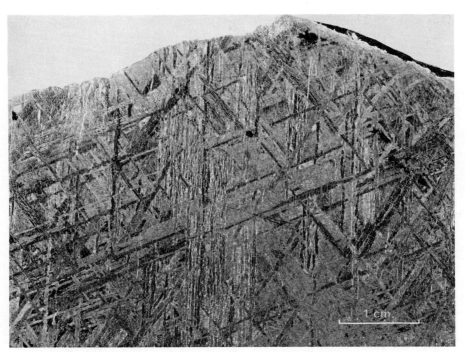

3.12 "Bya of Heaven": a polished section through a meteorite consisting of pure iron and nickel (octahedrite). The outer surface was somewhat rusty.

dynastic graves south of Cairo. At that time the Egyptians were using flint implements; bronze was unknown, copper objects were few and small. Chemical analysis of the beads showed that they consisted of 92.5 percent iron and 7.5 percent nickel, a sure indication that the metal had been taken from a meteorite, for terrestrial iron rarely contains nickel (Fig. 3.12).[56]

The ancient Egyptians, says Wainwright, were doing nothing unusual in obtaining scraps of iron from falling stars. The Sumerians, the Aztecs, the Eskimos, the American Indians did the same. This world-wide use of celestial iron is surely embedded in the present name for "iron science," *siderurgy*, which really means "the work on the stars."[57] Nor are meteorites so rare: up to 1932, those known and mapped were 634, of which 261 contained iron; and the rate of new arrivals actually seen as they were falling amounted to several per year.

The ancient Egyptians took bits of iron from meteorites, shaped them into blades, and used these for one of their most important ceremonies: the 75-step ritual of the Opening of the Mouth.[58] This was surgery at the mystical level: it meant "cutting open" the closed mouth of a mummy or statue and allowing new life to flow in (Fig. 3.13).

The name for iron was 𓌃 *b-y-a*. See how much we can learn from the word itself. In the first place, bya meant "iron" as well as "firmament"—surely no coincidence. It was written with the hieroglyph 𓇯 "a thing full of water" (the sky). When it meant iron, the spelling 𓇯 *bya* was usually

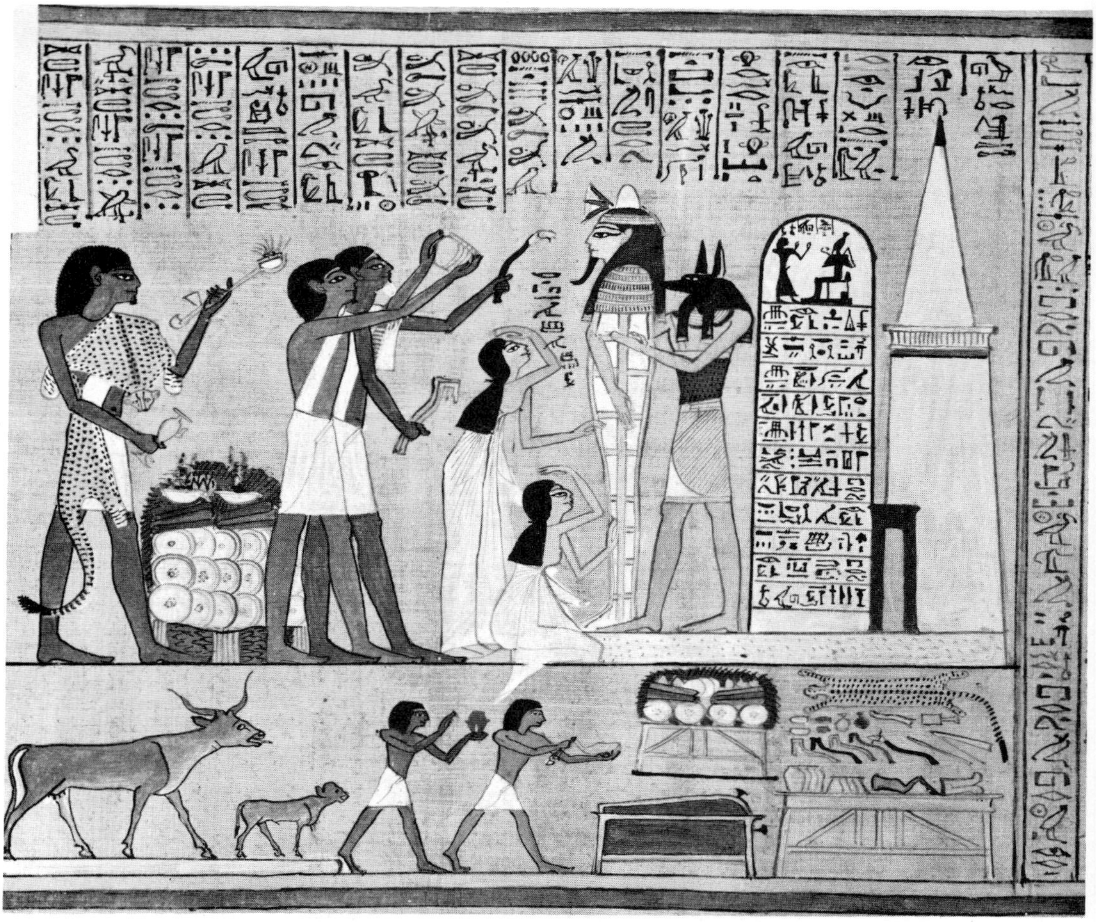

3.13 Metaphysical surgery: the ceremony of the Opening of the Mouth, performed on the mummy of the royal scribe Hunefer around 1300 B.C. Among the "opening" tools (lower right) are several shaped like the Big Dipper. Another object on the table is the foreleg of a bull, closely resembling the Big Dipper. The ritual amputation of the bull shown here is not as cruel as that in Fig. 3.19: the pedestal under the cattle at left suggests that live animals have been replaced by cheaper models.

reinforced with the letter *b* 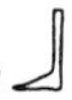 and determined with a block or something like it:

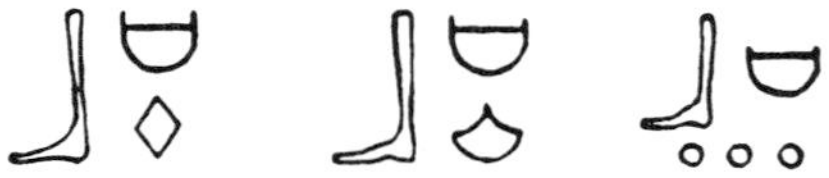

But bya could also be written with this astonishing combination: 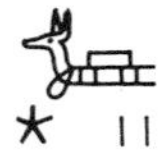 namely, a sledge carrying a meteorite and determined with a star;[59] the same ideogram was used to mean "marvel, astonishment." Which tells us that this particular marvel was something to take home (and notice, not yet on a cart, for there was still no wheel). Ultimately bya came to be called *bya-n-pt*, "bya of heaven":

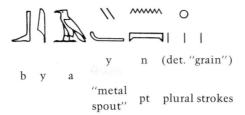

| b | y | a | | y | n | (det. "grain") |

"metal spout"   pt   plural strokes

This form passed into the Coptic **ϩⲉⲛⲓⲡⲉ** benipe, "iron."[60]

So the ancient Egyptians knew perfectly well where the bya came from. Perhaps this explains why some of the little gadgets used for Opening the Mouth were given the celestial shape of the Big Dipper, either this way:

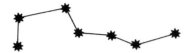

or straight up, as "the Foreleg of the Bull" (see Fig. 3.13):

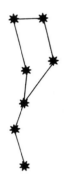

Clearly, no swnw in his right mind could hope to own a set of iron scalpels. Even in the treasure of Tutankhamun iron objects were few, small, and homely, including a set of paper-thin, symbolic blades (perhaps for Opening his own Mouth).[61]

Iron began to be "discussed fairly freely" in the New Kingdom, after 1500 B.C.[62] But in the meantime, Egyptian surgery had found another source of blades, cheaper than meteorites and almost as imaginative. It is mentioned in the Ebers papyrus, which refers to surgical incisions in this roundabout way:[63] "You shall give him the dwa [meaning the cutting treatment] with such-and-such a blade." The word dwa is written:

dw   a
   (det.)

There were four types of blades: the *ds*, the *shas*, the *khpt*, and the *swt*. Only the first is well known: it was a common household item, often determined with a knife plus a block of stone ▭ and therefore probably made of flint.[64] Now see how the four knives were spelled:[65]

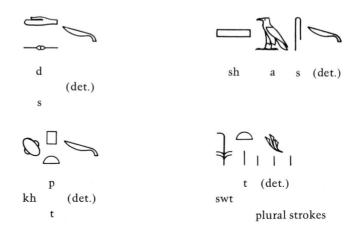

d		sh	a	s (det.)
(det.)				
s				

p		t (det.)		
kh (det.)		swt		
t		plural strokes		

Something looks terribly wrong. Three blades are determined, predictably, with a knife; but one with a reed. Mistake?

No: it was a disposable blade. "You shall give him a cutting treatment with the reed that is used to make cutting treatments."[66] Knives of this kind were quite current in antiquity. In the Egyptian "Tale of the Two Brothers," Bata castrates himself with a razor made from a reed.[67] In ancient India, surgeons used bamboo blades under special circumstances. And in the first century A.D. we find even the Romans using sharp reed knives for slitting ripe olives.[68]

Now, given these various kinds of surgical knives, it would be interesting to know what the cutting was about. Probably *not* for boring skulls; it is strange that this practice, so widespread in prehistoric times, encountered no favor in Mesopotamia and Egypt. Although trephined skulls from Egypt are occasionally mentioned in the literature, I have been unable to find an authenticated case.[69] The Ebers papyrus recommends the cutting treatment for three kinds of lumps, none of which can be safely identified; whereas certain "serpentine windings" are *not* to be operated on, because "that would be head on the ground [*upside down? deadly?*]." Perhaps these were varicose veins; but again I prefer to leave the matter open.[70] The difficulty of extracting modern medical terms from a hieroglyphic context is well illustrated by a passage of the Ebers papyrus, where one translator reads "prepuce [?]" and another, "acacia thorn."[71]

The Smith Papyrus, or How To Contend with Wounds

Before turning to read through this magnificent scroll, we should realize how lucky we are to have it. Egyptian papyri, left to their own, seem to navigate through time almost indefinitely; but like the astronauts, they face crucial dangers upon re-entry.

On January 20, 1862, in Thebes on the Nile, one Mustapha Aga happened to be the owner of an ancient Egyptian papyrus; that day he sold it to an American scholar, Dr. Edwin Smith. A couple of months later Mustapha Aga turned up with another papyrus. Dr. Smith was still around and bought that one too. The second papyrus, however, was—in the kindly terms of the buyer—"facticious," that is, made up of bits of three papyri, pasted together with glue.[72] Dr. Smith carefully removed the glue and discovered that two fragments were the remnants of a battered page one of the papyrus bought in January.[73] The reassembled scroll came to rest at the New York Historical Society as the Smith papyrus, waiting to be translated.

Finally, in 1920, James Breasted of the Oriental Institute in Chicago agreed to look at it. He was immediately absorbed—and in ten years of labor he produced an absorbing book, in fact the most elegant, thorough, critical version ever given of any ancient text. Thus was reborn the most ancient medical text of mankind.[74]

The text is tightly written. Sometimes a whole paragraph is merely suggested by a few catchwords. Breasted suggested that the original may have been a set of notes "of a lecturer or student."[75]

Through seventeen columns of elegant cursive hieroglyphs, the shadows of three men haunt the reader—three men so far off in time that the first two never even saw the wheel (Fig. 3.3). The first shadow is that of the unknown author, who spoke the language of the Old Kingdom and must have lived roughly between 2600 and 2200 B.C.[76] A man of vast experience and sound logic, he assembled dozens of surgical cases and arranged the descriptions so that they followed from the head downward, in order of severity within each group. He also gave each case one of three labels, depending on the chances of successful treatment:

> An ailment which I will treat.
> An ailment with which I will contend.
> An ailment not to be treated.

The second shadow, several centuries later, is that of the Commentator. By his time several terms of the papyrus had become so obsolete that apparently they could no longer be understood without the help of a scholar; thus, the Commentator inserted sixty-nine short explanations. Little could he guess that many of his glosses would serve their function as long as four  thousand years: to Dr. Breasted they were the only clues to the meaning.

Last, the Scribe appears, a rather careless fellow but with a beautiful hand (Plate 3.1), which was about average for Egyptian scribes. He keeps alternating between red and black ink, as was customary, without much method; he corrects in black the mistakes he makes in red, and vice versa; he inserts an asterisk (the world's first) where he forgets a word; but then—and this is a true heartbreak for the historian—halfway through the job, in the middle of a word, he just stops. From the waist down the Smith papyrus remains hopelessly blank. This happened about 1650 B.C.

Of the forty-eight clinical cases that the scribe was willing to copy, we will first consider case 10: a gaping wound of the eyebrow, penetrating to the bone (the subtitles are added by the translator).[77]

TITLE

Instructions concerning a wound in the top of his eyebrow.

EXAMINATION

If thou examinest a man having a wound in the top of his eyebrow, penetrating to the bone, thou shouldst palpate his wound, and draw together for him his gash with stitching,

DIAGNOSIS

Thou shouldst say concerning him: "One having a wound in his eyebrow. An ailment which I will treat."

TREATMENT

Now after thou hast stitched it, thou shouldst bind fresh meat upon it the first day. If thou findst that the stitching of this wound is loose, thou shouldst draw it together for him with two *awy*-strips, and thou shouldst treat it with grease and honey every day until he recovers.

We learn here that the swnw had two distinct techniques for closing a wound. The first is *ydr:*[78]

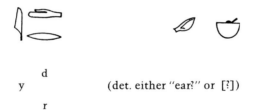

d	
y	(det. either "ear?" or [?])
r	

Ydr can be either a noun or a verb. Breasted's translation is "stitching," which he supports with four pages of argument.[79] If he is right, this is the world première of surgical suture. Breasted has to fight for his translation because, strangely enough, the ordinary Egyptian word for "sewing" has not come down to us; and the ydr itself (besides its thirteen appearances in the Smith papyrus) occurs only once in a very obscure text, then never again in the whole of Egyptian literature.

Here are the facts. In six of the forty-eight cases in the Smith papyrus, the surgeon is advised to "draw together the wound with ydr." So it must be something that would draw together the margins of a wound. A bandage? Probably not, for in one case (alas, its text is imperfect) the ydr is recommended, but with the additional advice "not to put on a bandage"; and in the follow-up of another case the ydr is found "sticking in the two lips of the wound," a wording that suggests some device quite other than a bandage.

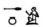

Now, in four of the six cases, the ydr "becomes loose" wnkh. If it is a suture, this makes good surgical sense: stitches in a contaminated wound would cause suppuration and give way. In fact, in case 47 the wound is "inflamed, open, and its ydr loose."[80]

A few years after Breasted, another Egyptologist wiped aside this translation and tried to prove that ydr was rather like a clamp. He was Ebbell, the translator of the Ebers papyrus.[81] It is just possible that both were right. Among primitive people, one of the earliest wound-closing devices is a combination of clamp and suture: a thorn or needle is stuck through both lips of the wound, and the protruding ends are tied together by a thread placed as a figure 8. Maybe this was the ydr. No surgical suture has been preserved in mummies. The oldest known stitches in human flesh are by the hand of the embalmer, and they were threaded about five hundred years later (Fig. 3.14).

The other technique for closing wounds is by applying "two awy[-strips]" "of" "cloth." The last sign is a strip of cloth with a fringe, combined with a folded cloth beneath it. The determinatives of the awy-strips vary, but they all imply tying, by either ropes (repeated, meaning "two") or the bowstring . The word is unknown outside of the Smith papyrus.

3.14 The world's oldest suture, placed by an embalmer on the belly of a Twenty-first Dynasty mummy about 1100 B.C. Usually embalming wounds were not sutured; sometimes they were covered with a plate of beeswax.

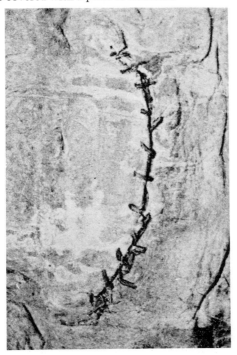

Luckily, the Commentator appended a gloss:

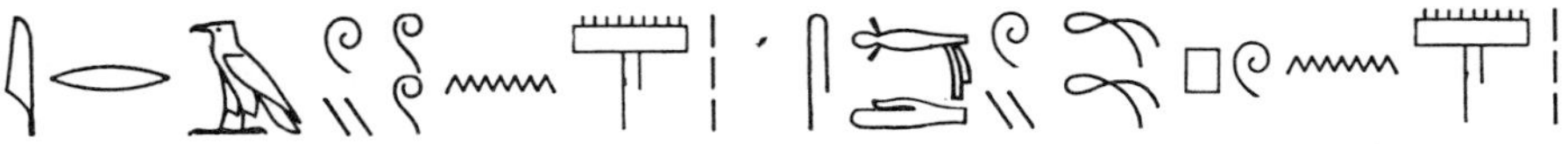

As for "Two strips of linen," it means two bands of linen

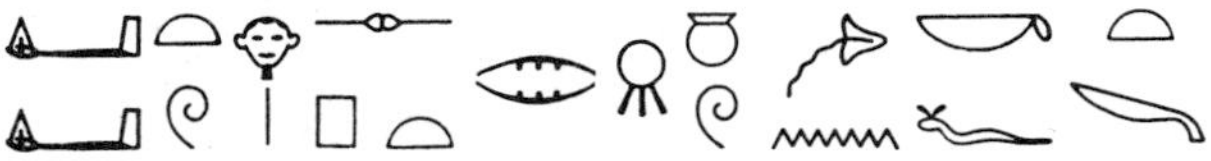

which one applies upon the two lips of the gaping wound

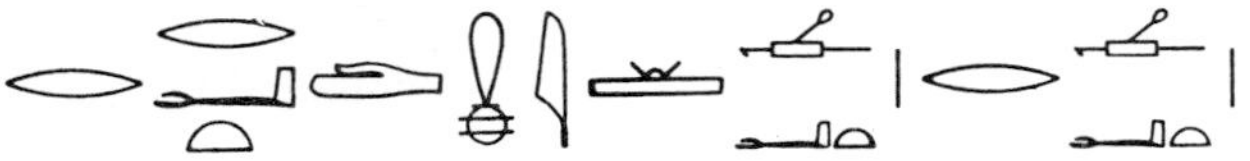

in order to cause that one (lip) join to the other.[82]

Breasted's translation, "adhesive strips," seems justified.[83]

Egyptian technology included plenty of adhesives, mainly gum from acacia trees and several types of resin.[84] Herodotos says that the Egyptians used gum, rather than glue, to fasten together the linen bandages in which the mummies were wrapped after embalming. In recent days such bandages were analyzed chemically, and they did in fact contain gum.[85] Its name was ḳmyt:[86]

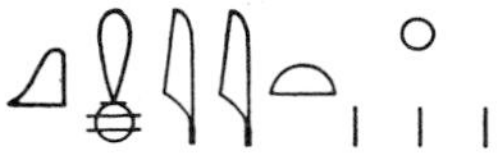

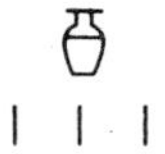

(det. "grain")	(det. "pot")
ḳ my y y t	sometimes with this other ending:
plural strokes	plural strokes

Note that tapes are better than stitches if the wound is infected: the margins of the wound are held in the right position without barring the exit to any pus that may need to escape; and the tissues are spared the presence of a foreign body (thread or clamp), which somehow favors infection.[87] This is why the technique of closing wounds with tapes became standard once again several millennia later, in the nineteenth century. By that time wound infection had become such a problem that it threatened to choke off surgery altogether; it was almost impossible to close a wound with stitches and hope that they would hold (Fig. 3.15). Another revival of tapes is taking place in this very day, not only because the rate of infection is lower, but because the pain is less, the scar looks better, and it holds just as well.[88]

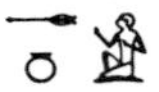

The following case describes a gaping wound in the head, penetrating to the bone and splitting the skull.[89] It belongs to the category with which the author is willing to "contend," implying an uncertain result:

TITLE

Instructions concerning a gaping wound in his head, penetrating to the bone, (and) splitting his skull.

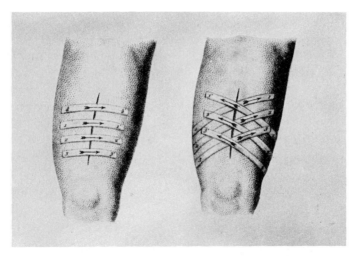

3.15 Closing wounds with adhesive tape may have been a current practice in ancient Egypt. It was current again, as shown here, in nineteenth century Europe. From a French manual of 1858.

EXAMINATION

If thou examinest a man having a gaping wound in his head, penetrating to the bone, (and) splitting his skull, thou shouldst palpate his wound. Shouldst thou find something disturbing therein under thy fingers, (and) he shudders exceedingly, while the swelling which is over it protrudes, he discharges blood from both his nostrils (and) from both his ears, he suffers with stiffness in his neck, so that he is unable to look at his two shoulders and his breast,

DIAGNOSIS

Thou shouldst say regarding him: "One having a gaping wound in his head, penetrating to the bone, (and) splitting his skull; while he discharges blood from both his nostrils (and) from both his ears, (and) he suffers with stiffness in his neck. An ailment with which I will contend."

TREATMENT

Now when thou findest that the skull of that man is split, thou shouldst not bind him, (but) moor (him) at his mooring stakes until the period of his injury passes by. His treatment is sitting. Make for him two supports of brick, until thou knowest he has reached a decisive point. Thou shouldst apply grease to his head, (and) soften his neck therewith and both his shoulders. Thou shouldst do likewise for every man whom thou findest having a split skull.

GLOSS   A

As for: "Splitting his skull," it means separating shell from shell of his skull, while fragments remain sticking in the flesh of his head, and do not come away.

GLOSS   B

As for: "The swelling (*tḫb*) which is over it protrudes," it means that the swelling (*šfw·t*) which is over this split is large, rising upward.

As for: "(Until) thou knowest he has reached a decisive point," it means (until) thou knowest whether he will die or he will live; for he is (a case of) "an ailment with which I will contend."

Faced with a very sick patient, the surgeon chooses to "moor him at his mooring stakes" (here are the mooring stakes ⟩⟩⟩). This extraordinary expression would be wholly unintelligible were it not for a gloss to the previous case, where the Commentator explains: "As for: 'Moor [him] at his mooring stakes' it means putting him on his customary diet, without administering to him a prescription."[90]

Now we understand the allusion: the bedridden patient, surrounded by healthy people, is being compared with a boat idling at its moorings, while traffic keeps moving up and down the Nile.[91]

The patient is also propped up with a support of bricks, and he is allowed to "reach the decisive point." What this means is spelled out in gloss C: the swnw is willing to "contend," but nature "decides."

Note also two major omissions, typical of the entire Smith papyrus. Washing the wound is ignored. Perhaps it was too obvious to mention, especially in a text such as this, written in a highly condensed, shorthand style. We are left hoping for a palm-wine rinse such as the embalmers used.[92] Hemorrhage is also ignored, except to note in passing that it happens. A century or so later the Ebers papyrus begins to show definite awareness of surgical bleeding. One paragraph deals with a "lump of ukhedu," described as a pocket full of gum-water: perhaps a cyst or abscess. "You should give it the cutting treatment; beware of the *mt* [*blood vessel*]!"[93] Another disease is described as a "vessel-tumor": "It comes from a wound of the vessel. Then you should give it the cutting treatment. It [*the knife*] should be heated in the fire; the bleeding is not great."[94] This is understood as prescribing the use of a red-hot knife to cut and burn at the same time, in order to check the bleeding. Five paragraphs later another nondescript lump, the *sft* of a vessel, has to be operated on with the reed for cutting treatments: "if it bleeds a lot, you must burn it with fire."[95] Thus the world's first recorded hemostasis was achieved by burning. Now think of a way of doing this *without metal and without a fire*. Case 39 of the Smith papyrus involves "One having tumors with prominent head in his breast, and they produce [pockets] of pus [*boils?*]. An ailment which I will treat with the fire-drill":[96]

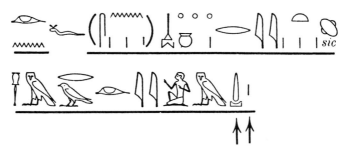

Note once again the little vertical stroke at the end: it means "the sign that precedes, the fire-drill *ḏa*, does not stand for the syllable '*ḏa*' but for the actual fire drill." The thrifty Egyptians, chronically short of fuel, had found a way to cauterize without having to light a fire.

A Hot Case

Case 47 describes five consecutive examinations of a single patient wounded in the shoulder. It is a very realistic case history, forming a crescendo of complications until the patient is appropriately moored at his mooring stakes, and winding up with final victory:[97]

TITLE

Instructions concerning a gaping wound in his shoulder.

FIRST EXAMINATION

If thou examinest a man having a gaping wound in his shoulder, its flesh being laid back and its sides separated, while he suffers with swelling (in) his shoulder blade, thou shouldst palpate his wound. Shouldst thou find its gash separated from its sides in his wound, as a roll of linen is unrolled, (and) it is painful when he raises his arm on account of it, thou shouldst draw together for him his gash with stitching.

Thou shouldst say concerning him: "One having a gaping wound in his shoulder, its flesh being laid back and its sides separated, while he suffers with swelling in his shoulder blade. An ailment which I will treat."

Thou shouldst bind it with fresh meat the first day.

SECOND EXAMINATION

If thou findest that wound open and its stitching loose, thou shouldst draw together for him its gash with two strips of linen over that gash; thou shouldst treat it afterward [with] grease, honey, (and) lint every day until he recovers.
If thou findest a wound, its flesh laid back, its sides separated, in any member of a man, thou shouldst treat it according to these directions.

THIRD EXAMINATION

If, however, thou findest that his flesh has developed inflammation from that wound which is in his shoulder, while that wound is inflamed, open, and its stitching loose, thou shouldst lay thy hand upon it. Shouldst thou find inflammation issuing from the mouth of his wound at thy touch, and secretions discharging therefrom are cool like *wenesh*-juice,

Thou shouldst say concerning him: "One having a gaping wound in his shoulder, it being inflamed, and he continues to have fever from it. An ailment with which I will contend."

FOURTH EXAMINATION

If then, thou findest that man continuing to have fever, while that wound is inflamed,

Thou shalt not bind it; thou shalt moor (him) at his mooring stakes, until the period of his injury passes by.

If, however, his fever abates and the inflammation in the mouth of his wound dissipates entirely,

Thou shouldst treat him afterward [with] grease, honey, (and) lint every day, until he recovers.

The swnw is struggling with infection. First he tries stitching, if Breasted is correct; when this fails, he tries adhesive tapes; when these also fail, he allows the wound to remain open, "until the period of his injury passed by"—actually, until the infection has abated. Note the matter-of-fact use of the term "inflammation;" here is one example, the word being pronounced something like *nesery*:

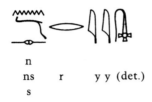

n
ns   r   y y (det.)
s

If the reader feels skeptical about the translation, I sympathize. For my part, encouraged by previous experience (the Mesopotamian word for inflammation had turned out really to be something "hot"), I left no stone unturned until it could be proven to my satisfaction that those seven archaic little signs— ∿∿ "water," ⌐ "ox tongue(?)," —o— "a bolt," ⟨⟩ "a mouth," ⎜⎜ "two flowering reeds," and ⎕ the determinative—could honestly be translated as "inflamed."

Breasted's answer dropped from the majestic heights of competence: ⌐⎜⎜⎕ *nsr-y*, "inflamed," is of course derived from the common verb *nsr*, "to burn," with its nouns *nsr* and *nsr-t*, "flame."[98] This, of course, is final.

There is nothing left to do but to take another look at the word itself. See the seventh sign, the determinative, which represents a flaming brazier, with stylized smoke rising from it and curving back to the ground. This was the common determinative for all things hot or flaming. See also the two other words for "pathologic heat", perhaps *shememet* and *seref*:

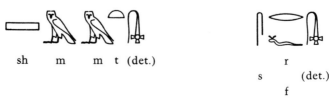

sh   m   m t (det.)

                          r
               s   (det.)
               f

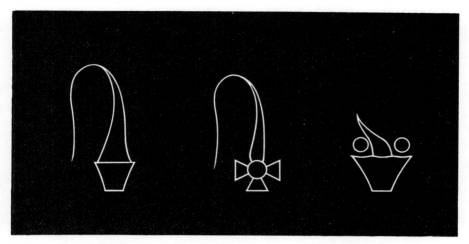

3.16 Three hieroglyphs portraying flames. An incense burner (right) stood for *sntr,* "incense," portrayed by the two grains on either side of the flame. The other two signs were used mainly as determinatives for "hot." One is an older form (left); perhaps this type of pot, full of burning oil, became so hot that later two handles and a foot were added (center).

The last sign is again a brazier. Both these words can be used for local or general heat, that is, inflammation or fever: one has to gather the meaning from the context.[99] Look also at this spelling for remedies that have to be applied to the skin at the

heat   of   finger[100]

If you are not yet convinced about the identity of the brazier—there were actually two forms of it (Fig. 3.16)—consider the following illustration from one of the many versions of the *Book of the Dead,* the beautifully illustrated papyrus of Ani dating from c.1250 B.C. (Plate 3.2). The theme is the underworld. The jagged lines are the conventional Egyptian way of representing water. This is the Lake of Flames, drawn in red and surrounded by four stylized braziers.[101]

Wounds Right and Wrong

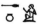

Case 41 of the Smith papyrus is a very sick man with two problems: a wound in the chest, complicated by infection:[102]

INSTRUCTIONS CONCERNING A DISEASED WOUND IN HIS BREAST

If thou examinest a man having a diseased wound in his breast, while that wound is inflamed and a whirl of inflammation continually issues from the mouth of that wound at thy touch; the two lips of that wound are ruddy, while that man continues to be feverish from it; his flesh cannot receive a bandage, that wound

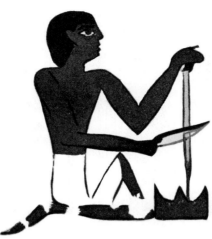

3.17 "A whirl of inflammation is in his wound"—perhaps this idiom referred to the fire-stick. A bow-string was wrapped once around the stick, which twirled under the stone cap held\in the left hand.

cannot take a margin of skin; the p'ys.t(?) which is in the mouth of that wound is watery, their surface is hot and secretions drop therefrom in an oily state,

Thou shouldst say concerning him: "One having a diseased wound in his breast, it being inflamed, (and) he continues to have fever from it. An ailment which I will treat."

Notice, incidentally, the typical bedside manner: touching the wound.[103]

Here are some of the glosses to this case:

As for: "A diseased wound in his breast, inflamed," it means that the wound which is in his breast is sluggish, without closing up; high fever comes forth from it, its two lips are red, and its mouth is open. The "Treatise on What Pertains to a Wound" [*lost!*] says concerning it: "It means that there is a very great swelling; and 'inflamed' is said concerning the height (of the fever)."

As for: "A whirl of inflammation in his wound," it means a whirl of inflammation which circulates through the interior of his entire wound. [*This does not help to understand the "whirl": Ebbell astutely suggested that the Commentator may have had in mind the twirling effect of the fire-drill (Fig. 3.17).[104]*]

As for: "His flesh cannot receive a bandage," it means that his flesh will not receive the remedies because of the inflammation which is in his flesh.

As for: "While heat continually issues (nšw) from the mouth of his wound at thy touch," (it means) that heat comes forth from the mouth of his wound at thy touch; as it is said that a thing which has come forth entirely, has issued (nšw).

The real nugget of this case lies in the first sentence, "One having a diseased wound in his breast":

Note the little man with blood streaming from his head. He stands for "enemy, death," and serves here as the determinative to the word "diseased," *shmay:*[105]

sh

ma   a   y

There can be no doubt about the reading: *shmay wbnw,* "diseased wound."

There are, indeed, two kinds of wounds. The simplest way to describe them is to call them sick and not sick. Today they would be called sterile and infected, that is, healing with and without pus. The clinical difference was noticed around 400 B.C. by Hippocrates, who is generally assigned the priority for the discovery. However, if there is a concept of good and bad wounds, its grandfather was definitely Egyptian. The Smith papyrus clearly states that wounds could become sick, develop $\;\;\;$ *ḥwa.t,* "the rots" (note the plural strokes),[106] and throw $\;\;\;$ *ryyt,* "pus."[107] And when a wound took a really bad turn, it was no longer called an *wbnw* but a *bnwt:*

b   n   w   (det.)
nw   t

The wbnw and the bnwt seem to have been a couple of notches lower than our twentieth century concepts of "good" and "bad" wounds. They certainly do not correspond to "wound" and "ulcer"; the wbnw alone appears to cover both, like the Greek *hélkos.*[108] The bnwt applies to particularly bad sores; although it could have no precise meaning, it seems to indicate complicated, perhaps gangrenous or cancerous ulcers.[109] A definition of bnwt comes from a late papyrus: "Bnwt, Brother of Blood, Friend of Pus, Father of the [smelly] Jackal."[110]

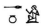

It would be interesting to know how much pus the swnw expected to harvest in the ordinary course of wound healing. Following is a relevant passage of the Ebers papyrus.[111] It must be read with special care, for it is a landmark in the history of medicine:

REMEDY FOR A WOUND, THE FIRST DAY

Fat from an ox so that it [*the wound*] may rot, or meat of an ox.
But if the wound rots too much then bind on it spoiled barley-bread, so that it may dry.

This is understood to mean that some pus is desirable as long as it is not excessive.

The text continues:

> But if (the wound) closes over its secretions, thou shouldst bandage it with grease . . . and crushed peas.
> If (the wound) beneath breaks open, then powder it with powder of green frit; then bandage it . . .
> If thereafter (the wound) has covered itself, then make an ointment to strengthen the blood vessels (*mtw*); therewith bandage it, so that it is cured.
> If thereafter it closes up over its secretions, then prepare: grease, [*a plant*]; therewith it is bandaged, so that it opens its mouth, so that it rots.

The thread of thought, from the beginning:

> It is good for a wound to rot a little.
> Some wounds may close too early, while there still is rot inside.
> Therefore, put something on the wound that will get out that rot.

I used the term "landmark" purposely, because if the above reading is correct, we have before us the first known statement of the dirtiest, messiest, most pernicious, and most persistent mistake in the history of surgery: *getting the badness out of the wound.* In practice, it means forcing a wound to suppurate. Though this procedure tends to make matters worse, it has been one of the catchiest concepts in the history of medicine. "Getting rid of something bad" has such a plausible ring, like modern drainage; and in fact there *is* a badness in wounds, only it is the bacteria instead of the pus. Trying to heal a wound by making it throw more pus is about as reasonable as getting more children to stop pregnancies. Yet rivers of pus flowed for another 3500 years, and the dreadful doctrine of good and laudable pus, *pus bonum et laudabile,* has only recently faded out.

Here we must pause briefly and analyze what we have been doing. We have just saddled the Egyptians with a very inglorious priority, and this on the faith of a few lines only, half sentences dropped just once. The reader should realize that I have quoted just about all the pertinent passages. Is this safe, or are we trying to weave a fabric out of a few bits of thread?

This is, I must admit, just what we have been doing, much like the archeologist who tries to squeeze a culture out of bits of pottery. But facts are facts, even if they are few—and I believe that our story is reliable. Besides, if the reader is not yet convinced that the Egyptians did expect some pus to flow in the ordinary course of wound healing, I will propose to dissect the only pertinent witness from ancient Egypt: the word for wound.

"Wound," *wbnw,* could be written in several ways.[112] Even the scribe of the Smith papyrus must have felt that the variations were cumbersome, because as he ground his way through the text, column after column, he gradually switched to the simpler forms:

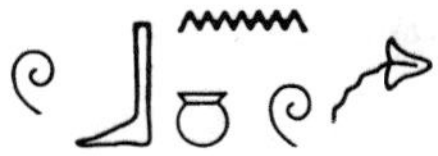

          n

w   b   (det.)

    nw w

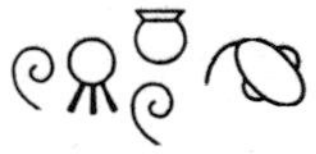

      nw

w wbn   (det.)

    w

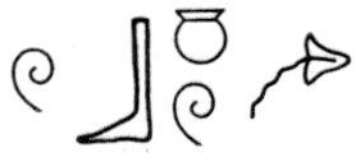

      nw

w   b   (det.)

    w

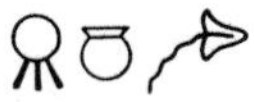

wbn nw (det.)

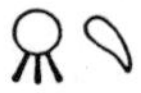

wbn (det.)

wbn (a precarious spelling because ⵕ wbn
also stands for "sunshine")

Note the three possible determinatives. One, ⵇ "a piece of meat," poses no problem. As to ⵏ "fluid issuing from lips," which suggests "effusion," it is used after "vomiting" and "spitting,"[113] and in ancient texts it also indicates putrefaction.[114] Thus, in connection with wounds it might refer to bleeding as well as suppuration. The third determinative ⵔ or ⵖ is generally used to convey the notion of smell and putrefaction.[115] It is also used alone thus ⵢ as a shorthand writing of ⵣ ḥs, "feces,"[116] or of ⵤ wḥdw, the basic cause of rotting. Obviously, the scribe's idea of a wound implies corruption.

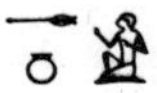

This third determinative, the strange object with two handles, deserves further study. It can be drawn ⵖ or ⵔ with or without the little curl, which appears to suggest "outflow" (by implication, "stinking outflow"); and indeed, the rare form is used when the preceding word is a liquid, as in *w s sh t*, "urine." It is also used after *wt*, "the embalmer." Gardiner interpreted it provisionally as "pustule or gland" and listed it with unclassifiable signs.[117]

The clue to its origin was found by R. Steuer on an old stele from about 2250 B.C.[118] The text reads in part, "A boon given by . . . Anubis, Who-is-on-his-Mountain, Who-is-in-the-place-of-Embalming (*wt*)"; and see the determinative for *embalming:*

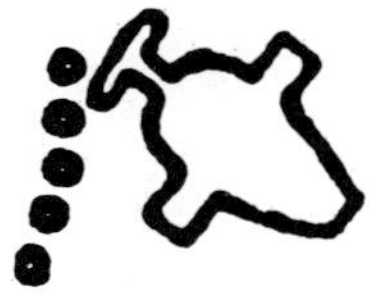

So the archaic form of was the pot of the embalmer pouring out the drugs of the trade. Here is where the Scribe came to seek his symbol for corruption.

To exploit the message of the determinatives to the extreme, we might follow Steuer one step further. Assume that we now have two kinds of wounds with two major determinatives: -wounds, the better kind, with a cleaner type of determinative that stands mainly for "clean outflow" (bleeding); and -wounds, the rotten kind, where the determinative stands for "stinking outflow," hence decay (pus). It might therefore be possible to gauge in a given text the prevalence of infection by the prevalent type of determinative. Now the Smith papyrus, a rational book of surgery dealing mostly with fresh wounds, has mostly or good wounds; the Ebers papyrus, replete with magic and quack-type remedies, has only or bad wounds.[119] Steuer suggested that this is not fanciful spelling but the expression of a real clinical difference.[120] To me, it seems almost too elegant to be true that the scribes were expressing clinical nuances by playing with the determinatives.

And now I feel free to confess one disturbing truth that I have been concealing. The precious, the divine, the life-giving *bya*, "iron," is sometimes spelled with the rotten determinative . Occasionally it also has two determinatives, both the star and :

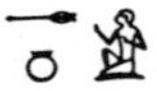

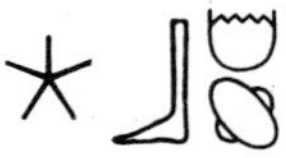

Wainwright, the expert on Egyptian iron, took this to mean that stands for "explosion." I would rather suggest that the ragged meteorites which drop on earth are being viewed as *excrement* of a *star:* of .

Lay Thy Hand upon It

The use of the hand in the Smith papyrus is impressive. Sometimes it has a precise purpose, such as searching for a fracture in the skull[121] or feeling a lump: "If thy puttest thy hand upon his breast upon these tumors, and thou findest them very cool, there being no fever therein when thy hand touches him . . . and they are bulging to thy hand . . . there is no treatment."[122] In another case the swnw's hand may be feeling for the heartbeat: "If . . . any physician puts his hands (or) his fingers upon the head, upon the back of the head, upon the two hands, upon the pulse, upon the two feet . . . he measures . . . the heart."[123] But most of the time the swnw is reaching right into the wound, and he does it so systematically that the world's first description of the human brain is "something throbbing and fluttering under thy fingers."[124] See the fingers (*) in the original text:

Hieratic

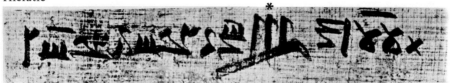

Hieroglyphic

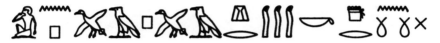

On a strictly surgical level, all this touching is of course very bad. The Greeks did away with it by replacing the finger with their all-purpose wound probe, though there is no proof that the one carried less bacteria than the other. How clean *was* the hand? The Egyptians are said to have been rather clean people, but data on their personal hygiene are few.[125] "Washerman's washing water" was used as a drug,[126] so that some kind of washermen must have existed. Soap, however, was unknown to them.[127] As detergents, they used fuller's earth, perhaps also the pounded lupins still used there today,[128] and above all their favorite chemical, *ntry*, a natural soda.[129]

But setting aside these purely hygienic considerations, I believe that we should read a deeper meaning into the gesture of touching the wound. It recurs so often, in a text that gives nothing but essentials, that it suggests an intrinsic value. In case 47, involving an open wound, the wording almost suggests a ritual: "Thy shouldst lay thy hand upon it."[130] Physical contact is reassuring; when a doctor touches the patient, both parties have the feeling that something is being done. Touching also means taking part; it means that matters are being taken in hand. The comfort of physical touch reaches deep down, to ancestral depths far older than mankind. Go back into the jungle with Jane van Lawick-Goodall and see how apes convey the message of reassurance: sometimes it is just the matter of a hand touching a hand (Fig. 3.18).[131]

Meat, Salt, and Shepenn

"Bind the wound upon fresh meat"—this backward advice is standard for wounds and bites on the first day.[132] One wonders what was expected of it. Were it not for the single passage quoted earlier, in which the meat was

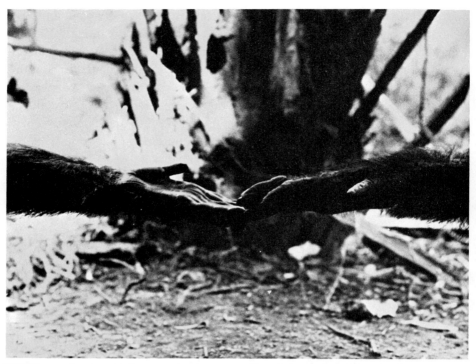

3.18 Reassuring by touch, a very basic gesture. Here it is employed by two chimpanzees in the forest.

supposed to transfer decay to the wound ("meat of an ox, so that the wound may rot"), one would guess the purpose to have been exactly the opposite. A slab of meat may have helped to check the bleeding as a mechanical plug, although nowhere in the Smith papyrus is any reference made to bleeding.[133] Meat, namely muscle, can also act as a clotting agent; crushed tissue in general works very well. An elderly neurosurgeon told me that in his younger days, before safe clotting agents had become available, it was standard practice to check very small hemorrhages on the surface of the brain by applying a tiny bit of muscle taken from the same patient (perfect hemostasis is crucial in brain surgery).

But this is not the wave length of the ancient Egyptians. A likelier rationale would be the simple, basic idea that flesh mends flesh. Lots of people  still bind a steak over a black eye; the practice is current among boxers. There is no particular theory about it, except that it is "good."

Now we are much closer to Egyptian thinking. In fact, see what kind of meat they used. The word for meat was *ywf*:

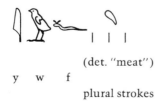

(det. "meat")

y   w   f

plural strokes

Sometimes a prescription says ywf of cow, or ywf of ox; and as such, the ywf is either *ywf wadj:*

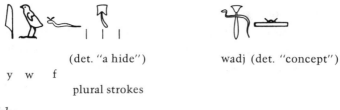

(det. "a hide")

y   w   f

plural strokes

wadj (det. "concept")

or *ywf ankh:*

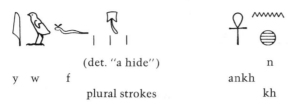

(det. "a hide")

y   w   f

plural strokes

n

ankh

kh

Wadj means "green," but luckily it also means "fresh," so we can assume that *ywf wadj* means "fresh meat." As to *ywf ankh*, everybody nowadays

seems to know that ⚲ *ankh* stands for "life, alive," but most of the learned translators have found a treatment with "live meat" too bizarre and, somewhat uneasily, have rendered *ywf ankh* as "fresh meat."[134] Others were sufficiently annoyed by the expression to suspect the sacred ankh of meaning, for the occasion, "goat."[135]

But after all, there is nothing wrong with the literal translation: *ywf ankh* = "meat alive," or flesh just cut off a living animal.[136] Inconceivable today, the idea was commonplace in Egypt. Priests were accustomed to cut off the foreleg of a young bull (Fig. 3.19)[137] as part of the ceremony of the Opening of the Mouth, which was precisely a matter of infusing life into mummies or statues. In that case the live meat was a very appropriate "refreshment for the dead."[138] On a wound, it made equally good sense: to heal *ankh* or "live" flesh, use *ankh* or "live" meat.

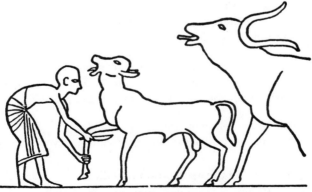

3.19 Ritual amputation of the foreleg of the bull, which was part of the ceremony of the Opening of the Mouth—perhaps also a way to obtain "live flesh" to put on wounds. From a tomb, c.1300 B.C.

And now for the wound drugs. Put yourself in the place of an Egyptian patient: here comes the swnw and smothers your wound with an unspeakable green mush. Would you not want to know whether the stuff has a fighting chance to do you good?

The first question, of course, is to determine whether we have a fighting chance to find an answer. The odds against making any sense of Egyptian pharmacy (or of ancient pharmacy in general) are huge. In the first place, what *did* they use? To choose one item from among the more studied, exactly what was

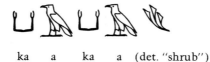

ka   a   ka   a   (det. "shrub")

"kaakaa"?[139] It was obviously a shrub; but was it really *Ricinus* (the plant that gives castor oil) as some of the experts suggest?[140] It is true that the Greeks had a vaguely similar name, *kíki*, for castor berries; but how safe is it to connect two words from texts that were perhaps one thousand years apart? And if we accept that kaakaa is *Ricinus*, what shall we do with the *dgm* plant, which also has very good reasons for being identified with *Ricinus*?[141] And regardless of which plant was *Ricinus*, what part was used, how was it prepared, how much was given, with what, and for what reason? Multiply these questions by some seven hundred "drugs," and the problem grows to such a size that one tends to brush it off by concluding that ancient Egyptian pharmacy was tremendously advanced—whereby what stands proven, rather than ancient wisdom, is modern confusion. Once and for all, beware: *next to nothing is known about the effectiveness of ancient drugs;* and even when the drug itself is known, experimental studies are almost nil.

In view of these dangers, I have chosen to analyze here only a few wound drugs, but those in depth. A good starting point is the series prescribed for the infected chest wound described earlier. It involves a three-phase program:[142]

I) Thou shalt make for him cool applications for drawing out the inflammation from the mouth of the wound:
    Leaves of willow, nbs-tree. . . . Apply to it.
    Leaves of ym'-tree, dung. . . . Apply to it.

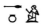

II) Thou shalt make for him applications for drying up the wound:
    Powder of green pigment . . . grease. Triturate; bind upon it.
    Northern salt, ibex grease. Triturate; bind upon it.

III) Thou shalt make for him poultices:
    Red shepenn, garden tongue . . . sycamore leaves. Bind upon it.

Breasted commended the application of willow leaves because "they contain salicin."[143] They contain very little of it; and anyway the treatment would amount to putting traces of aspirin on wounds, which would not be particularly effective.[144]

As for dung, I would have thought that no amount of enthusiasm could lead to praise it as a drug; but I was wrong. Breasted exclaims in admiration that dung is "ammoniacal."[145] Perhaps this was the most benign adjective that Breasted's medical adviser could supply (what about "natural" or "biological"?), but it is meaningless in this context. The only benign comment I can make is that the Smith papyrus is very light on dung; other papyri are much more "ammoniacal"—they recommend excrements from man and eighteen other animals, including flyspecks scraped off the wall.[146]

The "red shepenn" had no acceptable translation in 1930; now it seems to mean poppy, either the common corn poppy or *Papaver somniferum*.[147] If it was corn poppy, its alkaloids have no morphine-like effect.[148] If it was the opium poppy, it is conceivable that an extract applied to a wound might be absorbed in large enough amounts to work as a shot of morphine. There is some evidence that opium did reach Egypt sometime during the Eighteenth Dynasty (c.1590–1340 B.C.),[149] that is, a century or two after our present edition of the Smith papyrus. Opium, incidentally, is the dried sap that oozes from slits in the poppy capsules (Fig. 3.20). During the Eighteenth Dynasty, Egypt began to import tiny jugs made by hand in Cyprus, so distinctive in size and shape as to suggest a trademark. Nowadays they would stand a good chance of being seized at customs by the narcotics squad, for they are just too similar to poppy capsules (Fig. 3.21). Even their finish often recalls the buff-brown color of the dried capsules; and what could the parallel lines be if

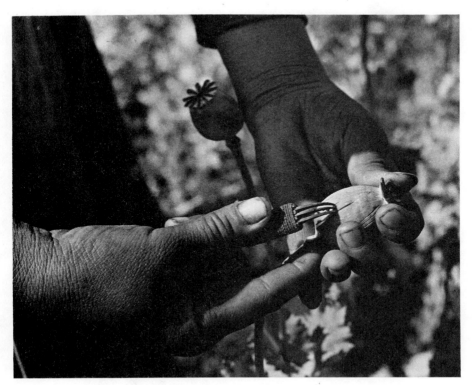

3.20 The basic technique for harvesting opium has not changed for millennia. The marks in this poppy capsule left by the three-pronged scraper (photographed in Laos in 1972), are very similar to those drawn on the "opium juglets" found in Egypt.

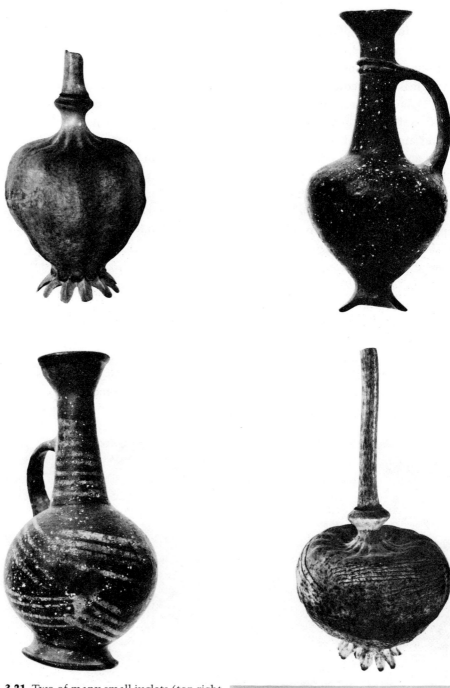

3.21 Two of many small juglets (top right, bottom left) that came to Egypt from Cyprus around 1600–1500 B.C., compared with poppy capsules (same scale). The similarity in size, shape, and surface pattern suggests that these juglets were full of opium. Insert at right shows scale.

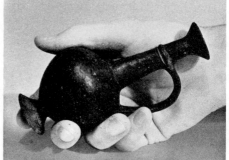

not the slits from which the opium trickled? The crafty Cypriotes had probably devised these suggestive juglets to export a costly drug, opium dissolved in wine or water.[150]

At this very time, about 1550 B.C., the Ebers papyrus suggests a fail-safe drink to placate a crying baby: an infusion of shepenn, improved with flyspecks scraped from the wall.[151] Again about this time, upstream in Thebes, death befell an architect by the name of Cha. He was laid in his grave with an alabaster pot full of ointment. In 1927 an Italian pharmacologist analyzed what was left of it and found, mixed in with the fat, something that behaved chemically and physiologically like morphine.[152] What opium would be doing in an ointment, again I do not know; but it seems very likely that the opium producers of the Greek islands had found customers in Egypt sometime between the Smith and the Ebers papyrus (Fig. 3.3).

In the second phase of treatment for the badly infected chest wound, several drugs were prescribed to "dry up the sore." I read this to mean "stopping suppuration," which suggests that antiseptics might be hiding here. The "Northern salt" was chiefly sodium chloride.[153] It could well have some antiseptic effect, as it does in salted meat or fish, but concentrations sufficient to kill bacteria would also hurt the tissues. The "green pigment" deserves a special treatment.

The Logic of Eye Paint

"Powder of green pigment . . . Triturate; bind upon it"—so goes the prescription. Thanks to the chemists, we are rather well informed about Egyptian green pigments.[154] They were called by the general name of *wadj*, which means "to be green." Here is one way to spell it:

dj
wad
(det. "concept")

But in most cases wadj referred to one particular green stone, malachite (Plate 3.3). This is copper carbonate. It lay about in the eastern desert and on the Sinai peninsula and, though very beautiful, was actually a copper ore.[155] Another ore designated as wadj was chrysocolla, copper silicate, which is a lovely blue-green (Plate 3.4). A third way to obtain a green powder was to grind up an artificial frit, that is, a kind of glass obtained by melting together sand, natron, and copper minerals.[156]

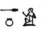

The Ebers papyrus also mentions a fourth kind, wadj "of boat":

n
(= "of")   "boat"

111

Being myself quite familiar with the blue-green patina that forms on the copper sheathing of old shipwrecks and on bronze fittings at sea, I found very attractive the interpretation of this "boat green"—published ten years ago—as "scrapings of marine hardware."[157] For safety, however, I wrote to the author—and almost wished I had not. Dr. Harris had since been seized by a reasonable doubt: what if the "boat green" were just some messy green stuff scraped off the bottom of a wooden boat? The original idea had been suggested in the nineteenth century, when copper-lined hulls were still within living memory; but the Egyptians did not build their boats that way.

Thus were shipwrecked the "scrapings of marine hardware." However, all is not lost. Somehow, *some* green pigment was being obtained from copper, because it appears to be implied in the expression wadj ḥmty, "coppery green" or "copper green," where 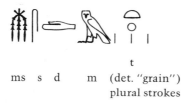 ḥmtyy is an adjective from ḥmt, "copper."[158] In summary, then, the Egyptians had at least four ways to obtain their wadj—green pigments from copper compounds.

Very often wadj also stands for green eye-paint;[159] and be prepared for surprises, for ladies' makeup, seen in the perspective of time, transcends cosmetics. Century after century Egyptian women kept painting their eyelids either black or green (Plate 3.5).[160] The black makeup was called:

ms	s	d	m	(det. "grain") plural strokes

pronounced something like *mesdemet*. So persistent were the ladies in using this makeup, over roughly five thousand years,[161] that its name passed into the Coptic **CTHⲗⲗ** *stim*, then into the Greek *stimmi*, and finally into the Latin *stibium*, "antimony." It was, in fact, antimony sulphide (stibnite). Its Mesopotamian equivalent had an equally brilliant philologic career. It was called *guhlu* and was either stibnite or "galena," lead sulphide. Guhlu lasted long enough for the Arabs to take it over as *kohl*. Being a powder ground to extreme fineness, the kohl—*al kohl*—came to mean something extremely subtle; hence, in the late Middle Ages Paracelsus applied it to the spirit of wine—yes, *alcohol!* Strangest of all is that the Arabs themselves now call alcohol by the Latin word, *sbirtu*.[162]

The little kits for grinding eye paint were an important item of Egyptian toilette. Their name happens to be written like the word for "to protect," possibly an allusion to averting the eye diseases that were then and still are a scourge all over the Near East. Eye paints were offered to the gods, the statues of the gods were painted with them, and they are often mentioned in connection with the eye of Horus.[163]

Green as a color was related to joy (think of the daily contrast between greenery and desert, almost synonymous with life and death).[164] In Ptolemaic times, another word for joy was *turquoise* (ideally turquoise is blue, but by the time it is found, it has often turned green from exposure to the light).[165]

Taking all this into consideration, I would conclude that whoever first decided to put green pigment on an ugly, infected wound must have had in mind something more than just a kind of paint. But could it have done any good? The intriguing fact is that every one of the four green pigments happened to be a copper compound. Copper is fairly toxic,[166] and what kills people should kill bacteria. Suspecting that one or the other *wadj* may have worked as an antiseptic, I set about procuring samples of green powders that would qualify as wadj, to test their capacity to prevent bacterial growth in cultures.[167] The first two samples were easy to make. I sacrificed small pieces of malachite and chrysocolla and ground them to a fine powder in a porcelain pharmacy mortar. A third sample, according to my original sources, might have been the patina from the copper sheeting of an ancient New England wreck (a precious specimen in my possession); but this plan, of course, had to be scrapped. The problem was to prepare an acceptable wadj directly from copper. Eventually I adopted the oldest method available, as described by Dioscorides in the first century A.D. In his day the copper-green powder now called verdigris was known in Greek as *iós xystós*, literally "scraped [copper-] rust," and in Latin *aerugo rasilis*: "But Aerugo rasilis is thus prepared. Pouring into an hogshead, or some such like vessel, ye sharpest vinegar, turn upon it a brazen vessel: it is good if ye hollow look downward, if not, let it be plane. But let it be made clean & having no breathing place. Then after 10 days take off ye cover & scrape off ye Aerugo that has come on it; or having made a plate of ye brass itself, hang it into the vessel, so as not to touch ye vinegar, and after ye like number of days scrape it off."[168] This last method works beautifully: we used strips of copper plate hung over vinegar in a tall, closed jar; overnight they became covered with a lovely blue-green wadj.

Using infected wounds as a source of pathogenic bacteria, the three powders were then submitted to a standard test. The results were fair for chrysocolla, good for malachite, and spectacular for verdigris; none of the bacteria resisted the onslaught of this last wadj (Plate 3.6, Figs. 3.22–3.23). Whatever the logic that prompted the use of wadj on wounds, I must conclude that the green wound-dressings—apart from their cheerful color—may well have beaten off some infections. Copper poisoning through a few local applications should not have been a major risk. If the test of time means anything, malachite and chrysocolla remained in use until the Greeks launched the variety that became most popular: verdigris (which is in fact corrupt Middle English for *vert-de-Grèce*). Dioscorides' concluding paragraph on chrysocolla rings distinctly true: "But Chrysocolla hath a faculty of wearing off scars, of repressing flesh-excrescencies, & of cleansing, & of binding & of warming & is gently corrosive with some little biting. And it is of ye number of those medicines that cause vomiting & are strong enough to kill."[169]

Skip another two thousand years: streptococci are being fought with copper to this very day. There is a streptococcal skin infection called impetigo. In France at least, a very popular—and, I am told, practically indis-

113

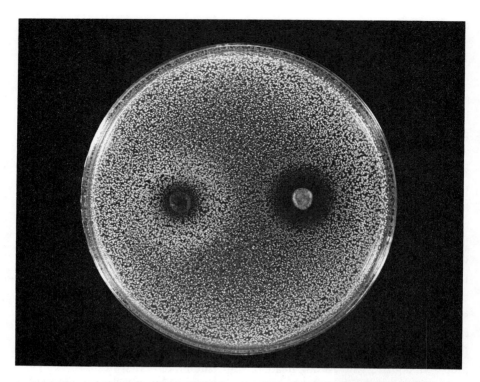

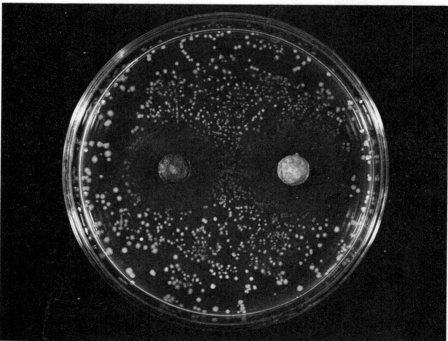

3.22 Two other experiments to test the bactericidal power of malachite and chrysocolla, this time against a pathogenic bacterium, *Staphylococcus aureus. Above:* The technique is the same as for Plate 3.6. This method gives the bacteria an unfair advantage, because the dry powder in the little wells has difficulty in diffusing out; hence, the inhibition of bacterial growth is not marked. *Below:* here the powder in the wells was moistened with water, which allowed more copper to diffuse out. Under these conditions, more comparable to those of a wound dressing, both minerals are very effective.

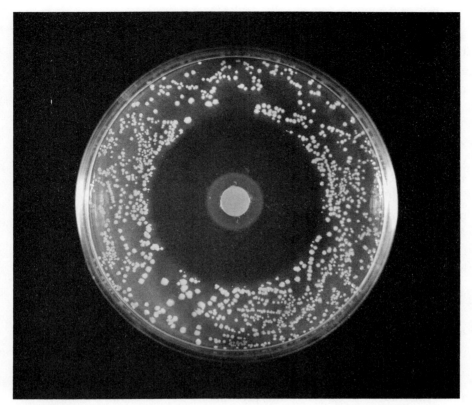

3.23 This time "green of copper" is in the center well: copper acetate scraped off copper plates exposed to vapors of vinegar. The bacterium is *E. coli.* "Green of copper" has a devastating effect on bacteria, as shown by the dark ring.

pensable—prescription against impetigo is the *Eau Dalibour*. It was devised around the year 1700 by Monsieur Jacques Dalibour, surgeon general to the army of Louis XIV. Its principal ingredients are copper and zinc, and it worked like a charm for "all Manners of Wounds, Cuts, Slashes by Sword or Sabre, and Injuries by all Cutting and Bruising Devices."[170]

Grease, Honey, and Lint

Mrht, byt, and *ftt*—this is the standard wound salve of the Smith papyrus:

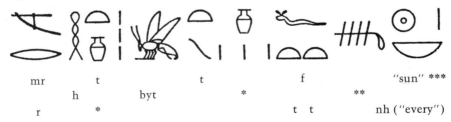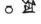

mr	t		t		f		"sun" ***
	h	byt		*		**	
r	*				t	t	nh ("every")

* Det. "pot" + plural strokes, meaning "stuff in pot"
** Det. "backbone and ribs" (fibers seen as backbones of a plant)
*** "Sun" means "day." The vertical stroke means "the preceding sign ('sun,' hence 'day') stands for the object drawn."

The lint, ftt, was some sort of vegetable fiber,[171] possibly a fluffy pad as shown in Plate 4.3; it was also used as a contraceptive.[172] To a bad wound in the throat that gives fever and drives the patient to his mooring stakes, ftt is applied alone and dry, without bandages, "perhaps to promote drainage" by capillary action.[173]

The grease, mrht, could be anything from vegetable oil to snake grease. The animal varieties come from at least twenty-two species.[174] Byt, or honey, was by far the most popular Egyptian drug, being mentioned some 500 times in 900 remedies. It came from wild bees, since the Egyptians did not practice apiculture.[175]

To visualize the salve, one should know the proportions of honey and grease. A single reference suggests $\frac{1}{3}$ to $\frac{2}{3}$.[176] Note here the improvement over Akkadian pharmacy: the Egyptians often specify the relative quantities of ingredients in their recipes, probably in volumes rather than weights.[177] They had several ways to indicate fractions. Here is one:

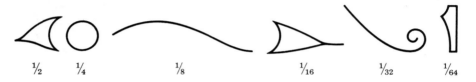

| $\frac{1}{2}$ | $\frac{1}{4}$ | | $\frac{1}{8}$ | | $\frac{1}{16}$ | $\frac{1}{32}$ | $\frac{1}{64}$ |

and if the reader will guess how this came about, he deserves an honorary Ph.D. in Egyptology (for the answer, see Fig. 3.24).[178]

Anyway, we prepared a mixture of $\frac{1}{3}$ honey to $\frac{2}{3}$ fat, using either beef fat or butter; and it turned out that $\frac{1}{3}$ honey is just right; more makes the paste too sticky. Despite the pleasant consistency, I thought at first that this would be dreadful stuff to put on an open wound. I visualized swarms of flies feeding on the honey, swarms of bacteria feeding on the sugar, and tissue reactions caused by the grease: when fatty substances are injected into the tissues, they produce a persistent lump called a fat granuloma. Today, looking back on this skepticism, I feel I should have paid more attention to one very unusual feature about this salve: the way it is recommended in the Smith papyrus. Egyptian remedies in general come with long lists of possible substitutes: "another . . . another . . . another . . ." often reinforced with

comments like 𓆓𓆓 "good, good," "really proven," "proven 𓆓 (= a million) times"—as is common with drugs that do not work. But the combination of "lint, grease, and honey" is recommended for twenty-two of forty-eight cases[179] with the bluntness of "penicillin," as if the author really knew that it worked.

One day, as my wife was spreading vaseline over a minor burn, I began to wonder. We still apply ointments to small cuts. Are vaseline or lanolin so very different from ox grease, ibis grease, lion grease, or grease from a hippo's foot?[180]

I looked up some literature, beginning with the bees. Bees are clean little beasts. If they are killed and dipped in a culture medium, bacteria rarely grow out.[181] Some years past a scientist worriedly noticed that honeybees were crawling "over the human excrement of the family privy" in Tennessee.[182] He tested the maximum survival time of bacteria in honey, using bacteria of the typhoid-colon group, and found much to his relief that all were killed within hours or days, as follows:

B. dysenteriae	10 hours
B. paratyphosus A	10 hours
B. paratyphosus B	10 hours–1 day
B. typhosus	10 hours–2 days
B. proteus vulgaris	3–4 days
B. coli communis	4–5 days

The honey was heat-sterilized, inoculated with the bacteria, then kept at room temperature (under these conditions the bactericidal activity is due mainly to the osmotic effect). The addition of 10 percent physiological saline to the honey often increased its effect; saline up to 50 percent did not decrease it appreciably.[183]

Thus honey does not support bacterial growth: if this were not so, the bees would have a hard time, and many housewives too. Honey is anti-bacterial for several reasons. The most obvious is a simple concentration effect: being extremely hypertonic,[184] it draws water from the bacterial cells, causing them to shrivel and die. This mechanism works so well that an offering of honey, piously buried in Paestum in a sacred chamber 2500 years ago,[185] never decayed and is recognizable to this day (Plate 3.7).

But honey can also prevent the growth of bacteria by an antibiotic mechanism discovered several years before the advent of penicillin, and active even in dilutions as low as 13 percent.[186] One of the active principles, inhibine, turned out to be an enzyme secreted by the pharyngeal glands of the bee: glucose oxidase.[187] The reaction is as follows:

$$\text{glucose} + O_2 \xrightarrow{\text{glucose oxidase}} \text{gluconolactone} + H_2O_2$$

where H_2O_2 is hydrogen peroxyde, the common household disinfectant, and gluconolactone equilibrates with gluconic acid, a mild antibiotic.[188] A convenient system indeed.

Inhibine is destroyed by light or heat. But a group of French workers discovered in honey yet another type of bacteriostatic activity that is resistant to both light and heat.[189]

The bee's antibacterial arsenal is not exhausted with honey. Cracks in the hive are patched with a sticky material called propolis, gathered from buds, and this too is antibiotic.[190] It even inhibits plant growth: if potato germs are introduced into the beehive, the bees quickly clean them up and cover them with a thin layer of propolis. Result: no growth.[191] Its main active principle is galangine, a flavonol, which now holds U.S. patent 2,550,269 as a food preservative.[192] During the Boer War, propolis was used successfully, it was said, for the treatment of wounds.[193]

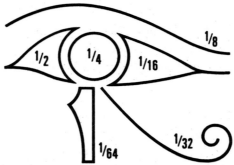

3.24 The eye of Horus, the falcon-god, was used as a device to express fractions. The whole story is very unmathematical. Horus and Seth became involved in a fight over the succession to their father. The eyes of Horus were pulled out and torn to pieces, and the physician-god Thoth put them together again. But the fractions for each part of the eye add up to only 63/64; presumably the last bit was supplied by Thoth.

Honey as a wound dressing never quite faded out. In Shanghai during World War II, hardship brought back the use of honey and lard for ulcers and small wounds. The results may not have been as "extraordinarily good" as claimed,[194] but like many other recent attempts they prove that honey is well tolerated and basically harmless, though it may sting for a while and cause some delay in healing.[195] The main advantage seems to be mechanical. Despite its own stickiness it prevents the dressing from sticking to the wound, because it draws out a large amount of fluid,[196] and this is said to have a cleansing effect, especially useful on dirty or infected wounds.[197]

In summary, *the swnw happened to choose an ingredient that was practically harmless to the tissues, aseptic, antiseptic, and antibiotic.* I should say *the* ingredient: nothing else, in ancient Egypt, could have begun to match these properties of honey. The nearest competitors would have been the resins, which were in fact used, but they were scarce and too sticky, or too dry, to use pure.

Now for the case of grease. On this score scientific literature was of little help. It was well known that fats and oils injected into the tissues produce untoward reactions, but it was not clear what would happen if fat were applied to the surface of a wound, which is reacting anyway. I suspected that the tissue reaction would be exaggerated, perhaps to the point of mushrooming into those exuberant growths once called by the Calvinistic name of "proud flesh." Several millennia of medical practice are worth the sacrifice of

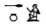

a few guinea pigs: we put Egyptian pharmacy to the test of science and compared wounds that had been treated with either beef fat or vaseline (the latter is said to be practically indifferent to wound healing). After eight days, both kinds of wounds had closed to a comparable degree, with no trace of "proud flesh" (Figs. 3.25–3.26).

A pessimist might still object that the grease-and-honey mixture could spoil. But actually it kills bacteria. To give the mixture the roughest possible test, we made it up with butter (apparently not known to the ancient Egyptians), which contains many bacteria of its own, including a group of coliform bacteria. Result: the bacteria initially present tended to disappear, and if

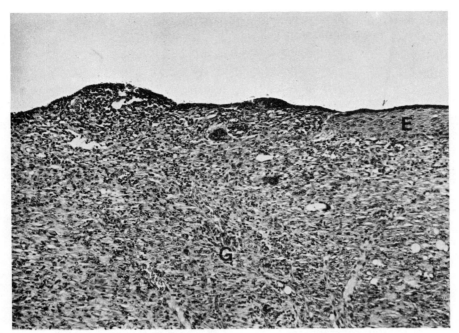

3.25 Microscopic section of the surface of an open wound in guinea-pig skin, left untreated for seven days except for a vaseline dressing. It was filled with granulation tissue (G), and the epidermis (E) is growing back over it. This is the normal course of events without any treatment.

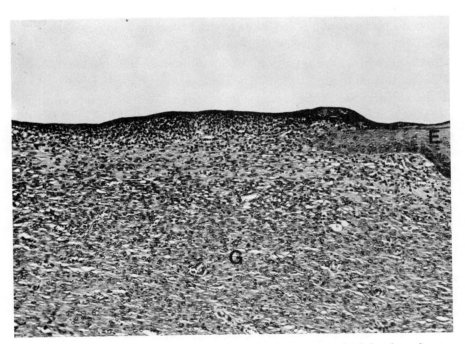

3.26 Microscopic section of a similar wound of the same age, which has been kept under a dressing of *byt* and *mrht*, "honey" and "grease." Compare with the preceding figure: no harm has been done.

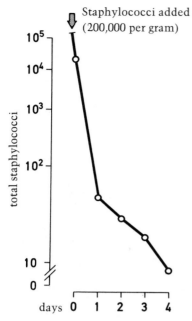

Staphylococci added (200,000 per gram)

total staphylococci

10^5

10^4

10^3

10^2

10

0

days 0 1 2 3 4

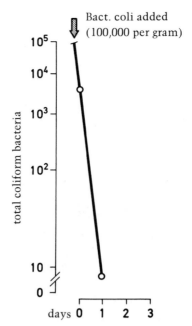

Bact. coli added (100,000 per gram)

total coliform bacteria

10^5

10^4

10^3

10^2

10

0

days 0 1 2 3

3.27 The self-sterilizing, antiseptic effect of the ancient Egyptian wound salve, $\frac{1}{3}$ honey and $\frac{2}{3}$ grease (here butter). The added staphylococci are rapidly killed.

3.28 The same experiment with another pathogenic bacterium, *E. coli.*

pathogenic bacteria were added, like *Escherichia coli* or *Staphylococcus aureus,* they were killed just as fast (Figs. 3.27–3.28).[198]

All this goes to say that, in view of the technology of Pharaonic days, it would be difficult to produce a more sensible ointment. One wonders how the ingredients were chosen. Perhaps there were some cultural reasons that escape us. Consider this hint from a charm: "I prepared for him . . . honey, which is sweet to men, but bitter to the dead."[199] But the truth is probably simpler. Both grease and honey would prevent the bandage from sticking; both have a soothing consistency; grease spoils little, oil and honey not at all. To a decay-conscious mind like that of the Egyptian, this last must have been an important consideration.

After this tribute to Egyptian acumen, it is only fair to remember that the bees, as embalmers, were actually ahead of the Pharaohs. When the hive is invaded and the intruder gets killed but is too large to be thrown out, the bees simply cover its corpse with propolis. After a while, all that is left is a harmless mummy (Fig. 3.29).[200]

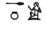

It must have taken a long time to work out this method; but insects had time. We had perhaps four million years. They had at least 400 million.[201]

The Drug That Came from Pwnt

It happened one day around 1370 B.C., when Egypt was running a huge empire, reaching all the way through Syria to the Euphrates and beyond.

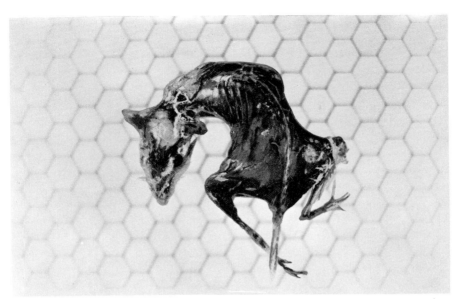

3.29 Mummy of a mouse found in a hive. The bees had covered it with antiseptic bee-glue (propolis), and it had dried out without obnoxious decay. The mummification is mainly due to drying, but the propolis surely helps.

Amenophis IV received a letter from Palestine. It came from Milkili, one of his lieutenants.[202]

Political affairs were a nuisance to Amenophis. He was a peculiar character, all wound up in a religious world of his own—the world of Aton, the Disc of the Sun. So great was his passion that, braving an irate clergy, he had the name of the ancient god Amun hammered off all the monuments he could reach. Eventually, to make the break more definitive, he stormed out with Nefertiti and all his court and founded a new capital of his own, Akhetaton (Fig. 3.30).

So Milkili's letter did not go to Thebes, but to the plateau that is now El Amarna. It was written in cuneiform characters on a clay tablet; deciphered by the palace cuneiformist, it must have read then as we can now read it among the "El Amarna Letters":[203]

> To the King, my Lord,
> my Gods [sic], my Sun,
> thus saith Milkili, thy servant,
> the dust of thy feet.
> At the feet of my King, my Lord
> my Gods, my Sun
> 7 times and 7 I fall.
> I have heard what the King, my Lord,
> has written to me.
> And let the King, my Lord,
> send troops
> to his servants, and
> let the King, my Lord,
> send myrrh
> for medicine.

121

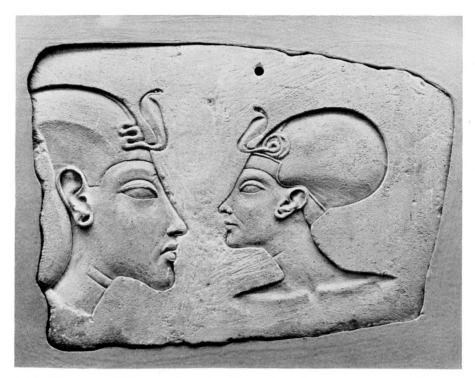

3.30 Akhenaton (?) (Amenophis IV) and his wife Nefertiti, c. 1370 B.C. Perhaps, when they posed for this portrait, they were perfumed with the oil of myrrh they had received as a wedding gift.

Milkili was no little lamb. In the past, the Pharaoh had received serious complaints about him; but since then they had made peace.[204] Now Milkili was sending three terse messages: "I have taken notice of your orders. Please send soldiers. Please send myrrh."

Asking for myrrh as a personal gift was not exactly modest. Myrrh, like frankincense and all the aromatic resins, was not a product of Egypt.[205] The Pharaoh himself had to buy his supplies from southern Arabia, from Abyssinia, and from what he called the land of Pwnt, probably the Somali coast. Perhaps Amenophis IV remembered the two stone boxes of myrrh that he himself had received as a gift from Tushratta, king of Mitanni, at the time of his wedding with Nefertiti: one had contained myrrh, the other oil of myrrh.[206] Perhaps another memory flashed through his mind: the old myrrh trees back in Thebes. Some one hundred years earlier one of his royal ancestors, the energetic Queen Hatshepswt, tired of depending on imported myrrh, had sent an expedition of five ships to the Land of Pwnt. They had returned triumphant, loaded with myrrh, dogs, baboons, and thirty-one myrrh trees (Fig. 3.31). The trees had been planted at Thebes and were supposed to have flourished thereafter. But even if they still existed, Amenophis would have had nothing to do with Thebes, let alone with trees that had been planted in the very garden of Amun,[207] so his only choice, to satisfy Milkili's request, would have been to draw on the palace supplies, being sure to leave enough reserves to embalm—Aton forbid—a royal mummy.

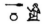

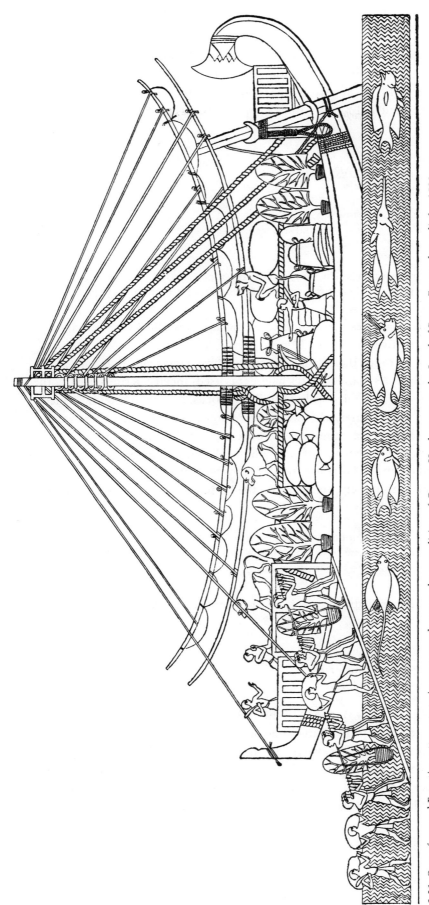

3.31 One of several Egyptian attempts to import myrrh trees: the expedition of Queen Hatshepswt to the Land of Pwnt. From a bas-relief, c.1500 B.C.

But what did Milkili have in mind? What ill did he plan to heal with "myrrh as medicine"—maybe some intestinal trouble? We will have to look at the sources. Myrrh appears in dozens of Egyptian prescriptions. It is unusually well identified, as Egyptian drugs go, under the name of *antyw*:[208]

a

tyw*

n   (det. "pot")

            plural strokes

 *Note that this is [bird] for *tyw*, not [bird] for *a*. The scribes must have had some training as birdwatchers, for there were at least fifty-four bird hieroglyphs.

The other major resin, used mostly as incense, was called *sntr*, perhaps the resin of the turpentine tree.[209]

 Now through the entire lot of the medical papyri, myrrh is applied externally in 63 of the 66 cases where it is used; incense resin is used in the same general way. Obviously Milkili was not asking for an internal remedy. Since he was a soldier, what we need to know next is whether there were wound salves based on resins. There are none in the great Smith papyrus, which must have been written by a honey-lover; but there are many plasters with myrrh in the Ebers papyrus, which was about 150 years old in the days of Amenophis (recent literature, on the Egyptian time scale). Here is one myrrh salve:[210]

> What is done for a wound in the neck:
> Myrrh, one part. Flour of the *djbt*-plant [*no amount given*].
> Work into a mass, bind on.

I would actually prefer this other salve for burns, also prepared with a resin:[211]

> *Sntr*-resin, one part.
> Honey, one part.
> Anoint with it.

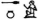

 Well, we know from Milkili himself that he did not need myrrh for offerings—or because he liked the smell of it. He wanted soldiers, and myrrh for medicine. I submit that everybody knew, at the time, that myrrh was good for wounds. So, going back to his letter, I read between the lines: "Amenophis— whatever people have been telling you about me, remember I am here to be skewered for your pleasure."

Magic As an Antibiotic

Magic, like penicillin, is directed against the cause of disease. The choice between drugs and magic depends on the current set of causes. In ancient Egypt, where evil forces caused a lot of trouble, magic was a perfectly logical therapy; an accepted science, with Isis as patroness. There was no clearcut distinction between so-called rational medicine and magic: drugs and incantations were administered in all possible combinations,[212] and by the same or by different practitioners.[213] Magic was especially indicated against the so-called "hidden diseases," or internal ones, as we now say; but oddly enough, it was used also for wounds.

What is a wound, anyway? To our way of thinking it is something out in the open, which should require nothing but ordinary, down-to-earth consideration. But read this extraordinary passage of the Smith papyrus, probably the world's oldest discussion of causes.[214] The text describes "a man having a smash of his skull, under the skin of his head . . . while his eye is askew because of it, on the side of him having that injury . . . Thou shouldst account him one whom something entering from outside has smitten . . . An ailment not to be treated." The Commentator explains: "As for: 'Something entering from outside,' it means the breath of an outside god or death; not the intrusion of something which his flesh engenders." He is obviously distinguishing between internal and external causes.

If even a wound implies "the breath of an outside god," treatment by magic is clearly indicated. It was used, for instance, in spells to accompany the acts of bandaging and of removing a dressing. Of the following examples,[215] the first occurs at the opening of the Ebers papyrus. As to the second, to be recited upon the removal of a bandage—think of the anxiety that this operation always induces; the soothing litany has real clinical merit. For burn wounds there is an oft-quoted, rather picturesque charm that has come down in several variants. It is a dialog between a messenger and the goddess Isis.[216]

To understand these incantations, it helps to know that Isis, the magician-goddess, had a good brother, Osiris, and a bad one, Seth. Seth killed Osiris and ripped him apart. Isis patiently reassembled him, lay over his body, and succeeded in conceiving Horus. Then she resuscitated her brother-husband. Every Egyptian hoped that after death he too might be as lucky as Osiris: extending this idea, every sick person was also Osiris and could be cured by Isis.[217] Then Seth, in another fit of dismembering rage, tore out the eyes of Horus and ripped them apart. It was Thoth, the ibis-god, who put them together again.

Incantations prevailed when the clinical situation was somber. For snake and scorpion bites, for instance, there were magic formulas but essentially nothing in the way of local treatment.[218]

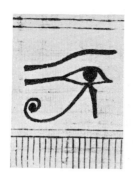

BEGINNING OF THE RECITAL
FOR APPLYING A REMEDY
ON ANY PART OF THE BODY
OF A MAN

I have come from Iwnw [Heliopolis]
with the Great Ones of the Great House
the Lords of Protection
the Rulers of Eternity

And yet I have come from Sais
with the Mother of the Gods
—I am in their safekeeping—

I know charms that the Almighty wrought
to chase away the spell of a God,
of a Goddess,
of a dead man,
of a dead woman . . . (continue at will)
that are in this mine head
in this mine nape
in these mine shoulders
in this mine flesh
in these mine limbs
to punish the Accuser, the Master of Those
who allow decay to seep
into this mine flesh
numbness
into these mine limbs
as Something entering
into this mine flesh
into this mine head
into these mine shoulders
into this mine body
into these mine limbs

I belong to Ra. Thus spoketh he:
"It is I who shall guard the sick man from his enemies.
"His guide shall be Thoth [*main patron of the physicians*]
who lets writing speak
who creates the Books
who passes on useful knowledge
to Those who Know, the Physicians
his followers,
"that they may deliver from disease
the sick man of whom a God wishes
that the physician may keep him alive"

I am one of those of whom a God wishes
that he may keep me alive

Spoken While Applying Remedies
to Any Sick Part
of the Body of a Man

REALLY OUTSTANDING,
MILLIONS OF TIMES

Loosened is he
who is loosened by Isis
Loosened was Horus by Isis
of the evil he felt
   when his brother Seth
   killed his father Osiris
O Isis, great in sorcery,
   mayest thou loosen me
   mayest thou deliver me
     from everything evil
       and vicious
       and **red** [*perhaps the swnw, while unwinding*
               the bandage, hoped the skin beneath
               would not turn out bloody and
               inflamed]
   from the spell of a God
   from the spell of a Goddess
     of a dead man
     of a dead woman
     of a fiendish man
     of a fiendish woman
     who will be fiendish within me
  the like of thine loosening
  the like of thine delivering
   thine son Horus
for I stepped into fire
 I stepped out of water
 I shall not be caught
   in this day's trap

      I spoke as if I were yet a child still small

Speak, Ra, of your belly
Mourn, Osiris, over that which seeped out of your body
         [*possibly the decaying corpse of Osiris*[219]]
Behold thou hast saved me
  from all things evil
    and vicious
    and **red**
  from the spell of a God,
  from the spell of a Goddess,
    of a dead man,
    of a dead woman . . . (continue at will)

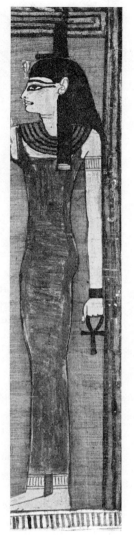

Isis

REALLY OUTSTANDING,
MILLIONS OF TIMES

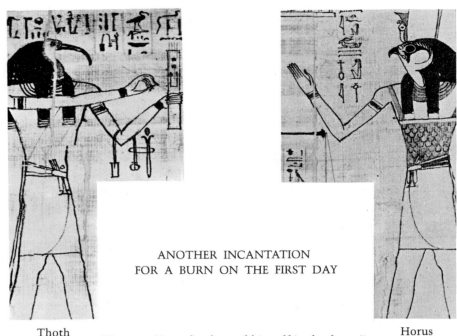

ANOTHER INCANTATION
FOR A BURN ON THE FIRST DAY

Thoth   Horus

"Your son Horus has burned himself in the desert"
"Is water here?"
"There is no water here"
"Water is in my mouth, a Nile is between my thighs,
    I have come to put out the fire.
        Flow out, burn!"

Recite [*this charm*]
over the Milk of a Woman
    who Gave Birth
    to a Male Child

Gum; hair of a ram; place onto the burn.

And here is a spell "against blood" (bleeding? redness?), with a perfectly
Egyptian ending:[220]

A CHARM TO DISPEL BLOOD

Retreat, creature of Horus!
Retreat, creature of Seth!
Dispelled be the blood that cometh by Wnw [*a city*]
Dispelled by the red blood that cometh by *wnw* [= *"by the hour"*]
You know not the dam; retreat before Thoth!

This Charm will be Recited over a Red Pearl of Cornelian
Placed in the Anus of the Man or Woman.

THIS IS TO DISPEL THE BLOOD.

Psychotherapy should help, no matter at which end it is applied.

Ukhedu—Not So Wrong

I have yet to see a psychiatric study about the Egyptian concern with the anus. One of the seven medical papyri, and 81 of the 900 prescriptions, refer only to the anus.[221] The Egyptians soothed it, refreshed it, smoked it,[222] and somehow even kept it from twisting and slipping.[223] Medically speaking, all this attention is difficult to justify; but philosophically the Egyptians had a point, because they apparently took the anus as the center and stronghold of decay.

Worry about decay must have slowly grown to a national concern. It governed daily life even in the time of Herodotos: "For three consecutive days in every month they purge themselves, pursuing after health by means of emetics and drenches; for they think it is from the food they eat that all sicknesses come to men."[224]

An explicit statement of the basic theory does not exist; but evidence from many sources, pieced together, suggests this reasoning: *decay is typical of death, disease, and wounds; decay also occurs inside the intestine; so this internal decay must be a source of disease.*

To live by this theory must have been uncomfortable indeed. Condemned to walk around all day with an internal load of deadly material, the Egyptians took whatever measures they could; and in so doing, they became all-time experts on enemas. Their enormous pharmacopoeia (close to 700 items) may have been almost worthless by modern standards, but if there was one effect it could definitely induce, that was probably diarrhea.[225]

The most frightening aspect of the feces was that they contained a very pernicious thing called *ukhedu*. Ukhedu lay there dormant, but might arise and settle anywhere else in the body.[226] The word *ukhedu* (actually *wḥdw*) cannot be translated, but it looks like this:

Sometimes it is shortened to the "rot" determinative only ⟨img⟩ as the rotten stuff par excellence.[227] The ukhedu was either male or female, caused disease and pain, and could be killed. It could work its way into the vessels and travel around, setting up disease (Plate 3.8). In essence, what bacteria can do, it could do.

And of course, ukhedu could turn up in a wound: "Another remedy to heal a wound in which the ukhedu have arisen. . ."[228]

The Egyptians' fear of ukhedu was justified in view of their amazing concept of the vascular system. Although the vessels were known to have their main center in the heart, they were thought to have a second rallying point around the anus.[229] Hence, my scheme of the Egyptian vascular system had to be drawn, uniquely, as viewed from the rear (Plate 3.8).

The vessels, incidentally, were called *mt*, plural *mtw* (*metw*):

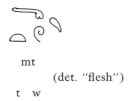

mt

(det. "flesh")

t w

The word is very ancient and indefinite. Sometimes it stands for hollow vessels; sometimes for tendons or "cords," and should perhaps be rendered as "sinews." Perhaps the spelling by means of the penis (also *mt*) helped to convey the multiple notion of a hollow tube as well as a cord;[230] but the Coptic *mut* preserved only the connotation of "solid strand, muscle." The metw contained blood, air, urine, tears, feces, depending on where they went. They seemed to have "mouths," so that they could take up drugs and disgorge disease under a magic spell. The heart spoke through them, and they could become dumb and die. They were subject to a goodly number of diseases[231] not well translatable: they could move, jump, tremble, become stiff or stretched; with given remedies they could be strengthened, soothed, cooled, or softened.[232]

"There are 12 metw," writes the scribe of the Ebers papyrus, then promptly gives a list of 22, just after having given another list of 50. Four or more led directly to the anus, into which they probably opened with little mouths,[233] but the six vessels going to the lower limbs passed so dangerously near the anus that they were exposed to becoming "flooded with excrements," which could rise even to the heart.

This was lowering the blood vessels to the status of sewers. The two lists of blood vessels that have come down to us are presented from exactly this angle. Instead of promising a beautiful vascular tree, the introductory sentence of each list suggests the map of a sewer system full of ukhedu:

[*Ebers papyrus*] Beginning of the book of the wandering of the ukhedu in every part of the man's body, as found in writings under the feet of Anubis . . .[234]

[*Berlin papyrus*] Beginning of the collected writings about the wandering of the ukhedu, found in old writings in a case with books under the feet of Anubis . . .[235]

Physicians reading these lines will have noticed that they are still fighting ukhedu, under different names: *Escherichia coli*, endotoxin, endogenous septicemia . . .

Embalmers Against Bacteria

When medicine could no longer help and the patient died, he had to face decay all over again, this time with the even greater danger of getting out of shape for the afterlife. Surely the Egyptians had noticed that if the body was buried in sand, decay was held down to a minimum. By this simple method people could be preserved (jackals and hyenas permitting) almost as well as papyri, simply by being dried up very fast. But that was not enough; religious pressure created a new art, embalming. This I will discuss in some detail, for I see it as a glorified struggle against bacteria; and in this sense, its technical aspects are of concern also to the living.[236]

Embalmers have two main enemies: the digestive power of bacteria (putrefaction) and to a lesser extent the digestive power of the tissues themselves (autolysis). Aside from freezing, both processes can be stopped either by removing the water, essential to the digestive action, or by stopping the action itself. The latter aim can be achieved rather brutally by soaking the tissues in a solution known as a fixative, which destroys all life, including bacteria, and leaves the tissues as a cemetery of wrecked molecules. This is the technique of modern undertakers. It turns the body into a firm lump that will discourage bacteria and molds for weeks and months; sealed aseptically in an airtight box, it might well defy centuries.

What fixatives were available to the Egyptian embalmers? Our modern list, with names such as potassium bichromate, formalin, picric acid, and mercuric chloride, sounds wholly irrelevant. One chemical available in large quantities was alum.[237] With one dubious exception, it seems that it was never used.[238] However, thinking of its virtues in tanning leather, I tried to use a saturated solution as a fixative. The result was disastrous: the tissues simply fell apart. Alcohol should work, but its concentration in wine, let alone beer, is too low. The only chemical possibility I see is vinegar. Owing to its 4–5 percent content of acetic acid, it is a good fixative and food preservative; and as such, it was certainly known to the Chinese as well as to the Romans.[239] But vinegar was never mentioned in the context of embalming. Moreover, the technique of fixing the body like a cabbage preserve would have been psychologically hard for the embalmer to recommend (I am now thinking of the embalmer's public relations) if the purpose was to keep the body fit for another life.

This is not loose talk: the embalmers also rejected two other techniques and far more obvious ones, drying and salting. Fish curing certainly antedates mummification (Fig. 3.32).[240] Yet here, too, I can see that nobody would like to step into a new life pickled like a sardine, any more than tanned like a shoe. I take it for granted that the embalmers ruled out salting without a second thought, as an insult to the deceased (and maybe also hard to sell among the living). This was perhaps in the mind of that Mesopotamian king who, after his archenemy had been slain, ordered that his body be brought to him "in salt."[241]

So, whatever else the embalmers did, they certainly used no salt solution and probably no fixing bath at all. Not much is left. The next best way to reach deeply into the tissues and stop decay would have been drying, either in the sun (not too practical), with fire (very expensive in Egypt), or just in sand, as in the ancient "natural" process. There is not the slightest evidence for any of these methods.[242] What the embalmers actually did was a bizarre compromise between drying and chemical fixing: they probably buried the body under lumps of their beloved, all-purpose natural soda: natron.

Although natron occurs in other parts of the world, Egypt gave it fame. It

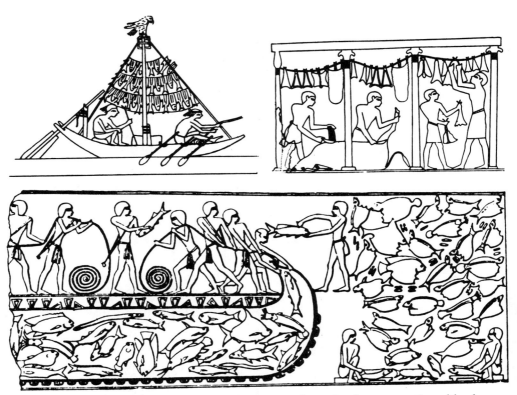

3.32 Man's first organized, successful fight against bacteria: the preservation of food by drying and salting. Both techniques are older than embalming. *Top left:* gutted fish hung to dry from a mast (c.1900 B.C.). *Top right:* meat hung up to dry (Thebes, c.1900 B.C.). *Bottom:* netting and cleaning sea-fish, whose flattened-out carcasses suggest drying (Saqqara, c.2500 B.C.).

is another gift of the Nile. River water seeps into the ground, especially during the floods, and works its way to distant flats, where it emerges to form shallow lakes, often below sea level. As the lakes evaporate, a yellowish or reddish crust forms on the shore and on the bottom: this is natron, long recognized as a national treasure, to the point that it eventually became a government monopoly. It is now found in Egypt in three places, including Wadi Natrun.

Its name, *ntry,* could be written with the simple ideogram ⌇ which combines the symbol of divinity ⌐ (a cloth wound around a pole) with ♉ "a bag of linen." It had lofty associations:

ntr (det. "god")   ideogram: t (det.
                                    ntr r "theoretical
                                          y concept")

god   *natron*   *divine*

Chemically, natron is a mixture of sodium carbonate and bicarbonate—its main components—with sodium sulphate and common salt as impurities, the latter in proportions varying from 0.5 to 50 percent.[243] One obvious difference with salt is that natron acts as a mild detergent, because when mixed with fats, it forms sodium soaps:[244]

Animal fat   Natron
(triglyceride)   (carbonate)   Water

$$2 \begin{array}{l} CH_2OOC(CH_2)_nCH_3 \\ CHOOC(CH_2)_nCH_3 \\ CH_2OOC(CH_2)_nCH_3 \end{array} \;+\; 3\,Na_2CO_3 \;+\; 3\,H_2O \longrightarrow$$

$$\longrightarrow 6\,NaOOC(CH_2)_nCH_3 \;+\; 3\,CO_2 \;+\; 2\begin{array}{l} CH_2OH \\ CHOH \\ CH_2OH \end{array}$$

Soap   Carbon   Glycerol
     Dioxide

Natron had a great many uses: prominently as a "soul detergent" for purifying the mouth before worship and for making incense, which was called s-nṯr:

n   (det. "grain")
ntr sn   ṯ
r   plural strokes

It was also used for making glass and glaze, for cooking, for compounding medicines, and for bleaching linen.[245]

Because of a mistaken translation from the Greek of Herodotos, it was once thought that the embalmers plunged the body in a solution of natron, like a fish in brine. This would have required large tanks or pots, and none of the kind were found.[246] The Greek verb was actually ταριχεύειν, "pickling," which does not imply the use of a solution.[247] It is now almost certain, thanks to chemical studies and actual trials, that the Egyptians used natron in bulk, which is a much easier process, not so messy—and far less effective. If this is true, it is possible to visualize what was going on in the "beautiful house"[248] (the pious name for the morticians' workshop) at the height of the embalming art: the embalmers removed most viscera, replaced them with

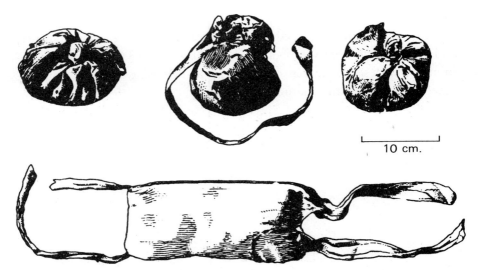

3.33 Small bags of solid natron from the mummy of Tutankhamun: the ancestors of mothballs.

lumps of natron either loose or in little packages, then covered the whole body for forty days with more natron (Fig. 3.33). In a well-aerated place, and perhaps in the sun, this combined—rather inefficiently—drying with chemical fixing. The natron surely made life unbearable to the bacteria and stopped decay at the very surface of the body, then diffused inward (together with its salt content, which could be high) to the depth of a few millimeters. But this diffusing process was very slow, and in the meantime, bacteria and insects could find safe corners to go on with their job. The evidence is still there to behold—beetles and maggots tucked away beneath yards and yards of wrappings.[249]

In essence, this was a mothballing technique with very weak mothballs. The reasons that made the embalmers prefer natron over salt were probably cultural, but to some extent chemistry too was on their side. Mothballing in natron was better than nothing. Dr. Lucas, the late Honorary Consultant Chemist to the Department of Antiquities, Egypt, gave it a try using pigeons—plucked, eviscerated, and then buried under lumps of dry salt or natron. After forty days he retrieved them hard and dry, "much emaciated," but essentially mummified. They were also in the company of many little insects, especially after being buried in natron; but both sets of pigeons were "practically free from disagreeable smell, of which there had been very little during the forty days of burial."[250] And both sets of animals were chemically salted, for the natron had been giving up its sodium chloride: so that the Egyptians were salting their mummies anyway.[251]

Dr. Lucas also tried a 3 percent natron bath, because in one case at least the embalmers had used it to preserve the organs of Queen Hetepheres.[252] After forty days the pigeon was bleached white, but "plump and in good condition, with the skin intact." It was laid out to dry and gave off a slight smell of putrefaction for some weeks. But another pigeon left in a 3 percent salt solution "was no longer recognizable as such." Thus, salt may be cheaper, but natron works in weaker concentrations.

134

To sum it all up, the embalmers used in the solid state a substance that would work fairly well if dissolved. The overall result needed a lot of retouching.

After the natron, there was another month of work: now was the time for treating with resins and gum resins, especially frankincense and myrrh, pure or mixed with fats and oils. Resin and pitch were sometimes melted over fire and poured on very hot, over the body, over the finished mummy, or even over the coffin itself. All this was very expensive, because none of these products was native to Egypt, not even the common juniper berries or the very important "cedar oil" of Herodotos, which is probably juniper oil;[253] both of these came from western Asia. In fact, you will recognize here Mesopotamia's favorite drug, burashu (juniper). And if it is true that cassia and cinnamon were also used on mummies,[254] the embalmers were importing their commodities from as far as China.[255]

A cheaper scent was onion. Onions were used freely—inside the body, between bandages, even over the eyes and in the ears.[256] Perhaps it was their name that counted, for the word hedjw, "onion,"[257] punned with hedjet, "damage [to the evil forces]."[258] Whatever the reason, their use must have had something to do with their smell. Now there is something about onion smell that needs a closer look. It has been claimed that onion paste emits vapors that are injurious to protozoa and to bacteria as well, and that it prevents the infection of wounds.[259] Antibacterial activity has been found in onion extracts.[260] A relative of the onion (*Allium cepa*), garlic (*Allium sativum*), has done even better: it has yielded an antibacterial substance that has about 1 percent of the activity of penicillin, but is also effective against Gram-negative bacteria, which are practically unaffected by penicillin.[261] In 1971, in the search for new pesticides as substitutes for DDT, garlic extracts were tested; they proved to be effective against mosquito larvae in concentrations as low as five parts per million.[262]

Two onions in the pelvis could at best discourage only a few bugs for a few hours. However, this episode anticipates a theme that will recur again and again: in his primordial struggle against bacteria, man had a trusty ally in his sniff.

Back to the embalmer. In the great days of the art, the finishing touches included packing handfuls of sand, mud, or linen pads under the skin to fill it out,[263] adding artificial eyes and nails, as well as other aesthetic improvements. The whole procedure was a major financial investment. There were  in fact, noted Herodotos, three types of service at increasing cost: the lowest-priced operation was rinsing out the intestines by way of the anus (the embalmers knew where the ukhedu was); next came the treatment of the body with natron; and last, the full treatment just described.

The achievements of the embalmers have been either extolled to legendary heights or debunked as poor craftsmanship. There is truth in both extremes, for the embalmer's method was a compromise, and its result was precarious. Some of the mummies, when exposed, gave off such a horrendous stench that they had to be destroyed without further ado.[264] A few others, face eternal sleep with a certain degree of humanity (Fig. 3.34). The head of

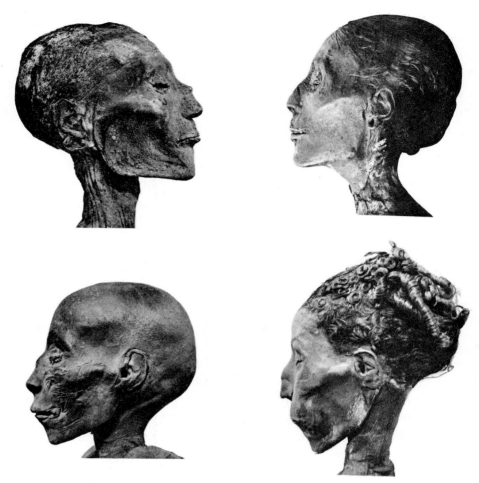

3.34 Four of the best royal profiles: Ramses V (top left), Thutmosis IV (top right), Thutmosis I (lower left), and an unknown lady. They were embalmed between 1550 and 1100 B.C.

Seti I is by far the masterpiece (Fig. 3.35). There is no reason to believe—Anubis forgive me—that the Egyptian embalmers had any particular secret. However, in view of the fact that they were trying to achieve "fixation" without any fixatives, they did very well. Placed in their position, a modern undertaker would consider the job impossible.

Psychologically, the embalmers proved to be extremely subtle in devising a preservation technique that was entirely their own, with no possible overtones of pickling. Technically, I believe that their major asset was the generous use of resins. Even if not fixed, a particle of tissue embedded in resin should be preserved forever, like the prehistoric insects embedded in amber. Add to this that resins, at the time, had a long tradition as agents of purification and as a link with the heavens. Lumps of resin were found buried in predynastic tombs, long before the practice of mummification, perhaps for use as incense; and even later, when 50 kg of resin were poured over a sarcophagus,[265] the purpose was not to preserve the marble. In any event, whether it was a matter of religion, magic, cosmetics, odor, or all these combined, resins

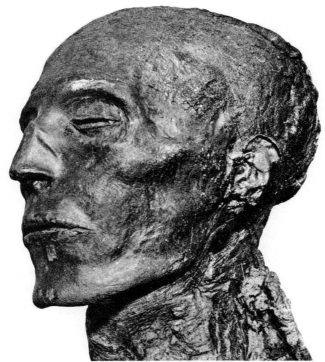

3.35 Seti I—perhaps the summit of the embalmer's art, c.1300 B.C. The body, much damaged by tomb robbers, is covered with resin-impregnated linen, now of stony hardness.

were a perfect choice as embalming material, and possibly the only one under the circumstances. They are wonderfully fitted to defy millennia. In his description of the "Royal Mummies," one of which I quoted above for its dreadful smell, G. E. Smith mentioned twice a "strongly aromatic odor" from powdered wood.[266] One such odor dated from the Seventeenth Dynasty, about 3500 years ago. And the body of Meneptah, son of Ramses II (Nineteenth Dynasty), was covered with very fine linen impregnated with a bright yellow, resinlike material, which when dissolved in alcohol, developed a pleasant odor "like Friar's balsam."[267] This odor came from the time of the Exodus, about 1230 B.C.[268]

But even resins could not operate miracles. Under the resin not much of the mummy is left, especially of the limbs, since the embalmers concentrated their efforts on the face. Consider the legs of Ramses II. They were encrusted  with a resinous mass 6 mm thick; beneath it, the limbs "seemed to consist merely of a layer of skin closely clinging to the bone."[269] And the thigh muscles of Tutankhamun, for all of the flamboyant looks of the mummy as seen from outside, were a couple of millimeters thick.[270] In this respect, it is ironic that all the labor of embalming—seventy days of it—led to no consistent improvement over the work of nature, for some of the best preserved bodies are from predynastic times and had been simply buried in dry soil.[271] So effective was this natural process that in one child, who died around 3500–4000 B.C., the intestine preserved the remains of the last

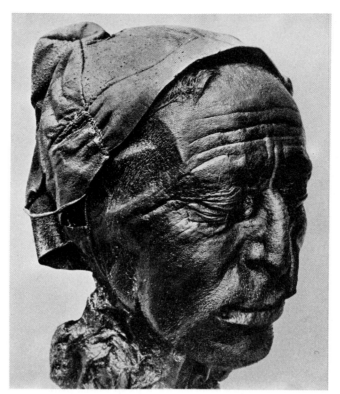

3.36 Nature alone accomplished this feat of embalming: a miserable Dane was strangled to death and thrown into a peat bog about two thousand years ago, where the tannic acid turned his skin into leather—perhaps the same method that he had used to make his leather cap.

medicine: a skinned mouse, young, well chewed, and mixed with vegetables.[272] It seems that mice were admired for their prodigious vitality: the swarms that appeared after each flood were thought to form spontaneously out of the mud, so that swallowing a mouse was something like taking a pill of life.[273]

Nature alone has produced mummies even more spectacular than these dried-up bodies. In the turf bogs of northwestern Europe it is not rare to discover bodies of human beings who fell in, or were thrown in, 500 to 3000 years ago.[274] Some are so well preserved that fingerprinting is possible (Fig. 3.36). In this case nature's secret is a chemical: the flesh is literally tanned, that is, toughened, by the same principle that turns fresh hides and skins into leather. Many substances can accomplish this, but the best natural agent is tannic acid, obtained since time immemorial from oak galls, oak bark, and other plant products.[275] It is odd that the tanning principle, so ancient and so well-known, was never put to use for the preservation of bodies. Perhaps, once again, the obstacle was psychological: shoe technology and religion do not mix.

Too much has been said about lessons that medicine may have learned through embalming.[276] The points of contact are more theoretical than real. It has been noticed, for example, that in the *Book of the Dead* "treating" and "embalming" are sometimes expressed with the same word, *srwkh*:[277]

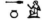

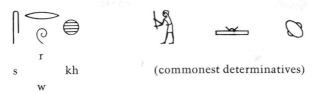

r

s   kh   (commonest determinatives)

w

This calls for two comments. First, four thousand years from now, someone may notice that in the backward 1900s people spoke about curing patients as well as sausages. Second, Egyptians actually had two different words: *srwkh*, "to treat," and *sdwkh*, "to embalm." However, the ⌐ *r* and the ⌐ *d*, in their cursive, hieratic form, are very similar; and the scribes who copied and recopied the *Book of the Dead*—which was to be buried with the corpse—did not pay much attention to such details.[278]

Certainly the bandages that were prepared for embalmers could be used on live people, and sometimes they were.[279] The major antidecay drugs, especially natron and the resins, were the same, but there was one major exception. Honey, the standard antiseptic of the Smith papyrus, was not currently used in Egyptian embalming.[280] If it is true that the body of Alexander the Great was carried to Egypt in honey, this embalming was done in Babylon.

Another instance of embalming in honey occurred in the Near East when a Hasmonean ruler of Judea was poisoned, and "his dead body also lay, for a good while, embalmed in honey, till Antony afterwards sent it to Judea, and caused him to be buried in royal sepulchre."[281] To test the feasibility of embalming in honey, we ran a few experiments using rat and mouse tissues. It seems that very small pieces might be preserved almost indefinitely. But with larger pieces, deep down where the honey cannot reach, putrefaction is rampant, gas develops, and the result is a terrible waste of work, especially for the bees. They must have buried that Hasmonean in a hurry.

I see no evidence that the embalmer's crude handling of organs advanced the knowledge of anatomy any more than did the butcher's. In the long range, however, his approach probably helped medicine indirectly. It may have accustomed the Greeks to the notion that the body can be manipulated after death, and thus helped to establish the practice of human dissection in Greco-Egyptian Alexandria.

After the Swnw

Twice as long as Christianity, almost: this is how long the swnw's civilization lasted. Its ways and its medicine had time to soak into Western life to an extent difficult to fathom; but here again words help. *Na*, our symbol for sodium, is a living fossil of *natron*, the maker of mummies; just as Nefertiti's eye shadow, *msdmt*, slid over into our *Sb* for antimony; and *gum* is straight from *ḳmyt* through the Greek *kómmi*. Tradition derives *ammonia* from the stench of camel urine around the temple of Amun.[282] One of the many theories on the origin of the word *chemistry* holds that it comes from *Kmt*, the original name of Egypt (in Coptic *Chemi*):[283]

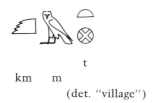

km m
t
(det. "village")

And the pharaoh is embedded for good in our *paper*. The word for pharaoh
(which came down through the Hebrew) was *pr-aa* ⟷ literally "the Great
House"; and *pa-pr-aa* meant "that of the pharaoh": papyrus was indeed a
royal monopoly.[284]

Those "beaten" sheets of papyrus probably influenced the history of
medicine more than any ancient drug. The genius required to create them is
beyond belief. It is a sobering exercise to take a stem of papyrus (not from
Egypt, however, where it is extinct except in the far south) and try to make a
sheet from it following Pliny's instructions. It does not even look as if it
should work. Yet the sheets represented only one use of the plant. I like to
think what a native Egyptian might have been able to accomplish if
abandoned on an island overgrown with papyrus. He could have used some
parts of the plant for food, while using others to equip himself with clothes
and sandals. He could have built a whole ship, with sails and ropes, and even
caulked it. He could have loaded it with food and fuel in baskets, plus articles
for sale—mats, wicks, sieves—and he could have sailed away while making
paper to write up his story.[285]

As regards the treatment of wounds, besides a vast number of uninterp-
retable or unwholesome plasters, the swnw dreamed up two great salves,
possibly the best of antiquity and certainly the ones that I would choose:
honey with grease, and honey with aromatic resins. He produced some
excellent anatomoclinical correlations; probably the first tapes and sutures;
the beginnings of hemostasis by the cautery; the beginnings of antisepsis with
copper salts, in the form of green eye shadow (what was there about Egyptian
eyes that made them so influential? ?);[286] and a theory about infection
and contaminated blood that was bound to change form but never died. The
concept of bad blood (and getting rid of it) later became the main excuse for
venesection, and contributed to wasting more innocent blood than many
wars have spilled.

If fame is a measure of success, we can only congratulate the swnw. In
the Mediterranean world his art was unsurpassed, until it was absorbed and
replaced by Greek medicine. We shall bid him farewell in his own words—as
live Egyptians hailed the dead:[287]

> May his *metw* flourish . . .
> May his *metw* be sound . . .
> May his *metw* be excellent . . .
> May his *metw* be comfortable . . .

Ἰατρός

4   The Iatrós

Athens, 400 B.C. Two physicians are discussing their patients, in a language now listed as dead. Here are some of their professional terms: "arthritis . . . epiphysis . . . rheuma . . . crisis . . . asthma . . . tetanos . . . anthrax . . . opisthotonos . . . mesocolon . . . epiploon . . . dysenteria . . . sepsis . . . ataxia . . . stranguria . . . pleuritis . . . hypochondria . . ."[1]

Every one of these words is essential in today's medical jargon. Suddenly, we feel among modern men.

Greek Medicine: The Sources

There is a good reason for lifting the curtain so abruptly on Athens of the golden age: the beginnings of Greek medicine, which should fill a library, are mostly blank pages. Surely the medical terms used in 400 B.C., the time of Hippocrates (460–380 B.C.), were not an instant product. Famous physicians had already come and gone,[2] and if Xenophon was accurate in reporting the words of his master, Socrates, medical treatises made "a large collection."[3] But alas, not one of these ancient books has survived; and after the Hippocratic works there is another blank of four centuries.[4] What is left of the beginnings adds up to fragments, quotations, pots and shards, and a few stones.

And poetry, from about the ninth century B.C.: the oldest witness of Greek medicine is Homer.

Ἰατρός

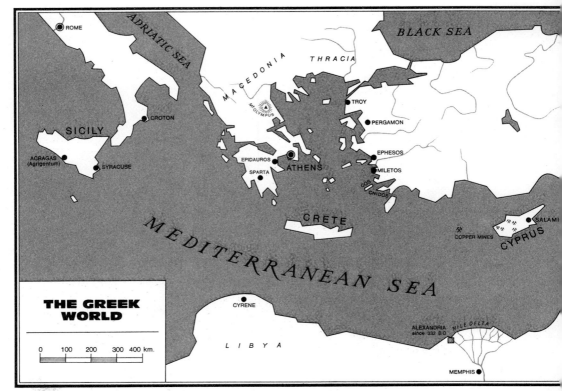

4.1 The Greek world: from Asia Minor to Sicily.

Wounds in Verse

There are 147 wounds in the *Iliad*—31 to the head, all lethal. The overall mortality rate was 77.6 percent.[5] The single nicety about this bloodshed, besides the poetry, is that for the first time in history one hears of the wounded being carried off the battlefield and tended in barracks, *klisíai,* or in the nearby ships.[6]

Wound care itself was just above rock bottom. Once, a iatrós was wounded: he was Machaon, the very son of Asklepios. The first attentions that he received in the *klisía* were a seat, lots of storytelling, and a cup of Pramnian wine sprinkled with grated goat cheese and barley meal, served by a beautiful woman.[7] Plato finds that even this treatment was too much—not the woman, but the cheese and the barley, which, he says, are surely inflammatory.[8] Later, Machaon's wound was washed with warm water by the same woman;[9] others, less fortunate, had this service performed by fellow warriors.[10] Nothing was done to stop the bleeding, which may account for the high mortality. In fact, bleeding must have been considered hopeless, for the one and only type of hemostasis mentioned in Homer is an *epaoidé,* which means that somebody sang a song or recited a charm over the wound.[11] Whether it worked or not, the poet does not say:

> Then . . . the wound of noble, god-like Odysseus
> They bound up skillfully, and checked the black blood
> With a charm.

'Ιατρός

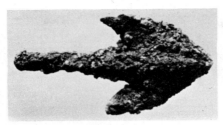

4.2 Bronze arrowhead with two barbs from Homeric Troy. It was lying in the rubble, in the middle of a street. Slightly enlarged.

Arrowheads were made of iron[12] or bronze. Some were *tricuspids*, "with three barbs";[13] but most had two, thin enough to break off if pulled back through a leather belt.[14] One of these, just one, was actually found in the ruins of Troy VII-a, the Homeric level (Fig. 4.2). Arrowhead barbs have always been a curse of battlefield surgery. For the wounded at Troy there was no way around the problem except by enlarging the wound with a knife[15] or possibly by pushing the arrowhead through.[16] In later Greece, around 400 B.C., Diokles of Karystos invented a gadget that eased out the arrowheads very neatly (Figs. 9.14–9.15).

Drugs were also applied to the wound. They came only from plants, apparently raw, the more complex Egyptian and Akkadian poultices being either ignored or forgotten. The only detail available is that the wound of Eurypylos was sprinkled with "bitter root," possibly onion.[17] Its purpose was to cool and dry the wound.[18] Both of these concepts reappear in the Hippocratic books, where it is explained that wounds should be kept warm, unless inflamed, and dry, because the dry state is the natural one.[19] Perhaps there is another message, now lost, in the bitterness, for Galen notes that the bitter taste is typical of counterpoisons.[20] Even in a medical classic of ancient India it is said that "The Bitter taste is so disagreeable as to produce disgust for itself, but . . . it destroys the action of poisons."[21] I take this to be a variation on the universal theme that a good medicine must be unpleasant.

Binding is mentioned only twice in Homer, so it is possible that some of the braves walked or lay about with their sores exposed rather than dressed. When an item that seems obvious today is omitted in an ancient text, the historian's attitude is necessarily skeptical: the omission could mean "item unknown" just as well as "item obvious."[22] However, some four hundred years after Homer, Hippocrates actually states that not all wounds should be dressed or bandaged: which is not as bad as it may sound, because the dry scab that forms over a noninfected wound is now recognized as a natural dressing.[23]

Ἰατρός

One of the two bandages mentioned was needed for Agenor, whose hand had been pierced by a spear. He bound it with a sling, *sphendóne*, of wool, which his squire held ready,[24] presumably something like an eye patch. Hippocrates, too, mentions a sphendóne.[25] It must have looked like the woman's hairband of the same name (Fig. 4.3) and was undoubtedly the most economical form of bandage.[26]

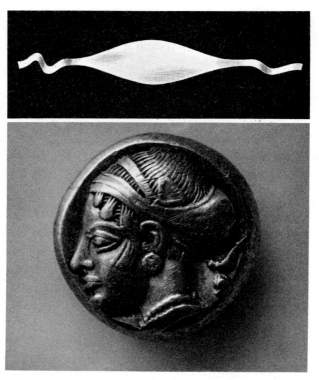

4.3 The Homeric bandage (above)—called *sphendóne*, "sling"—was probably shaped like the hairband of the same name (below), worn by a young woman of Phókaia around 500 B.C.

The pain of a wound was supposed to be soothed by drugs put on it[27] and maybe also by a drink of wine.[28] A sip of opium, though never mentioned, should have been within easy reach: with the Egyptians importing Greek opium before the war of Troy, surely some of that opium stayed home. The evidence is compelling. A woman's pendants in the shape of poppy capsules were found in Sparta.[29] This precise shape recurs in objects found all over Greece: pottery, jewels, even clay models that may have been offerings to the gods (Fig. 4.4).[30] Often the capsules are represented with several slits. These are the knife marks: they shed the tears of sap that dry into crude opium (Fig. 4.5).[31] Finally, in 1937, Greek archeologists exploring Crete dug their way down into a secret room, doorless and windowless, where they were greeted by the raised arms of an ancient Minoan goddess. She had strange eyes, perhaps closed. Before her were the remains of a heap of coals and some pottery; and she wore three hairpins shaped as beautiful, well-slit poppy capsules (Fig. 4.6).

The goddess of the poppy dates from 1300–1250 B.C., precisely the time of the war of Troy. This coincidence supports the tradition whereby opium was the active principle of Helen's famous Egyptian potion, *nepenthes*, which relieved the deepest sorrows.[32] It may seem bizarre that a Greek lady would need an Egyptian recipe to use Greek opium, but one has to remember that when Homer wrote his lines, the best trademark for a drug was "Made in Egypt" and had probably been so for one thousand years.

Ἰατρός

144

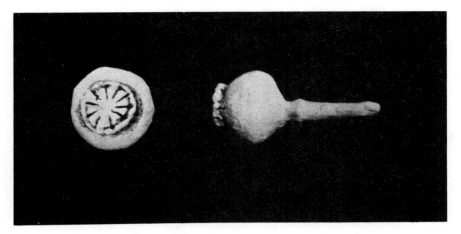

4.4 Clay model of a poppy capsule found in a sanctuary. It was probably a votive offering to Hera, eighth–fifth century B.C. The "asterisk of Dioscorides" on the top of the capsule and the "knee" in the stalk just below leave no doubt as to the identification. Slightly reduced.

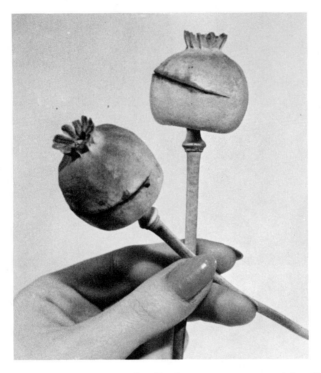

4.5 Real poppy heads or capsules, artificially slit. Juice oozes out of the slits and dries, forming opium. Its morphine content is on the order of 5–10 percent.

Ἰατρός

Of one casualty Homer says that the wound was "sucked out."[33] Experts have haggled over this word, some trying to interpret it as "pressed out."[34] Yet it is clear that something had to be taken out of the wound: perhaps just dirt, but more likely an abstract "bad influence," a concept typical of primitive medicine.[35] It might also have been arrow poison. Although this kind of treachery never occurs in the tales about Troy, the *Odyssey* mentions a voyage of Ulysses all the way to Epiros to get some arrow poison.[36] It would be

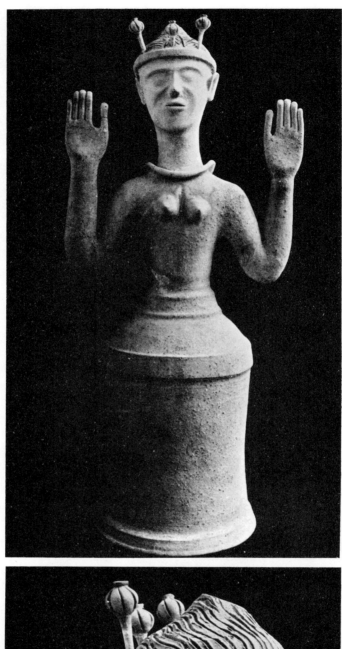

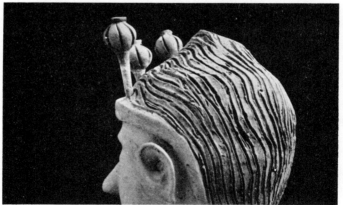

4.6 A Minoan goddess wearing poppy capsules as hairpins; the vertical slits in the capsules are stained brown like opium. This little statue (78 cm) was found in a secluded setting highly suggestive of opium smoking (c. 1300–1250 B.C.).

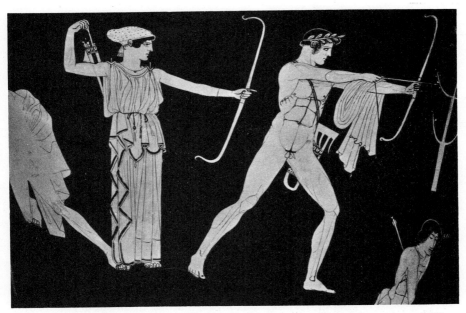

4.7 The Greek bow, *tóxon*, gave the word *toxic*. Here Apollo and Artemis are killing the sons and daughters of Niobe.

interesting to know what poison this might have been. If it came from a plant, Greece had perhaps two dozen candidates, the likeliest being *Helleborus orientalis Lam.*,[37] black hellebore—the very same root that was to become the pet prescription of the Hippocratics!

The drug sought by Ulysses in Epiros was called a *toxic*. However, *toxic* then did not mean poisonous at all; it meant "for-the-bow-and-arrow," from *tóxon*, "bow" (Fig. 4.7). Think how many poisoned arrows must have flown to change the meaning of toxic.

Arrow poison, wrote a Greek physician of the first century A.D., was used by the *bárbaroi*.[38] That word, too, has changed. It meant strangers. The author must have forgotten about Ulysses.

Surgery Without Surgeons

To return to the year 400 B.C., at that time Hippocrates should have been in his sixties and perhaps practicing in his home island of Cos. He had lived through the age of Pericles, the building of the Parthenon, the Great Plague of Athens, the fall of Athens to the Spartans, many a première of Sophocles, Euripides, and Aristophanes, and the last years of Socrates (Fig. 4.8). In Plato's dialogs Socrates speaks of him with utmost respect, and so does Aristotle:[39] at least we can be sure that he really existed. But we do not know for sure anything that he really said, let alone discovered. The Hippocratic Collection represents not his collected works but rather the remains of a library, possibly that of his medical school at Cos.[40] It is a potpourri of about seventy anonymous essays and fragments varying in length from one to a few pages, and very uneven in value. A few contain passages worthy of the master; others are poor, incomplete, or even contradictory.[41] The voice of Hippo-

'Ιατρός

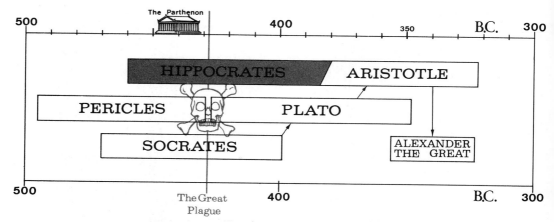

4.8 The life span of Hippocrates, in the context of two centuries. Arrows run from master to pupil.

crates, that voice which guided men for 2200 years, comes through as blurred as if it arose from the bottom of a well. But let there be no misunderstanding: if medicine was not born here, it was certainly reborn here.

The Hippocratic Collection is at its best in matters surgical, and has a lot to say about wounds. It also gives a picture of the iatrós that is a far cry from the homely asu. In those days, Greek physicians spent much of their time traveling[42]—or to use their term, doing *epidemics*: the word has radically changed its meaning, for it meant "visits to places" (several Hippocratic books are titled *Epidemics*). However, the iatrós also had a permanent working place in town, called the *iatréion*. This was a truly professional establishment, roomy, with "two kinds of light, the ordinary and the artificial . . . either direct or oblique,"[43] and equipped with surgical instruments, drugs, apparatus, and perhaps scrolls of medical literature. The physician himself, though not aseptic, was spotless, neat, and reassuring—even perfumed[44] (one book discourages the use of "elaborate" perfumes[45]). By today's standards he probably had rather long nails, since they had to be "neither longer, nor shorter than the fingers"[46]: perhaps he could not have trimmed them any better using shears instead of scissors, but Galen comments that this nail length was just right.[47] His skill in bandaging had been acquired in formal exercises, using one end of the bandage, or both ends, and "with both hands or either separately"[48] (Fig. 4.9). Even his posture in operating had to be elegant: "If he stands, he should make the examination with both feet fairly level, but operate with the weight on one foot (not that on the side of the hand in use) . . . When seated, his feet should be in a vertical line straight up as regards the knees, and be brought together with a slight interval. Knees a little higher than the groins and the interval between them such as may support and leave room for the elbows. Dress well drawn together, without creases, even and corresponding on elbows and shoulders."[49]

Since the daily practice in the iatréion was mostly surgical, the word itself has been translated with the old English expression "the Surgery."[50] This is misleading: to the mind of the Greeks the medical art was one,

'Ιατρός

148

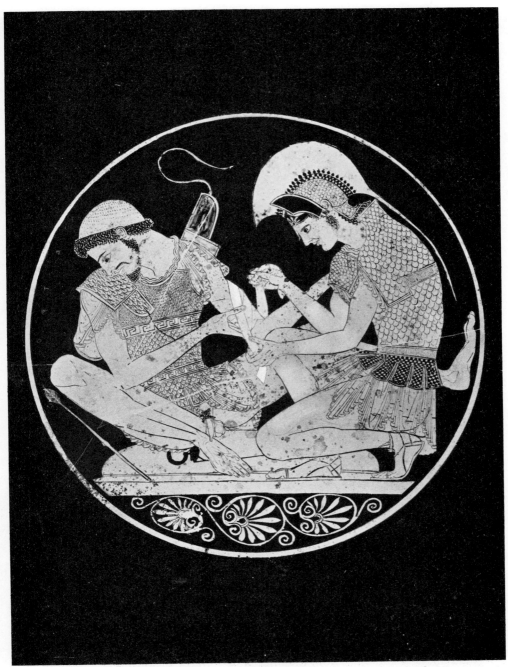

4.9 Achilles trying to employ a favorite style of Greek bandage: a left-handed and right-handed spiral, intertwined. It should be easy to finish off the bandage with a knot—but here Achilles has a problem, because he has turned both spirals the same way. From a vase of about 490 B.C. (just before Hippocrates).

without distinction between medicine and surgery.[51] It is significant that the Greek language of the time ignored the word *cheirurgós*, "surgeon," but used the name *cheirurgía*, "hand-work," and the verb *cheirurgéin*, "to work with the hand";[52] surgery was one of the physician's techniques, not a separate way of life.

Outpatient Care, Hippocratic Style

Now we shall try to step into the iatréion and see what happened there in real life. Detailed descriptions of clinical cases, complete with treatment, do not exist in the Hippocratic books. However, there are many bits of cases, sometimes even with the name of the patient: Thrinon, Billos, Dislytas. Those bits that are alike can be fitted together, and Hippocratic theory can be used to bind them. So, as an archeologist might rebuild ten acceptable amphorae out of a seabottom covered with shards, I rebuilt ten patients—and we may assume that they stand for men, women, and children who really sought help at the iatréion. In the case studies that follow, every medical fact and most words of the physician are lifted from the original text.[53]

The mood in the iatréion is set by a special hospital smell: smoke from the brazier where the cauteries are kept red-hot, fumes of boiling drugs, the aroma of herbs, resins and spices on the shelves, and a soupçon of roasted human flesh. In a corner, it looks as if a man were being pulled apart in a horrendous machine: actually he is being "treated" in the Hippocratic bench for a supposed dislocation of the hip. The iatrós and two male apprentices are working around him.

Patient No. 1: Severe Hemorrhage

Two men run in carrying a carpenter: his axe had slipped and cut his foot deeply. He is very pale and bleeds a lot. While the men lay him on a couch, the physician sees to it that the wounded leg is raised.[54] Then he dips a towel in cold water and wraps it loosely around the ankle. This will help to check the hemorrhage, because "cold water is to be applied not *to* the spot, but *around* the spot whence blood flows"[55]—a Hippocratic aphorism that stood the test of experiment in 1970.[56] Another towel is dipped in warm water and wrapped around the patient's head:[57] the idea is evidently to draw blood up there and away from the injured foot. In the meantime, an assistant has stepped outside and gone to a fig tree, where he is breaking off leaves and gathering the drops of white sap on a plug of wool.[58] The plug goes onto the wound.[59] Then—surprise—a beautiful white bandage, rolled from both ends, is soaked in red wine and applied dripping, with an adroit play of both hands.[60]

Ἰατρός

As for the juice of the fig tree: to the mind of the iatrós, it was a very good means to stop bleeding.[61] The reason was obvious to every Greek. Hear this passage from the *Iliad*.[62] The brazen Ares has been speared and immortal blood flows from his wound. Paieon spreads simples thereon, and "even as the

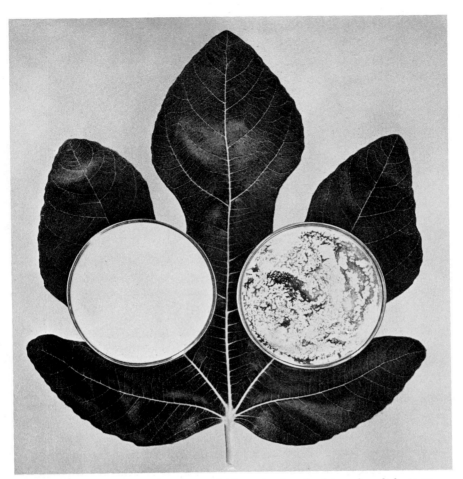

4.10 Confirming Homeric chemistry. The bottom of each of two glass dishes was covered with milk; three drops of latex from a fig tree were dropped into the dish at right; and the photograph was taken within a couple of minutes. Curdling is already obvious.

juice of the fig speedily maketh to grow thick the white milk that is liquid, but is quickly curdled as a man stirreth it, even so swiftly healed the furious Ares." Evidently Homer knew, or thought, that the sap of the fig tree caused milk to clot. From this, in Hippocratic logic, it was only a short step to conclude that what clots milk should also clot blood.

Therapy has changed so much since the *Iliad* that I found myself unable to assess either of these biological statements. So, with the help of two assist- ants, I scoured the Genevan countryside for a suitable fig tree and eventually procured a syringeful of latex. A drop of the latex mixed in a small dish of fresh milk made it curdle unbelievably fast (Fig. 4.10), just as Homer said. Our surprise was great. Then we went back to the literature (more of a task than doing the experiment) and found that this effect of fig-tree juice was current knowledge throughout antiquity. It is also mentioned casually in a Hippocratic treatise, which takes for granted that the reader is so familiar with the phenomenon that he can use it by analogy (as in the *Iliad*) to under- stand a medical theory: disease causes bodily humors to clot, just as rennet

'Ιατρός

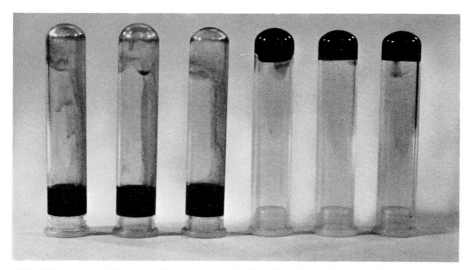

4.11 Disproving a Hippocratic treatment for bleeding. First, six test-tubes were aligned, right side up; the three at left received two drops of fig-tree latex; and one ml of blood was added to each of the six tubes. Then three minutes later they were all turned upside down, as shown. In the "blood-only" tubes (right), clotting had occurred normally; in the others, the blood ran down, because the latex, far from speeding up the clotting, had prevented it altogether. (Until the sap is tried on a bleeding wound, however, Hippocrates still has a chance to be correct).

causes milk to curdle.[63] The word for rennet is *opós*, "the juice," and the curdling juice par excellence was that of the fig tree.[64] We had stumbled upon a fact of elementary dairy technology at least as old as Homer.

Thus far our experiment had confirmed the first part of the physician's reasoning: "Opós will clot milk; therefore, opós will clot blood." Opós did clot milk. But the second and critical step of the reasoning proved a total failure: when we added the fig-tree juice to blood, clotting was prevented altogether (Fig. 4.11). Chances are that fig-tree latex as a styptic should be written off to psychotherapy.

Back to the iatréion. The physician is planning what to do next, in case the hemorrhage should continue; and he might explain it to the carpenter in these terms: "If the milk of the fig tree will not stop the bleeding, I can apply a ligature around your leg. If you have ever been bled from the arm, you will know that a gentle tie will increase the flow of blood; and that a stronger one will stop it.[65] But I will not leave the ligature on too long, because the part of the leg below it might become gangrenous."[66] In the meantime, more cold water is poured over the ankle.

ʼΙατρός

The bleeding stops; but beware. Shortly the iatrós reaches for a sharp blade, ties a band above the carpenter's knee, slits a vein in his ankle, and makes him bleed again! Quite a letdown after the brilliant beginning. This is the product of too much theory and too little anatomy. Muddled by notions that he takes for facts, the Greek practitioner has to live and work by this dilemma:

Hemorrhage kills, but bleeding helps.

So he compromises by stopping the hemorrhage and causing more bleeding. A dangerous game, especially in the hands of one who does not yet know how to tie off a spouting vessel.

Still, the iatrós had already worked out the main principle of the tourniquet, and even its built-in danger, gangrene: toward saving lives, this was a major step. Or rather, it should have been so: because this basic principle of first aid, the tourniquet, somehow failed to gain general acceptance. In the Hippocratic Collection it was clearly mentioned only once; it reappeared incidentally in the first century A.D. by the pen of a second-rate Roman writer, who ridiculed it.[67] And then it was lost. To this day, the credit for discovering the principle of the tourniquet is assigned to Ambroise Paré, who staunched bleeding in the mid-1500s "with a strong and broad fillet, like that which women usually bind up their hair withall."[68]

It is difficult to understand how a statement of this importance in the Hippocratic Collection could have been so consistently overlooked, even by modern commentators.[69] One reason may be that the tourniquet is mentioned in the context of a theoretical principle, in relation to surgical bleeding (venesection), not as a practical technique useful in first aid. Also, it appears in a book that rates fairly low in the traditional scale of excellence: category 5 in Littré's 11-point classification, under the heading "a mere collection of notes and extracts."[70] In fact, this book was never translated into English. Here is the passage, which comes after a short note on a woman suffering from quartan fever: "In case of profuse bleeding, one must find the appropriate position; in general, if [*the part*] is low, it should be brought high. In venesection, ligatures increase the flow of blood; if strong, they stop it."[71] The danger of gangrene by ligature is stated twice, but even more laconically; the clearest of the two passages reads: "Causes of gangrene of the tissues are: constriction in wounds with hemorrhage, compression in fractures of bones, and mortification from bandages."[72]

But whatever the reasons that drowned out the message in modern times, in the days of Hippocrates the tourniquet was bound to fail: the ligature of bleeding vessels was not yet known. After three or four hours, anyone who had applied a ligature faced a desperate choice: either leave it on, and cause gangrene; or remove it, and run the risk of more bleeding. The discovery had come too early.

Patient No. 2: A Round Ulcer

Ἰατρός

Next comes a plump woman, with bad varicose veins and a typical complication thereof: a stubborn ulcer on the ankle, which is bandaged. The iatrós begins by taking a pot from the burner and pouring some water, first over his own hand to check the temperature,[73] then over the woman's hand, because it is the patient who must decide whether it is comfortable.[74]

The bandages are removed while the ankle is showered with the warm water.[75] This is primarily a wash, but in the intention of the iatrós the warmth itself is essential, for two reasons. First, he believes that it will keep the sore "relaxed," thereby preventing "spasms" (anything from chills to tetanus, as we shall see). Second, he has been taught that heat favors bleeding[76] (which is true), and he believes that this will be good for the ulcer.

As for the woman's bulging varicose veins, they will remain untouched. The books recommend puncturing them once in a while, "as circumstances may indicate," but also warn that large sores may follow:[77] perhaps a more scientific way to restate, 1200 years later, the warning of the Ebers papyrus that it is wrong to cut into "snakelike swellings."

Now the ankle is sponged with hot vinegar,[78] very carefully, because the smell of vinegar was supposed to be "harmful, especially for women"[79] (this I cannot explain). The ulcer turns out to be almost perfectly round and hollow—one of many possible shapes (a detail of no relevance today).

"For an obstinate ulcer, sweet wine and a lot of patience should be enough,"[80] says the iatrós; "but this one is round, and it will not heal unless I change its shape into a long one. I could burn it out with a caustic,[81] but it will be faster to use a knife." So this is the treatment: carving the circle into an oval. The pain is made more bearable by allowing the patient to rest after each cut.[82]

After this astonishing procedure comes the dressing: a pad of wool dipped in an énaimon, a "drug for fresh wounds" (usually anglicized as enheme):[83]

Copper acetate (verdigris)[84]
Copper oxide, red (flower of copper)[85]
Lead oxide (molýbdaina)[86]
Alum, Egyptian, roasted

Myrrh   equal parts, dilute in wine
Frankincense

Gall nuts
Vine flowers

Grease of wool[87]

As a wound drug, this medicated wine might be better than nothing. The four inorganic salts would probably sting but would also kill any bacteria within reach. Myrrh and frankincense would add a touch of perfume to the proceedings and join the fight against bacteria. No harm is likely to come of the vine flowers; tannin from the gall nuts may be hemostatic. The only dubious ingredient is the grease of wool, essentially a crude form of lanolin smelling strongly of sheep and probably not too clean. The Greeks loved it. Its texture, smell, and taste seem almost real in the lines of Dioscorides.[87]

The bandage over the ankle is drawn tight, probably too tight for modern standards. The purpose is to apply pressure over the swelling, so as to squeeze out dangerous blood and humors.[88]

Finally, the woman is sent home with the inevitable purge and the very appropriate warning that standing, walking,[89] or even sitting will cause her sore to heal more slowly.[90]

There is one especially bizarre procedure in this case, namely, changing

'Ιατρός

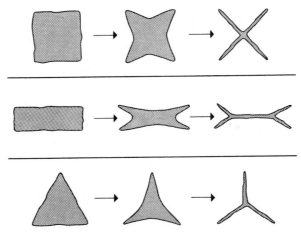

4.12 Gaping wounds heal by the inward movement of their margins, called wound contraction; hence the branching shapes of the scars.

the shape of a round ulcer. It is mentioned only once in the Collection, but thereafter the bad reputation of round ulcers grew into a surgical axiom. Ambroise Paré took it for granted,[91] and Francis Adams, the learned surgeon and commentator on Hippocrates, agreed in 1849 that "circular sores are particularly difficult to heal. Every experienced surgeon must be aware of the fact, however it may be accounted for."[92] If Adams says so, we have to think twice before brushing it off.

There is indeed a fair amount of truth in the lore of the round ulcers. All gaping wounds close, to a large extent, by contraction: the raw surface becomes lined with a contractile tissue that draws the opposite margins together. Hence, square or triangular wounds heal with star-shaped scars (Fig. 4.12). As for a round wound, in theory, if it were to remain round and heal by pure contraction, it would have to reduce itself to a point: ultimately its margins would have to pile up into a vanishing space, which is not conceivable. The phenomenon is more intuitively obvious than scientifically understood; but the final result is well illustrated by the analogy with two sets of imaginary turtles. One set is laid out in a square, the other in a circle. Instruct the turtles to crawl toward the center, and see what happens (Fig. 4.13).[93]

In practice, a round wound does not heal as well as an irregularly shaped wound, unless some force is present that draws it into an oval.[94] Wounds with a surface of 30 square centimeters, produced experimentally in rabbits, took on the average 18.82 days to heal if they were triangular, 25.46 days if they were circular.[95]

The ulcers that develop in legs with varicose veins are difficult to heal (round or not), because their blood supply is bad. Long-standing ulcers also develop thick, firm, fibrous edges that resist the centripetal pull. Hence, the ancient practice of carving them out was dangerous—indeed heroic—but not entirely irrational.

If patient no. 2 heeded the advice not to walk after the surgery (she probably had little choice) this alone should have helped her ulcer. Her dressing was antiseptic. Perhaps she gained something at the iatréion.

'Ιατρός

155

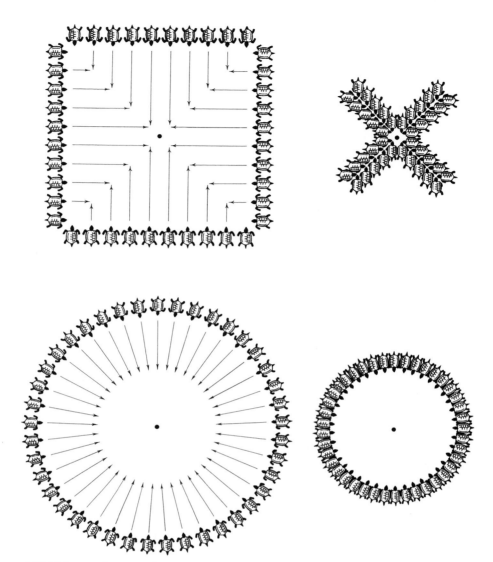

4.13 Using turtles to understand the rules of wound contraction. A formation of crawling turtles laid out in a square (above) shows how the inward motion of the margins leads to an X. A circular formation of turtles (below) can never close: this resembles the behavior of round wounds, which cannot heal except by changing shape.

Patient No. 3: Pus in the Chest

'Ιατρός

This feverish young man is directed to sit on a stool, facing away from the light.[96] On the back of his chest, rather low, there appears a broad, soft lump. To the iatrós the correct diagnosis is obvious: there is so much pus in the pleural cavity (empyema) that it is ready to come out through the skin. Empyema so far advanced as to bulge under the skin is rare nowadays, but it was common in antiquity. Celsus recorded that "it is common for fistulae to have their exit between ribs."[97]

To confirm his diagnosis, the iatrós seizes the patient by the shoulders, shakes him, and listens closely,[98] expecting to hear "a wave and a noise . . .

like [*shaking*] a skinsack."[99] But this time there is no noise at all. This he takes to be a bad sign.[100] Pus is definitely there, since it is ready to come through the skin, so it must be "too thick, or too abundant," to splash around in the pleura.[101]

In any event, the correct conclusion is that pus must be removed from the chest, and this calls for surgery. Although the painful spot indicates where to incise, the iatrós prefers to double-check. He and his aide dip their hands into a jar full of wet potter's clay and quickly smear it all over the back of the patient. Then they watch attentively. The first patch to dry up will indicate the hottest point of the skin and therefore the best place for cutting.[102] The back of the patient is now washed with a lot of hot water, and the operation is performed. The style of the text suggests that this was routine surgery:[103]

Cut as low as possible so that the pus may flow out more easily. Cut between the ribs, the skin first, using a knife with a rounded blade. Then take a pointed knife, wrap its blade in a cloth so that only the point will protrude as much as the length of a thumb's nail, and cut through [*to the pleural cavity*]. Let out as much pus as you think best, then put in a tent[104] of raw linen attached to a thread [*presumably to retrieve the strip of linen, should it slip beyond reach*]. Let out the pus once a day. On the tenth day, having removed all the pus, put in a tent of fine linen; then inject warm wine and oil through a small tube, so that the lung, accustomed to be moistened by the pus, may not remain suddenly dry. Remove in the evening the oil and wine injected in the morning; that injected in the evening, remove it on the following morning. When the pus becomes as thin as water, slippery to the finger, and scanty, put into the wound a hollow tin drain. When the pleural cavity becomes dry [*i.e. ceases to produce fluid*] cut the drain shorter little by little, and allow the incision to heal as you retrieve the drain.[104] Signs that the patient will escape death: if the pus is white and pure and contains streaks of blood, there are good chances of healing. But if pus . . . on the next day flows thick, greenish and fetid the patients die after the pus has run out.

Oil was still being injected into the pleural cavity some years ago in the treatment of lung tuberculosis;[105] drainage with a rigid tube is an important world première (Fig. 4.14). The overall procedure is quite advanced. But once again, postoperative treatment is just about disastrous. To stop the formation of pus the patient is bled from the arm, purged, and given a starvation diet: thin barley gruel and dilute *oxymel*, a mixture of water with a little honey and vinegar.[106]

Ἰατρός

Obviously, some of these patients came out alive. Daring as the operation may seem, it was probably suggested by the natural course of events (that is, the spontaneous exit of the pus) and by familiarity with holes in the chest due to stabbing with "spears, daggers and arrows."[107] Survival from such wounds was not unusual.

The patients were operated while sitting "on a firm stool"[108] (the firmness of the patient being taken for granted). Afterwards, they probably went home. It has often been claimed that the iatréion had facilities for inpatients. I checked the evidence and found it to be unbearably thin: one court

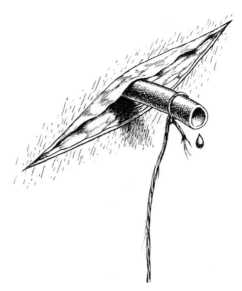

4.14 Surgical drainage of pus with a piece of tin pipe—another Greek practice that sank into oblivion.

case in which the defendant, a citizen of peculiar habits, was accused of sleeping at the iatréion *with the physician!*[109]

Not enough to make a ward.

Patient No. 4: A Fallen Lung

This young woman has been operated on for empyema several weeks before. The wound has begun to close, but now she complains of what she calls pleuritis. Doctors tend to be irritated by patients who offer their own diagnoses, but the young woman is not doing that. *Pleurón* meant "side," and *pleuritis* was vaguely "the thing of the side."[110] The ending *-itis* was still far from taking the turn it took with appendicitis, where it now means "inflamed." Athena Ophthalmitis had no red eyes; she was just the goddess "with the [big] eyes." Hepatitis was not a disease, but a vein connected with the liver, and steatitis was "the thing like fat," a stone.[111]

So the iatrós directs the young woman to sit on a stool, kneels behind her, lifts her chitón, and applies an ear to her back. Yes, auscultation! His gesture was just like ours (Fig. 4.15).

He hears an abnormal sound, "a creaking sound like leather."[112] Today we know what this means: the surface of the lung, roughened by infection and inflammation, is rubbing against the rib cage. As the iatrós sees it, the lung "has fallen against the side,"[113] and he has an answer to the problem. On a shelf are stored several pieces of tubes and dried animal bladders of various sizes, his disassembled syringes (Fig. 4.16). He attaches a bladder to a small tube and inflates it.[114] Then he slips the free end of the tube into the wound, pushes it into the pleural cavity, and blows in the air. Finally he withdraws the tube and plugs the passage with a solid rod of tin. He thus obtains an ar-

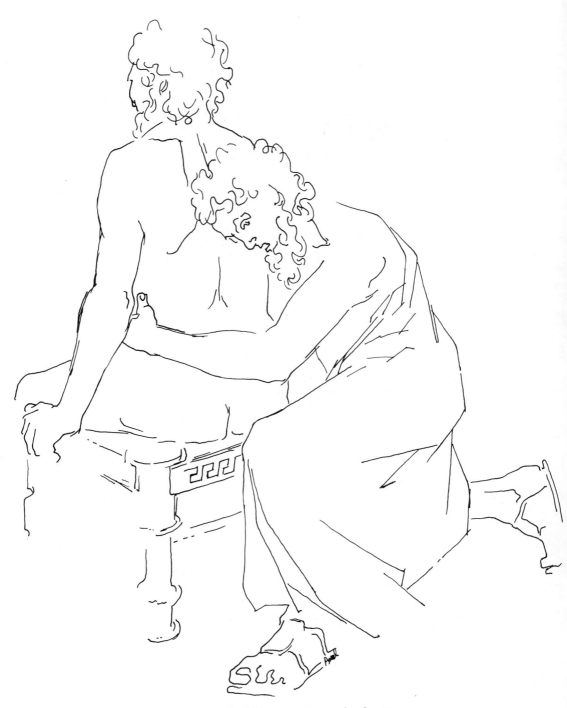

4.15 A iatrós listening for lung noises, of which he understood at least two.

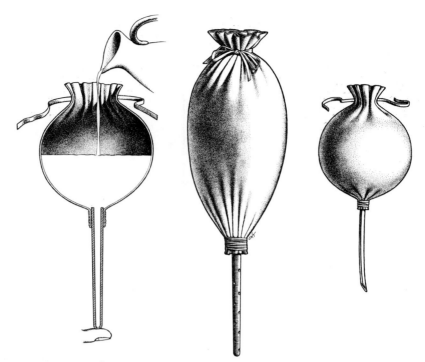

4.16 Greek syringes: an animal bladder tied to a pipe was filled with fluid or air. The largest pipe (left) was for enemas; the finest, a feather shaft (right), was for the urinary ways. The middle one, made of silver, was for gynecological use. About one-third actual size.

tificial pneumothorax—a nineteenth century invention! But why did *he* do it?

To solve the mystery we will have to analyze that phrase "fallen lung," which seems to make no sense at all. Commentators have either ignored it or found it bizarre.[115] Having first repressed all modern knowledge of anatomy, we will step into the sandals of a iatrós who is trying to learn something about the lung, perhaps by standing next to a butcher as he opens the chest of a slaughtered animal.[116] As the knife plunges into the rib cage, there is a faint wheeze: normally, the lungs are in contact with the inner surface of the chest, being held there by the negative pressure in the pleural cavity (Fig. 4.17a). The instant that a blade reaches the pleura, air is sucked in, and the lungs—while they are still out of sight—recoil inward and upward to their point of attachment (Fig. 4.17b). This is the position in which the Hippocratic physician finally sees them, and he necessarily takes it to be normal. If the normal lungs are perched high up in the chest, in order to come and rub against the lower rib, they obviously have to fall (Fig. 4.17c).

Now the purpose of the operation becomes clear: it was a matter of blowing back into place a lung that had fallen down, just like air blown into the vagina was used to straighten out a "displaced uterus,"[117] or the wind of the blacksmith's bellows to pop an intestinal obstruction.[118]

As a result of the operation, the creaking noise has disappeared. For the pain in the side, a beef bladder or skin bag full of hot water will help. But the young woman is no better off. The pain in the side is still there, because the iatrós has given her an acute pneumothorax (air in the chest)—luckily not

Ἰατρός

160

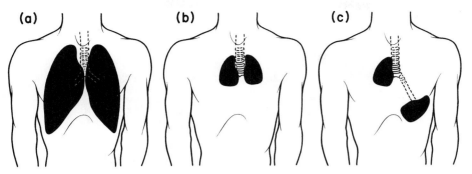

4.17 The Greek misconception of a "fallen lung": when a physician heard the lung rubbing against the chest wall, he thought it had dropped against it.

severe, but enough to cause discomfort, to speed up the heart rate, and to make breathing difficult. And her pleural infection has been increased. She would have been well advised, I fear, not to seek help.

Patient No. 5: A Cut in the Face

A youngster comes in accompanied by a slave. He has a clean slash on the nose, where a playmate hit him with an *óstrakon*, a piece of broken pot.[119] The wound is washed with a generous shower of white wine,[120] then patted with a sponge and pieces of clean, dry linen.[121]

"This is a sharp cut," says the iatrós. "Had there been any bruised flesh, I would have helped the wound to produce pus, for pus makes the bruised flesh melt away.[122] Since there is no bruise, I can make the wound close fast, without the formation of pus." He takes a bronze needle, threads it, stitches the flesh, and covers the suture with a mixture of copper oxide and honey.[123] The dressing is a double pad of cloth soaked in wine, then a slice of clean sponge, rather dry, and a handful of leaves.[124] The sponge under the bandage is to apply pressure. The leaves have not been understood,[125] but I assume they served the purpose of today's gutta-percha or plastic sheet, namely, to prevent rapid evaporation from the dressing. The bandage is an artful *semi-rhómbos* (Fig. 4.18),[126] its end being sewn in place with thread and needle.[127]

Greek physicians took great pride in sending away their patients with tricky and aesthetic bandages. The Hippocratic Collection has much to say on the art of bandaging, but also warns that some turn it into "a foolish parade of manual skill,"[128] and that a stupendous bandage is not equivalent to excellent medicine.[129] "Leave aside theatrical bandages that serve no purpose; this is miserable and fit for charlatans, and often hurts the patient. Indeed the patient is seeking not ornaments, but help."[130]

ʼΙατρός

To a modern patient, the end of the bandage ritual brings a sigh of relief. But a Greek patient still had lots of trouble ahead. The physician might caution the child: "Now that your wound is sutured, we must prevent it from throwing pus, or it will open again. We will have to purify the body from below (*hypocatharsis*).[131] So drink this potion." The scrolls at the iatréion list over sixty drugs claimed to be cathartics (*catharsis* meant "puri-

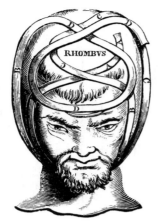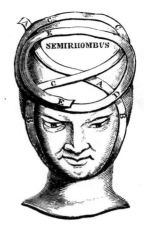

4.18 Rhómbos and semirhómbos bandages. Bandaging the head was an art; Galen's book *On Bandages*, based on Hippocrates, has at least seventy varieties. To apply these bandages, follow the letters.

fication"), and some are indeed very powerful.[132] Then, turning to the slave, the iatrós says, "See to it that he drinks hydromel, seven parts water to one part honey,[133] but allow very little food and absolutely no cheese until I tell you." The Greeks made a great fuss about the dangers of cheese. They were probably alarmed by the resemblance between cheese, mainly coagulated protein, and the whitish fibrin that coagulates in sores—which they called *phlegm*: "cheese is phlegmatic."[134] Finally, the patient is instructed to come back "the day after tomorrow," for it was standard practice to change the dressings every other day.[135]

These sutures, with their Indian counterparts, are the first definite examples after the Egyptian *ydr*. In view of the tendency of nonaseptic sutures to become infected and drop off, it is not surprising to find that stitches in the flesh are mentioned only three times in the Collection,[136] and then only in relation to the nose and the eyelids. Modern surgeons are well aware that wounds about the face heal "more kindly," with less risk of infection.[137] Perhaps the iatrói, too, had discovered that wounds in the face stood a better chance of tolerating sutures.

So far so good—except for the purge and the diet. If infection does not cause the suture to break down (young people are good patients in this respect), the iatrós will have performed a useful function.

Ἰατρός

Patient No. 6: Recurrent Dislocation of the Shoulder

The next patient is a sleek *éphebos* still oily from his last wrestling match in the gymnasium (Fig. 4.19). He is clutching his left arm, obviously dislocated at the shoulder; the pain is not great, and it is the fourth time it has happened anyway. The treatment is routine to him. In principle, all dislocations were supposed to be treated on the contraption that is now called the Hippocratic bench or *scamnum*, basically a device for stretching the patient with winches (Fig. 4.20).[138] But a humerus that kept slipping out of its sockets

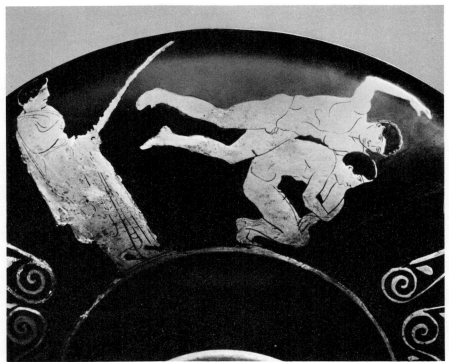

4.19 A Greek throw, the *se-oi-nage* of modern Judo, which will cause a heavy fall. The emphasis on dislocation of the shoulder in the Hippocratic books was certainly related to the popularity of wrestling.

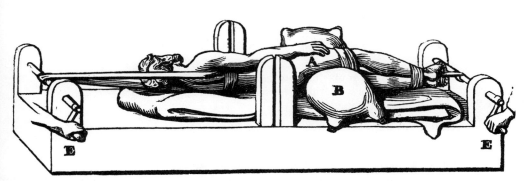

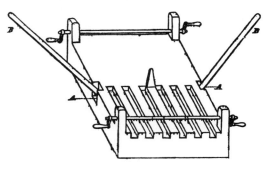

4.20 The Hippocratic bench at work (above). Here the upper end of the femur (A) is supposed to have been luxated inward, so the inflated skin bag (B) eases it outward, while the limb is submitted to traction and counter-traction. Note the crankshafts (E); the screw had not yet been invented. This is a very dangerous machine, which could have helped only rarely, if ever. In a later interpretation of the bench (right), with two lateral levers (AB), the patient lay astride the central pin (*priapískos*).

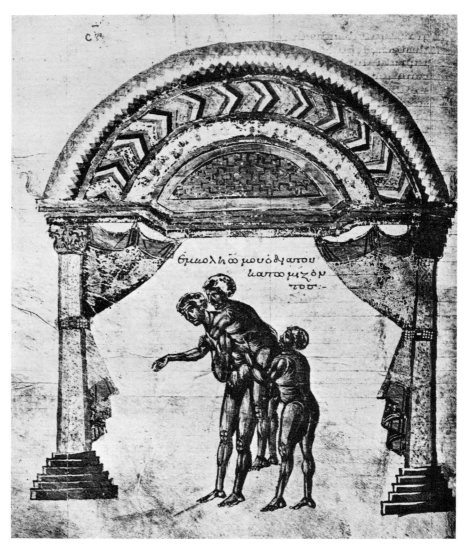

4.21 One of nine ways to reset a dislocated humerus. The physician, if tall enough, pulls the patient's arm over his shoulder. This method was "very convenient at the wrestling school." From a Byzantine manuscript of the Hippocratic book *On Joints*, c.950 A.D.

could be reset by simpler means. Thus, the éphebos lies down on the bare floor; the physician sits down beside him, puts a little ball of sewn leather in the patient's armpit, and tugs at the arm while pushing the ball with his heel—a technique still recommended.[139]

Ἰατρός

The main problem is solved once again; and if the maneuver had failed, the iatrós had eight other ways to go about it, like pulling the patient's arm over a door or over a chair (Figs. 4.21–4.22). This time, however, the young man is served a sermon. His humerus has been slipping out too often. What if someday it slips out during a real battle? It has happened to others, and that was their last time.[140] Since the joint is too loose, the remedy will be to poke a cautery through the skin of the armpit (Fig. 4.23). This will cause the tissues to retract and keep the bone in its place.[141] Gritting his teeth, the éphebos accepts the new challenge.

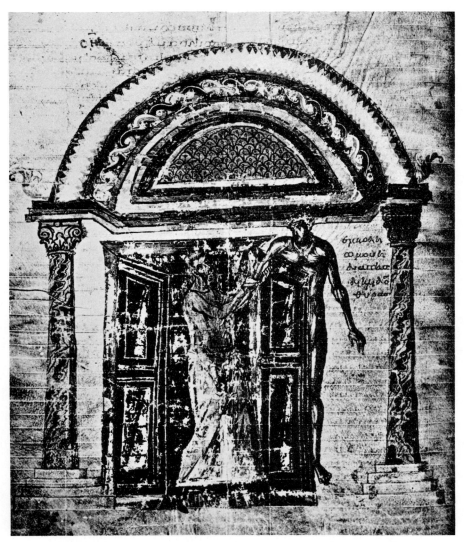

4.22 Another method to reset a dislocated humerus—over a door. From the same manuscript.

Before decrying the iatrós for suggesting this dreadful procedure, consider his grasp of matters surgical. He knows, in fact he applies the phenomenon of wound contraction, which is so powerful in burn wounds ("in this way the cavity, into which the humerus is mostly displaced, is best scarred over and cut off"). He also knows the basic surgical anatomy of the axilla and devises the operation accordingly, for the text mentions the "glands that everyone has in the armpit" and even the neurovascular bundle. Here is the physician's warning to the patient, transcribed almost literally: "I will heat the cautery until it glows white: that way it will be faster in going through the fold of skin; but be sure not to move, for deep down there are some nerves and a large vein, and at all cost they must not be touched."

The operation, extremely painful, leaves three black sores. Each one is covered with a lump of greasy wool. The iatrós is again worried that they

'Ιατρός

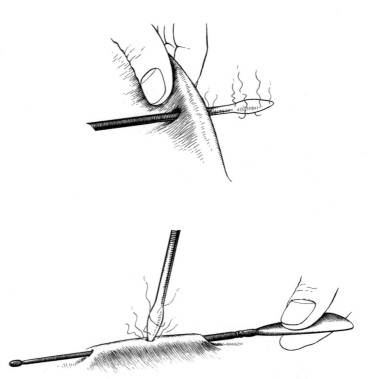

4.23 Triple cauterization of the armpit in cases of recurring luxation of the shoulder. The contracted scar left by the burns was supposed to hold the bone in place.

might catch cold, especially since they are burn wounds.[142] This obsession with cold may be connected with the specific choice of unwashed wool for the wounds. A seventeenth century Italian commentator refused to believe that the Divine Master himself could have recommended such filth,[143] but after all, if warmth is the purpose, greasy wool is warmer.

My guess is that in the long run the operation worked—by keeping the patient away from the palaestra, and maybe from the battlefield as well.

Patient No. 7: Carpentry on the Skull

This boy aged eleven is mentioned in the fifth book of the *Epidemics*. While grooming a horse, he received a kick in the forehead.[144] The iatrós explores the wound with a probe (Fig. 4.24)[145]—no fingers—trying to determine whether there is a fracture or maybe only a shallow dent left by the horse's hoof (Fig. 4.25). He calls such a dent by the name of *hedra*, literally "chair" or "seat." The Greeks were so concerned with the fate of bruised bone that they developed this special name for dents in the skull un-accompanied by fracture. It is one of the few Greek medical terms that died out, because the underlying concern has also disappeared: bruised bones heal perfectly well if left untouched and sterile (hedrae still happen, but they are absorbed into the general notion of contusion).

To the iatrós, this preliminary probing is essential. If there *is* a fracture, he will *not* operate further; if there is no fracture, he will drill a hole in the

'Ιατρός

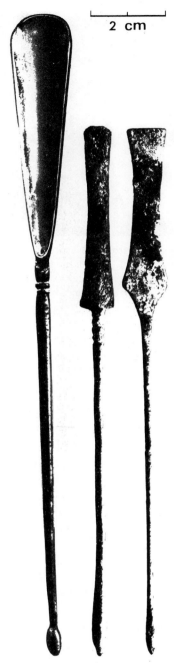

4.24 Multipurpose probes, with which Greek physicians touched and treated wounds, rather than using their fingers, as had their Egyptian predecessors. Whether probes were better or worse than fingers depends on how clean they were kept.

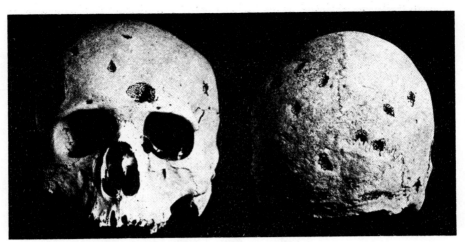

4.25 Dents or notches in the skull, without fracture, caused by blows. The Greeks called them *hédrae*, and worried physicians scraped them away. How wrong they were is shown by the skull of this miserable prehistoric Peruvian, who had about seventeen hedrae (from sling-stones?), all presumably unscraped, and all healed.

skull; and if there is just a hedra, he will scrape it away. Here he runs into a diagnostic problem: how is he going to distinguish a thin crack from a normal joint between two bones?

The answer is a hair-raising bit of carpentry *in vivo*.[146] First he shaves the head.[147] Then he enlarges the wound, lifts the scalp all around it, and packs the space with lint. Then he plugs the wound itself with a plaster made by boiling vinegar and barley flour, and covers the whole with a bandage. That is all for the day. The next day he removes everything, smears the skull with something that looks like black shoe polish;[148] and covers it again with oil, linen, and more barley plaster. The third day he scrapes the blackened skull with a sharp knife: experience has shown him that the black will come off everywhere except from cracks and dents (Fig. 4.26). He goes on scraping until all the black is gone. To the Hippocratics this horrible procedure was very important. Perhaps they thought that bruised bone would decay and slough off, as soft tissues do, and therefore preferred to scrape it out from the start.

The most perplexing part of the story is that if the iatrós had found no fracture or hedra at all, he would have felt compelled to drill a hole with one of the several gadgets at his disposal (Fig. 4.27). In essence, *if you find no hole, make one*. Rivers of ink have flowed over this riddle. But again, it made good sense in the context. To the mind of the Greek physician, a blow must cause blood to spill beneath the skull or humors to accumulate there; all this material has to be given a way out before it turns into pus. If there is a way out already, such as a fracture, fine; but if not, it will be necessary, as Francis Adams put it, to "slacken the tightness of the skull."[149]

Drill slowly, recommends the text, because the bone may heat up and burn.[150] The unknown writer was well acquainted with this problem, because similar hand-drills were used to start fires,[151] much as in ancient Egypt.

'Ιατρός

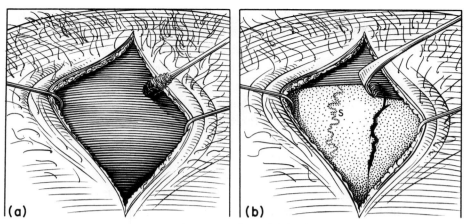

4.26 Greek method for distinguishing a crack in the skull from a normal suture (s): just smear a black paste on the bared skull (a) and scrape (b). Only cracks will show up.

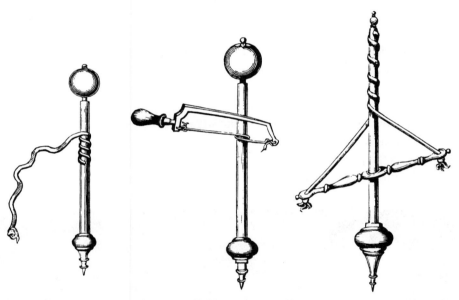

4.27 Three types of Greek bone-drill (*trýpanon*). Drills like these were also used on wood for starting fires, as in Egypt.

Twenty days after the operation the little groom is shaking with fever, his face red and swollen beyond recognition.[152] The bacteria have taken over. His trouble is diagnosed as erysipelas and is treated with a cathartic,[153] besides plasters on the face and a burn with the cautery. He will survive; but it is somewhat startling to read that "his wound had nothing to do with these accidents."[154]

Ἰατρός

Patient No. 8: A Chest Like Boiling Vinegar

Fighting a fit of cough—a long, rumbling cough—a withered old woman staggers in and takes a seat. She is out of breath and obviously feverish. When she has quieted down a bit, the iatrós kneels down behind her, puts an ear to her back, and listens for a long while. If it was a surprise to see him practice auscultation, there is no word for what will happen now. This ancient Greek is about to draw conclusions worthy of a modern treatise of pathophysiology—except, alas, for the therapy.

To him, it sounds "as if it were boiling inside like vinegar."[155] He takes this to mean, quite correctly, that there is fluid inside the lung.[156] Then, unlike many of today's physicians, who leave their patients in the dark, he tells the old woman the complete story as he sees it. This is actually a calculated display of insight, on the principle that it impresses a patient to be told his own symptoms before he has a chance to describe them himself.[157] His speech might run: "You must have been coughing like this for a long while. I can tell from your fingernails. Remember how they used to be curved only sideways, like mine; now see how they are curved also the other way (Fig. 4.28). Your toenails must look the same. This means that your lungs are sick. You will probably have more fits of coughing and fever like this one, and the tips of your fingers might even become swollen. Then perhaps the water in your lungs will seep out and pour into the space all around. Should this happen, I will be able to help you by drilling a little hole in a rib and tapping that water, a little at a time.[158] In the meanwhile, I will keep studying your urine, which tells me how your disease progresses.[159] I shall give you some fumigations, and a diet that will dry up your body."

Note how this talk has improved the situation. The patient is greatly relieved to know that she is in the hands of a doctor of obvious competence, who knows the present as well as the past and the future; he even guessed about the fingernails. She has also escaped the knife. If she gets worse, she can

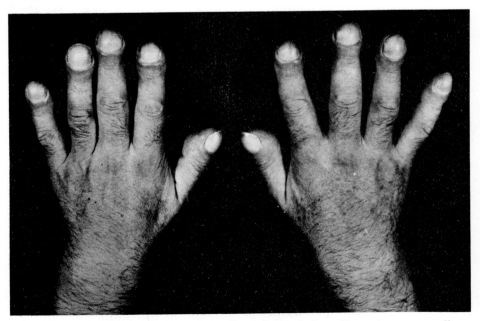

'Ιατρός

4.28 "Hippocratic fingers." This strange effect of chronic lung disease is not yet well understood.

hope for a treatment; and in the meantime her medicine is not too unpleasant. It was worthwhile going to the iatréion.

The physician, too, is gratified. He may not have spelled out the diagnosis in modern terms (chronic bronchitis on bronchiectasis with recurrent bronchopneumonia), but this is not at all his concern, for almost anybody can tell what is going on right now. What counts most is to be able to anticipate what is going to happen—*prognosis* rather than diagnosis. In his eyes, he should be congratulated for making what he calls a good prognosis; good, that is, primarily for his ego. Today's physicians behave somewhat alike when they speak of a good diagnosis after having discovered a hidden cancer.

To understand the peculiar lack of interest in diagnosis in ancient Greece, remember also that disease, in general, was always viewed as the same: an imbalance. The author of *On Breaths* goes so far as to say, "Of all diseases the fashion is the same, only the seat varies."[160] The satisfaction of a beautiful diagnosis was therefore minimized, and the iatrós replaced it with a "beautiful prognosis." Here is a rather shocking example: "If convulsions do appear, death is likely, and there is a chance for a beautiful prognosis."[161]

As to the curving nails and swelling fingertips, they belong to the category of strange but true: they are common effects of chronic lung disease. Although theories abound,[162] on the whole the phenomenon is not understood much better today than in the days of the iatréion. French clinicians still record it as *hippocratisme digital.*

Note also that the iatrós has been able to recognize the presence of fluid bubbling in the bronchi by placing his ear on the chest. But what can he be hearing that is *boiling like vinegar?* Other readings have been proposed for this passage, such as "smelling like vinegar"[163] or "seething like sour wine,"[164] which is chemically impossible; none improves the meaning. The answer is probably the simplest. It occurred to me one day that it might help to pour some vinegar into a pan and heat it. As it started to boil, it produced a very special rushing, crackling noise, quite unlike that of boiling water, and comparing very well with the sound heard over a lung when fluid obstructs the finest bronchi, a sound called "fine moist râles" in modern terminology. The iatrós was familiar with the procedure of boiling vinegar, a common step in preparing drugs and plasters.[165]

Patient No. 9: Punches in the Head

Ἰατρός

The next patient looks like a nightmare: a giant, with scarcely any face, just a bloody mess of black eyes, swollen ears, and a broken nose. This is the new breed of professional boxer.[166]

Boxing had degenerated by 400 B.C. In the old days it had been a game like all others, practiced by gallant young amateurs whose fists were protected by soft leather thongs (Fig. 4.29). Then over-competition bred professionalism, which spoiled the game.[167] Boxing was taken over by huge brutes, "pot-hunters," who wandered from city to city in search of a bloody fight to the finish (Fig. 4.29). They wore a new kind of sharp, cutting gloves called *sphái-*

4.29 Greek boxing scenes. *Below:* These sporty young men wearing soft leather thongs about 490 B.C. are amateurs. The aim is typically at the head. *Right:* Later boxing scene, about 336 B.C. The athletes have changed to the professional type: heavyweights, wearing vicious cutting gloves (*spháirai*).

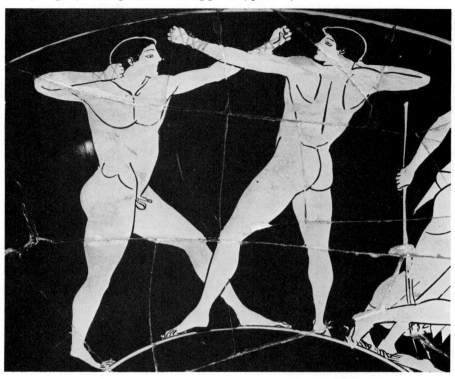

rai: no less a man than Plato had just recommended them for use in his ideal state, as part of the people's training for "the greatest of contests," war.[168]

The iatrós feels very much at ease before this patient. He knows that the ugly sight actually corresponds to a rather benign situation.[169] Complications are unlikely, and soon the monster's face will be improved by an elegant bandage (Fig. 4.30). This type of client must have been quite common, for it is discussed in considerable detail in one Hippocratic book.[170]

A good wash with wine shows, under the wound, a break in the nasal bone. With a special bronze spatula introduced into a nostril, the depressed fragment is raised, while fingers help from outside, pushing downward. "I am glad you came just after the fight," the iatrós might say; "Later it would have been more difficult to reduce the fracture. To hold up the bridge of your nose, I will now slip into your nostril a little roll of soft leather, containing fluff scraped off a linen towel.[171] It may bother you a little, but it does not smell. Once, having nothing else at hand, I stuffed in a piece of sheep lung. Now the two ends of the bone are aligned, but they will not stay in place unless you work for it. You will have to hold it in place yourself, if you have the will and the patience. No physician is worth your own two index fingers, held naturally on each side of the nose as long as possible, preferably until the bone has set. If you cannot do this yourself, ask the help of a child or a

Ἰατρός

172

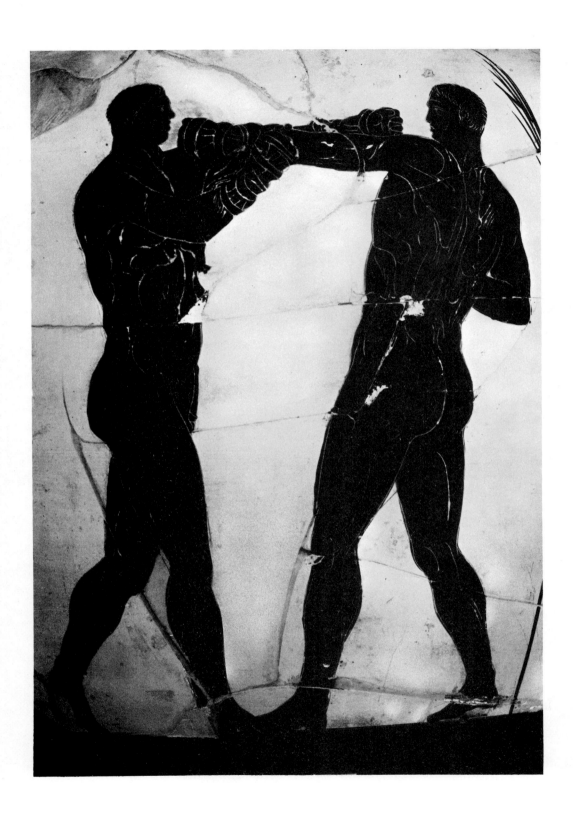

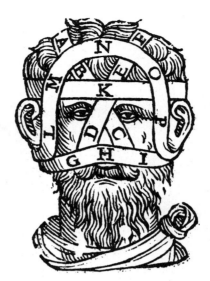

4.30 Bandages for the nose, like this one, were the most spectacular types: "Those who practice dexterity without judgement look forward to meeting with a case of fractured nose, that they may apply the bandage. For a day or two, then, the physician glories in his performance, and the patient . . . is well pleased, but speedily . . . he complains of the incumbrance."

woman, for the fingers ought to be soft. But I know you will find it difficult. *Although men would give a great price to escape being deformed, at the same time they will not pay attention or take care unless they experience pain or fear death.* Anyway, straight or crooked, the parts will be consolidated in about ten days."

On the wound is placed a sticky plaster of wheat, *kómmi* (gum), and an aromatic resin, held in place by a cloth. This is a sticky mixture, but not stiff enough to serve as a support.

Next come the crumpled, or as we now say, cauliflower ears (Fig. 4.31).[172] Ears were a prime target in Greek boxing. Despite the covers (*amphotídes*) sometimes worn in practice,[173] broken ears recur often in Greek and Roman literature as a badge of the athlete. Aristophanes even coined the term *oto-kátaxis,* "ear-breaker," for boxer.[174] When Athens was occupied by the well-trained Laconians, some citizens advertised their political sympathies by adopting Spartan tastes and took to boxing, so that in Plato's time "the fellows with broken ears" came to mean "the sympathizers" or "Laconizers."[175]

'Ιατρός

"As to your ears," the iatrós might continue, "almost anything I could do would make matters worse. *It is sometimes a good remedy to apply nothing at all, and this is true not only for the ears.* Even a bandage would hurt. Later on, if pus forms, I may have to cut, and maybe even burn a hole in the ear with the cautery, though that would leave you with one ear smaller than the other. In the meantime we will work at preventing suppuration: take this purge, which will remove matters from below; and if you know how to vomit easily, I will also purge you from above with the mild method called *syrmaism,* according to which you load your stomach with a large amount of salt, water, and radishes, then throw it up.[176] After that you can go home, and do not sleep on your ears."

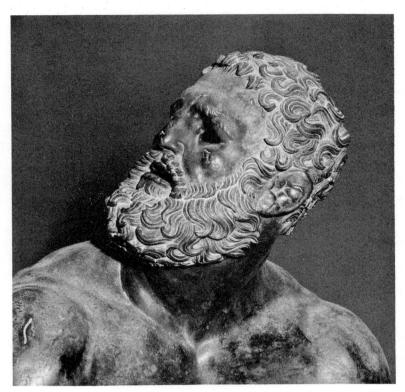

4.31 Head of a professional boxer, with injuries to the nose and cheeks and a typical "cauliflower ear." Hellenistic, first century B.C.

Note that the physician does not bother to examine the rest of the body. There was no need to do so, because Greek boxers—for some strange reason— aimed only at the head (Fig. 4.29).[177]

Patient No. 10: Stripes

The last patient is a taciturn slave named Xanthias because of his blond hair.[178] He comes from far-away Scythia and speaks little Greek; but once he has bared his back, there is not much need for words. It is a cruel sight: his skin is crisscrossed with sores from a whipping.[179] One of them looks particularly bad—red, hot, and swollen. This vicious infection draws a frown even from the detached iatrós.

'Ιατρός

"One of your sores, Xanthias," he might explain, "has gone into a state of orgasm.[180] I will cool it down for you with a plaster of boiled celery,[181] and then you will take a purge." There are finesses in this little talk that unfortunately are lost on Xanthias. "Orgasm" was a medical term perhaps more congenial than inflammation; it was also applied to the turgid state of ripening fruit, and it required immediate purging.[182]

The wild celery, too, left Xanthias indifferent. To Greek ears it would have had a noble ring, like laurel. It would have recalled the winners of the Isthmic and Nemean games, who were crowned with celery.[183] "He needs celery" meant "he is in danger," for *sélinon* was also used for chaplets to hang

175

over tombs. It also gave the name to the lovely city of Selinunte and to its river (Fig. 4.32).

The cool celery plaster will have to be renewed as often as possible, because once warm, it is supposed to be harmful.[184] This happens to be an exception: the usual injunction is to keep wounds warm, but it is allowable to cool them down when they are inflamed.

The other sores call for a different approach. The iatrós reaches for a pot of whitish, greasy ointment; and while he spreads this soothing paste onto the back of Xanthias, he explains: "After all, you are lucky, because sores can go four ways: deeper by gnawing into the body, outward by building new flesh, sideways by becoming larger, or inward by becoming smaller. All but one of your sores are moving inward, which is the natural way of healing."[185] Here is the formula of the salve he applies:

Goat grease ⎫
Swine grease ⎪
             ⎬   add zinc oxide[186]
Oil ⎪
Frankincense ⎭

Note again the frankincense, libanotós. The salve is in fact a perfumed zinc oxide ointment, fit for twentieth century use. Greasy applications such as this one were kept for clean wounds near healing.[187] They were supposed to make the flesh grow, and so strong was the belief that it required a special verb, sarcophyésai or "making-the-flesh-grow."[188]

Nature was doing it, of course, in those days as well as today; but some still think they are doing it. They can use a verb from the Oxford dictionary: to incarn.

Wounds As Diseases: Hippocratic Theory

The gist of these ten cases is that Hippocrates scored 50 percent on the two basic questions about wounds, questions now too elementary to ask: should a wound be allowed to bleed, and should a wound give pus? The answer in both cases was a shaky yes and no, after a lot of thinking.

It was a peculiar, or shall I say non-ripe way of thinking, typical of the time. While the Greeks had been training their bodies for the Olympic Games ever since 776 B.C., [189] their mental gymnastics began to gather momentum only with the first great philosopher, Thales of Miletos, around 600 B.C., barely a century before the birth of Hippocrates. In the Golden Age, logic was still a new technique and little understood, so that a Greek might well accept for a fact what we would instantly recognize as an hypothesis.[190]

The word hypothesis itself occurs for the first time in the Hippocratic book On Ancient Medicine, a book in which the author, possibly Hippocrates himself, starts out with an argument against hypotheses and in the same breath sets forth a new one of his own.[191] Testing by experiment was not felt to be a necessity. The few experiments worthy of the name in the Hippocratic books are mostly analogies with irrelevant facts, which are

Ἰατρός

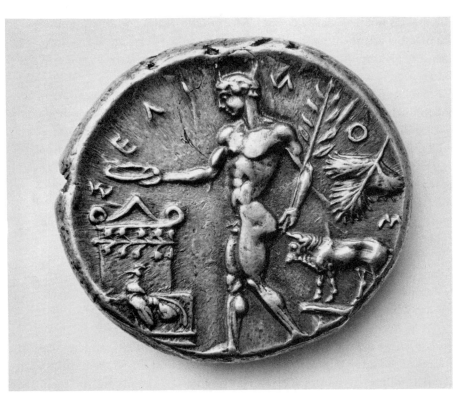

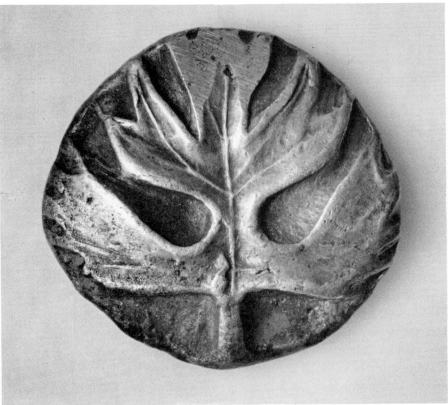

4.32 Wild celery (*sélinon*) was a wound drug and a noble plant. Here it appears on two coins from Selinunte, c.467 and 520 B.C., where it still grows. Enlarged about four times.

themselves not necessarily correct. An example: water coming from melted ice or snow is unhealthy, having lost its lightest parts. Proof: in winter, measure an amount of water; let it freeze; the next day thaw it, and you will find a good deal less.[192]

I mention this to explain the feeling of frustration that may come from the following few pages of medical theory. Intelligence without method could not lead far; the results might be rational, but not scientific. Indeed, Greek medicine, great as it was as an art, was a failure as a science.[193] The Hippocratic books are usually at their lowest when they would be scientific; their peaks are abstract thoughts. One of the loftiest is the very definition of thought: utterly Greek, it extends the idea of exercise from the body to the soul: "Thought is the soul's walk abroad" ("La réflexion est l'exercice de l'âme").[194]

Impressed as they were by the possibilities of the "soul's walk," the Greek physicians studied disease primarily by giving it a lot of thought. Nobody expressed this better than Charles Daremberg: "they tried to explain Nature while shutting their eyes."[195]

The result was an overall, synthetic, but wholly imaginary theory of disease, in which the basic disturbance, and therefore the treatment, was always of the same kind, even in the case of a wound.[196] The reasoning went about as follows. In nature everything is balanced. "Too much" or "too little" causes an imbalance, which is disease. The actual components of the body that may go out of balance are the celebrated four humors: blood, phlegm, yellow bile, and black bile. In the normal body these humors are harmoniously mixed; disease ensues if they are mixed in the wrong proportions, or if they become unmixed. Something like it happens when the Scythians shake milk in a pot, and the part that they call "butter" gathers on top;[197] or when one adds the juice of the fig tree to milk, and the curdle separates out.[198] How these four particular principles were chosen by the Greeks is not clear, and even the origin of the theory is uncertain, except that it was just one of the many schemes that the Greeks had been devising since roughly 600 B.C. in their quest for fundamental laws and symmetries. Nowadays, these schemes look naive and worthless (Fig. 4.33); but we must beware of taking them too lightly, for they may mean more than at first appears. The pentagram of Pythagoras, for instance (Fig. 4.33 bottom), which became the secret pass-sign and symbol of the Pythagorean sect, contains the geometry of the golden section, the secret aesthetic formula of Greek architecture, which was rediscovered only during the Renaissance.[199]

Ἰατρός

As to the scheme of the four humors, its success suggests that it was perfectly suited to the needs of mankind. Its fourfold symmetry had the appeal of an order that could also embrace the whole of nature: the four humors could be made to fit the four seasons,[200] four winds, four states of matter, four tastes, four temperaments (the word means "blends") with all the temperaments in between. There was no truth to speak of in the scheme, but it could serve as a framework for many truths. So it stood as the basic theory of medicine for over two millennia, and slowly grew to swallow the entire macrocosm—including, when their time came, the Four Apostles.[201]

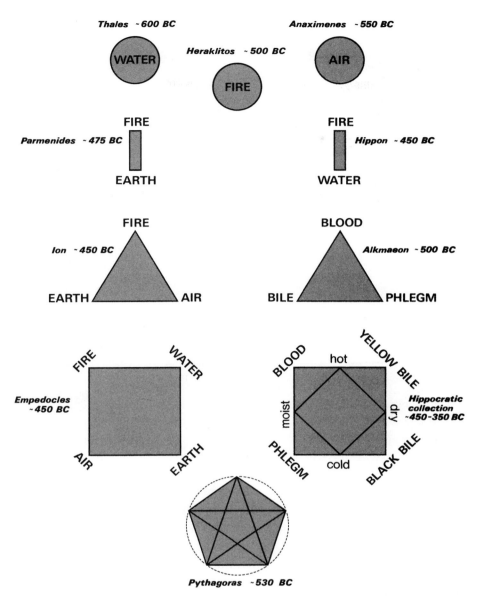

4.33 The search for universal laws and symmetries in Greek philosophy and medicine, during the two centuries in which Hippocrates lived.

Greek aesthetics had a penchant for fourfold symmetries. Law is to gymnastics, says Socrates, what justice is to medicine: almost a credo of the Greek physician (Fig. 4.34).[202]

᾿Ιατρός

Thanks to the theory of the four humors, any pain or lump could be explained as a "distemper" or disharmony of the blend, the likeliest humors to misbehave being phlegm and bile. The treatment followed logically. It was the triple, indefensible commandment:

Bleed, to get rid of bad humors.
Starve, to prevent new ones from forming.
Purge, to get rid of the rest, "from above and from below," or from any other exit.

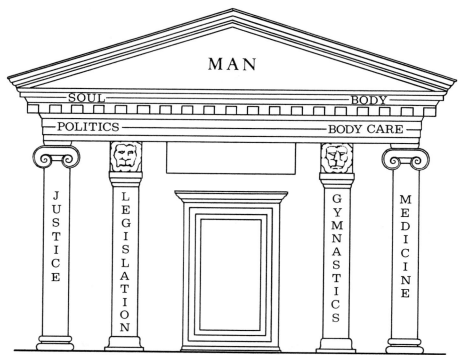

MAN

SOUL — BODY

POLITICS — BODY CARE

JUSTICE | LEGISLATION | GYMNASTICS | MEDICINE

4.34 Another fourfold symmetry, explained by Socrates. The scheme shows the importance of gymnastics for the Greeks, its position relative to medicine, and the parallel between medicine and justice.

Nobody seemed to worry that the good humors might go out with the bad ones.

There were other theories as well; we are less informed about them, perhaps because they were less popular. One maintained that sickness is due to undigested "residues"; [203] another, that all diseases are due to "breaths" or winds, a concept that we shall find also in India and China. In practice, however, the treatment must have been similar, whatever the school of thought of the physician.

All this is well known; but there is a forgotten part of the story, equally interesting, which explains how disease happens at the microscopic level. [204] Of course, the Greeks had no such instrument as a microscope, but they had a much more powerful and dangerous one: "what escapes the sight of the eyes can be seized with the sight of the mind." [205] The result was a story so well knit that it would be acceptable even today to many a layman.

'Ιατρός

Imagine, to begin, the soft parts of the body as they were conceived at the time: a solid mass called flesh, penetrated by the very fine roots of a dead-end plumbing system, the small veins (*phlébia*, "venules"). So there were at least three things that could go wrong: the blood, the venules, and the flesh. [206]

Of the three, blood was regarded as the worst offender, because it was liable to spill out easily and therefore to "stagnate." This was supposed to be dangerous, because one of the key propositions in Greek medicine maintained that stagnating blood will decay.

There was an easy comparison here (though never stated) with the fresh water of a brook and the smelly water of a marsh. Blood was not thought to "circulate," of course, but it was supposed to move back and forth in some obscure fashion; if spilled out, it would have to stagnate. In decaying, it might even become pus.[207] Galen, writing five hundred years later, was not sure that he could accept a full transformation of blood to pus, but the decay of spilled blood was "certain."[208] The ounce of truth here is that blood clots left in a wound do tend to become pastures for bacteria, and thereby induce pus.

The second possible source of disease was the flesh. If irritated, it could undergo spasms. Spasms covered a large family of symptoms, ranging from shivering to cramps to convulsions and tetanus: the Greek craving for synthesis could not fail to see them all in the same light.[209] The stated causes of spasm were cold,[210] excessive bleeding,[211] and drastic purging with hellebore,[212] which did throw people into agonizing convulsions. When the flesh went into spasm, it could either attract blood out of the venules[213] or simply squeeze it out, whereupon the "out-veined" blood would decay (Plate 4.1).[214] Therefore, spasms were an important mechanism of disease. In pleurisy, for example, "the chill is considered to be the cause and the beginning of the disease."[215]

The third possible site of disease were the venules. They could spill out their blood by several mechanisms, either by sheer fatigue[216] or by falling into a spasm themselves. A convulsing venule could either tear itself apart and bleed,[217] or trap the blood into a sort of cul-de-sac, whence it would seep out and decay (Plate 4.2).[218] Chills after a wound were thought to come from the vessels,[219] presumably because the exposed vessels caught cold and convulsed.

I mention these apparently wild theories because the venules were too small to see except with the *gnómes ópsei*, "the sight of the mind." Yet one part of the guess was exceedingly good. Small vessels do have spasms, and in 1969 the electron microscope showed that irritated venules do, in a sense, tear themselves apart (Fig. 4.35).[220]

Now apply all this to a wound. Normally the flesh is kept warm under the skin. Once exposed to the outer world, however, it is bound to catch cold and suffer:

> Wounds love warmth; naturally, because they exist under shelter; and naturally they suffer from the opposite; and naturally the veins too, which live in warmth.[221]

'Ιατρός

> The bones, the teeth, the tendons have cold as an enemy, warmth as a friend; because it is from these parts that come the spasms, the tetanus, the feverish chills, that the cold induces, that heat removes.[222]

From this comes the refrain about keeping wounds warm.[223] If chilled, the parts *around* the wound will develop spasms, attract blood, become soaked with it, and decay. The beauty of this thought (corruption originates *around* the wound), however wrong it may sound today, is that it shows how the Greeks struggled to explain the mechanism of what we call infection—or in their terms, corruption. They could have no idea that the cause was

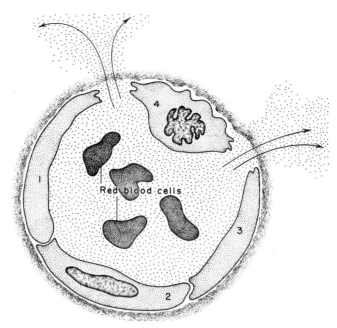

4.35 "Spasm in a venule" as it really occurs. This drawing shows a microscopic vein, in cross section and enlarged about 5000 times, as it would appear in the electron microscope. The inner surface of the vessel is lined with flat cells (1–4) applied against a supporting membrane. Chemical agents, such as histamine, cause some of these cells to contract (top right) and pull away from each other, thereby creating gaps through which fluid escapes. The escaping fluid causes the swelling typical of inflammation.

something deposited on the surface of the wound. Therefore, using their principle that "stagnating blood decays," they rationalized that the trouble had to arise all around the wound: *blood was attracted there, and turned into pus.* This thought is stated or hinted many times in the Collection; for instance, "all wounds draw their inflammation and swelling from the surrounding parts, because of the blood flowing into them."[224] The mistake here is that the inflamed surrounding parts are not *causing* any trouble to the wound; they are suffering from infection just as much as the wound itself, indeed they are fighting it off *with the help of the blood.* But if we accept the Greek way of thinking, at this point the absurd conclusion becomes perfectly rational:

'Ιατρός

Bleed the wound

either by encouraging its hemorrhage, or by slitting an appropriate vein elsewhere. "In every recent wound . . . it is expedient to cause blood to flow from it abundantly, and as may seem seasonable; for thus will the wound and the adjacent parts be less attacked with inflammation . . . When the blood flows they become drier and less in size, as being thus dried up. Indeed what prevents the healing . . . is the decay of the blood."[225]

This notion of drying up the wound explains also the dangerous practice of bandaging tightly, as well as the ultimate aberration: "and in a word, the greater the wound, the more severe and protracted should the regimen be."[226]

All this must have been on the mind of the Hippocratic author (or was it the master himself?) who dropped the loaded remark: "The wound, I believe, is a disease."[227]

Pus or No Pus

A key fact about wounds in ancient Greece is hidden in the very word for wound: *hélkos*. It just cannot be translated accurately. The title of the treatise about wounds, *Perí Helkón*, is translated by Adams *On Ulcers* and by Littré *On Wounds*. Both are right, for the word *hélkos* covers both situations.[228] Today this is shocking, because we associate the notion of ulcer with delayed healing and the foul look of infection; but in ancient Greece that was precisely what happened to most wounds. There was no need to make a distinction. It is even more shocking that this was still largely true for both translators, Adams and Littré, who lived during the first half of the nineteenth century. The situation had been summed up a short time earlier by a commentator who failed "to recognize any difference between wounds and ulcers, except that which was contributed by time."[229]

Infection being almost inevitable, and therefore almost "natural," the Greek physician had ambivalent feelings about pus: it could not be something entirely bad. Sometimes he took it as corrupted blood, and as such it was definitely bad: this was the turbid and smelly variety which he called *ichór*.[230] But other times he interpreted it more benevolently as phlegm, "ripened" by a process of "coction," *pepsis*, never clearly defined, which I visualize rather like the ripening of Camembert. This kind of pus was odorless; it flowed "pure and white," and it was a good omen.[231] Something to hope for.

Today, of course, the meaning of the two kinds of pus is obvious: severe infection versus more benign infection. But the Greeks, mistaking the benign infection for the "good and natural" course of events, did their best to encourage it: a fatal mistake, which survived as surgical gospel until the nineteenth century. Not until Lord Lister did it become apparent that encouraging "good and laudable pus" was playing the game of the bacteria. In defense of the iatrós, I must say that he had several reasons for believing that pus was a good thing; and there is some deceptive truth in each of his reasons.

Ἰατρός

First, patients with white and "pure" pus had a better prognosis than those with "bad" pus. This is true.

Second, in a bruised wound suppuration helps because it cleans out the dead tissue.[232] This is defensible. Bits of dead or doomed tissue prevent the wound from closing. Modern surgeons prefer to pick them out, by a painstaking operation called toilette or débridement of the wound. The Greeks cut out the major pieces[233] and let the pus destroy the rest—a cunning use of natural processes (Fig. 4.36).

Third, "if swellings do not appear on severe wounds, it is a great evil."[234] This is true: in a wound, total absence of swelling and pus *may* mean that the

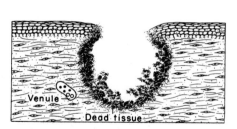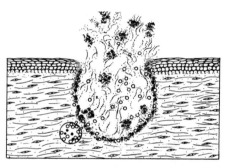

4.36 *Left:* A bruised wound. Before its margins can join again, the dead, bruised tissue (black) must be removed, either by natural processes or by surgery. If such a wound becomes infected (*right*) the dead tissue can be removed incidentally by the pus: that is, by the white blood cells (small circles) that have swarmed in to destroy the bacteria. This cleaning operation was a practical, but dangerous use of wound infection in ancient Greece.

body is incapable of defense. By the shaky logic of the iatrós, this proposition could be restated: "no pus is bad, so pus is good."

Fourth, the Greeks believed that "good, white pus" actually prevented more dangerous complications.[235] This, too, was the result of their peculiar logic; it was somewhat like arguing that foggy weather prevents rainy weather. You have either one or the other. Nowadays one would say that "white pus" is the least of evils.

Fifth and last, the concept of "good pus" was necessary to fill a slot in current medical theory. There had to be a process whereby bad humors could be eliminated, by "ripening" and a final "setting aside," *apóstasis* (hence the ancient English term *apostem* for "abscess").[236]

Still, despite these arguments in favor of pus, the Greeks could not fail to notice that many wounds healed perfectly well without suppuration. Therefore, every wound posed a dilemma: was it one that could heal directly, or one that should be "helped" to suppurate?

It is generally easier to help infection than to fight it. I suspect that the iatrós was more successful in the first task. His decision depended on the presence of bruised tissue. If there was any, he tried to clean it out "by taking the wound rapidly through suppuration."[237] A typical drug placed on the wound for that purpose was:

'Ιατρός

Wool as greasy as can be procured,
dip it in very little water,   boil to good consistency[238]
add ⅓ wine

I would not be surprised if greasy wool, stuffed in a wound, did indeed help it to suppurate. Note that this "taking the wound through suppuration" was to be done "rapidly." The recommendation to keep wounds open and oozing for a long time to extend the supposed drainage of bad humors was a later aberration; it is never advised in the Hippocratic Collection. However, it is already mentioned in a fragment by Diokles of Karystos, a younger contemporary of Hippocrates, as "making the wound last" after dog bites.[239]

To prevent suppuration, there was that special set of drugs called enhemes, used especially on fresh wounds. Several enhemes were dry powders to be sprinkled on the wound. They could be washed off with vinegar or wine. Here are four:[240]

Lead oxide (*flower of silver*)

{ Lead metal powdered together with
  Zinc oxide (*? ashes from Cyprus*)[241]

{ Copper oxide, black (*copper scales*)
  Copper sulphate (*chalcitis*)[242]

Alum

These powders are crude antiseptics, in that they kill bacteria at the price of killing tissue cells[243] (some also carry the danger of lead poisoning). Specific antibacterial weapons would not come until the twentieth century.

Other enhemes were moist, like this one, which must also have had antiseptic properties:[244]

White vinegar, strong
Honey
Alum from Egypt   } boil together
Sodium carbonate, roasted (*nitron*)
Bile, a little

Note that two of these five ingredients came from Egypt; a third, honey, was an Egyptian favorite. Another antiseptic enheme based on honey is recommended after various operations on the nose:

Honey
Copper oxide, red (*flower of copper*) } boil together[245]

The fascination with copper, used in so many forms, may also betray Egyptian influence; it will carry over into Roman medicine. Some copper compounds existed in nature (remember malachite and chrysocolla, sources of the Egyptian *wadj*); others could be prepared fairly easily. The mines of Cyprus, famous since the third millennium B.C.,[246] supplied the metal in such large amounts that the island itself, Kypros, gave its name to copper. Cyprus was also a source of zinc. Its zinc ores, heated in water, produced zinc carbonates and hydrosilicates, called "cadmian earth" or simply cadmia. When the mixture was stirred with a reed (calamus), these hydrosilicates stuck to it; hence the name "calamine," which is still applied to zinc lotions. Cadmia, when heated, gave off a vapor of zinc oxide, which condensed on the wall of the furnace. This was scraped off and called *spodium* ("ash"), another favorite wound drug of antiquity[247]—and a favorite drug of modern dermatology.

'Ιατρός

185

Wine and Vinegar As Antiseptics

Vinegar owes its sting to acetic acid, which is a powerful antiseptic.[248] A 5 percent solution—about the same strength as in vinegar—was tested recently in Makerere, Uganda, on a series of patients suffering from burns and superficial wounds. Some bacteria proved resistant, but infections with *Pseudomonas* did very well. As expected, the dressings were painful; but the pain did not last.[249] Vinegar is definitely a rational wound-wash.

As for wine, it has been the commonest item in wound treatment since the Greeks. This record alone suggests that there should be something effective in it. The first question to arise is whether this something could be alcohol.

The 9–11 percent concentrations of ethyl alcohol in ordinary wines have very little effect on bacteria. The optimal strength of alcohol-water mixtures against *E. coli* and staphylococci is 70 percent by weight.[250] Yet most experiments with wine as an antiseptic have proven successful (Fig. 4.37). The first were published in 1892 by Alois Pick, an Austrian military doctor. They came in the wake of an epidemic of cholera in Paris, during which a Dr. Rabuteau had noticed that wine drinkers were relatively spared by the disease, and he therefore advised everybody to mix wine into the water.[251] To test this theory, Dr. Pick took cultures of cholera and typhoid bacilli, and added 1 cc of each to each of five flasks containing either water, wine (red or white), or 50–50 water-wine mixtures. In the two flasks with water, the bacteria flourished; whereas the wine, straight or diluted, killed all cholera vibrios within ten or fifteen minutes. Although some of the typhoid bacilli were still alive at that time, they too had disappeared after twenty-four hours. Dr. Pick concluded that during cholera or typhoid epidemics it was advisable to drink water that had been mixed some time earlier with wine.

This forceful, one-page article was followed by many others. Despite the variety of wines and authors, a review of the results in 1951 showed consistent data: wine kills cholera vibrios in 0.5–10 minutes, *E. coli* in 25–60 minutes, and *E. typhi* in 5–240 minutes.[252] Rhine wines, both red and white, kill staphylococci in one hour, or in two if they are diluted with equal amounts

4.37 Bactericidal power of two wines (alcoholic content 9.8 percent); compared with that of 10 percent ethyl alcohol, as tested on the bacterium *E. coli*.

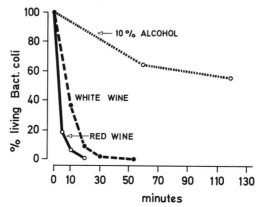

of water.[253] In Bordeaux, Prof. Ribéreau-Gayon found his strain of staphylo-cocci so sensitive that he had to dilute the wine in order to obtain any bacter-ial growth after fifteen minutes.[254]

This long list should be convincing enough; but I resorted once again to my bacteriological friends for first-hand confirmation, using Greek wine. Two samples of white wine—one resinated, one not—were obtained from a farmer in Crete; they were tested against bacterial cultures on agar plates, by the "center well" method that had also been used to test copper compounds. Both wines behaved as if they contained an antibacterial substance, yet this could not be the 10 percent alcohol, because tests with the latter proved to have no effect. Thereafter, four bottles of red wine were sacrificed to science: a Chianti, a Beaujolais, a Dôle du Valais, and a Rioja from Spain. Samples were infected with *Staphylococcus aureus*, *Streptococcus pyogenes*, *E. coli*, *Proteus mirabilis*, and *Pseudomonas aeruginosa*. After six hours no live bacteria could be recovered, except a few staphylococci, but they too failed to grow after twelve hours.[255]

The antiseptic power of wine is no myth. Since it cannot depend on alcohol alone—in fact, it persists when the alcohol is removed[256]—it was thought for some time that it depended on a mutual reinforcement between alcohol and the organic acids of which wine is rich.[257] Recent studies from Bordeaux have taken an entirely new departure. They pin down the mechanism to the anthocyanes, a subgroup in the large group of polyphenols present in wine.[258] The most important member of this group of compounds, as regards antibac-terial effects, is also the principal pigment of red wines, malvoside or oenoside; there is a colorless equivalent for white wines (Fig. 4.38). This pigment is al-

4.38 A relative of phenol, the historic antiseptic—in wine: malvoside or oenoside, a polyphenol.

ready present in the grapes, but combined with a carbohydrate and thus not antiseptic; during alcoholic fermentation it splits free and becomes activated. This hydrolytic cleavage cannot take place unless the solution is acid; but all the steps in the sequence work out as if prearranged, because wine is very acid. The average pH for red wines is 3.6, which is also the degree of acidity that corresponds to optimal solubility of the red pigment.[259] One would there-fore expect the bactericidal power of wine to increase with age; and so it does, in unison with the behavior of the pigment, as shown in the following tabula-tion. The bactericidal index was obtained by finding the maximum dilution of wine in water that would kill a given strain of *E. coli* in no more than ten minutes but no less than five minutes. For example, an index of 17 means that the maximum active dilution was $\frac{1}{17}$:[260]

Ἰατρός

Age of wine	Bactericidal index (dilution factor)
Fermented must	0
Wine of same year	11
3-year wine	14
4 " "	16
5 " "	16
6 " "	16
9 " "	19
10 " "	19
14 " "	17
23 " "	16
29 " "	16
36 " "	16
46 " "	12
56 " "	9
82 " "	6

The effect of wine is thus truly bactericidal, not bacteriostatic. Red and white wines are about equal in this respect. Most effective are the strong southern wines like port, among which the palm goes to a Greek wine from Samos, which kills E. coli within three minutes.[261] Other polyphenols in wine may help, but their concentration is small.[262] It is pleasing to know that the bacteria are killed by substances really present in native wine, not by the sulfurous anhydride that is now almost universally added to prevent acetic fermentation.[263]

So the Greeks were quite right to pour wine into wounds and over dressings. Wine has to be used generously, however, because its power is short-lived: the active principles are rapidly bound and inactivated by proteins,[264] which explains why wine is not currently sold with first-aid kits.

By cleansing wounds with wine the Greeks were actually disinfecting them with a polyphenol, a more complex version of Lister's phenol—the pioneer drug of antiseptic surgery. And the polyphenol of wine, malvoside—weight for weight and tested on E. coli—is 33 times more powerful than phenol.[265]

The Reverse of the Coin: Cures That Made Matters Worse

Ἰατρός

All in all, Greek care for the wound itself probably did little harm and some good. It is quite another story when one comes to the general treatments, aimed at "helping the wound" more indirectly. They range from bad to hair-raising. Imagine cutting the veins of a patient who has already half bled to death through his wound, plus the combined effects of enemas, purges, and vomiting, plus the side effects of poisoning with hellebore, and all of this on a starvation diet. These were times when medicine worked for evolution.

Hellebore alone could claim a long chapter in the history of human error. Even the name applies to two wholly unrelated plants: "black" hellebore, which is now identified with *Helleborus*, better known as Christmas rose (Fig. 4.39), and "white" hellebore, which is *Veratrum* (Fig. 4.40).[266] All they have in common is an almost perverse endowment with poisonous principles, so irritating that they will do something wherever applied. Armed with roots of either kind of hellebore, the iatrós could raise blisters; evoke sneezing, vomiting, and diarrhea; induce delirium, muscular cramps, asphyxia; even cause the heart to stop. Scientifically these effects are fascinating, but too dangerous to be harnessed.

In essence: both hellebores tend to kill, but before doing so, they have a few side effects, including nausea and diarrhea—which is all that the Greek physician really wanted. One might as well shoot a gun blindly in order to enjoy the noise and the smell. It is no wonder that some patients chose the wrong effects, convulsed, and died.[267] The saving grace of hellebore was that it caused vomiting so fast that the patient stood a chance of getting rid of it before absorbing a lethal dose.[268] In the words of Herophilos the Alexandrian, it behaved "like a powerful general: it sets up a great stir inside, and then gets out with the first."[269]

Having survived the hellebore, the patient had to contend with his diet. The attending physician made a strong point about it, for the proper choice of food was supposed to be the foundation of the medical art.[270] Normal food, for the sick, was supposed to be as bad as the food of wild beasts would be for normal human beings.[271] The safest item was a sort of watered-down porridge, barley slops, with much ado about the proper dilution. There was a whole book about it, surnamed *The Ptisan*.[272] It is often said that the ancient Greeks recognized the importance of diet, which is true; but whatever diet they prescribed was unwholesome even for the healthy. They thought that there was something wrong with almost every vegetable; fruit was even worse; the safest foods were meat and cereals. This expensive regimen retained its authority for a couple of millennia. Many of those who could afford it certainly headed toward vitamin deficiency.[273]

And finally, the Greeks thought they could help a wound to heal also by working on it locally with whole families of drugs: *sarcotics* to make flesh grow, *epispastics* to attract humors, *catheretics* to excite the tissues, *mundifiers* to clean sordid ulcers, *emollients* to produce supple scars, and so on. With the exception of a few antiseptics, all this was wishful thinking. But so intense was the wish, so true was the need, and so great the authority of Hippocrates, that the use of such drugs lasted until World War I. They should have died out about 1920. Some are still for sale.

This is a thorny subject. People want to be healed, and industry has responded with healing drugs and salves. Some are even advertised in French as *cicatrisants* or "scar-inducers." Yet I am not aware of a single substance that can make a wound heal faster. In experimental animals it is possible to improve certain properties of the wound, such as its tensile strength; but a proven, reliable accelerator of wound healing is not yet available.[274]

Ἰατρός

189

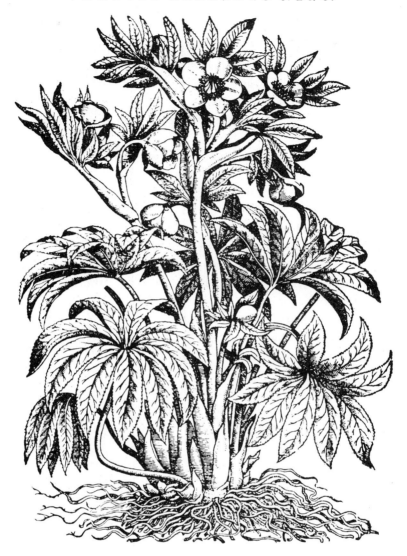

Dell'Elleboro nero .   Cap. CLIII.

LO ELLEBORO nero si chiama Melampodio : percioche si dice , che Melampo pastore di ca-
pre fu il primo , che purgò , & sanò con esso le figliuole di Preto diuentate furiose. Produce le
frondi uerdi , simili à quelle del platano , ma minori , & quasi simili à quelle dello sphondilio,
ruuidette , piu nere , & assai piu intagliate . Produce il fusto aspro : & i fiori , che nel bianco porpo-
reggiano , racemosi : & il seme simile al cnico , il quale chiamano in Anticira sesamoide , & usanlo
per le purgationi . Le radici ha l'elleboro nero sottili , & nere , le quali hanno origine da un capo
quasi simile alla cipolla , delle quali è l'uso . Nasce nelle colline , & luoghi aspri , & secchi . Il piu
ualoroso è quello , che si porta da gli infrascritti luoghi , come d'Anticira , doue nasce il nero uera-
mente ellettissimo. Debbesi elleggere quello , che è ben carnoso , & ben pieno , che ha poca midol-

4.39 Black hellebore (Christmas rose, a Ranunculacea), the all-purpose drug of
the Greeks. It produced centuries of diarrhea and vomiting, some deaths, and
presumably no cures. The plant is about one foot high.

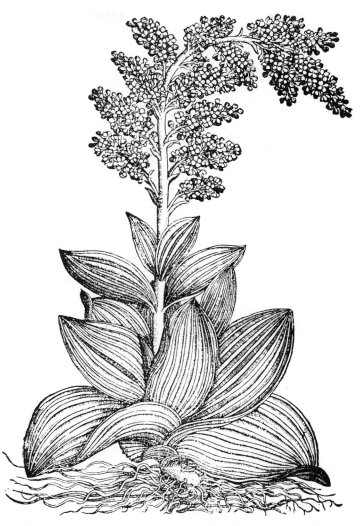

4.40 White hellebore (*Veratrum*, a Liliacea), another favorite Greek drug. A much taller plant and quite unrelated to black hellebore, it too is loaded with poisons.

The Limits of Greek Surgery: Amputation

The Hippocratics did not know how to amputate. However, in private practice they had to deal with amputation happening by itself. Poor circulation can lead to gangrene of a whole limb; if the dead part dries up fast enough, bacterial infection is held in check, the tissues become mummified, and they eventually fall off. This process is relatively benign, though horrible to see. The Greeks called it "blackening" (*melasmós*). Here is what they did about it:

> With regard to the gangrene of fleshy parts . . . when the forearm and leg drop off, the patients readily recover . . . Those parts of the body which are below the

Ἰατρός

191

boundaries of the blackening are to be removed at the joint, as soon as they are completely dead and have lost their sensibility; care being taken not to wound any living part; for if the part . . . which is cut off give pain, and if it should prove not be quite dead, there is great danger lest the patient may swoon away from the pain, and such swoonings often are immediately fatal [*the swooning was called* lipothymia, *literally "soul-leaving"; it was rather the effect of blood loss*]. I have known of the thigh-bones . . . to drop off on the eightieth day; the parts below the knee were separated at the knee on the twentieth day, and as I thought, too early for it appeared to me that this should be done more guardedly.[275]

In another case, "the bones of the leg . . . separated at its middle on the sixtieth day."[275] The account concludes that "such cases . . . are more formidable to look at than to treat . . . for they come to a crisis for themselves; only the diet must be attended to . . . and the body is to be placed in the proper positions."[276]

In essence, the iatrós just stands by while the limb slowly drops off, and nature has time to plug the large vessels, by a beautiful, built-in mechanism. He helps now and then by removing bits of dead tissue, but he will not even saw off the dead bone, which, as explained in the text, sometimes sticks out alone long after the flesh has gone. His wise, conservative attitude was justified: he did not have the know-how, and nature usually did.

Links with Egyptian Medicine

Wound care in ancient Greece was based on ten salient techniques (Plate 4.3). When these are compared with their counterparts in the Smith papyrus, it turns out that the two basic Egyptian methods are not being used by the Hippocratics. The slab of fresh meat is reserved for very special situations (a piece of meat bigger than the big toe, six fingers long, treated with oil of roses, etc., and attached to a thread, went to soothe ulcers of the matrix[277]); the honey-and-grease ointment has disappeared, and honey alone is rarely used.[278]

However, several drugs came from Egypt, and some Egyptian ideas must have traveled with them. Among the materials specifically mentioned as Egyptian are nitron, alum, perfumes, thread, and leather.[279] A heritage of ideas is more difficult to prove, but certainly present.[280] The Hippocratic texts constantly refer to humors that "fix" themselves somewhere in the body and cause disease processes, such as suppuration.[281] The Ebers papyrus had spoken of fixation 1200 years earlier.[282] Even the *ukhedu* may have crossed the Mediterranean; some scholars see it hinted in the theory whereby disease is caused by "undigested residues."[283] The Greeks would amply repay their Egyptian medical heritage by founding Alexandria of Egypt, which became a beacon of medical science.

Ἰατρός

Authentic Clinical Histories

We are now more ready to appreciate a very unusual gift of history: original notes about Greek patients. Although there are no complete clinical histories of the time, there do exist several sets of short notes that traveling physicians took during their *epidemics* or "visits abroad" to various islands and cities of the Greek world. These epidemics make up seven books of the Hippocratic Collection. Most of them read like personal memos, jotted down in haste; the iatrós recorded only a few facts that he thought to be especially important and probably never meant them to be published in this form. At times one wonders why they were preserved at all.

I have chosen some cases dealing with wounds from Books IV and V. The author may not be Hippocrates himself, because the style is not so elaborate as in Books I and III, traditionally believed to be from the hand of the master. As a result, none of these cases, so far as I know, has been considered worthy of an English translation. Yet the text is gripping for its ability to convey the essential and for its obvious interest in truth. We shall use these notes as a practical seminar in Greek pathology, in which we will try to guess what the iatrós had in mind when he chose to record a given fact.[284]

> Billos had been wounded in the back; much air came out of the wound, with noise; he bled; he was treated with enhemes and healed.
> The same happened to Dyslytas.[285]

Survival from war wounds such as these must have encouraged physicians to cut their way into the chest.

> Aristippos was hit high in the abdomen by a powerful and dangerous arrow. Terrible belly pains. Soon there was inflammation. He did not void from below; he retched; dark bile; and when he vomited he seemed relieved; but a little later the terrible pains returned. Abdomen like in ileus [*intestinal paralysis*]; heat, thirst. He died within the seven days.[286]

Clinically this must be a perforation of the stomach or colon, with peritonitis resulting in intestinal paralysis. Note the implications between the lines: not voiding is bad; vomiting helps. Another undercurrent is evident in the "seven days"; there is a whole Hippocratic book called *On Sevens*.[287] This emphasis reflects the preoccupation with detecting patterns of events in time, patterns that may help future prognoses.

> The man of Aenos, in Delos, wounded by a javelin in the back, on the left side, the wound was not painful.
> On the third day, sharp pain in the belly; no stools; an enema in the night brought some feces. The pain did not relent.
> On the fourth day it was in the loins and invaded the pubis and belly. He could not stay still. He threw up some dark bilious matter; eyes like those of people who faint.
> After five days he died; there was a little heat [*fever*].[288]

'Ιατρός

Probably another intestinal perforation, this time from the rear, ending in peritonitis. Note again the preoccupation with "days," and the standard treatment of wounds by voiding the intestine.

At Larissa, a man was wounded from behind by a broad lance held in the hands; the point came through under the navel, a long path. Livid, swollen. After the wound he felt at first a sharp pain, and the belly swelled up. The next day this patient was given a purge; he passed some bloody stools and died. It seemed that something was wrong with his intestine, and that blood filled the abdomen.[289]

Again a penetrating abdominal wound, but here the internal bleeding takes its toll before the peritonitis. "It seemed that his intestines were unwell," reads the text literally. To judge from the bloody stools, the intestines are perforated. The purge given under these conditions may have been the coup de grâce.

The following cases show that purging and inducing vomit belonged practically to first aid. To understand the first case, note the shape of Greek anchors at that time (Fig. 4.41).

In Salamina, the man who fell on the anchor was wounded in the belly. He suffered a lot. He took a potion and could not evacuate, neither from below, nor by vomiting.

The woman who cut her own throat was choking. She was given a purge much too late; it did loosen the belly.

The woman slave. A potion made her evacuate little from above, with choking, but a lot from below. She died in the night; she was a barbarian.[290]

4.41 An anchor from the time of Hippocrates. This shape, which was relatively new, may explain the case of the "man of Salamina" who fell on an anchor and was wounded in the belly. Greek coin, c.400 B.C.

Ἰατρός

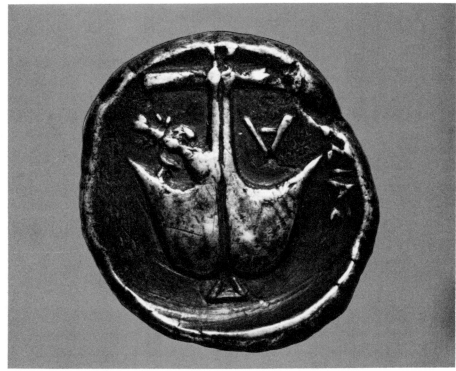

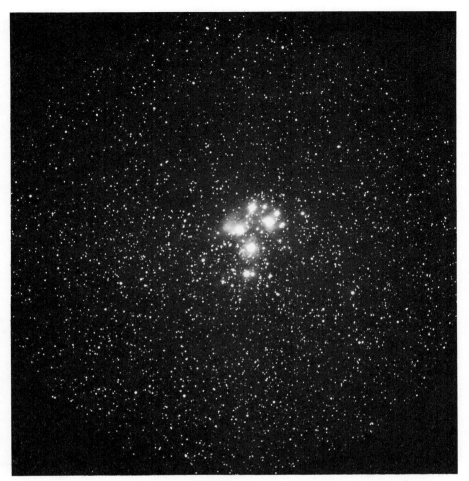

4.42 In trying to explain disease, the Greeks took into consideration even the stars, such as the Pleiades. Here they are today, minus one cluster that has faded away since the time of Hippocrates.

The last case, not a wound, shows the mental workings of the iatrós. His closing remark is not xenophobic; he is trying to find explanations by putting things together, including the fact that this particular woman, who reacted in this particular way, was a barbarian.

What were the relevant facts to put together? The dilemma was overpowering:

> Even for good physicians . . . it is difficult to work out, with insight, the right paths: [*a patient may have*] a pointed head, a flat nose, a hooked nose, a bilious nature, he may vomit with difficulty, or be atrabilious, or young, or having led a heedless life—it is difficult to put all these different things together into one sense.[291]

'Ιατρός

One important factor in any illness could be the weather. A good clinical history included a *katástasis* or "constitution" of the weather and stars at the time of illness.[292] Here is a brief example related to surgery (Fig. 4.42).

> About the time when the Pleiades set, the son of Metróphantos—wounded in the head with a shard (*óstrakon*) by another child—had fever. It was the twelfth day.

[*The reason:*] while washing himself, he hurt the edge of the wound, and caught cold. Soon the lips of the wound swelled up, and all around it the skin became thin. He was promptly trepanned. No pus came out, nor was there any relief. Pus seemed to form near the left ear (the wound was on that side). But then this abscess did not form, and the left shoulder filled up fast with pus. He died about the twenty-fourth day.[293]

This was a deadly infection spreading downward from a relatively minor wound of the head. The implications: maybe the stars had something to do with the malignant course, but the wound definitely caught cold. And disappointingly, the crown drill (Fig. 4.43) found no pus; perhaps there was some difficulty in the formation of pus (this is, indeed, the case in certain very severe infections).

Another patient taken away by infection:

The man of Malia, a loaded wagon passed over his chest and broke his ribs. After some time pus formed, low on his side. Cauterized below the spleen, and carrying a wound dressed with a tent, he went on for ten months. An opening appeared going from both sides into the epiploon [*a membrane inside the belly*] and leading, through a corrupt passage, from the open skin to the kidneys and bones.

It had not been recognized that this man's body was of bilious habit; and there was corruption in the body as well as in the disease: advanced corruption of the epiploon and other flesh, to be eliminated at once by means of a dry drug, while the man still had some strength. In fact, moist means, far from helping him, made the corruption worse. Moisture being retained by the tents, he was taken by shivering and fever; the corruption advanced; there dripped a putrid, blackish, stinking matter, of the same kind that flowed out before the beginning of the treatment; it did not come easily. It was recognized that the main disease was farther than beneath the skin. Even if all had been done in the best possible manner, it seemed that he could not have been saved. Diarrhea took him.[294]

Treatment poor; insight and honesty great. The bizarre notion that not only the body but the disease itself had become corrupt may be a way of

4.43 The crown drill (*prión*), sometimes used on the skull instead of the pointed drill (*trýpanon*). About one-half actual size.

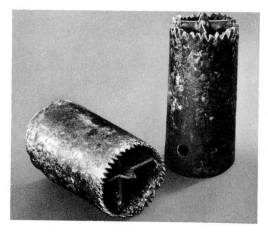

saying that the course had become "malignant." The "dry drugs" are the antiseptic enhemes.

Several histories relate to osteomyelitis in children—a reminder of what life can be like without antibiotics. Patches of bare bone, exposed by infection, were so common that they had a special name, now forgotten: *psíloma*, "a bareness":

The child of Phile, who had the bone laid bare in his forehead, had fever on the ninth day; the bone became livid; he died.

The same happened to the child of Phanias and to the child of Euergetes. The bone becomes livid, there is fever, the skin comes off the bone, and no pus appears.[295]

The cases of osteomyelitis reappear in *Epidemics VII*, slightly modified, and with this addition:

Trepanation brought out of the bone itself a thin ichor, serous, yellowish, stinking, deadly. In such cases vomiting may also occur, and spasms towards the end, and sometimes loud cries, and sometimes paralysis, on the left if the wound is on the right, on the right if it is on the left.

The child of Theodoros exposed himself to the sun on the ninth day. Fever came on the tenth day from a bareness of the bone which was, as one might say, nothing at all. During the fever the part became livid, the skin came off; many loud cries; on the twenty-second day the belly swelled up, especially toward the hypochondria; on the twenty-third he died . . .

The child of Isagoras was wounded in the back of the head, the bone was injured and became livid on the fifth day. He was healed, and the bone did not slough off.[296]

The next, appalling case of osteomyelitis can scarcely be the result of just a caries and infection; bad nutrition may well have interfered:[297]

At Cardias, the son of Metrodoros, after a toothache, had gangrene of the jaw; terrible overgrowth of flesh on his gums; he gave a moderate amount of pus; the molar teeth and the jaw fell out.[297]

But infection was unpredictable, then as now (Fig. 4.44):

The cobbler, while piercing a sole, stabbed his thigh with the awl, above the knee, to the depth of about a finger.

No blood came out and the wound closed fast, but the whole thigh swelled up, and the swelling gained the groin and the flank. This man died on the third day.

But the one who was wounded by an arrow in the groin, and whom we saw ourselves, was saved most unexpectedly: because neither was the point extracted (it was lying too deep) nor was there any hemorrhage worth mentioning, nor inflammation, nor lameness. When we departed he still had the point, and that was after six years. It was thought that it lay between the tendons, and that no vein or artery had been severed.[298]

ʼΙατρός

Note the unbiased report. The first man had a typical stab wound with practically no bleeding, and died, which fits the writer's scheme of things,

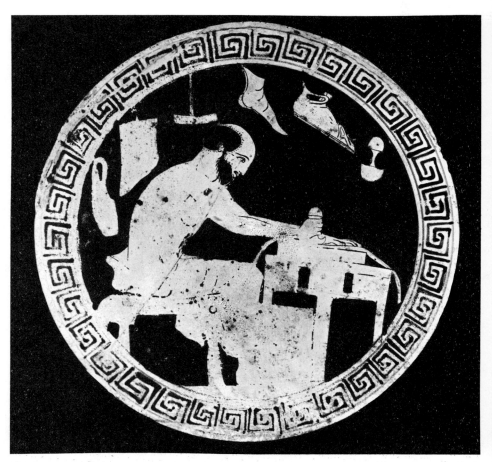

4.44 "The cobbler, while piercing a sole, stabbed his thigh . . ."

since bleeding helps. But he also tells that the second healed beautifully, though his hemorrhage "was not worth mentioning." The passage is also remarkable as being the only one, as far as I can ascertain, in which arteries and veins are clearly mentioned in a proper anatomical context[298] (the tendons, however, are still called *neura*; to this day some are called apo*neuro-ses*).

The next case is a war wound with something strange about it:

> Tychon, at the siege of Datos, was hit in the chest by a catapult, and after a while he was taken by convulsive laughter. It seemed to me that the physician who drew out the shaft left a piece of the lance in the diaphragm. Because he was in pain, the physician gave him an enema and a purge. He went through the first night very uncomfortably. When day came it seemed to the physician and to the others that he was better.
>
> Prognosis: with spasm developing, he will die promptly.
>
> The following night he was in pain and could not sleep; he lay mostly on his belly. On the morning of the third day he was seized by spasm and died.[299]

Ἰατρός

To the writer this case was important because he had observed, or believed he had observed, a strange kind of laughter (Littré rendered it as *rire plein de trouble*). It also seemed to him that a piece of the missile (Fig. 4.45) had been left in the *diaphrágma*. The diaphragm, also called *phrénes*, was currently thought to be the site of the soul and probably also of laughter (*phrenítis* meant "madness," hence the modern words *phrenetic* and *frantic*). This belief was certainly held five hundred years later when Pliny wrote his *Natural History*: "To this membrane unquestionably is due the subtilty of the intellect; it consequently has no flesh, but is of a spare sinewy substance. In it also is the chief seat of merriment, a fact that is gathered chiefly from tickling the arm-pits to which it rises . . . On this account there have been cases in battle and in gladiatorial shows of death caused by piercing the diaphragm that has been accompanied by laughter."[300] In the Hippocratic books, opinions vary. One book maintains that the diaphragm can scarcely be the seat of the soul, because . . . it has no hollowness in which to receive the good and the bad; but in another book the diaphragm can become delirious.[301] As the question remained open, it was worthwhile remarking that a piece of lance stuck in the diaphragm was associated with strange laughter.

The "spasms" in this case are possibly terminal convulsions, but in the next cases the spasms tell a more precise story:

> The one who was hit by a sharp arrow in the back a little below the neck had a wound that seemed barely worth mentioning, because it did not go deep. But before long, after the arrow was pulled out, he was arched back by convulsions like those of opisthotonos; and the jaws locked; and if he took some fluid into the mouth and tried to swallow it, it came back through the nostrils; and the other signs became worse, and on the second day he died.[302]

This must be tetanus, with its typical symptoms, opisthotonos (Fig. 4.46)[303] and "lock-jaw." Between the wound and the first symptoms, the incubation period is on the average six to seven days; an incubation period of one day, though not unheard of, is extremely rare. Hence, death "on the second day" should rather be understood as "on the second day since the onset of spasms." This also applies to the next two cases:

> The watchman of the big ship had the index and lower bone of the right hand crushed by the anchor. Inflammation developed, gangrene, and fever. He was purged from below, moderately; heat and pain mild; a bit of the finger came off. After the seventh day there came some pus, of passable quality. After this [*he complained*] of the tongue, he said he could not pronounce all [*words*].
> Prognosis: opisthotonos will come.

4.45 A tricuspid spearpoint, probably fired from a machine. About 348 B.C.

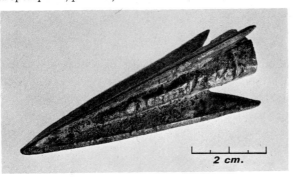

2 cm.

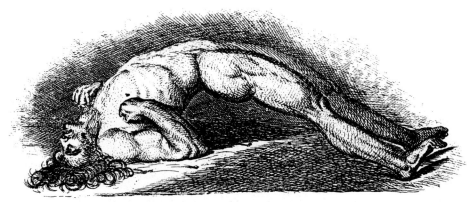

4.46 Opisthotonos ("the backward spasm") and lockjaw, the terrifying symptoms of tetanus. For the Greeks, spasms in general were diseases, not symptoms; the simplest was shivering.

> The jaws began to come tightly against each other, then the neck [*was taken*]. The third day the whole body arched back in a spasm, with sweat. On the sixth day after the prognosis he died.

> Telephanes, son of Harpalos and of the freedwoman, sprained his thumb.[304] It became inflamed and painful. And after this was over he went to the country. When he returned he had pains in the loins; he took a bath; during the night the jaws locked, and opisthotonos appeared; his spittle was frothy and could scarcely come through the teeth; he died on the third day.[305]

Peace to the watchman, he surely died of tetanus. As to Telephanes, it may seem strange that he caught tetanus by a simple sprain; but modern statistics allow it. In some series, less than half of the cases have a visible injury of the skin.[306] Besides, in another book the case of Telephanes is written up again, and that time he "hurt" and most likely "pricked" his thumb.[307]

Tetanus could also be the doctor's fault:

> Thrinon, son of Damon, had a wound at the ankle near the tendon, already mundified; it was irritated by a drug, and he came to die with opisthotonos.[308]

The spores of tetanus thrive in the feces of domestic animals. A clean folk, with plenty of animals and no soap, was well qualified to hand down the name of *tetanus*, "the stretches," and of *opisthotonos*, "the backward spasm."

Ἰατρός

The iatrós tended all these wounds the best he could. In the back of his mind, however, he knew that he was not alone. Witness these two thoughts, recorded in the *Epidemics:*

> Nature, without instruction or knowledge, does what is necessary.
> Natures are the physicians of diseases.[309]

The word for nature was *physis*. There is this message in the word *physician*.

The Drakon

When all else had failed; when the wound simply refused to heal, and no iatrós in town could think of a new and different plaster; when Gorgias had carried the arrowhead in his lung for a year and a half and filled sixty-seven pots of pus[310] and nobody could help him—there was still one hope: the temple of Asklepios. It was called the Asklepieion. Asklepios, the patron god of physicians (his name was Latinized as Aesculapius), did some healing of his own; and since his mortal pupils were loathe to take on a hopeless case,[311] his practice must have been a large one. It was an aid, not a competition, for official medicine. There is no evidence that the lay physicians ever objected to the assistance offered at the Asklepieia;[312] and besides, doctors have always welcomed help in hopeless cases. The two approaches were basically different, and could be well integrated in a society in which patient and physician alike firmly believed in the existence of the gods, with physicians themselves offering sacrifices to Asklepios.[313] "Prayer indeed is good—is written in a Hippocratic book—but while calling on the gods one must oneself lend a hand."[314] And in another book: "The gods are the real physicians, though people do not think so."[315]

The crowd of hapless beings who flocked to the temples of Asklepios knew that there would be no knife, no cautery to fear. The ritual would be simple: relax on the holy grounds, take in the beauty of the surroundings, listen to the hymns, and wait for the night.[316] Then each patient would be required to lie down in the sacred hall called the *ábaton* ("place of no walking") and wait for the god to appear and give advice in a dream. The priests would assist, receive a small gift for the god (perhaps a cheese cake or a votive tablet), and maybe act as guides to the amenities that came with the temple: the baths, the theater (Fig. 4.47). But all the medical gestures would be up to the god.

The god appeared sometimes in person, sometimes in the disguise of his sacred animals, the snakes and the dogs, which were tended in the temple.[317] Where were these creatures kept? How did they reach the patients? What did the sacred hall look like? Unfortunately, no artist has left us a picture, although at least one hundred shrines of Asklepios existed in ancient Greece.[318] But the priest saw to it that the results were recorded.

In Epidauros, in the ruins of the most celebrated Asklepieion, a large marble stele was found (Fig. 4.48), together with the remains of three others.[319] It preserves the case histories of seventy patients who came to the temple with a problem and shed it there, plus one who misbehaved toward the god and came away with a problem.[320] One of these cases is that of Gorgias.[321] Written in very simple style, about 350 B.C., with no punctuation or separations between the words, it reads like this (the opening phrase is a title):

'Ιατρός

GORGIAS OF HERAKLEIA WITH PUS IN A BATTLE HE HAD BEEN WOUNDED BY AN ARROW IN THE LUNG AND FOR A YEAR AND A HALF HE HAD SUPPURATED SO BADLY THAT HE FILLED SIXTY-SEVEN BASINS WITH PUS WHILE SLEEPING IN THE TEMPLE HE SAW A VISION IT SEEMED TO HIM THE GOD EXTRACTED THE ARROWHEAD FROM HIS LUNG WHEN DAY CAME HE WALKED OUT WELL HOLDING THE ARROWHEAD IN HIS HANDS

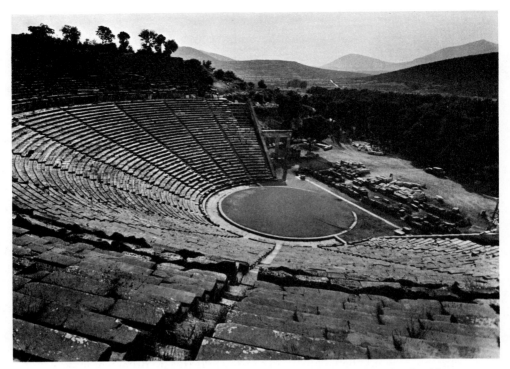

4.47 The plays offered in this amphitheater, on the grounds of the temple of Asklepios at Epidauros, were surely of value as psychotherapy.

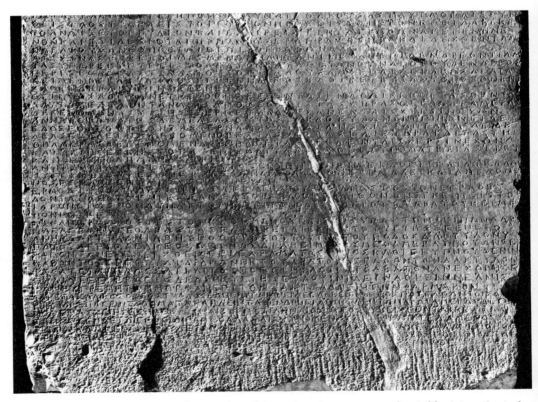

4.48 Marble stele, found at Epidauros, describing miraculous cures at the Asklepieion. Several of the cures concern wounds. About 350 B.C.

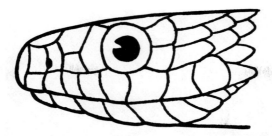

4.49 Head of *Elaphe longissima longissima*, the snake of Asklepios. It is a tree climber and a constrictor, harmless to man.

When Asklepios used a drug, it was a dream drug:[322]

> TIMON [*fault in the stone*] WOUNDED BY A SPEAR UNDER HIS EYE WHILE SLEEPING IN THE TEMPLE HE SAW A DREAM IT SEEMED TO HIM THAT THE GOD RUBBED DOWN AN HERB AND POURED IT INTO HIS EYE AND HE BECAME WELL

Asklepios also practiced dream surgery. Note that the pupils of the eye are called "the so-called pupils," as if the readers were assumed to be rather simple-minded laymen:[323]

> ANTICRATES OF CNIDOS EYES IN A BATTLE HE HAD BEEN HIT BY A SPEAR IN BOTH EYES AND HAD BECOME BLIND AND THE SPEARPOINT HE CARRIED WITH HIM STICKING IN HIS FACE WHILE SLEEPING HE SAW A VISION IT SEEMED TO HIM THAT THE GOD PULLED OUT THE MISSILE AND THEN FITTED INTO HIS EYELIDS AGAIN THE SO-CALLED PUPILS WHEN DAY CAME HE WALKED OUT SOUND

The next patient was lucky enough to receive also the attention of the snake, the *drakon*;[324] his case combines the three main therapeutic themes, the snake, the god, and a drug. Descendants of the healing snake are still quite common: *Elaphe longissima longissima*, Europe's only constrictor, can be five feet long but is quite harmless to man (Fig. 4.49). Its reputation as a healer was tremendous: the Romans imported it from Greece in 291 B.C., even before they had imported a regular Greek physician (Fig. 4.50).[325]

> THE MAN WHOSE TOE WAS HEALED BY THE SNAKE THIS MAN MUCH SUFFERING FROM A DREADFUL WOUND OF HIS TOE WAS CARRIED BY DAY ON A STRETCHER BY THE SERVANTS OF THE TEMPLE AND LAID OUT IN THE OPEN AIR AND HE FELL ASLEEP THEREUPON A SNAKE HAVING EMERGED FROM THE ABATON HEALED HIS WOUND WITH ITS TONGUE AND HAVING DONE THAT RETURNED TO THE ABATON WHEN THE MAN UPON WAKING UP FOUND HIMSELF TO BE HEALED HE SAID IT SEEMED AS IF HE HAD HAD THE VISION OF A FAIR YOUNG MAN SPREADING A DRUG ON HIS WOUND

Ἰατρός

The man was rather vague about the facts because he had been asleep, and also was probably blindfolded, just in case. We know this from Aristophanes, who is no believer in the system and tells of patients who peeked from beneath the bandage and saw the servants making off with their goods:[326]

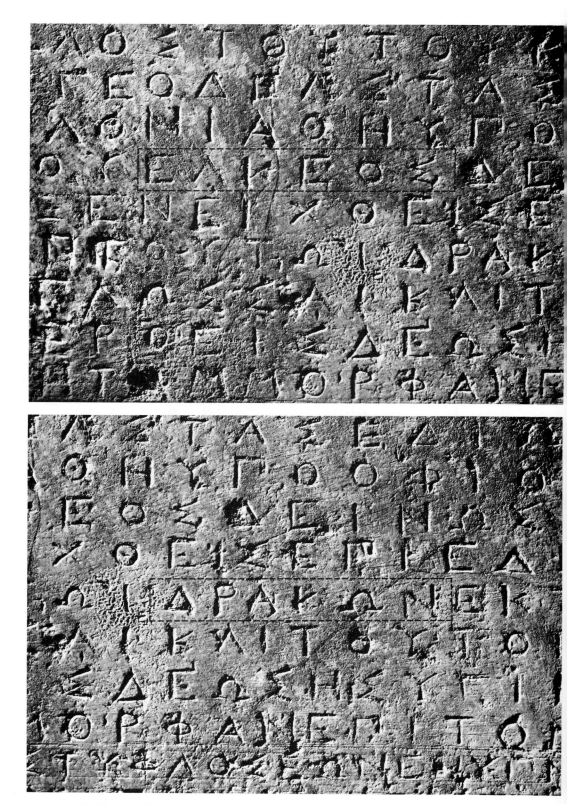

4.50 Details of the text on the stele at Epidauros: this man suffered "of a wound," ΕΛΚΕΟΣ (above, box), and was healed by the touch of "the snake," ΔΡΑΚΩΝ (below, box).

Then, glancing upwards, I behold the priest
Whipping the cheese-cakes and the figs from off
The holy table; thence he coasted round
To every altar, spying what was left.
And everything he found he consecrated
Into a sort of sack.

Anyway, the wound was healed.

After Hippocrates

With respect to the treatment of wounds the Hippocratic legacy left
much to be desired. But it would be unfair not to acknowledge the unique
insight of those physicians. Their natural ease with the abstract led them to
guess a number of rules before the game was ready to be played. They spoke
of sepsis[327] without knowing of bacteria, of spasms in vessels that they could
not see, of *diuretiká* with no diuretics to speak of. Two millennia later we are
still hunting for facts to fit their concepts. The notion of *rheumatism*,
although exasperating in its vagueness, remains the title of university courses.
Even that ghastly theory of blood, bile, and phlegm was so well adapted to
human nature that, instead of dying, it became permanently embedded in
our language. When we say that someone is sanguine, or bilious, or melan-
cholic, or phlegmatic, we are still blaming, in turn, each one of the four
humors (Fig. 4.51).[328]

In dealing with wounds, the antiseptic enhemes were a discovery, and
they caught on. The Greek emphasis on cleanliness and the generous
affusions with wine survived with ups and downs. Hemostasis with the tourniquet, though dangerous alone, was a good beginning; but it faded away and
was lost for some 1500 years. The surgical drain, like auscultation, was not
resuscitated until the nineteenth century.

The tight bandages were a step in the wrong direction. So was the notion
of encouraging suppuration, which became standard practice. And worst of
all, the three basic general "treatments"—bleeding, starving, and purging—
spread like wildfire all over the Western world. In today's jargon one would
say that they had been very well sold. Anybody could see how true they
were—with the eyes of his mind.

After Hippocrates, the first major advance had to be the ligature of blood
vessels. It came soon and was lost again, not to be retrieved until the 1500s.
Apart from this, the tale of the wound becomes one long, dull parenthesis,
broken by a few bright episodes; the pace will change abruptly in 1865,
with Lord Lister and antisepsis. It took that time, some seventy generations, to find out how the body works. Greek philosophy had thrown open
the door to the abstract; but to understand the ways of the flesh, a different
approach was required: the experimental method. To produce real science,
remarks Joly, it is not enough to free oneself of magico-religious concepts;
other demons have yet to be conquered, and these will be all the more
difficult to exorcise in that their link with reason is closer.[329] Here the iatrós

'Ιατρός

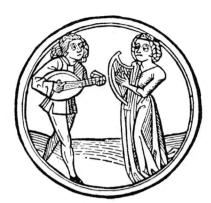

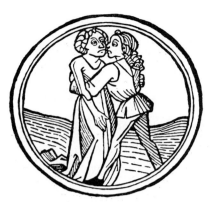

Flegmaticus.
Vnser complex ist mit wasser mer getan
Darumb wir subtilikeit nit mügen lan.

Sanguineus.
Vnser conplexion sind von lustes vil.
Darumb sey wir hochmütig one zpl.

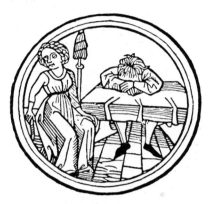

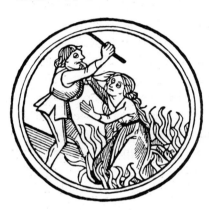

Melencolicus.
Vnser complexion ist von erden reych
Darüb sey wir schwärmütigkept gleich

Coleticus.
Vnser complexion ist gar von feüer
Schlahē vñ kriegen ist vnser abentreüer.

4.51 The four temperaments, illustrated in a German calendar about 1480 A.D.

stopped short. His basic science should have begun with anatomy, and he knew some, but he preferred the anatomy of thought. He had freed himself of religion to become the prisoner of philosophy.[330]

Hence it is appropriate to close this chapter with words of wisdom from a Greek philosopher—medical wisdom, which will last as long as men will care for men. In one of Plato's dialogs, a young man—Charmides—complains about a headache. He would like a certain drug; but Socrates explains to him at length that this simple treatment is not adequate. "To treat the head by itself, apart from the body as a whole," he says, "is utter folly." The ideal approach had once been described to him by a Thracian physician:

Ἰατρός

> You ought not to attempt to cure eyes
> Without head,
> Or head without body,
> So you should not treat body
> Without soul.[331]

206

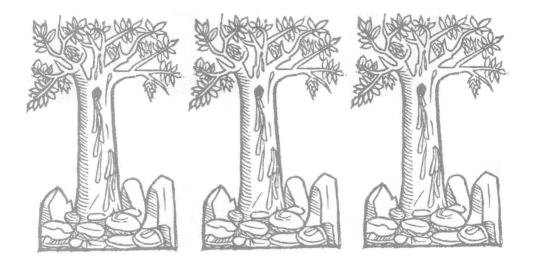

5 The Perfumes of Arabia

There is a lost fragrance about ancient drugs. A disconcerting fragrance of incense, roses, and cinnamon, which keeps luring the mind out of medicine into the church, the kitchen, and the beauty parlor. But these contrasts are entirely a matter of custom. Our ancestors, who liked to smear themselves with cinnamon oil, might have marveled at cinnamon bread as we would at incense pie.[1] Besides, perfume for them was a far broader concern, with broader implications than it has today. What was good to breathe, or eat, or drink was also good for the gods, for disease, and for wounds. So the Greeks had one lovely word, *arómata*, to cover much of what we would now break down into incense, perfumes, spices, and drugs.[2] Aromata were the zest of life. That is what the Romans meant when they said "my myrrh, my cinnamon" as we would say "my darling."[3]

It is difficult to grasp the importance of perfumes in the history of mankind.[4] More than a luxury, they have been one of the basic necessities of life. In ancient Egypt, around 1180 B.C., laborers on a necropolis went on strike because the food was bad and "we have no ointment."[5] In the Old Testament, "ointment and perfume rejoyce the heart."[6] Good and bad smells have always enjoyed the loftiest associations: Good and Bad, God and the Devil. Part of Alexander's greatness, according to tradition, was his personal fragrance;[7] and I have before me a list of Christian saints who smelled good, either alive or dead: it is thirty-five pages long.[8]

Doubtless these associations have a deep biological meaning, rooted in

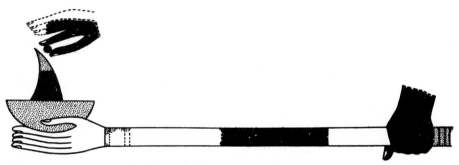

5.1 Egyptian censer in the form of a human arm, c.1900 B.C.

evolution. By recognizing the smell of decay as "bad," we automatically shun danger and death. On the other hand, the sense of smell may have been of help in recognizing plants of medicinal value: substances that have a strong smell are also likely to have a physiological effect. This may have been the manner, for instance, in which the South African natives narrowed down their available nine thousand plant species to perhaps two or three hundred.[9] So the quest for good smells has always been pursued with the intensity of a need. The sense of smell, after all, is not just a luxury: it has a survival value.

The spiritual role of perfumes is bound up with sacrificial fires. It was smoke that carried aloft the fragrance of man's gifts to the gods.[10] In fact, the word perfume comes from *per fumum*, "by smoke."[11] Incense was the perfect gift to the gods, because it was not shared by man, being consumed by fire to the last grain (Fig. 5.1).[12] The smoke of sacrificial fires was regarded as actual food for the gods, who would starve without it.[13] There is a comedy of Aristophanes in which birds stir up trouble by preventing the sacrificial smoke from reaching the heavens; and in a satirical work of the second century A.D. the workshop of Zeus is depicted as a sort of attic, with trapdoors covered by a lid, one of these being reserved for sacrificial smoke.[14]

The first sacrifices of the ancient Greeks, wrote Theophrastos, were fires of aromatic bushes.[15] Eventually the Greeks developed a whole line of aromatic gum-resins, their favorite being obtained from *Pistacia terebinthus*, the turpentine tree; but none of these home products could match Arabian frankincense and myrrh, whose reputation was already at least two thousand years old by the time of classical Greece. An Egyptian inscription from the Fifth Dynasty, about 2500 B.C., records the purchase of "80,000 measures" of myrrh; whatever the measure, this was a lot of myrrh (Fig. 5.2). A thousand years later another Egyptian bas-relief shows that the grains of myrrh, those precious grains that had been gathered one by one, were hoarded in heaps (Fig. 5.3).

The Perfumes of Antiquity

A few perfumes of antiquity, like musk, were animal products. Of these, the most used in medicine was castoreum, which has nothing to do with

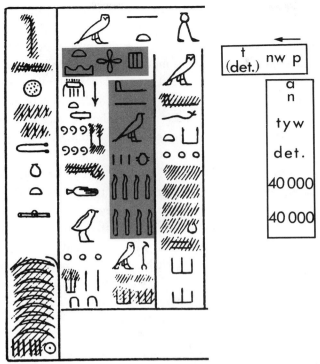

5.2 The earliest reference to myrrh (shaded), about 2500 B.C., when its trade was already on a wholesale scale. The pharaoh Sahurê was importing "Pwnt antyw 80,000": *Pwnt* was probably Somaliland; *antyw* was myrrh.

5.3 About one thousand years later myrrh was still used by shovelfuls at the court of Queen Hatshepswt, as shown by part of a relief commemorating the queen's own expedition to Pwnt, to get myrrh and myrrh trees.

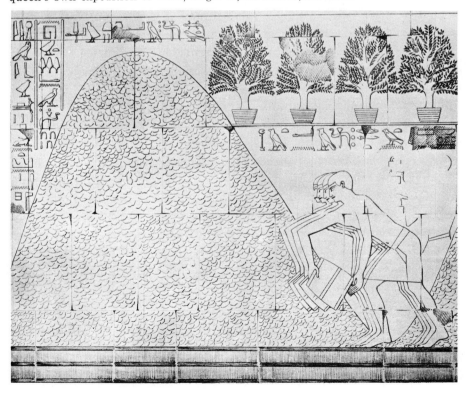

castor oil, being obtained, against all odds, from the rear end of the beaver. According to all ancient treatises on drugs that I have seen, castoreum was obtained from the testicles, but it seems that some information was lost between the beaver and the market: a modern chemical analysis of castoreum specifies that it was extracted from the scent glands, which lie between the anus and the genital organs. It contained, among other aromatic substances, hydro*cinnamic* acid; and it may also be the only animal product known to contain salicin and salicylic acid: aspirin in disguise![16]

Many other perfumes were obtained from herbs; still others were the product of trees, sometimes of wounded trees. Of special importance was (as it still is) the group of substances that ooze out of trees. Some of these trickle straight out of an incision, like blood (though they are not to be confused with sap, which is the real "blood" of the tree); others are pathologic: they develop some time after an injury, as if a "gathering" had formed around a bruise in the bark.[17] Chemically they are highly complex and varied mixtures, which can be broken down into three main groups of components, not all perfumed: *resins*, the sticky materials that are insoluble in water but often soluble in alcohol; *gums*, which are insoluble in alcohol but capable of taking up water to form a mucilage, like gum acacia; and *oleoresins* and *balsams*, the syrupy liquids that contain resin dissolved in volatile oils and are responsible for the perfume, like Mecca balsam or the ooze of the turpentine tree. Balsams also contain a high proportion of *balsamic acids*, which are partially soluble in water.[17]

The whole family of resins, gums, and balsams that were prized in antiquity would be too tedious to review, but even a partial list suggests the variety of the trade. The two most important were frankincense and myrrh. Then there was mastich, obtained from a shrub, the lentisk. The best specimens came from the island of Chios. As it "speedily softens in the mouth, and may be easily masticated and kneaded between the teeth,"[18] I assume it was the principal chewing gum of antiquity. The history of turpentine, queen of resins, would easily fill a volume; the best also came from Chios. Ladanum—not laudanum—was the strangest of all. This resin, which rubbed off onto sheep as they brushed by the plants, was combed off the sheep's fleeces with a special gadget, called *ladanisterium*;[19] not surprisingly it had a musklike perfume. Galbanum, mentioned in Exodus 30:34, was an ingredient of incense; with Hippocrates it dropped to pessaries, in which it shared its fate with incense.[20] There was ammoniacum, which had nothing to do with our ammonia.[21] Pliny mentions, without further details, a resin from a sort of olive tree, sold by the Arabs, which was excellent "for contracting the scars of wounds."[22] Then there were bdellium, two kinds of storax, and opopanax. The black sheep was asafetida, a condiment in India, but definitely not a perfume. And I leave out many, many others.[23]

Nor shall I dwell on the uses of all these aromata; but just consider that the gums were chewed long enough to give the verb *to masticate*, from gum mastich (the Egyptians, however, chewed papyrus[24]). The resins were precious as adhesives, though Pliny, who tends to find reasons for complaint, writes in the first century A.D., "I am ashamed to confess that the chief value

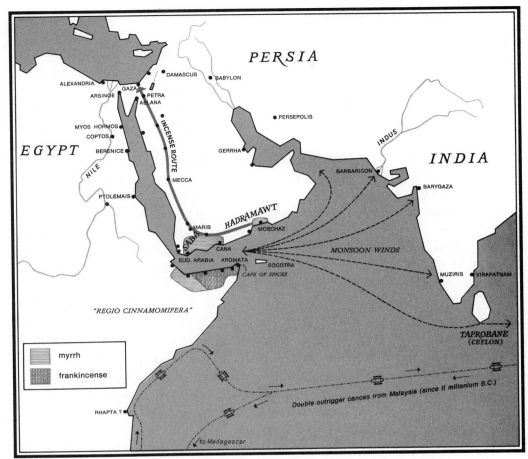

5.4 The home of myrrh and frankincense: a small area, but in a key position. The Roman name of *Regio cinnamomifera* for East Africa proves the success of Arab merchants in hiding the true source of cinnamon, India.

now set on resin is for use as a depilatory for men."[25] The volatile oils were chiefly responsible for the medical uses. When we read that their fragrance is plainly detectable today in some Egyptian mummies,[26] we can begin to understand why the ancients felt so strongly about them, even to the point of fighting pitched battles in defense of a single shrub.[27]

Twice-Happy Arabia and Its Trees

In view of the fame of myrrh and frankincense, it is hardly conceivable that they came, as they still do, from a very small corner of the world: part of the South Arabian coast—the main source—and the Horn of Africa just opposite (Fig. 5.4). That is where the right trees have chosen to grow:[28] two genera belonging to the family of Burseraceae.

In Greek and Roman times, Arabia was a shifting mosaic of small states, including the Biblical Saba, strung around the desert.[29] It was about 950 B.C. when the Queen of Saba paid her famous visit to Solomon, third king of Israel. Although the precise motives of her trip are not recorded, it certainly included commercial interests, and tradition relates it to the incense trade.[30]

211

Saba itself was the main producer of myrrh; most of the incense came from the kingdom of Hadramawt, farther east (Fig. 5.4).[31] Until the first century A.D., part of the precious harvest found its way to the southern harbors to be shipped as far as India; but the supplies for the Mediterranean countries went mainly overland, heading north by the Incense Route.[32] The caravans threaded their way through the various states, paying duties all along, so that by the time they reached their destination, the price of a camel load had soared.[33]

It was largely because of the generous Burseraceae that this semidesert region rose to such legendary wealth. The area now called Yemen earned from the Romans the name of *Arabia felix*, "happy Arabia," and eventually attracted Roman greed in the form of a military expedition, which ended in total failure.[34] In the meantime, the southern harbor of Aden, lying midway between India and the Mediterranean, grew to such importance that it earned the Greek name of *Eudáimon Arabía*, "Happy Arabia" again, until the jealous Romans destroyed it.[35] Regardless of whether myrrh and frankincense ever soothed any wounds, they surely caused a lot of bloodshed.

The peculiar feature of these trees, which raised them to such historical status, was revealed by the microscope over one hundred years ago. In and beneath the bark are small canals and larger cavities, full of an oleo-gum-resin, which is a specialty of the family (Fig. 5.5). A typical incense tree of South Arabia is shown in Fig. 5.6. Its product, known also as *frankincense* (archaic for "choice incense"), is still collected as described in 1848 by a British surgeon, in somewhat surgical terms:

> The gum is procured by making longitudinal incisions through the bark in the months of May and December, when the cuticle glistens with intumescence from the distended state of the parts beneath; the operation is simple, and requires no skill on the part of the operator. On its first appearance the gum comes forth white as milk, and according to its degree of fluidity, finds its way to the ground, or concretes on the branch near the place from which it first issued, from whence it is collected by men and boys employed to look after the trees by the different families who possess the land in which they grow.[36]

The lumps of fresh, milky sap (Fig. 5.7) gave incense its Arabic name, *al lubán* (from the Semitic root *lbn*, "milk"), which has been Anglicized to "olibanum."[37] In a week or two the white lumps dry into an amber-colored oleo-gum-resin, which ignites easily and smolders, giving off a pleasant smell. *Incense*, in fact, means "that which is lit."[38]

Myrrh is tapped from a scraggy, unfriendly tree of "crippled appearance," with a grey-white bark, and usually gathered from thickets not over three meters high. It is leafless most of the year, and its rough branches end in thorns (Fig. 5.8). The bark tends to crack spontaneously letting the myrrh trickle out even without man-made wounds. Eventually it hardens into reddish-brown masses (Fig. 5.9). The old name of *bitter myrrh*[39] refers to the characteristic taste—in fact, twice so, because the word *myrrh* itself comes from the Hebrew and Arabic *murr* for "bitter."[40]

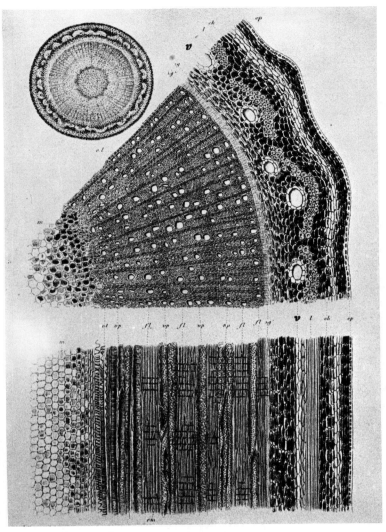

5.5 The secret of the myrrh tree as seen through a microscope: the oleo-gum-resin collects in and beneath the bark, especially in the canals marked *v*.

5.6 Frankincense trees in Hadramawt, South Arabia.

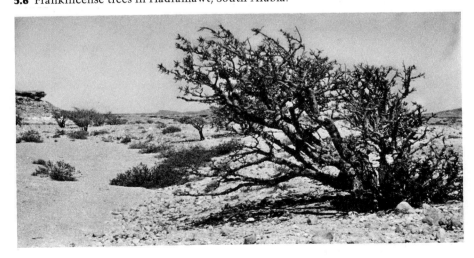

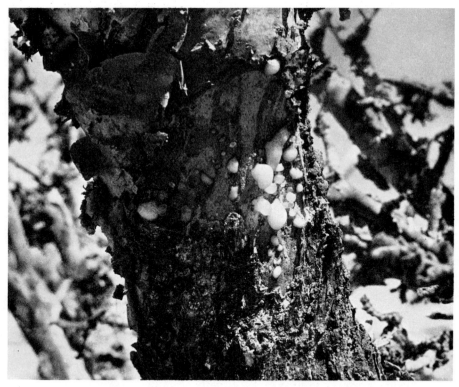

5.7 Milky-white drops of frankincense oozing out of a wounded tree, *Boswellia carterii*, in South Arabia.

5.8 The thorny branch of a myrrh tree, *Balsamodendron myrrha*.

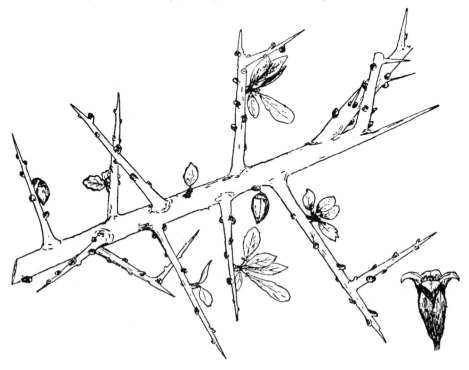

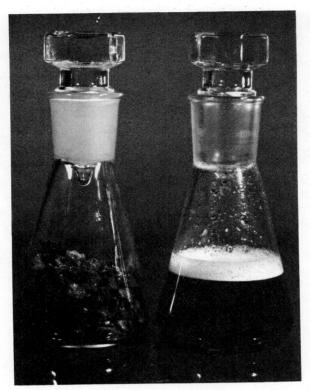

5.9 Grains of myrrh (left). In water (right) they easily form an opaque suspension, with many impurities.

From Tree Wounds to Human Wounds

The use of tree sap for treating injuries must be older than man's oldest documents. About 3000 B.C. the Egyptians were barely starting to write, yet in 2500 B.C. they were already importing huge loads of myrrh. Whether any of that lot went for medical purposes is not known for sure, but a few centuries later there are records of excellent wound-salves in the Smith and Ebers papyri, based on resins. About 1370 B.C. Milkili made his cryptic request for myrrh, most likely to use for battle casualties. Eight hundred years later, around 480 B.C., in the eastern Mediterranean Greeks and Persians happened to fight a fierce naval battle. According to the account of Herodotos, the captain of a Greek trireme "bore himself very gallantly; for his ship being taken, he would not give over fighting till he was all hacked about with wounds; and when he fell, yet was not slain but had life in him, the Persian soldiers on the ships were at great pains to save him alive for his valour, tending his wounds . . . with myrrh."[41] In the Hippocratic books, myrrh is by far the favorite resin, being prescribed fifty-four times.[42] The Romans kept up the trend. A lotion of wine and myrrh for burns is one of the many uses mentioned by Celsus in the first century A.D.,[43] and about the same time, a Roman doctor in the military camp at Vindonissa, Switzerland, lost his stamp for DIAZMYRNES, a rather poorly spelled myrrh-medicine "for old scars" (Fig. 5.10).

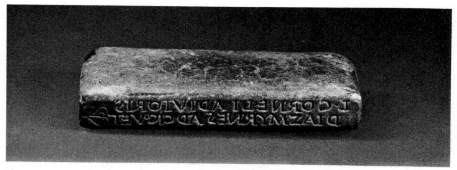

5.10 Stone stamp with which L[UCIUS] CORNELIUS ADIUTOR, a Roman physician, marked his little sticks of myrrh medicine, DIAZMYRNES, for old scars, AD CIC[ATRICES] VET[ERES]. Such sticks, called collyria, were dissolved in milk or eggwhite, especially to make eyedrops. Enlarged almost three times.

This is only a part of the evidence to prove that myrrh and other resins were among the commonest drugs used on wounds. But there is better yet:

> I am wounded at the sight of my people's wound;
> I go like a mourner, overcome with horror.
> Is there no balm in Gilead, no physician there? . . .
>
> Go up into Gilead and fetch balm,
> O virgin people of Egypt.
> You have tried many remedies, all in vain;
> No skin shall grow over your wounds.[44]

In the language of the Old Testament, the surgical use of balsams has an overtone of salvation. There could be no better proof that the sap of wounded trees was the treatment par excellence of human wounds.

Why did balsams come to be used as "balm"? I can suggest four reasons. First, the ancients might have been guided by a conscious or subconscious analogy, namely, that what fills gashes in plants should also heal gashes in people.[45]

Second, wounds used to smell. There was nothing perfumed that was not called upon for help, spices included. One of the countless examples appears in Theophrastos (from the third century B.C.). In his treatise *Concerning Odors* (who would write such a treatise nowadays?) he gives the formula of *megaléion*, a perfume "believed to relieve the inflammation caused by any wound." It was composed of burnt resin, cassia, cinnamon, and myrrh, all more or less fragrant.[46] Since we have been blessed by Listerian antisepsis, this smell problem can no longer be fully appreciated. It was memorialized by Homer in the sad case of Philoctetes, whose festering wound was so unbearable that the Greeks left him stranded alone on an island. In the tragedy of Sophocles, when Neoptolemus finally came to look for him, the ailing hero wailed:

> Alas, my son! I fear thy prayers are in vain
> For once again upwelling from the wound
> The black blood trickles auguring a relapse.

Out, out upon thee, damned foot! Alack!
What plague hast yet in store for me? Alack!
It prowls, it stalks amain, ready to spring,
Woe! Now ye know my torture, leave me not . . .
Raise me thyself and spare thy men this task,
Lest they be sickened by my fetidness
Before the time; they'll have enough to bear
With me for messmate when we are aboard . . .[47]

The ancient gesture of spreading perfume on a wound was as logical, in its context, as putting out a fire with water. The most offensive-smelling sores (the gangrenous) were also the most lethal: the obvious cure was perfume.

A third reason for using resins on wounds must have come from observing that resins are among the few products of nature that never decay, and from the hope that they might transmit this property to wounds. In this the sense of smell was truly prophetic, for antisepsis is a "transmissible" property almost by definition: antibacterial substances do not themselves decay, and applied to organic matter they can preserve it too from decay.

The fourth and probably most important reason for the surgical use of resins is that they actually improved the course of wound healing. A modern study of the effect of resins, balsams, or spices on wound healing does not seem to exist; hence, I cannot support my statement with scientific proof. However, indirect evidence is powerful. Let us first consider the case of myrrh. As a wound drug, myrrh has lived past its fourth or fifth millennium: we can therefore conclude, at the very least, that it does no harm to the tissues. Second, myrrh is said to have antiseptic properties (I am obliged to use this cautious expression, because the modern treatise from which I quote this statement gives no supporting reference).[48] A drug that is harmless to the tissues as well as antiseptic should be useful in the treatment of wounds.

The flaw in my argument thus far is that it hinges on textbook authority rather than on scientific proof. I therefore set about to find a kindly and competent bacteriologist who would be willing to test the effect of myrrh on bacteria (almost as hard as finding the myrrh itself). The first surprise was that the hard, resinous lumps of crude myrrh dissolve quite easily in water (Fig. 5.9). The fluid was tested against a selection of bacteria, including a typical wound bacterium, *Staphylococcus aureus.* The result was clearcut: myrrh acts as a bacteriostatic against *Staphylococcus aureus* and other gram-positive bacteria (Fig. 5.11).[49]

I conclude that the ancient use of myrrh as a wound drug was fully justified. Doubtless the same holds true for the many other resins and balsams that have been traditionally used for the same purpose. Indeed, I believe that the antiseptic properties of myrrh may be among the lowest in the entire family of drugs, because it has almost no perfume, suggesting that it has a low content in antiseptic volatile oils (this may explain the limited use of myrrh in present times: it is still burned with incense, but its only medical use is as a mouthwash[50]). Some of the most popular resins and balsams came from the New World, as gifts of the American Indians; and they, too, are

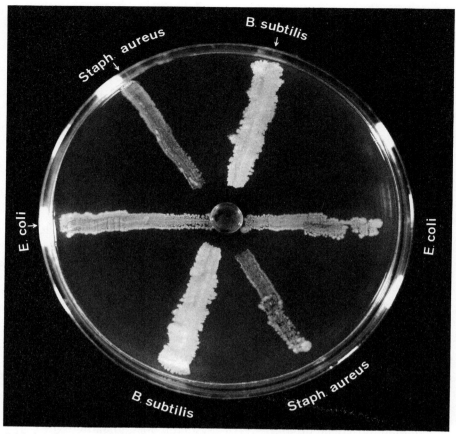

5.11 Antibiotic effect of myrrh. Cultures of three different species of bacteria were streaked across the whole plate, to form a star; a suspension of myrrh was placed in the center well. After incubation at 37°C for twenty-four hours, two of the three bacteria failed to grow in the vicinity of the myrrh.

currently listed as antiseptics. Brazilian Indians treated their wounds with copaiba,[51] an oleoresin that enjoyed thereafter a formal career as a urinary antiseptic.[52] The balsam of Tolu was "muche esteemed amongst the Indians" of Colombia and Venezuela, because "it healeth all freashe woundes, comfortying the partes, and joynyng them without makyng any matter."[53] The balsam of Peru is a pathologic secretion of *Myroxylon pereirae*, which the Indians of Central America obtain by beating the bark and then charring it a week later.[54] It soon became part of the U.S. Pharmacopoeia and is still used as an antiseptic; I found it at work as late as 1967 in a routine study of wound healing in a U.S. Army hospital.[55] Among its constituents are two that echo the names of spices, *cinnamate* and *vanillin*.[56] In Russia, a very successful wound salve is the *Unguentum Vishnievskii*, made of resin, mineral oil, and bismuth.[57]

Really, the antiseptic power of resins and balsams needs no pleading. One can go a step further and include certain plant perfumes that are not necessarily resins or balsams. A good example is thyme. The Hippocratic books, surely guided by the fragrance, prescribe it for several infectious diseases.[58] In that context, and in that low dosage, it was probably used in vain;

but today, its essence—crystalline thymol—adds a fragrant touch to laboratory life, where it floats on solutions to preserve them from bacteria and mildew. Industry uses it to preserve meat, and it is an all-round, pleasant, aromatic antiseptic.[59] In this case, then, the use of an aroma was not yet a discovery; but it was, if I may say so, the aroma of a discovery.

Someone spread the rumor that burning incense, the prototype of all aromata, gives off carbolic acid, the magic, odorous drug with which Lister opened the era of antisepsis.[60] Startled by this overlap of bodily and spiritual health, I had the statement verified. It turned out to be chemically true, but medically irrelevant. In the words of the chemist, "The amount of phenols set free in the atmosphere of a church should be far from having a purifying effect, at least on a material level."[61] It is nevertheless perfectly true that the chemical formula of many scents given off by balsams and spices are variations on a theme: the skeleton of carbolic acid (Fig. 5.12).

The trail of aromata has kept its promise.

Two Spices from Nowhere: Cinnamon and Cassia

Like myrrh and frankincense, there was another twin set of drugs that had a special appeal to the nostrils of antiquity: cinnamon and cassia. They tend to be treated as a couple because they taste alike and because they come from the same botanical family, the Lauraceae. The best cinnamon nowadays is the variety *Cinnamomum zeylanicum* from Ceylon; cassia comes from *Cinnamomum cassia*. Although cinnamon is considered the finer of the two, their similarity has caused much confusion. Because the bark of cassia is rougher, its name was often used for "low-grade cinnamon." The confusion continues: Americans order "cinnamon toast" but eat cassia toast.[62]

Nobody will ever know the cost of cinnamon and cassia in human lives, for they had to sail west a record distance, on double outrigger canoes: cinnamon came from India, cassia from North Vietnam and southern China.[63] The Cinnamon Route, based on the two-way sweep of the monsoons, ran from India to East Africa. It may have been open as early as 1500 B.C.[64]

One can only marvel at the impact of these gentle perfumes. I cannot even say spices, for there is no evidence that they were used on food before the ninth century A.D.[65] One of the oldest records on the subject is again the Bible. Thus spoke the Lord to Moses: "You yourself shall take spices as follows: five hundred shekels of sticks of myrrh, half that amount (two hundred and fifty shekels) of fragrant cinnamon, two hundred and fifty shekels of aromatic cane, five hundred shekels of cassia by the sacred standard, and a hin of olive oil . . . This shall be the holy anointing oil for my service in every generation."[66] And to quote from a Hippocratic book: "If there is inflammation and pain in the womb, take rose leaves, cinnamon, cassia . . . fumigate therewith, and it will sooth the pain."[67]

The actual spices came, and still come, as little rolls, being the bark of trees, stripped and sun-dried into little quills or hollow canes; hence the

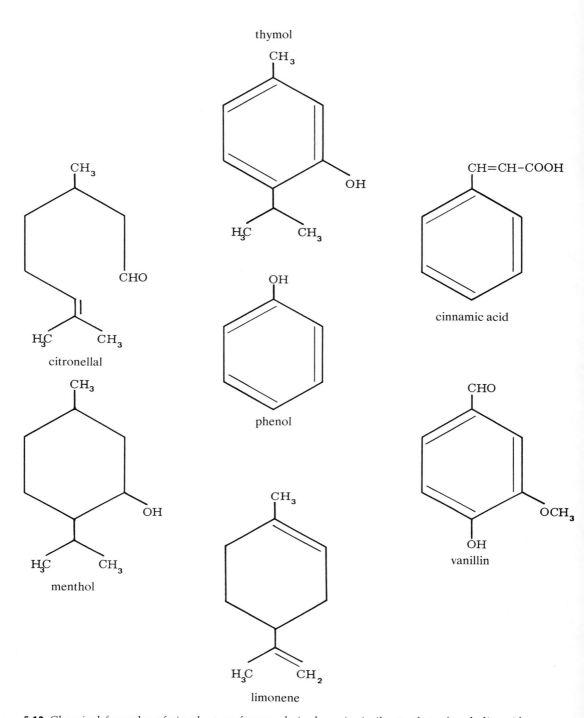

5.12 Chemical formulas of six plant perfumes: their shape is similar to that of carbolic acid or phenol, the pioneer antiseptic (center).

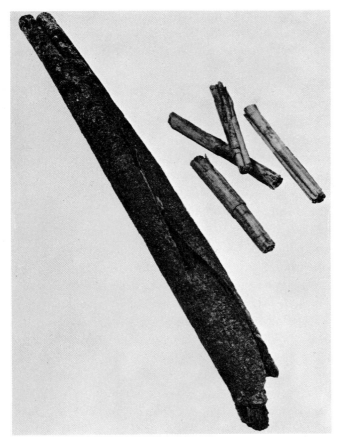

5.13 Four quills of Ceylon cinnamon and one of the coarser cassia: little rolls of sun-dried bark. About half-size.

French name *cannelle* (Fig. 5.13). The laurel family to which they belong is a very scented collection of trees, all aromatic, and growing in the warmer parts of the world. Some of these trees carry eugenol, an antiseptic,[68] and smell like cloves. Others contain camphor, another wound drug, which did not come West until the Middle Ages.[69]

Concerning the effect of cassia and cinnamon on wounds I have no personal data, but a recent treatise on pharmacognosy reports that oil of cinnamon is a powerful germicide.[70] Another germicidal aroma.

Wounds, Wine, and Bacteria

The jump from spices to wounds to wine is not as long as it may seem. For wounds and wine, to begin, have the same problem: bacterial infection. And both can be cured by aromatic substances.

The main infectious disease of wine is vinegar. So, while the people of antiquity were trying to prevent their wounds from developing what they called "corruption," they were also spending enormous amounts of energy in trying to keep their wine from turning into vinegar. The villains, be they staphylococci or acetobacteria, were always microorganisms, and they had to be killed with antiseptics.[71] Consciously or not, our ancestors did make the connection between the two problems, for they discovered that many of the substances that kept wounds clean, also kept wine from becoming vinegar, especially the aromata. And I would venture to say that they came closer to a final solution with their wine problem, perhaps because of the amount of research that went into it: "there is no department of man's life on which more labour is spent."[72] Although this statement comes from a Roman, Pliny the Elder, it probably applies to many other peoples of antiquity. The following pages deal mostly with the Romans only because they have left more documents on their struggles against vinegar.

Most of us amateur wine-lovers do not realize this paradoxical fact: wine is not the natural end-product of must fermentation.[73] Left to its own means, must will usually give vinegar. Granted, wine will form first; but the wine stage can be very short. A Roman expert of the first century A.D., Columella, mentions wines that "scarcely kept sound for thirty days."[74] The reason is that lurking in must are the seeds of its own destruction: the bacteria of acetic fermentation. It follows that the very first problem of wine making is to stop the bad bacteria that produce vinegar, without disturbing the good yeasts that produce alcohol. This is a tall order, for the two microorganisms swim side by side (Fig. 5.14).

The problem has not changed in the last two thousand years, nor is a perfect solution yet at hand. Since the early 1800s, however, the answer has been sulphur: more precisely, SO_2 or sulphur dioxide.[75] It is generally added to the must (and wine) as a concentrated solution of sulphur dioxide in water, and sometimes also by burning sulphur in a sort of spoon suspended in the air space of the vat, over the wine. The spoon contains a wick (*mèche* in French) soaked with sulphur; its fumes are literally asphyxiating, and the wine can become too *méché*. Fine noses can apparently detect the typical smell of sulphur when the dose is excessive, whereas the smell of regular doses has now become so much a part of the establised bouquet that its absence, I am told, may rather be recognized as "something wrong." To the public at large the smell of sulphur dioxide is therefore not an issue, so wine makers are free to enjoy its special property, which is to inhibit acetic fermentation without significantly affecting alcoholic fermentation. The must goes on to wine, then graciously stops there, unless the wine is exposed to air.[76] This is the magic whereby it is possible, nowadays, to open almost any bottle of wine with near-mathematical certainty that it will not be a bottle of vinegar.

The magic, however, comes at a price. When dissolved in water, sulphur dioxide becomes sulphurous acid, which is said to be "not very toxic" (and even "good for allergies")—but still, it is not comfortable to hear that the average bottle of wine contains—besides the friendly poison, ethyl alcohol— about $1/30$ of a lethal dose of sulphurous acid.[77] This is a constant worry for wine makers, who are trying hard to get away from sulphur; yet nothing better has been found. One has only to leaf through the issues of the most important journal of wine making, the *Bulletin de l'Office International du Vin*, to realize how much effort is going into the search for alternatives.[78]

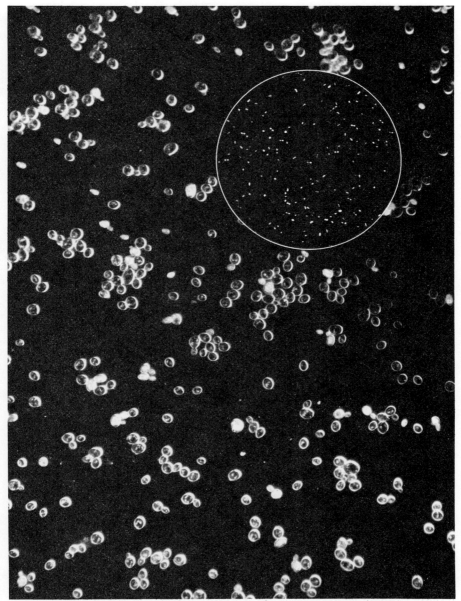

5.14 Friend and foe: yeast cells, which turn sugar into alcohol, and acetobacteria (circle), which turn alcohol into vinegar. Wine inherits both these organisms from the grapes. Pure cultures, enlarged about 1250x.

So this is where we stand. But how did the ancients fight off *acetobacter*, the maker of vinegar? The most sophisticated method, described in detail by Columella, was to make up a *medicamentum*, literally a "medicine;" today one would say a preservative. Here is the recipe, containing a selection of the world's best aromata.[79] Boil some must, not in a bronze vessel, which would impart a bad taste, but in a leaden vessel (!) well rubbed with oil. When the volume of the must has boiled down to ¾ or ½, add liquid pitch and turpentine resin; then sprinkle on myrrh, cassia, cardamom, saffron, six other spices, and more resin. Only small amounts of this preservative could be used, for if its flavor was noticeable, it "drove away the purchasers."

Many other techniques were also used. Pliny reports that whole volumes had been written on how to prevent wine from turning into vinegar.[80] He mentions turpentine and all sorts of resins, pitch, honey, spices, perfumes, salt, even sea water. Between spices and perfumes there was no clear-cut boundary. Myrrh was the veteran preservative: "The finest wines in the early days were those spiced with the scent of myrrh."[81] Remember the myrrh wine offered to Jesus before he was put on the cross: "He was offered drugged wine, but he would not take it."[82] The great variety of aromatic wines was probably a matter not only of choice or taste, but also of preservation.[83] "Aromatic wine is constantly made from almost the same ingredients as perfumes (*unguenti*)—first from myrrh . . . next also from nard, reed," horehound, sweet rush, costus, cardamom, cinnamon, saffron, marjoram, dittany, mint, thyme, mandrake, hazelwort, lavender, pepper, and many others, including Pontic wormwood[84] (*wormwood*, incidentally, is the word—and the substance—that gave *vermouth*). Another possibility was to treat the must with certain berries, or to boil it with chips of sweet-smelling woods, like cedar, laurel, and terebinth, added in the amount of about "ten drachms per congius," or about 13 grams per liter.[85]

The barrels themselves were coated inside with hot pitch and fumigated with myrrh.[86] Pliny makes a tantalizing reference to "adjusting wine with sulphur," with no further details.[87] Fumigations of sulphur were used to purify homes, but only in religious ceremonies.[88] So here is another mysterious crossroads for antiseptics, cookery, cosmetics, and religion.

After all this, I cannot vouch that the Romans produced wines that would suit our taste; but their methods worked, at least sometimes.[89] Pliny mentions wines that increased in value for twenty years, and only then declined.[90] One priceless vintage was about to score two thousand years when it was dug up in France. A far-sighted Gallo-Roman gentleman had taken with him several sealed glass containers of his favorite drink. When found, all were broken but one, which contained a yellowish fluid that smelled like wine and tasted a bit sour. Analysis found it to be 0.12 percent acetic acid and a surprising 4.5 percent alcohol.[91]

Ultimately, man's consuming interest in wine paid off. Much wine had to flow—and much vinegar—until the catharsis came in the nineteenth century. One great day Napoleon III, heeding the call of distressed French wine makers, looked around for a scientist who could solve their problems, and chose Louis Pasteur. That was July 1863. Within three years, Pasteur had earned a gold medal for proposing a cheap remedy that was later called pasteurization. Thus, pasteurization was born in wine, not milk.[92] Pasteur's classical book on the *maladies du vin*, published in 1866, contains many lovely drawings of bacteria in "diseased wines" (Fig. 5.15). The work on human infections that eventually made of Pasteur one of the saviors of mankind, the work that inspired Lister's antisepsis, grew from Pasteur's earlier studies on what makes sugar turn to alcohol, and alcohol to vinegar.[93]

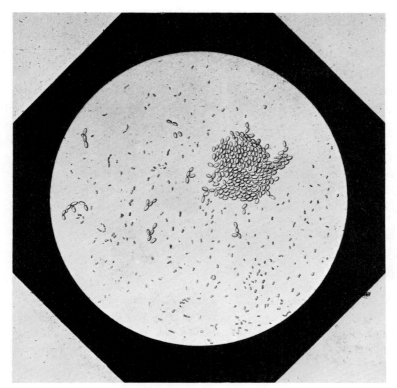

5.15 The good yeasts and the vinegar-making bacteria swim side-by-side in wine, as drawn in 1866 by Pasteur.

The Spice Curtain

The many roles of aromata in human affairs created a near-global network of commercial interests and led eventually to an Arabian monopoly, which may have had far-reaching effects on all cultural exchanges between ancient East and West. Look first at a map of the Red Sea, with the names of antiquity (Fig. 5.4). The Horn of Africa is called the Cape of Spices; on it is a city bearing the very name of Aromata. Clearly this city was a major trading post between East and West, and the trade was based largely on spices.

Look also at the strategic position of the Arab merchants, placed naturally as middlemen between Europe, Africa, and the East. The "happiness" of Arabia depended as much on this situation as on the fabled trees. Something had to be done to protect this advantage—perhaps not from the Egyptians, who let themselves be outsailed by almost everybody else,[94] but certainly from the other great Mediterranean powers.

But how could one keep these seaworthy customers from sailing directly to the sources? Fighting off their ships would have been bad for business. The Arabian merchants therefore chose the psychological approach, and they knew how to handle it. When they resold their cassia or cinnamon, imported from the East, they made up tall tales about the tremendous risks they had faced in order to obtain these goods, so that no Greek or Roman in his right mind would ever bother to try his own luck at it; or if he did, his informers made sure that he wound up in the wrong place. Covered by the screen of nonsense were also Arabia's domestic products, incense and myrrh.

The Arabs' tales were highly imaginative. Yet they were swallowed even by Herodotos, the Father of History, for he wrote that Arabia was "the only country which yields frankincense and myrrh and cassia and cinnamon."[95] Just read the facts of the Arab spice trade as he understood them. On frankincense:

> The spice-bearing trees are guarded by small winged snakes of varied colour, many round each tree; these are the snakes that attack Egypt. Nothing save the smoke of storax will drive them away from the trees [*whereby the Arabs were also raising the price of storax*] . . . They gather frankincense by burning that storax which Phoenicians carry to Greece . . . The Arabian winged snakes do indeed seem to be many . . . these are all in Arabia and are nowhere else found.[96]

On cassia:

> The Arabians get their frankincense as I have shown: for the winning of cassia, when they seek it they bind oxhides and other skins over all their bodies and faces, leaving only the eyes. Cassia grows in a shallow lake; round this and in it live certain winged creatures, very like bats, that squeak shrilly and make a stout resistance; these must be kept from the men's eyes if the cassia is to be plucked.[97]

The spiciest account of all is on cinnamon:

> As for cinnamon, they gather it in a fashion even stranger. Where it grows and what kind of land nurtures it they cannot say, save that it is reported, reasonably enough, to grow in the places where Dionysus was reared. There are great birds, it is said, that take these dry sticks which the Phoenicians have taught us to call cinnamon, and carry them off to nests built of mud and attached to precipitous crags, to which no man can approach. The Arabian device for defeating the birds is to cut into very large pieces dead oxen and asses and other beasts of burden, then to set these near the eyries, withdrawing themselves far off. The birds then fly down (it is said) and carry the pieces of the beasts up to their nests; which not being able to bear the weight break and fall down the mountain side; and then the Arabians come up and gather what they seek. Thus is cinnamon said to be gathered, and so to come from Arabia to other lands.[98]

Even Aristotle mentions the cinnamon birds.[99] Much later yet, about 77 A.D., Pliny repeats the "fables" of Herodotos, adding sourly they have been "invented by the natives to raise the price of their commodities."[100] But he concludes: "all these stories being false . . . inasmuch as . . . cinnamon grows in Ethiopia."[101] So the Arabs had won anyway.[102]

But not for long. Just as Pliny was writing, the Spice Curtain was being ripped apart. Greek and Roman ships were learning to use the monsoons, another well-kept secret, and were trading directly with India.[103] Gold kept flowing directly east, to the discomfiture of the middlemen. In the end, however, nobody laughed. The imbalance of payments, largely due to the trade of spices and perfumes, was one of the forces that brought about the downfall of the Roman Empire.[104]

The Arabian states withered. Many of their cities vanished altogether. Even the magnificent dam at Marib, capital of Saba, which was one of the wonders of antiquity, returned to the desert.[105] The caravans that used to carry aromata now carry rock salt.[106]

Thus ends the tale of the Spice Curtain.[107] It had lasted perhaps 1500 years, a success of connivance unmatched, except perhaps by the secret of the silk trade. In relation to the history of medicine, this commercial barrier may well have played a role in restricting communications between East and West: it let the spices through, but no information with them, except for the bare names.

We will now see what was going on beyond the Spice Curtain.

Arabia . . . airs wondrous sweet blow from that land.
Herodotos[108]

Her good fortune has been caused by the luxury of mankind.
Pliny the Elder[109]

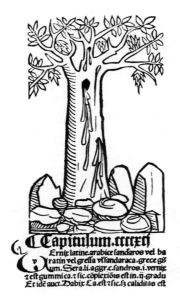

6.1 The world as Hippocrates knew it: China did not yet exist. Mapped about 500 B.C. by Hekataios, a Greek of Miletos surnamed "the Father of Geography."

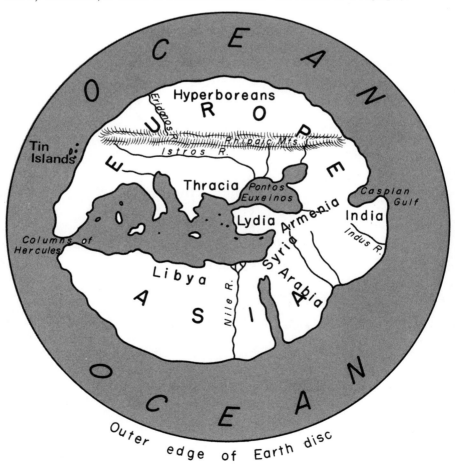

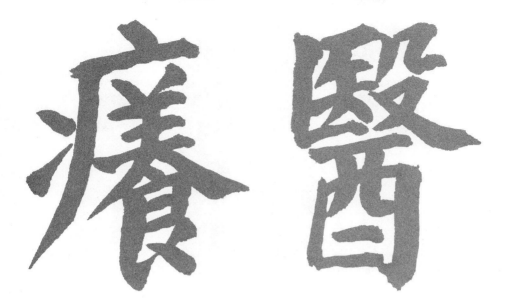

6   The Yang I

It is again 400 B.C. About this time Hippocrates, clad in his woollen tunic, was sailing among the Greek isles. If his skipper owned a map of the world, it must have looked more or less like the map of Hekataios (Fig. 6.1).

In the meantime, great things were happening beyond the eastern border of that map, in a world so isolated that it might almost have been on another planet. Somewhere in that never-never land, a black-haired scholar, clad in shining silk, was busily compiling the chronicles of his king.[1] He kept the records in booklets made of wooden tablets and on bamboo strips, writing vertically (Fig. 6.2).[2] The beautiful characters that he was tracing were already more than one thousand years old (Fig. 6.3).[3]

Books of the Chou

We have landed at the court of the Chou, a Chinese dynasty that lasted from about 1030 to 221 B.C. and ruled a small area south of the Yellow River. Chou was just one of some twenty-five small states, all clustered in a fraction of modern China (Fig. 6.4), nominally bound as a feudal empire under the Chou, but actually building walls against each other and fighting for supremacy; in this process they were gradually merging into larger and larger units, on the way to becoming unified in 221 B.C. as the great empire of Chhin (221 B.C.–1912 A.D.).

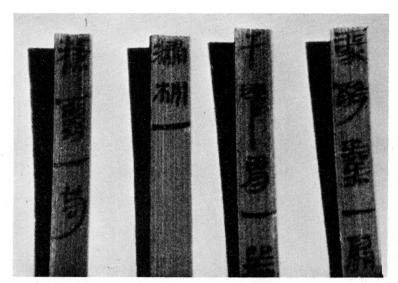

6.2 Ancient Chinese writing on bamboo strips: an inventory of treasure deposited in a Han tomb, about 180 B.C.

6.3 The character *ts'ê*, for "book." *Left:* the ancient form (slips of wood or bamboo held together with two lines of cord). *Right:* the modern printed form.

This was the period of Chinese history known as "The Warring States." Despite the political turmoil, it was also the intellectual golden era of ancient China. Two of its greatest minds were Lao Tzu, spiritual father of Taoism, and Khung the Master or Khung Fu-tsu, whom we know as Confucius, adviser to the Chou emperor and contemporary of Buddha (c.552–479 B.C.). Strangely enough, this flowering almost paralleled that of Greek philosophy, to the point that the Academy of the Gate of Chi, founded about 318 B.C. in the state of Chhi, came into being between the two Athenian academies, the Peripatetic and Stoic.[4]

So the court library at the disposal of the Chou historian, if it was anywhere near complete, was probably as large as any that Plato could muster at the time in Athens. Let us look among the shelves, with the help of an expert, and see what we might find.[5] Among the medical books would probably be the works that a couple of centuries later were to be compiled into the *Huang Ti Nei Ching*, the great medical classic that already deals extensively with acupuncture. There would be books of poetry, like the *Shih Ching* or "Book of Odes," at least as old as the *Iliad* and the *Odyssey* and not devoid of medical interest; as well as books on music, like the *Yo Ching* or "Music Classic," now lost.[6] Also on the shelves would be vast numbers of chronicles and histories, especially works of philosophers, for that happened to be the time of the "Hundred Schools of Philosophy."[7] We would surely

6.4 China about 400 B.C., when it was a loose feudal empire of warring states, partly separated by walls and occupying a small part of present China. Note the mountain barrier toward India and the distance from Greece. The march of Alexander, 334–323 B.C., is shown by a solid line. There were many more walls (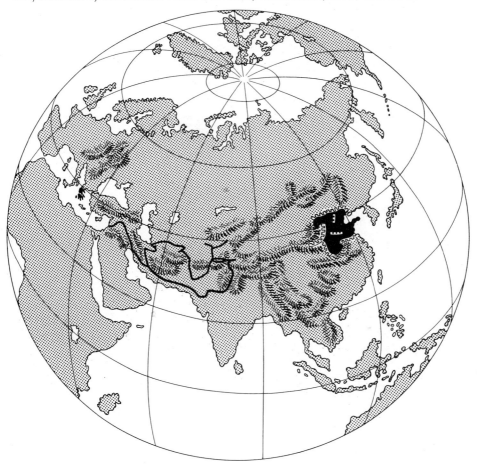) than indicated.

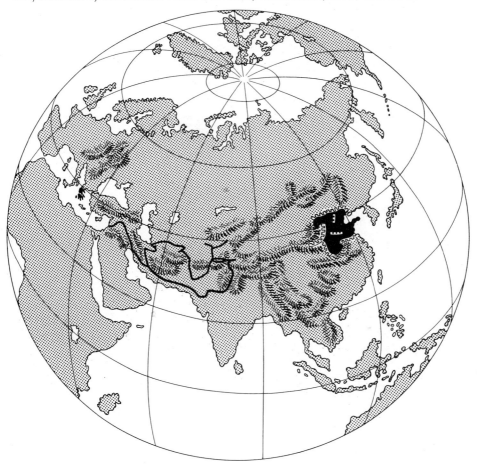

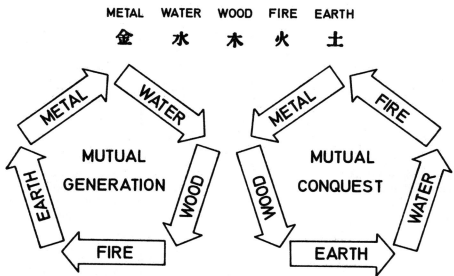

METAL WATER WOOD FIRE EARTH
金　　水　　木　　火　　土

MUTUAL
GENERATION

MUTUAL
CONQUEST

6.5 The five elements and their interrelations.

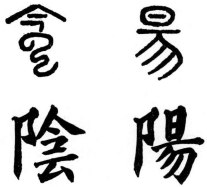

6.6 Origin of the signs *yin,* the female, moist principle, and *yang,* the male, dry principle. *Above left:* ancient form of *yin,* a cloud beneath a roof-shaped sign, "cloudy weather." *Below left:* modern form, with the radical ⻖ for "hill." Hence, one of the original meanings of *yin* was "shady side of a hill" (a *radical* is a part of a character that gives the general meaning of the word, much like the Egyptian determinative). *Above right:* ancient form of *yang,* sun above the horizon and sunrays. *Below right:* modern form again with the radical ⻖ for "hill." Hence, *yang* also meant "sunny side of a hill."

find the *Lun Yü* or "Conversations and Discourses" of Confucius, and leafing among tablets and bamboo strips, we might find hints of the five-element theory that was about to crystallize.[8] It held that everything was made of water, fire, wood, metal and earth, bound by an "order of mutual production" and an "order of mutual conquest" (Fig. 6.5).[9]

Somewhere we would run into the characters 侌 and 昜, the archaic versions of yin and yang (Fig. 6.6). The two inseparable forces had already been a theme of Chinese philosophy for some time. One can envision Chou scholars discussing yin and yang at the time the Parthenon was going up.[10] Yang was the bright, dry, masculine aspect; yin the dark, moist,

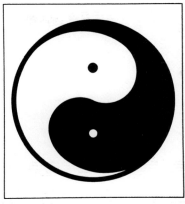

6.7 This figuration of yin and yang implies that the two principles are inseparable: there is yin in yang, and yang in yin.

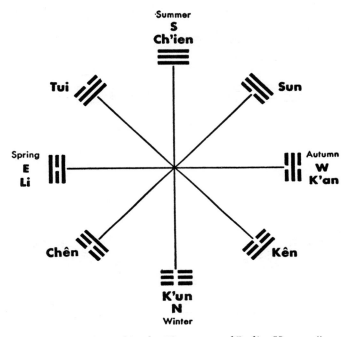

6.8 The Eight Trigrams, arranged in the "Sequence of Earlier Heaven," one of several possible patterns. Each trigram has a name and correlates with a season, a cardinal point, and many other notions (note that the south, Chinese style, is at the top).

feminine. They were not opposed as "good" and "bad,"[11] but were complementary, and both were necessary for proper balance, so that pure yang and pure yin could not exist. There is always yin in yang and yang in yin. Nowadays everybody knows the visual symbol of this ancient scheme, made of two figures shaped as tadpoles inscribed in a circle (Fig. 6.7). Less familiar is the linear representation, which was probably already known at the time of the Chou scholar. Three continuous yang lines ☰ and three broken yin lines ☷ were diversely combined to produce eight (*pa*) trigrams (*kua*), each combination having a name, a special meaning, and a long list of associations (Fig. 6.8).[12] The number of lines could also be doubled to form a

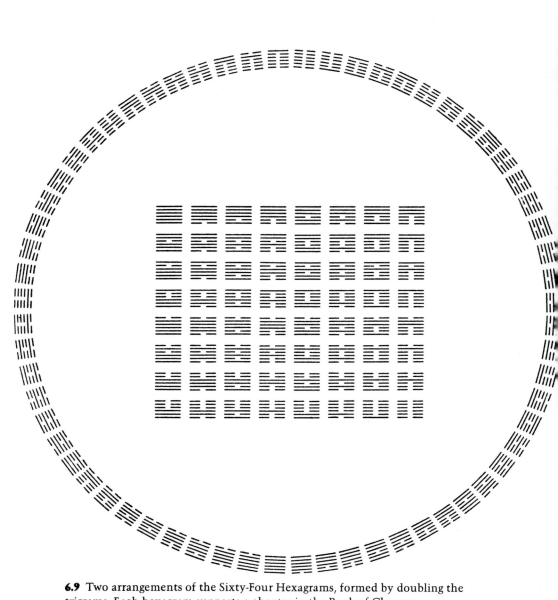

6.9 Two arrangements of the Sixty-Four Hexagrams, formed by doubling the trigrams. Each hexagram supports a chapter in the Book of Changes.

hexagram. This gave birth to a series of sixty-four combinations, from the purely yang-line set ≣ to the purely yin-line set ≣ ≣, each one of the symbols again having a name and an abstract significance, like "coherence," "slow advance," "corruption," "inspiration" (Fig. 6.9).

These sixty-four hexagrams formed the basis of another great classic available in the Chou library, the *I Ching* or "Book of Changes," which also began to take shape long before the Golden Age of Greece.[13] This is an oracle book of tremendous reputation, especially the reputation for giving the right answer.[14] It has been consulted throughout Chinese history until recent times.[15] Unlike any other oracle book, the *I Ching* attracted a vast amount of comment and scholarly work, which mingled with the original "irrational" element to form something not known in other cultures: an oracle book with high ethical overtones.[16]

The *I Ching* consists of sixty-four short texts, one per hexagram, written in a style that is both lofty and obscure.[17] It works like this. The reader who needs advice performs certain manipulations with fifty little sticks; in this way he obtains a series of six lines, whole or broken, that build up a hexagram. This is the key to the proper place in the *I Ching*. For example, for the hexagram ䷘, which stands *wu wang*, "innocence," he would find:

> Use no medicine in an illness
> Incurred through no fault of your own.
> It will pass of itself.[18]

From there on the reader has to decide for himself what to do.

The success of this book is difficult to grasp for Western readers. It was discussed not long ago by C. G. Jung, the Swiss psychologist, who interpreted the use of the *I Ching* as a subtle technique for exploring the unconscious.[19] The idea is fascinating, although it would apply as well to any other oracle book, for it simply means that the reader is unconsciously guided to search for his own solution.

One of the statements in the *I Ching* is that "the great-souled man always meditates on trouble in advance and takes steps to prevent it."[20] The same thought is expressed in many other books, political as well as medical, and even in an old geography treatise on the shelves of the Chou library, the *Shan Hai Ching* or "Classic of Mountains and Rivers," which mentions in passing a number of herbs and drugs "good for preventing" this or that ailment.[21]

Prevention is better than repression: why would this particular thought keep reappearing, like a tune played in different keys? A likely reason is that it came about at first as a political principle, reflecting the strains of a feudal society in which forethought and prevention were means of survival. Then the same concept was applied to bodily illness. There is nothing strange about this shift from politics to medicine, for in the Chinese view of the world, everything was correlated: a healthy state depended on a balance of individuals, the health of individuals depended on the world around, and the health of each organ depended on all the others—so that nothing could change without changing the whole. A fifth century A.D. commentary on the *I Ching* actually states that this is the basic idea of the book; it "can be expressed in one single word, *Resonance* (Kan)."[22]

I will stop here, for it is uncomfortable to browse in a dream library. But the point of this survey is that the Chou scholar had at hand a vast and ancient literature, utterly unknown in the Mediterranean world, and utterly unaware of that world. The actual records that the Chou scholar himself was compiling were used about two hundred years after his death by historians of the early Han Dynasty (2nd century B.C.), to compile a book on the organization of the Chou state as they saw it.[23] Called the *Chou Li*, or "Institutions of the Chou," this book is a document of great interest, because it portrays the ideal state as the Han imagined it. It also contains a few nuggets about things medical.

The Institutions of the Chou

For those who wrote it, the table of contents of the *Chou Li* was a purely technical list of palace administrators; to us it reads as if it came from a fable: Chief of the Palace, Cooks for the Interior, Cooks for the Exterior, Workers of the Extracts, Workers of the Ice-room, Chief of the Writings, Imperial Concubines, Director of the Silk, Officer of the Feathers, Superintendent of Violence . . .[24] Each service was assigned a specific staff, so that one can assess its relative importance. The personnel assignments for the five medical services ran as follows, arranged here as in the original text, after the turtle-catchers and officers of dried food, and before the wine-people:[25]

Service of the Turtle-Catchers

Third-class graduates	4
Warehouse-wardens	2
Scribes	2
Apprentices	16
	24

Service of the Officers of Dried Food

Third-class graduates	4
Warehouse-wardens	2
Scribes	2
Apprentices	20
	28

Service of the Chief of Physicians

First-class graduates	2
Third-class graduates	4
Warehouse-wardens	2
Scribes	2
Apprentices	20
	30

Service of the Physician for Simple Diseases

Second-class graduates	**8**

Service of the Ulcer Physicians (Yang I)

Third-class graduates	**8**

Service of the Food Physician

Second-class graduates	**2**

Service of the Physician for the Animals

Third-class graduates	**4**

Service of the Superintendent of Wines

Second-class graduates	4
Third-class graduates	8
Warehouse-wardens	2
Scribes	8
Aides	8
Apprentices	80
	110

Service of the Wine-Men [sic]

Eunuchs	10
Wine-women	30
Convicts	300
	340

It is obvious from these lists that the employees of the Chou were fitted into a system of degrees, much like that of today's state administration.[26]

The specific duties of each employee are listed in Book 5 of the *Chou Li*. Quoted below are the main duties of the physicians, with explanations contributed by ancient commentators in brackets.[27] Note the recurring "established sets" of items, usually five, six, or eight, and the persistent references to seasons in human affairs.

Chief of Physicians (I Shih)

He is entrusted with the overall direction of the physicians. He collects the powerful drugs [literally "poisonous drugs;" these are "the bitter substances used as medicines. According to the *Chou-king*, a drug cannot heal unless it is disagreeable"] used in the art of healing. All the people belonging to the administration of the kingdom, who suffer from ordinary diseases, head diseases, or wounds, come to him. Thereupon he orders the various physicians to share among them the treatment of these diseases. At the end of the year he examines the work of the physicians, in order to settle their appointments. The first degree corresponds to ten complete recoveries, or to ten complete treatments. One mistake out of ten cases is the second degree. Then, two mistakes out of ten cases; three mistakes out of ten cases; the last degree is four mistakes out of ten cases. [According to one commentator, there were five degrees below the maximum. Two other commentators disagree about the requirement of complete recovery, for "there are incurable diseases. The Chief of Physicians only verifies whether the treatment has been applied with knowledge of the disease. One cannot demand recovery"].

Food Physician (Shih I, "Dietician")

He must arrange for the regular preparation of the six vegetable foods, the six types of drinks, the six main foods, the one hundred delicate foods, the one hundred dressings, the eight choice dishes for the Emperor. In general, for the regular preparation of the vegetable foods, he considers spring. To prepare juices or sauces, he considers summer. To prepare dressings, he considers autumn. To prepare drinks, he considers winter [meaning of the seasons: "vegetables must be warm, sauces hot, dressings cool, drinks cold"].

Physicians for Simple Diseases (Chi I)

They treat the minor ailments and the diseases of the people.

There are special diseases for each season. In spring, there are headaches and troubles with the head. In summer there are ulcers and sores. In autumn there are fevers and colds. In winter there are coughs and troubles of breathing.

They look after and treat these diseases with the five tastes [vinegar, wine, honey, ginger, and salt], with the five kinds of grain, with the five kinds of drugs [herbs, trees, insects, stones, and grains].

They test by the five kinds of breaths, by the five kinds of sounds, by the five colors, whether the patients are alive or dead.

They test a second time by changes in the nine orifices of the body. They test a third time by movements of the nine viscera.

They treat separately the men of the people who are sick. If death occurs, or end of life [death applies to the young, end of life to the aged], then each physician writes the causes whereby this happened, and hands over this note to the Chief of Physicians [The Chief of Physicians collects the death-notes; he uses them to fix the level of appointment, or even to forbid a physician from treating any further].

瘍醫

Ulcer Physicians (Yang I)

They are in charge of treating swollen ulcers, ulcers that drip, ulcers caused by metal ["wounds caused by cutting weapons"; Fig. 6.10], ulcers of fractures ["those caused by falling"]. They apply drugs to them. They cleanse them and destroy them [the comments suggest that the "destruction of bad flesh and of spoiled blood" is accomplished by the drugs applied].

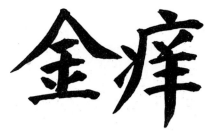

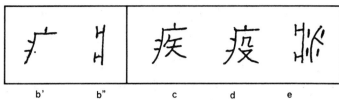

a   b'   b"   c   d   e

6.10 "Metal ulcer," *jin yang*, the term used in the *Chou Li* for wounds caused by weapons. Some older, related signs appear below: (a) "metal," probably a mine-shaft with a cover and lumps of ore; (b', b") "bed," the radical *ni* contained in the character for "ulcer" (most diseases were later classified under this radical; see Fig. 6.15, for example); (c) "epidemic disease," a man on a bed; (d) "epidemic fever," a hand and stick over a bed, symbolizing a man belabored by disease (the same hand and stick as in the character for "physician"; see Fig. 6.11); (e) "itching scabies-like epidemic" (presumably an infectious fever with a skin rash), a man with spots lying on a bed.

     In general, to heal the ulcers, they attack them with the five poisonous substances; they fortify them with the five emanations or with the five kinds of grains; they heal them with the five medicinal substances; they temper them by the five flavors.

     In general, when they apply drugs, they fortify the bones with the acid principle; they fortify the nerves with the stinging principle; they fortify the pulse with the salty principle; they fortify respiration with the bitter principle; they fortify the bodily openings with the oily principle.

     All those that have ulcers receive their drugs.

Physicians for the Animals (Shou I, *"Veterinarians"*)

     In general, to heal the simple diseases of the animals, they sprinkle them and make them walk ["Diseases of animals are difficult to recognize. The animal is sprinkled with an infusion of medicinal plants, so as to make it feel comfortable." "When the animal has walked at a moderate pace, its pulse is examined: this way its disease is recognized"] . . .

     In case of death, the number of lost animals is counted, so as to raise or lower the physician's level of appointment.

[*The duties of the Superintendent of Wines, which follow, are quite a bit longer and more complex.*]

     Dissected by the historian's scalpel, these pages of the *Chou Li* reveal more than they say. First of all, they show that medicine—as in Greece—had

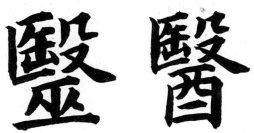

6.11 A step in the evolution of Chinese medicine, reflected in the evolution of the character *i* for "physician." The lower part changes from "sorcerer" (bottom left) to "wine" (bottom right).

slipped out of the hands of the priests and sorcerers, whose duties are listed separately. This evolution must have fully occurred by the time of Confucius, who said around 500 B.C. that "a man without persistence will never make a good magician (*wu*) or a good physician (*i*)."[28] The birth of professional Chinese medicine corresponds to an interesting change in the character *I* for "physician."[29] Its ancient form consists of three parts (Fig. 6.11). At the top left is the radical for "quiver of arrows" or "chest of arms," on its right is a hand grasping a weapon 殳 and below is the symbol for "sorcerer" or "priest" 巫. The complete character conveys that the priest uses strong weapons to fight off the demons of disease. Later, the lower part of the character changes to the symbol for "wine" 酉—indicating that the practice of medicine is in the hands of professionals, who are now giving drugs—indeed "wine-drugs."

A second message of the *Chou Li* is the low status of surgery, since it was limited to a small group of "third-rate graduates." Things were quite different in China's great neighbor India, where surgery was a noble art.

Third, the practice of medicine was a tightly organized state system, in which the physicians were graded according to achievement, like everybody else. The grading of state employees remained a typical feature of Chinese administration from the Chou onward. At first the criterion was achievement; then came regular exams. On this subject the Chinese claim to priority is unbeatable: objective techniques for measuring the ability of a candidate for service in the government was devised as early as the fourth century B.C., and the earliest formal written examination of which there is an unimpeachable record, anywhere in the world, was given at the Chinese court in 165 B.C.[30] Slowly the idea diffused West, via Baghdad and the Islamic world. It reached Europe early in the twelfth century and was applied first in the medical field: the practice of examining physicians, required in Sicily by the statute of Roger II the Norman in 1140, was in all likelihood a distant reflection of Chinese standards.[31] Classical Greece had no such rational system for selecting its public physicians. What little is known about it suggests that if there was any test, it was rather a matter of delivering a good speech.[32]

瘍醫

The Cornerstone of Chinese Medicine

The most important medical text of Chinese antiquity, indeed of Chinese medicine altogether, is by far the *Huang Ti Nei Ching*, or *Nei Ching* for short, comparable for its impact to the Hippocratic Collection. Scholars, Chinese or not, agree on one point: although its basic principles are relatively simple, the *Nei Ching* is an extremely difficult book to translate, and often also to understand. The difficulties begin with the title, usually translated as "The Yellow Emperor's Classic on Internal Medicine." Huang Ti was in fact the Yellow Emperor (his yellowness, however, had nothing to do with skin color: yellow stood for "centrality," hence "majesty," doubtless because of the color of the cradle of Chinese civilization—think of the Yellow River[33]). According to tradition, Huang Ti lived between 2629 and 2598 B.C., and it was he who wrote the *Nei Ching*. It is now known that Huang Ti belongs to legend, and in any event Chinese history cannot be pushed farther back than about 1500 B.C.[34] *Nei* means "inside," and by extension everything "this-worldly," rational, practical; as opposed to *wai*, "outside," and by extension "other-worldly," having to do with gods and spirits. *Ching* may be rendered as "classic" or "manual." Therefore, the best translation of *Nei Ching*—to use an old English word—might be "Manual of Physic."[35]

One basic difference with the Hippocratic Collection is the certainty of dates. The Collection unquestionably took shape between 450 and 350 B.C. As for the *Nei Ching*, Huang Wên believes that the original text was probably put together between 479 and 300 B.C. (which would make it almost exactly contemporary with the Hippocratic corpus) and then recast or reedited four times, the last between 1068 and 1078 A.D. According to Lu Gwei-Djen and Joseph Needham, the text had probably reached its present form—or nearly so—by the first century B.C.[36] In any event, it is certain that in the course of successive editions the original message lost some of its purity. How much it lost, nobody knows. Part of the problem is that in ancient manuscripts the comments were written into the text and therefore became practically indistinguishable from it. In this respect, a special debt of gratitude is owed to the ancient Egyptian commentator who inserted his glosses into the Smith papyrus, but always labeled them with the formula *yr . . . pw . . .* , "As for . . . it means . . ."[37] Thus, his own text and the original cannot be confused.

To someone who cannot read any of the 49,000 Chinese characters, a complete translation of the great Chinese medical classic is available only in French, and that only since 1957. It is a book of average size and reads rather like a catechism, being written in the form of a conversation between Emperor Huang Ti and his prime minister, Ch'i Po, who speaks like a wise logician and never presents himself specifically as a medical man. If the book originally had a plan, not much of it is left; the discourse runs unpredictably about disease mechanisms at a physiophilosophical level. On the whole, what would be called practical advice is left in the shade. The author seems much more concerned about guiding the patient back to *Tao*, "The Way," than about specifics for his diarrhea (Fig. 6.12). The single form of treatment

瘍醫

240

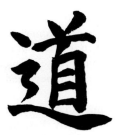

6.12 *Tao*, "The Way" or "The Way of Nature." The bottom stroke and the left part of the sign are the radical for "treading a path;" the right part means "head."

discussed in some detail is acupuncture; even treatment by drugs is just hinted.

A book that presided over the health of one quarter of the people on this globe for 2500 years is not to be taken lightly. However, an overall judgement on the *Nei Ching* is very difficult to give. The English translation is incomplete and tentative;[38] as a layman, I have my own doubts about the French version too, for it uses expressions such as "epidermis" and "violin strings."[39] The Chinese original is said to be in parts very obscure; and there is always the risk of mistaking obscurity for profundity.

It is safe to say that the book has a definite coherence, in that it is based on the yin-yang concept, on the five elements, and on the maze of correlations so typical of ancient Chinese philosophy. Inevitably, to anyone who does not share these premises, the beauty of the system becomes vagueness and irrelevance. A German scholar has recently undertaken to explain the inner logic of the yin-yang world using Latin terminology:[40] to the average reader the result is thoroughly forbidding.

Yet, even in translation, and even if its literal message is partially lost, the *Nei Ching* is a document of great human interest; the very fact that it is more philosophical than strictly medical may contain an important message for physicians of the Western world. I will quote below a few paragraphs that I find especially pertinent, although I feel obliged to warn the reader once again that the *Nei Ching* in English garb may come as close to the original as dream to reality. I should never have tried to compare the translations. For example, consider Su Wên 14. In the French version, the Emperor asks: "Comment doit-on soigner le malade?"—"How should one look after the patient?" In the English, he asks: "How can one prepare soup?"[41] In Su Wên 16, the Emperor is inquiring, in French, about "the examination of the patient;" in English, about "the rules of death."[42] I find this unnerving. On the whole, however, the topics and the "atmosphere" remain similar enough to warrant the following quotations.[43]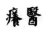

The first one shows that some problems have not changed in two millennia:

The Yellow Emperor once addressed T'ien Shih, the divinely inspired teacher: "I have heard that in ancient times the people lived (through the years) to be over a hundred years, and yet they remained active and did not become decrepit in their activities. But nowadays people reach only half of that age and yet become decrepit and failing. Is it because the world changes from generation to generation? Or is it that mankind is becoming negligent (of the laws of nature)?"

Ch'i Po answered: "In ancient times those people who understood Tao patterned themselves upon the Yin and the Yang and they lived in harmony with the arts of divination.

"There was temperance in eating and drinking. Their hours of rising and retiring were regular and not disorderly and wild. By these means the ancients kept their bodies united with their souls, so as to fulfill their allotted span completely, measuring unto a hundred years before they passed away.

"Nowadays people are not like this; they use wine as beverage and they adopt recklessness as usual behavior . . . They do not know how to find contentment within themselves; they are not skilled in the control of their spirits. They devote all their attention to the amusement of their minds, thus cutting themselves off from the joys of long (life). Their rising and retiring is without regularity. For these reasons they reach only one half of the hundred years and then they degenerate."[44]

The next two examples, though typical of the *Nei Ching*, develop the same theme as the Hippocratic treatise *Airs Waters Places*—disease depends on geography and the seasons:

The Yellow Emperor asked: "When the physicians treat diseases, do they treat each disease differently from the others and can they all be healed?"

Ch'i Po answered: "Yes, they can all be healed according to the physical features of the place where one lives . . . The people of the regions of the East eat fish and crave salt; their living is tranquil and their food delicious. Fish causes people to burn within (thirst), and the eating of salt injures (defeats) the blood . . . Their diseases are ulcers, which are most properly treated with acupuncture by means of a needle of flint. Thus, the treatment with acupuncture with a needle of flint has its origin in the regions of the East."[45]

Those who disobey the laws of Spring will be punished with an injury to the liver. For them the following Summer will bring chills . . .

Those who disobey the laws of Summer will be punished with an injury to the heart. For them the Fall will bring intermittent fevers.[46]

And here is the case for preventive medicine. Note the arguments drawn, typically, from politics:

The superior physician helps before the early budding of the disease. He must first examine the three regions of the body and define the atmosphere of the nine subdivisions so that they are entirely in harmony . . . Therefore he is called the superior physician.

The inferior physician begins to help when (the disease) has already developed; he helps when destruction has already set in. And since his help comes when the disease has already developed, it is said of him that he is ignorant.[47]

Hence, the sages did not treat those who were already ill; they instructed those who were not yet ill. They did not want to rule those who were already rebellious; they guided those who were not yet rebellious . . . To administer medicines to diseases which have already developed and to suppress revolts which have already developed is comparable to the behavior of those persons who begin to dig a well after they have become thirsty, and of those who begin to cast weapons after they have already engaged in battle. Would these actions not be too late?[48]

The following is an example of yin and yang theory. It, too, is related to the seasons:

Thus, mankind should correspond to this system: the Yin and Yang of man are (arranged in the order) that on the outside there is Yang, and inside there is Yin. Yin and Yang of the human body (are arranged) that Yang is in back and Yin is within the front part. Yin and Yang of the (five) viscera and the (six) bowels are (arranged) that the viscera are Yin and the hollow organs are Yang. All of the five viscera—liver, heart, spleen, lungs, and kidneys—are Yin; and all of the five hollow organs—gall-bladder, stomach, lower intestines, bladder, and the three burning spaces [*imaginary organs*]—are all Yang.

The reason why we must know (the rule of) the Yin within the Yin and (the rule of) the Yang within the Yang is that the diseases of Winter are located in (the region of) Yang and the diseases of Summer in (the region of) Yin; the diseases of Spring are located in the (region of) Yin and the diseases of Fall in the (region of) Yang. We must know the location of all these diseases for (the purpose of) acupuncture.[49]

Now hear an interesting statement on acupuncture, one that may contain a profound truth—cure depends on the patient's will:

The Emperor asked: "When the body is worn out and the blood is exhausted, is it still possible to achieve good results?"
Ch'i Po replied: "No, because there is no more energy left."
The Emperor inquired: "What does it mean, there is no more energy left?"
Ch'i Po answered: *"This is the way of acupuncture: if man's vitality and energy do not propel his own will, his disease cannot be cured."*[50]

More about acupuncture, the seasons, and wind as a cause of disease:

If one perspires while (physically) weary, one is susceptible to (evil) winds which cause eruptions of the skin; and those, if irritated, will develop into sores . . .
If the atmosphere of the (main) "ducts" is not harmonious with the system of the flesh, it will cause ulcers and swellings. Then the perspiration of the animal spirit is unable to reach out . . . the "(acupuncture) spots" will be closed, and there arise winds and intermittent fevers.
Thus, wind is the cause of a hundred diseases. When people are quiet and clear, their skin and flesh is closed and protected. Even a heavy storm, afflictions, or poison cannot injure those people who live in accord with the natural order.

If a sickness lasts a long time, there is danger that it might spread, then the upper and the lower (parts of the body) cannot communicate; and even skillful physicians are then not able to help.
If Yang accumulates excessively, one will die from the (resulting) disease . . .
If one does not drain it thoroughly and guide away the rough matter [with acupuncture], there will be destruction.[51]

And finally, here are some thoughts on the soul, the body, and disease:

When the spirit is hurt, severe pains ensue; when the body is hurt, there will be swellings. Thus, in those cases where severe pains are felt first and the swellings

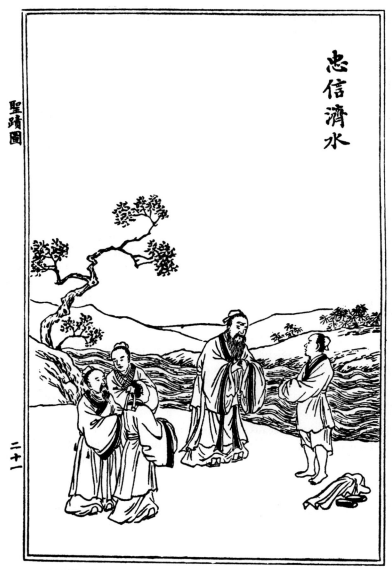

6.13 Confucius on the bank of the Yellow River. This is an episode of his life, drawn by an artist of the Yüan Dynasty, 1260–1368 A.D. Confucius died in 479 B.C., a few years before the birth of Hippocrates.

appear later, one can say that the spirit has injured the body. And in those cases where swellings appear first and severe pains are felt later, one can say that the body has injured the spirit.[52]

Ch'i Po answered: "The utmost in the art of healing can be achieved when there is unity."

The Emperor inquired: "What is meant by unity?"

Ch'i Po answered: "When the minds of the people are closed and wisdom is locked out they remain tied to disease. Yet their feelings and desires should be investigated and made known, their wishes and ideas should be followed; and then it becomes apparent that those who have attained spirit and energy are flourishing and prosperous, while those perish who lose their spirit and energy."[53]

Life itself is the beginning of illness.[54]

244

The Yang I Approach to a Sore

Surely, about 400 B.C., some prince at the Chou court in Loyang limped from a varicose ulcer on the ankle, a bad case, complicated with infection and inflammation. How would he have been treated, compared with a similar patient in an Athenian infirmary?

I have not forgotten the warning of Calvin Wells about imaginative insight having to stop short of delirium; but defeatism is a crime, too. I shall therefore attempt to answer my own question, using the *Nei Ching* as a guide, as I have done with the Hippocratic books. If Huang Wên is right, the core of the *Nei Ching* appeared at the time of our story, around 400 B.C.; some of its content, like the yin and the yang, is even older, and if some is later, it still refers to ancient Chinese practice. So here is a sequence of medical gestures, reconstructed from the *Nei Ching*.[55]

Upon meeting his patient, the yang i would begin—as we do today—by asking questions, though not quite the same as we would choose: was he rich or poor? had he seen better times? had he noticed any change in appetite? had there been any change in his comfort of living? was his disease affected by changes in the weather? Failure to ask any of these questions was one of the "five errors" and "four mistakes."[56]

Then he would feel the pulse on both of the patient's wrists and compare it with his own, in an elaborate ritual, which could take hours (Fig. 6.14). He was supposed to recognize dozens of subtle changes, poetically described in the *Nei Ching*. The pulse could be:

> . . . sharp as a hook
> fine as a hair
> taut as a music string
> dead as a rock
> smooth as a flowing stream
> continuous like a string of pearls
> slightly indented in the middle
> the front crooked
>   and the back delayed
> soft and fluttering
>   like floating feathers
>   blown by the wind
> elastic like a bending pole
> taut as a bow when first bent
> following up delicately
>   like a cock treading ground
>   or lifting a foot
> sharp as a bird's beak
> like water dripping
>   through the roof
> resonant like striking a stone
> rapid as the edge of a knife
>   in cutting
> vibrating as when one stops the strings
>   of a musical instrument

245

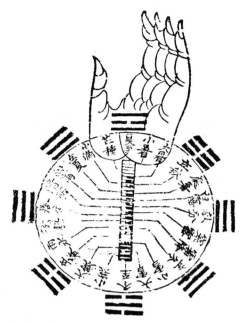

6.14 Instructions for feeling the pulse during each of the twenty-four seasons of the year.

> light as flicking the skin
>   with a plume
> arriving like a suspended hook
> multiple as the seeds
>   of the flower blossom
> like burning firewood
> like leaves scattering
> like visiting strangers
> like a dry mud-ball
> like mixing lacquer
> like spring water welling up
> like sparse earth
> like being stopped
>   by a horizontal partition
> like a suspended curtain
> like a sword lying flat ready to be used
> like a smooth pill
> like glory . . .[57]

If the translation is correct, one can visualize the yang i holding the wrist, closing his eyes, and trying to decide whether the throbbing beneath his fingers felt like any one of the items listed above, or even like the colors red, white, green, yellow, or black.[58] The purpose of this exercise was to extract from the pulse the whole picture of the disease, which is about as hopeless as trying to gather the contents of a page—or of a whole book—from a single line. Thus, it is inaccurate to say that these or any other ancient physicians developed a great "mastery" of the pulse.[59] However, it must be remembered that while little information was passing—through the pulse—from patient to physician, much comfort was surely flowing the other way.

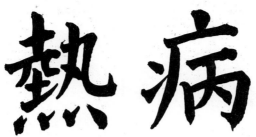

6.15 The "hot disease," mentioned in the *Nei Ching,* presumably a variety of feverish conditions, including inflammation. Note the flames (bottom left).

Next, the yang i would examine the hot, inflamed skin around the ulcer. He might conclude that this was a form of the "hot disease," as indicated by the flames in the Chinese character (Fig. 6.15; there were also a cold and a lukewarm disease).[60] Now it was thought that heat developed when yin was wanting and yang prevailed. Remember: yin is cold and moist; yang is hot and dry. To bring back the balance, there were at least two maneuvers of the kind that we would call "local treatment": piercing the skin with one or more needles (acupuncture), and burning it with small lumps of smoldering material, a procedure known today—outside of China—as *moxa.*

Drainage, Chinese Style

Drainage: this was, indeed, the basic meaning of acupuncture. It was not a mild form of Chinese torture, dreamed up by a sadist; nor was it an Eastern fantasy, created out of thin air. It was a different solution to the problem of restoring the balance. The Greeks had the same general idea; but their imbalanced four humors were all in the blood, so their response was to draw out blood. The Chinese solution was much more subtle. It seems that the barbarous procedure of slitting veins was totally unknown in ancient China[61] (though a few drops of capillary blood were drawn at times by acupuncture). Instead, the Chinese conceived a set of imaginary, or spiritual, vessels or "meridians," containing not blood but *ch'i.* This principle was something like the Greek *pneuma* or "energy."[62] It could be either drawn out or replenished (inward), simply by needling the right ch'i vessel. Thus, the needling could be called a form of drainage—of "energy" rather than blood.

This dual "inward" and "outward" purpose of needling is evident throughout the *Nei Ching.*[63] The terms used in the translations are "extraction," "purging," "draining."[64] It is possible that the use of the needle as an "energy drain" may have had its roots in true surgical drainage; at least it is often said—on what authority I do not know—that acupuncture began in prehistoric times, with the practice of piercing to let out pus or blood.[65] However, an advantage of spiritual drainage is that it can go both ways. The needles could let "energy" out as well as in and thus replenish it from the outside (Fig. 6.16). Even today's acupuncturists sometimes "disperse" and sometimes "tonify."[66]

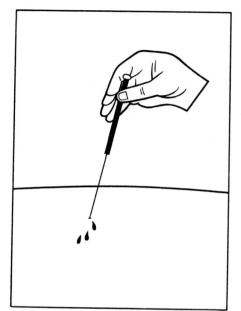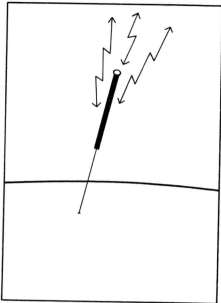

6.16 Scheme of the ways in which a needle can "drain in the intention of the acupuncturist: letting blood out (left), letting energy in and out (right).

Yin and yang were seen then, as they are still, not as bodily juices—like black bile and yellow bile—but as cosmic forces present everywhere. Yang gives the heat of fever and inflammation, but also the warm air of the south; and the clammy excess of yin is also responsible for the chills of the north. In the words of a modern scholar-acupuncturist, "the vital energy of the body is the same energy that fills the cosmos."[67] All this adds up to a beautiful, universal scheme, easily explained to any patient, and perfectly designed to suit the needs of men and women who firmly believed in the need to be tuned to the outside world.

So the yang i, having first established that the season, the day, the hour, and everything else was right, took a sliver of flint from his set of nine needles and stabbed it into the skin along a certain line. Of the 365 possible points, only one would do (Fig. 6.17).[68] What was the effect on the varicose ulcer? I transcribe this astonishing statement from the modern preface to the French version of the *Nei Ching:* "[It is here again] that we found, as regards technique, that sensational novelty—the handling of the triangular needle. With it, the most rebellious varicose ulcers disappear in a short time."[69]

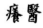

However, accidents were also possible. Even the *Nei Ching* admits that sometimes the condition worsened, and that needles "wrongly applied" could cause abscesses and even death.[70] "Wrongly applied" means that if an infection developed, the yang i could not write it off to bad luck or accident; he would be guilty of having hit the wrong point. Hindu surgeons reasoned the same way in cases where an abscess developed after piercing an ear lobe.

The next step of the treatment for the ulcer might be to rekindle the fiery yang—of course, not on the leg, where it had been drawn by the ulcer,

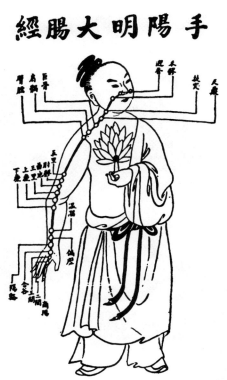

手陽明大腸經

6.17 One of the vessels or "meridians" of acupuncture, none of which follow the blood vessels. This one, for instance, runs from the tip of a finger to the nose.

but at some other distant spot. To do so, the yang i would ask the patient to lie on his bed, face down. Then he would reach into a bag, pull out two or three pinches of a gray, powdery fuzz, roll it into a little cone, and balance it on the back of the patient, at one precise spot.[71] After carefully setting fire to the tip of the cone, he would let it smolder until nothing was left but ashes, and—presumably—a blister.

This method is still used widely today as an adjunct to acupuncture (Fig. 6.18). The material consists of powdered leaves of *Artemisia vulgaris* or *alba* (mugwort, a relative of wormwood); its active principle is supposed to be the down of these leaves. Basically, this treatment is a cautery, but a discreet, even thrifty one, typical of a culture closer to plants than to minerals.[72] Its Latin name of *ignipuncture*, literally "stinging with fire," implies the link with acupuncture. The more common name, however, is a word of Japanese origin, *moxa*. Fire being yang, the theory seems to be that moxa is indicated when there is an excess of yin.[73]

It goes without saying that the moxa hurts, though less than did the red-hot irons of the Greeks. Nowadays, a slice of onion, garlic, or ginger may be placed beneath the smoldering cone; or the cone is removed before it has burned down to the skin.[74] Otherwise, patients grin and bear it. The Chinese approach to pain is epitomized in the traditional story (perhaps 1800 years old) of the surgeon Hua T'o operating on General Kuan Yü, whose arm had

醫療

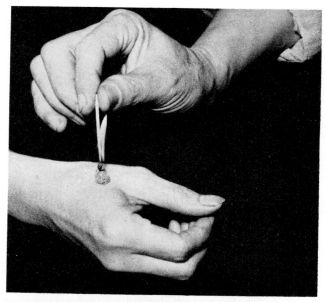

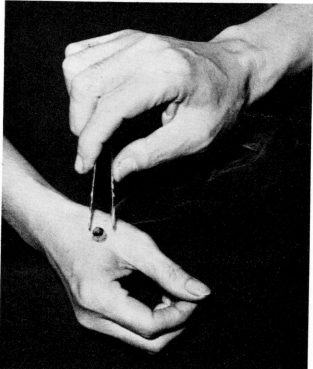

6.18 Chinese ignipuncture or *moxa* as practiced today. A cone of *Artemisia* fluff is placed on the proper point and lit (above), then allowed to smolder. According to this particular modern scheme, the cone is removed just as it begins to cause a reddening of the skin (below). In this mild version, the moxa can no longer be considered a cautery in the ordinary sense; however, the burning *Artemisia* fluff is supposed to produce curative effects of its own, independent of cauterization.

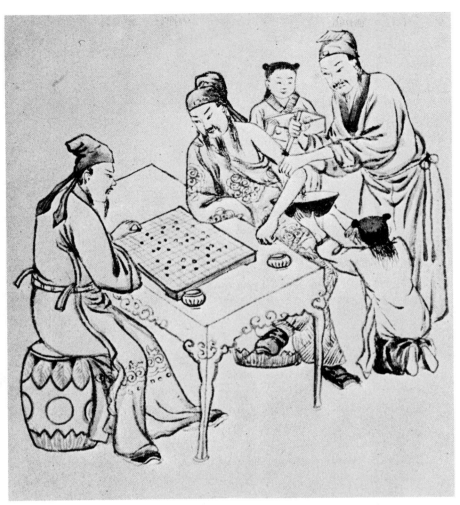

6.19 Ancient Chinese anesthesia: stoicism and a game of oriental chess. Hua T'o, a surgeon, is operating on General Kuan Yü for a poisoned-arrow wound.

been pierced by a poisoned arrow. While the knife went *hsi, hsi,* scraping the bone, the general played chess—and drank cups of wine (Fig. 6.19).[75]

After the use of the needle or the burn to treat an ulcer, there would come some medicine, possibly also a purge,[76] and the prescription of a diet. On these I cannot comment,[77] except to say that if the yang i was really to observe his five-fold correlations, I doubt that he could do so without a book. In the tables of correlations that eventually grew out of Chinese medico-philosophical thought, everything was linked to everything else (Fig. 6.20). To make the "correct" move in that maze today, one would need a computer; and even then the answer would be nonsense, or the computer would jam, because the tables were contradictory. In one catalog, for example, the correlations add up to more than one hundred categories.[78]

In the end, if the patient did not improve, the yang i had the perfect excuse: he had been called in too late. In the words of the sages, who would wait to be thirsty before beginning to dig his well?

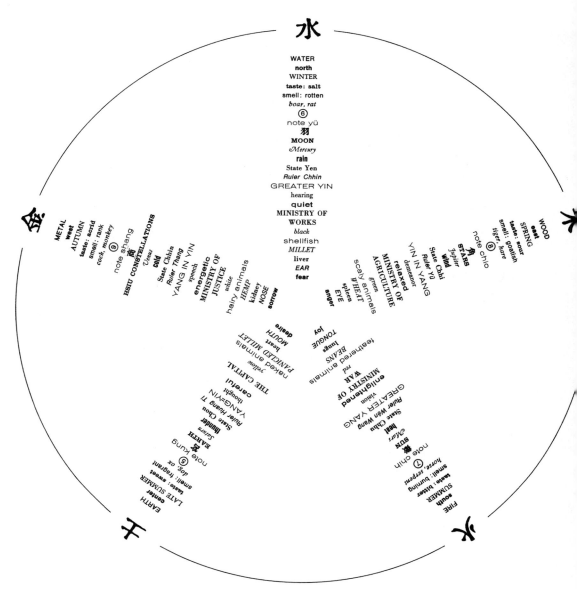

水

WATER
north
WINTER
taste: salt
smell: rotten
boar, rat
⑥
note yü
羽
MOON
Mercury
rain
State Yen
Ruler Chhin
GREATER YIN
hearing
quiet
MINISTRY OF
WORKS
black
shellfish
MILLET
liver
EAR
fear

金

METAL
west
AUTUMN
taste: acrid
smell: rank
cock, monkey
⑨
note shang
商
Gold
State Chhin
Ruler Thang
YANG IN YIN
speech
energetic
MINISTRY OF
JUSTICE
white
hairy animals
HEMP
kidney
NOSE
sorrow

HSIU CONSTELLATIONS

木

WOOD
east
SPRING
taste: sour
smell: goatish
tiger, hare
⑧
note chio
角
STARS
Jupiter
Wind
State Chhi
Ruler Yü
YIN IN YANG
demeanor
relaxed
MINISTRY OF
AGRICULTURE
green
scaly animals
WHEAT
spleen
EYE
anger

TONGUE
joy
lungs
BEANS
feathered animals
red
MINISTRY OF
WAR
enlightened
Ruler Wen Wang
State Chhu
GREATER YANG
vision
Mars
SUN
熒
note chih
horse, serpent
taste: bitter
smell: burning
SUMMER
south
FIRE

火

heart
desire
MOUTH
PANICLED MILLET
naked animals
yellow
THE CAPITAL
careful
YANG-YIN
thought
Ruler Huang Ti
State Chou
Saturn
塡
note kung
宮
⑤
dog, ox
smell: fragrant
taste: sweet
LATE SUMMER
center
EARTH

土

6.20 Some of the fivefold correlations. Within each of the five categories, everything "fits." For instance, "spring" (top right) brings "wood," the mood is "relaxed," the color is "green," and the time is good for the Ministry of Agriculture. It must have been impossible to live according to the letter of this bureaucratic philosophy, but certainly some of the correlations were observed. For example, the Ministry of Justice (under the sign for "metal," top left) did in fact postpone all executions until autumn.

One Surgical Operation

Yang i has been translated as "ulcer physician"[79] or "Physician-in-Ordinary for External Medicine."[80] "Surgeon" might be too much, at least until we know more about the type of "external medicine" that the yang i performed. It is usually said that the yang i operated rarely; but his status being low, his labors were not liable to be mentioned. It is possible that he knew how to sew up a wound; surgical sutures are well documented for Hua T'o (this famous surgeon of the second century A.D. was a contemporary of Galen), and there is evidence for sutures as far back as the second century B.C., which brings them close to Hippocratic times. Soporific drugs are also mentioned in ancient texts; their sociological importance in ancient China went beyond surgery, because physicians used them at times to alleviate pain caused by the severe physical punishments inflicted by the law. It is now certain that neither opium nor hemp were used, whereas several drugs of the so-called anticholinergic group were known (including henbane, *Hyoscyamus*, known also in Greco-Roman antiquity).[81]

Until further research provides more data on Chinese surgery as it was about the time of Hippocrates, the wound practice of the yang i rather recalls the type of surgery prevailing in Egypt at the time of the Smith papyrus, a practice that dealt broadly with matters surgical, but only on wounds that were ready-made or on sores.

The "surgical" Smith papyrus never mentions the knife; the *Nei Ching* mentions surgery only twice,[82] and then very much as a side issue. Most revealing is a passage that lists the five kinds of treatment, in this order:

PSYCHOLOGY ("cure the spirit")
DIET ("give proper nourishment to the body")
DRUGS
ACUPUNCTURE
CLINICAL MEDICINE ("examine and treat the bowels, the viscera, the blood and the breath" [?]).[83]

Surgery does not even fit into this picture. It did far better with the Hindus, with the surgically-oriented Hippocratics, and even more so with the down-to-earth Romans. Celsus says that there are three ways to treat a patient—through diet, medicine, and surgery—but that only surgery gives definite help.[84]

瘍醫

The single act of surgery that the ancient Chinese surely performed was not a treatment for disease. Many court employees were eunuchs. The *Chou Li* takes this situation for granted, without explaining the procedure. If the surgical method was the same in ancient days as under later dynasties, it was dangerous, because all the external genitalia were removed.[85] According to tradition, when Hua T'o was jailed by order of the emperor, he entrusted his manuscripts to the jailer, who burned them all except the improved castration technique.[86] Today the method of Hua T'o is lost. Yet a method that was practiced in 1929 cannot be very different:

When about to be operated on, the patient is placed in a semi-supine position on a broad bench. One man squatting behind him grasps his waist, and another is told to look after each leg. Bandages are fastened tightly round the hypogastric and inguinal regions, the penis and the scrotum are three times bathed in a hot decoction of pepper pods, and the patient, if an adult, is solemnly asked, whether he repents or will ever repent his decision. If he appears doubtful he is unbound and dismissed, but if his courage has held out, as it usually does, all the parts are swiftly swept away by one stroke of a sickle-shaped knife, a pewter-plug is inserted into the urethra, and the wound is covered with paper soaked in cold water and is firmly bandaged. The patient, supported by two men, is then walked about the room for two or three hours, after which he is permitted to lie down. For three days he gets nothing to drink nor is the plug removed from the urethra. At the end of this period the dressings are changed, and the accumulated urine is allowed to escape. The parts generally heal in about one hundred days . . . About two percent of all cases prove fatal, some by hemorrhage, some by extravasation, and some doubtless by sepsis . . . For a long time there is incontinence of urine.[87]

Note that the blood vessels are only compressed, not tied, just as in Hippocratic surgery. Perhaps there was some anesthesia with drugs taken by mouth—or just wine, since it was built into the character *i* for physician.[88]

This barbaric practice was not unique to China. In Mesopotamia, judicial castration and the employment of castrated domestics were perhaps two thousand years older than Hua T'o. In Syria, during a certain religious festival, young men would work themselves up to such a state of exaltation that they would seize a knife, castrate themselves, then run naked through the streets and fling the amputated parts into some house; those who lived there were obliged to provide them with clothes.[89] In the Roman Empire castration was forbidden, but it was performed all the same despite severe penalties. The emperors set a bad example by importing eunuchs at high prices.[90] This trade was legal as long as the operation had been performed abroad; but it also encouraged a sordid, clandestine industry in Rome. According to an official report from the sixth century A.D., after a series of ninety operations, only three of the victims survived.[91] A satire of Juvenal mentions the castration of slaves as a matter of fact. It also gives the name of a physician who took the dirty job away from the barbers; some of his clients were in high demand among women, but they paid for it by being objects of general curiosity at the public baths.[92]

 Eunuchs in China were offered an odd sort of compensation in public life: open doors at the court. Because they were unable to found competitive dynasties, they were particularly welcome there. It was under the Han that eunuchs first began to play an important role in politics.[93]

Chinese Wound Dressings and the Message of the Han Lady

In one way my surgical curiosity remains dissatisfied. What were the wound-dressings of the yang i? Not a word about it appears in the *Nei Ching*, in stark contrast to the Hippocratic books, where this is a major issue. In the *Chou Li* is that single sentence, "In general, to heal the ulcers, they attack them with the five poisonous substances."

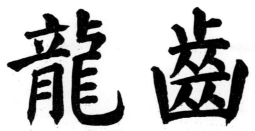

6.21 The characters for "dragon teeth," a common Chinese drug—actually pounded fossilized mammoth teeth.

A commentator of the second century A.D. explains the "poisons" as follows: "Nowadays, physicians prepare them in a special yellow clay pot. They put in this pot some "bile stone" (Chi-than), cinnabar [*mercuric sulphide*], sulphur, magnetic stone, and a poisonous stone called Yü [*arsenolite, an oxide of arsenic*[94]] . . . They heat this mixture three days and three nights. When vapor rises, they collect it on a little brush of cock feathers, and with it they wipe the suffering part. The bad flesh and broken bones come out completely. They cleanse, corrode, and fortify the sound flesh."[95] All five "poisons" are minerals. The analogy with the Greek antiseptic *énaima* based on inorganic salts is obvious, though the inorganic materials are different—with the possible exception of cinnabar.[96]

Chinese pharmacy after the *Nei Ching* grew to huge proportions, involving some 2000 items, especially plants, and 16,000 prescriptions.[97] It would use anything at all as a "drug," including old drum-skins and toad secretions; but there is nothing particularly Chinese about this. Pliny mentions Greek gymnasium-keepers who made a fortune by selling, as a drug, the scrapings from the skin of athletes, consisting of sweat, oil, and sand.[98] And if the strange Chinese used "dragon teeth" as a drug—actually fossilized mammoth teeth (Fig. 6.21)[99]—the Europeans used fossilized shark teeth until the seventeenth century at least, thinking that they were snake tongues (Fig. 9.3).

It would be interesting to discover, some day, whether the Chinese knew about the antiseptic properties of resins and balsams. Certainly they knew of incense; in fact, they burned it before consulting their favorite oracle book, the *I Ching*.[100] Like the Mediterranean peoples they did a lot with resins, though again in a different way.[101] Their favorite balsam was storax, which was most unusual for the Chinese, as it was imported. It came at first from wounds of a tree in the Greek Levant, *Styrax officinalis*,[102] and later from *Liquidambar orientale*. The latter happens to be very rich in cinnamic acid and balsamic acids,[103] both of which we have already encountered as powerful antiseptics. The high prices that the Chinese were willing to pay for storax led to another curious parallel with the Mediterranean situation: the Indian middlemen made up outrageous tales about the danger of obtaining it, just as the Arabs did about cassia and cinnamon: they tried to pass storax off as lion dung.[104]

Guessing is not a respected historical approach, about antiseptics or anything else. However, there is the provocative new fact of the Han lady. In 1972, Chinese archeologists discovered a tomb of the early Han period,

癰醫

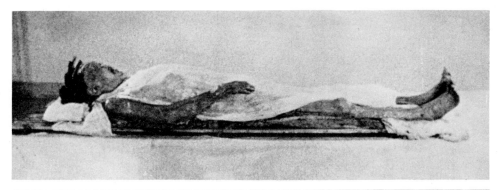

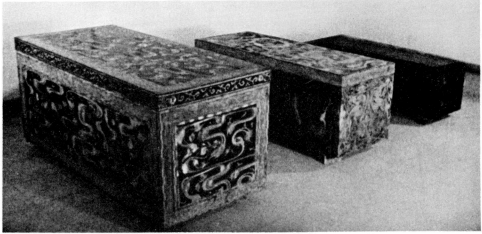

6.22 The only known preserved body from ancient China, about 180 B.C. It had been submerged in a pink fluid and sealed inside the triple coffin.

dedicated by a feudal lord to the body of his wife who died about 180 B.C. At a depth of sixteen meters they found three huge coffins, one inside the other; priceless treasures of silk and craftsmanship were stacked in the free spaces. In the innermost coffin, half bathed in a pink fluid, was the body of a woman, preserved in a manner that had never before been witnessed (Fig. 6.22). Since the ancient spell had been broken, the noble lady had to be taken to a hospital for injections of modern preservative drugs; and European television audiences gasped at the sight of her soft arm, resilient under the finger of a physician.[105] Shortly thereafter the *Peking Review* released the first scientific data: "Chemical analysis proved that the fluid inside the intermost coffin contained various organic acids and mercurial compounds and was slightly antibacterial."[106]

癢醫

If one of the organic acids was acetic acid, my guess is that the pink fluid was mainly vinegar. The *Chou Li* describe a whole staff of Employees of the Vinegar, "in charge of preparing the Five Pickles [*marinades*], the Five Vegetable Preserves, and all that is [kept in] vinegar."[107] So the Han, who followed the Chou, had vinegar and knew how to use it. Note also the presence of mercury, which appeared among the five "poisons" used on wounds. Mercury is more toxic than lead (a favorite drug in Roman wound dressings) but also more bactericidal;[108] a property exploited in many modern antiseptics.

All this means that by the second century B.C. the Chinese had learned a great deal about decay. Somebody, at the time of the early Han, knew enough to stop decay for 2100 years.[109] I venture to suggest that people who had discovered a "pink fluid" to preserve corpses had also invented some "pink fluid" to fight the infection of wounds.

East and West of the Headache Mountains

In the hands of the yang i, then, an ulcer patient was punctured, blistered, probably also purged, and put on a special diet. None of this did him much good, which placed him on a par with a comparable Greek patient. His dressings were fairly safe, also as in Greece. And his treatment was well rooted in philosophy, as in Greece.

And yet, while the basic therapeutic themes were the same East and West, they were developed quite differently in the East, and more gently. The Chinese diet, for all of its intricate rationale tied to geography, the weather, and almost everything else, was not a starvation diet. The single use of starvation that I found in the *Nei Ching* was in the treatment for "madness and rage."[110] So it seems that the Chinese were spared this particular medical aberration—starvation as a wound therapy. This is confirmed indirectly by the report of a Chinese Buddhist who went to India in the seventh century and commented on its medical science: "In it, the most important rule is fasting . . . Most of the Chinese were not accustomed to such a practice, and consider it as a separate religious fast."[111]

The cautery, too, was toned down in China: it was made not of iron but of fluff from a plant. More important yet, the patient did not run the risk of having his veins slit and being bled to a faint: a truly enormous advantage over his fellow-sufferers in the West. There was, in fact, no theoretical reason to draw large amounts of blood: Chinese medical theory did not include any "peccant humors" requiring to be drained out. Bleeding was reduced to little punctures, and most of the time the punctures drew no blood at all, just energy. Nothing of this kind ever saw the light in Mediterranean countries. The only possible relative of acupuncture, I believe, may be the Indian doctrine of the vital points.

As regards theory, the mental pathways of the yang i were bound up with yin and yang, the five elements, and number lore. All this was far more complex, rigid, and demanding than any Greek system.[112] A Greek iatrós, 瘍醫 whether he believed in the two-, three-, four-, or five-element theory, did not have to worry about such concepts as resonance and correlations. His acts remained basically the same: bleeding and purging to "restore the balance." It has been said that Greek medicine became the prisoner of philosophy; Chinese medicine came close to being identified with philosophy. An eleventh century commentator of the *Nei Ching* made this clear when he deplored the old mistake of considering the *Nei Ching* as a "medical" text: "How could they give the most essential and the most delicate methods to the lowest and most humble men"—the physicians?[113] It was obviously a book for

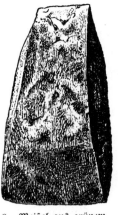

Südamerika, welche Fundstellen

:tracht kom=
ı und spär=
und Steier=
man allein
den erften
:nn 6¹/₂ Fuß
ırlithügels,
ırg. Gelb=
:er Nephrit
veißer nur
bietet uns
Werkzeuge
ſchon in

9. Meißel aus grünem
Nephrit
(natürliche Größe).

6.23 A prehistoric Chinese export: one of twenty-seven green or white jade axes found by Heinrich Schliemann at Troy (Hissarlik). Being extremely hard, jade was much prized for making tools in prehistoric times. The white jade could come only from China. Slightly enlarged from a German book on Schliemann's excavations.

the sages. This may explain the relatively slow progress of Chinese medicine from the *Nei Ching* on, whereas other Chinese sciences flourished.[114]

The real question, therefore, is how ancient China came to share some healing *ideas* with Europe, yet developed a healing *art* so distinctly its own. The reasons are both geographic and human. Prehistoric contacts across the Eurasian continent surely existed, on what might be called a capillary level.[115] The idea of the wheel did seep eastward from Mesopotamia, and a Chinese jade axe found its way to prehistoric Troy (Fig. 6.23). Perhaps it passed from hand to hand, and its last owner never even heard of its homeland. But despite these subtle contacts, on the whole, isolation prevailed. During the great upsurge of Egyptian and Mesopotamian cultures, China was still living in prehistory; it joined the Bronze Age only around 1600 B.C.[116] When a Chinese civilization eventually began to take shape, it was largely bound to agriculture rather than to the sea, and was therefore land-oriented.[117] And because the land produced practically all that the people needed, there was no compelling reason to look elsewhere. While the Chinese had items that other people wanted badly, like silk, they had little to ask in exchange.[118] Gradually, the Chinese people developed a "marked disinclination to travel far outside what they felt to be their natural geographical boundaries," and the Chinese sages possessed a certain "psychological disinclination . . . to believe that other countries could have anything valuable to add to the sciences that they had so far developed in their own country."[119]

The first major "tunnel" from China to the West was the adventurous eleven-year expedition of the Chinese ambassador Chang Ch'ien, who never got very far and spent most of his time abroad as a prisoner of the Huns, but who still managed to bring back information from far-away Syria, Mesopotamia, and perhaps even Egypt.[120] This led to the opening of the Old Silk Road across the two continents in 106 B.C.[121] But to grasp the meaning of geographical difficulties, consider this passage from one of the Chinese annals, the *T'ung Chien Kang Mu*.[122] It is in the report of Tu Ch'in, a high official, telling the prime minister what he thinks about the prospect of communicating with the country of Chi-Pin, somewhere north and northwest of India:

> Friendly intercourse with barbarian nations is advisable only where communications are reasonably easy . . . (In order to reach Chi-Pin) after passing the P'i-Shan mountains, our envoys would have to traverse four or five countries, each of which is full of robbers. Then one must cross the Greater and the Lesser Headache Mountains, chains of naked and burning rocks, so named because they cause headache, dizziness and vomiting . . . Then comes the Shan-Ch'ih-P'an gorge, thirty *li* long, where the path is only 16 or 17 inches wide, on the edge of a precipice, and where the travellers have to be tied together with ropes . . . Such useless enterprises should not be the policy of an enduring dynasty.[123]

Tu Ch'in was obviously describing the symptoms of mountain sickness, an eerie malady that might have carried the message "stay at home."[124]

Such were the basic obstacles that prevented Hippocrates from trying his luck with acupuncture.

Oddly enough, the geographic gap men found so difficult to bridge—or not worth bridging—the gap that slowed down so effectively the diffusion of ideas, was easily overcome by homely little bundles of spices. Cassia, *Cinnamomum cassia*, was a Chinese specialty.[125] Hippocrates used it. And there is a faint chance that when Hippocrates prescribed *kasía*, or *kassía*, he was speaking two words of garbled Chinese,[126] the only two that had spread across the seas and beyond the Headache Mountains—*kuei shu:*

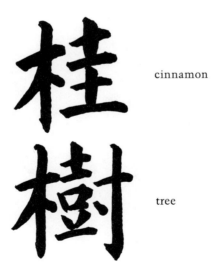

桂　cinnamon

樹　tree

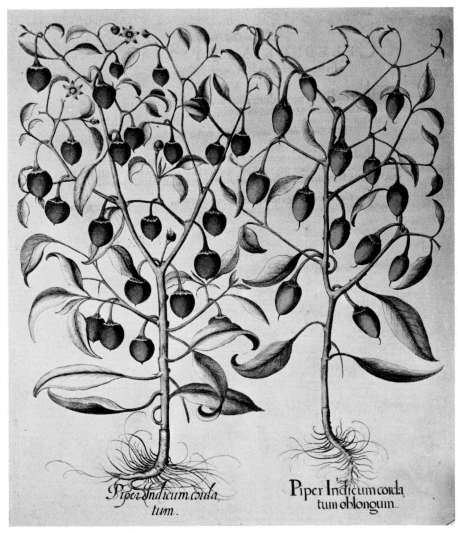

7.1 Pepper, one of the first Indian ambassadors to Greece.

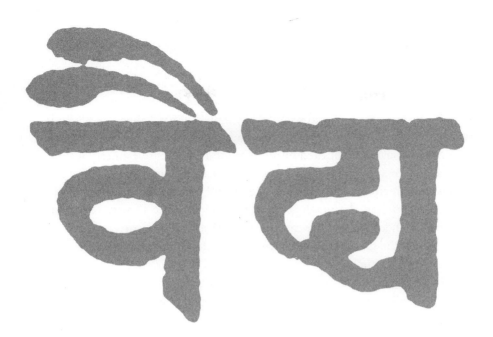

7 The Vaidya

South of the Headache Mountains, at the foggy fringe of the Greek map (Fig. 6.1), was India. Just how foggy, judge from the plans of Alexander the Great: when he drove his troops east through Persia, barely two generations after Hippocrates, he was hoping to discover the sources of the Nile! It is true, though, that when he realized his mistake, he went back to a letter he had just finished to his mother and "deleted what he had written about the Nile."[1]

On the evidence of the Hippocratic books, all that India meant to their authors was pepper and a mouthwash for bad breath.[2] Even the pepper sounds unusual, for it is "the Indian substance that the Persians call *pépéri*" and "the Indian drug for the eyes, that is called *pépéri*"[3] (Fig. 7.1). After all the tribulations of a 6000-mile trip—escaping robbers, pirates, and storms at sea—*Piper indicum* was used by the Greek physicians merely as an ingredient for pessaries: miserable tokens indeed to represent a highly civilized Hindu world that was over a thousand years old.

वैद्य

Indian civilization itself was even older. The original, dark-skinned inhabitants of India, the people who built the city of Mohenjo-daro, now famous for its beautiful baths, had a writing of their own in 2500 B.C. About 1500 B.C. they were overrun by lighter-skinned people who called themselves Aryans, a name perhaps connected with their origin, Iran.[4] Their language came from the same stem as Greek and Latin, and from it evolved, with many dialects, the literary language that came to be known as Sanskrit: a word made of two parts, *san-skrit*, like the Latin *con-fectus*, meaning "put together," hence "finished," hence "elegant," and thus the language of the elite.

The newcomers brought with them, or produced as they settled, a huge body of literature: primarily the four Vedas, sacred books in Sanskrit reputed to have arisen by divine inspiration. They may well have appeared without ever having been written down, because according to Indian custom, they were meticulously transmitted by word of mouth—the investment of time being approximately twelve years to memorize one Veda.[5] The chant of a Hindu vedic reciter—a highly controlled blend of melody and staccato—can be heard to this day. Although Sanskrit may sound quite abstruse, being an Indo-European language it has many familiar roots. The word *Veda*, for instance, has the same root as *wisdom*; and so does the word for physician, *vaidya*, "he who knows."[6]

Another product of Hindu culture was a system of medicine that was eventually called *Ayurveda*, literally "knowledge of life" or "science of life."[7] It was fitted into the stream of tradition as part of the fourth Veda, the *Atharva Veda*: a collection of magic and spells representing the lore of the Atharvan priests. Ayurvedic medicine is based essentially on two treatises by Charaka and Sushruta, composed in verse and prose: the *Charaka Samhita*, mainly on medicine, and the *Sushruta Samhita*, mainly on surgery (*samhita* means "collection").[8] Both were preserved in full: oral reciters have their advantages!

These two great classics of Ayurveda are not actually volumes of the *Atharva Veda*; rather, they developed, in a general sense, the basic theme of the Atharvans: warding off trouble, including disease. The spells of the Atharvans included formulas for almost any need: stopping hemorrhage, curing snakebite, ensuring success in warfare, or even extolling a cow. Charaka had no quarrel with Atharvan magic; his ideal lying-in room, for instance, is equipped (besides an ox, a mule, and much else) with "Brahmans conversant with the *Atharva Veda*."[9]

The dates of these literary works, and the dates of ancient Indian history altogether, are distressingly uncertain. The climate and the people of India have conspired to erase them, perhaps forever. Most of the annals of the rajas—kept on birchbark in the north, on banana leaves in the south—have succumbed to rain, war, and insects,[10] under the indifferent eyes of the Brahmans, who shrugged at such frivolities: life being an illusion, a mere step to reincarnation and nirvana, biographies and histories were part of human vanity.[11] This attitude, combined with two other cultural traits—worship of the ancient and an aversion against committing texts to the written form—drives modern scholars to despair: dating an Indian classic is almost hopeless. Sushruta, for instance, has been thought to live anywhere between 1000 B.C. and 1000 A.D.[12] The first definite date for all of Indian history is Greek—326 B.C., the year that Alexander crossed the Indus River.[13] As for the first Indian writings that can be approximately dated, they are the edicts that King Ashoka began to carve in rock half a century later.

A map of India as it was at about the time of the Golden Age of Greece

वैद्य

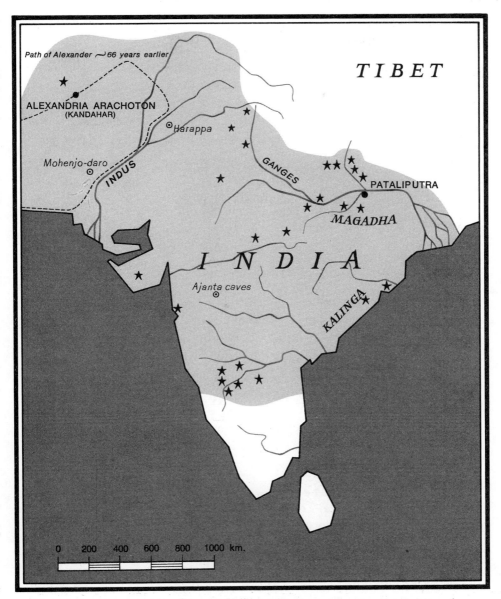

7.2 Map of the Maurya Empire about 260 B.C. (shaded), showing the distribution of Ashoka's inscriptions (★).

shows that the two great valleys of the north were following separate destinies. The Indus Valley, in the west, was part of the Persian Empire (to become with Alexander a Greek dominion), while the valley of the Ganges, in the east, was subdivided among many small kingdoms fighting for supremacy, much as in China. The vast Indian triangle to the south was almost entirely absent from the mainstream of history.

Among the kingdoms of the east, Magadha became the most powerful and eventually took over most of India (Fig. 7.2). Its kings were converted to Buddhism by Buddha himself.[14] One of them was Ashoka (c.269–c.232 B.C.), third of the Maurya Dynasty. No history of the wound would be complete without a page about this great king, whom the horrors of war turned into an apostle of peace.

वैद्य

Nonviolence Carved in Rock

Ashoka's dynasty bursts into history with an odd assortment of writings. One of them is, in plain words, a revolting book: the *Artashastra*. It is a treatise on government, written under the first king of the dynasty, Chandragupta (the one who probably met Alexander the Great). Suffice it to mention that the art of governing is called *dandaniti*, "the science of punishment," and included among its practices is a horrible list of eighteen kinds of torture to elicit confessions from citizens accused of theft.[15] In essence, the *Artashastra* is a cynical version of Machiavelli's *The Prince*.

The second book is by the hand of an exceptional visitor, Megasthenes, a Greek ambassador, who was pacing the streets of Pataliputra, the capital of Magadha, at the time that the *Artashastra* was being written. This sophisticated outsider was much impressed with what he saw and wrote a report on his mission, the *Indiká*, most of which is unfortunately lost. It is also unfortunate that while on duty Megasthenes never fell so ill as to use an Indian physician, for his account of Indian medicine, though laudative, is vague.[16]

The third set of documents is unique. King Ashoka himself, "the Beloved of the Gods," laid bare his soul on India's rocks in words that no other king has used. His "edicts," some carved in boulders, others in pillars, are strewn all over the country (Fig. 7.2). One of the earliest stemmed from remorse. Shortly after rising to the throne, Ashoka had decided to unleash his massive army against Kalinga on the eastern border. The campaign was victorious, but at the price of tremendous slaughter. Such was Ashoka's remorse that he turned to Buddhism for relief, and he told his people about the experience in Rock Edict XIII:

> Kalinga was conquered by His Sacred and Gracious Majesty when he had been consecrated eight years [261 B.C.]. 150,000 persons were thence carried away captive, 100,000 were there slain, and many times that number perished.
>
> Directly after the annexation of the Kalingas began His Sacred Majesty's zealous protection of the Law of Duty, his love of that Law, and his giving instruction in that Law [*Buddhism*]. Thus arose His Sacred Majesty's remorse for having conquered the Kalingas, because the conquest of a country previously unconquered involves the slaughter, death, and carrying away captive of the people. That is a matter of profound sorrow and regret to His Sacred Majesty . . .
>
> Of all the people who were then slain, done to death, or carried away captive in the Kalingas, if the hundredth or the thousandth part were to suffer the same fate, it would now be matter of regret to His Sacred Majesty . . . For His Sacred Majesty desires that all animate beings should have security, self-control, peace of mind, and joyousness.[17]

Ashoka's conscience never recovered from this war. Later edicts portray him as a fatherly, hard-working monarch and as a fervent Buddhist (Fig. 7.3). Here are two more excerpts, from Rock Edicts III and I, to set the tone of India under his rule:

> Thus saith His Majesty King Priyadarsin [*"of pleasing mien," one of Ashoka's designations*[18]]:

वैद्य

264

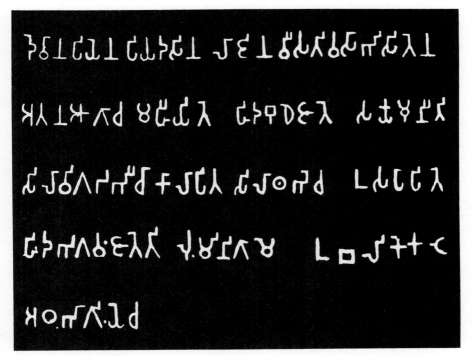

7.3 One of Ashoka's inscriptions, on a pillar in Rummindei, 249 B.C. It declares the village tax-free, being the birthplace of Buddha.

In the thirteenth year of my reign I issued this command:

Everywhere in my dominions . . . the Commissioners, and the District Officers must every five years repair to the General Assembly, for the special purpose, in addition to other business, of proclaiming the Law of Piety, to wit, "Obedience to father and mother is good; liberality to friends, acquaintances, relatives, Brahmans, and ascetics is good; respect for the sacredness of life is good; avoidance of extravagance and violence of language is good" . . .

Here [*in the capital?*] no animal may be slaughtered for sacrifice, nor may holiday-feasts be held, for His Majesty King Priyadarsin sees manifold evil in holiday-feasts. Nevertheless, certain holiday-feasts are meritorious in the sight of His Majesty King Priyadarsin.

Formerly, in the kitchen of His Majesty King Priyadarsin, each day many thousands of living creatures were slain to make curries.

At the present moment, when this pious edict is being written, only these three living creatures, namely two peacocks and one deer, are killed daily, and the deer not invariably.

Even these three creatures shall not be slaughtered in future.[19]

Presumably King Ashoka of the Maurya Dynasty had to have his daily peacock because *maurya* meant "peacock."[20]

Rock Edict II is often quoted as representing the world's first reference to hospitals.[21] Much as I regret to cast doubt on this aspect of Ashoka's heritage, I find that it hinges on a single word, *chikisakâ*, which one translator renders as "hospitals," but most others as "remedies."[22] Sanskrit words are notorious for their multiple meanings; I looked up *svastika* and found "well-being,"

वैद्य

265

"cross," "cake," "demon," "mode of sitting," and "libertine," which is just average. Here is the edict in question, which has been given the modern title of "Provision of Comforts for Men and Animals":

> Everywhere in the dominions of His Majesty King Priyadarsin, and likewise in neighbouring realms such as those of the Chola, Pândya, . . . the dominions of the Greek King Antiochus, . . . have two kinds of remedies [*hospitals?*] been disseminated—remedies for men, and remedies for beasts. Healing herbs, medicinal for man and medicinal for beast, wherever they were lacking, have everywhere been imported and planted.
>
> In like manner, roots and fruits, wherever they were lacking, have been imported and planted.
>
> On the roads, trees have been planted, and wells have been dug for the use of man and beast.[23]

However this edict is read, the concern for life under the Maurya Dynasty should not be overestimated. Much of that concern was for animals, as Ashoka's edicts show.[24] Although the *Artashastra* remarks that the army had an ambulance service, with well-equipped surgeons and women to prepare food and beverages,[25] compassion was definitely not the slogan of state administration. Care for the wounded in the Maurya army, as in most armies, was first of all a matter of economy.

Now, returning to the history of wounds, I will invite my reader to visit some ancient Hindu patients. Using the treatises of Sushruta and Charaka as I used the Hippocratic books, I have reconstructed ten case histories. For ease of comparison with Greek medicine, I chose the time that our ten Greek patients were queuing up at the Athenian infirmary—about 400 B.C. I assume that Sushruta had just lived,[26] and that the patients all came from the outskirts of Benares, where Buddha had lived and taught (Fig. 7.4), and where Sushruta had acquired his knowledge, or so the legend goes, by divine dictation.[27]

Nine of the ten Hindu patients will be men: not only because men were more likely to be wounded, but also because there are not enough data to reconstruct a likely relationship between vaidya and female patient. Sushruta and Charaka rarely mention women except in relation to childbirth and gynecologic diseases. Two patients could have been women (those with earring problems), but I chose males to bring out other cultural traits, such as that men wore earrings. Hindus loved their women but were far from considering them as equals. Charaka speaks of their "state of dependence and ignorance"[28]: enforced ignorance, for women were not allowed to learn Sanskrit!

वैद्य

The Home of the Arrow-Doctor

A messenger was running along the bank of the Ganges. Two men had been wounded by arrows in a skirmish with outlaws,[29] and he was going to get the vaidya.

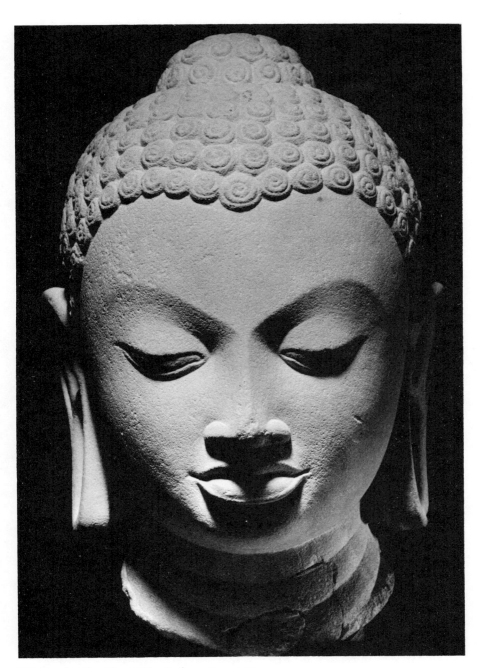

7.4 Head of Buddha. Fifth–sixth century A.D.

A Greek on a similar mission would have just headed for the nearest
iatrós, but the ancient Hindu, for better or for worse, had the privilege of
being able to choose among a whole array of specialists.[30] In this particular
case, however, there was no real choice: neither the internist (*rogahara*), nor
the poison expert (*vishahara*), nor the demon expert or magic expert
(*krityahara* and *bishag-atharvan*) would be of any help; but only the
surgeon, *shalyahara. Shalya* meant "arrow," "sword," "lance," in fact almost
any weapon, and ultimately any foreign body embedded in the flesh; *hara*

267

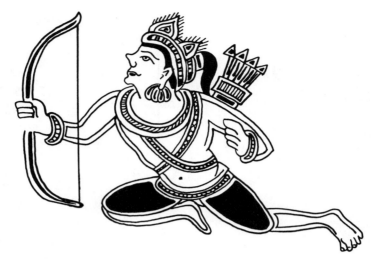

7.5 Indian hunter, redrawn from an ivory carving. Note large earrings and the typical Indian weapon, a bow and arrow. About second century A.D.

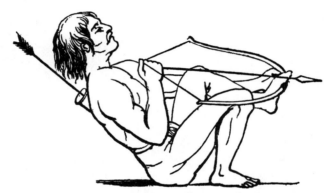

7.6 A special Indian style for firing arrows with great force, noticed by the ancient Greeks and still in use in 1860, at the time of this drawing. Perhaps it was a shot of this kind that pierced the breastplate of Alexander the Great, bowled him over, and almost killed him.

meant "remover." So the name of the vaidya who specialized in surgery meant something like arrow-remover—an appropriate term in India, where the bow and arrow (which did not enjoy great favor in Greece) had been the traditional weapon (Figs. 7.5–7.6).[31]

वैद्य 　　When the messenger reached the house of the surgeon, he recognized it by the neatly kept garden of medicinal herbs,[32] and by the scene taking place before the front door.[33] A Greek might have thought that he had come upon some bizarre religious rite, which would not have been far wrong. Seated on the ground on his ritual sand cushion, "measuring a cubit in length and breadth" and plastered with cow dung,[34] was the vaidya, wearing a white cloth and turban. At his side was the sacred fire of cow dung. Before him sat three young men, each wearing a yellowish cloth.[35] The vaidya chanted verses of the Ayurveda, in a precise, monotonous rhythm; the young men repeated them. These were from the surgeon's part of the Ayurveda, the

Sushruta Samhita. No amount of gold could have bought that precious text, for it was not for sale: the only way to become an acceptable surgeon was to learn it all by heart, from someone who had done the same. Nor did the young apprentices understand what they were saying, for they spoke only a dialect, whereas Sanskrit was a literary language. They were taught, at first, just the rhythm of the syllables, word by word, forward and even backward; explanations would come later.[36]

The vaidya rose to greet the newcomer, listened to the message, and prepared for his mission of mercy. In the house, the two appropriate walls (north and east) were studded with wooden pegs,[37] from which hung bunches of herbs and leaves collected within the year.[38] Shelves bore earthen pots, little linen bags, and wooden containers shaped as tubes. The vaidya gathered half a dozen items into a bag, together with a box of instruments made of the excellent Indian steel.[39] A servant was handed the lot, with instructions to run ahead.[40] Then the vaidya took his umbrella and stick, gave last-minute instructions to his pupils, picked three fresh bamboo sprouts while studiously facing north,[41] and followed the guide.

The three apprentices, left to their own means, set to work as directed. They were a dainty group, hand-picked to meet Sushruta's requirements: "initiation should be imparted to a student, belonging to one of the three twice-born castes [*those whose members were born first into ordinary life, then again, ritually, into one of the higher castes*], such as the Brahmana [*priests*], the Kshatriya [*warriors and nobles*], and the Vaishya [*free men*]."[42] The motivation to practice medicine was different for each one of these castes, as explained by Charaka: Brahmans, to do good; Kshatriyas, for self-preservation; Vaishyas, for gain. But all three could derive religious merit, wealth, and pleasure from the practice, in that order.[43] The apprentice, Sushruta continues, "should be of tender years, born of a good family, possessed of a desire to learn, strength, energy of action, contentment, character, self-control, a good retentive memory, intellect, courage, purity of mind and body, and simple and clear comprehension, command a clear insight into the things studied, and should be found to have been further graced with the necessary qualifications, of thin lips, thin teeth and thin tongue, and possessed of a straight nose, large, honest, intelligent eyes, with a benign contour of the mouth, and a contented frame of mind, being pleasant in his speech and dealings, and usually painstaking in his efforts." Hippocrates was far less exacting, having no requirements as to social origin, although the tone was similar: the iatrós "should look healthy, and as plump as nature intended him to be" and "let him be of a serious but not harsh countenance."[44]

वैद्य

The efforts that the three Indian apprentices were about to undertake would now be called experimental surgery, of a kind unique in the world.[45] One of the youngsters, armed with a sword-shaped knife, began to practice making incisions of peculiar shapes in a watermelon. Another waited for his cautery to become red-hot in the hearth; he was going to practice with it on a small piece of fresh meat. The third threaded a curved needle of triangular

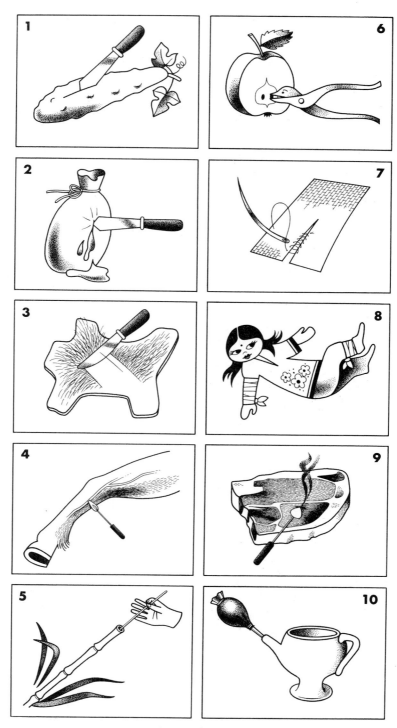

7.7 Hindu experimental surgery. For practice in the various surgical techniques, Sushruta recommends the following: (1) *incising* on a cucumber or the like, (2) *lancing an abscess* on a leather bag full of slime, (3) *scraping* on a piece of fur, (4) *venesection* on the veins of a dead animal, (5) *probing* on a bamboo reed or worm-eaten wood, (6) *extracting* by picking seeds out of fruit (here with the appropriate butcher-bird forceps), (7) *suturing* on cloth, (8) *bandaging or tying* (for snake bite) on a full-sized stuffed doll, (9) *cauterizing* on a piece of meat, (10) *injecting* on a pitcher.

section;[46] his assignment **was** to practice surgical knots on a piece of hide. These were only three of the many established exercises (Fig. 7.7).

In the meantime, the vaidya was on his way with the messenger, trying to reconcile the professional duty of having a friendly chat[47] with the serious business of studying the omens. He had memorized dozens of verses on this topic, because "the favorable or unfavorable termination of a disease may be predicted from the appearance, speech, dress and demeanour of the messenger sent in to call the physician, or from the nature of the asterism and the lunar phase marking the time of his arrival, or from the direction of the wind blowing at the time, or from the nature of the omens seen by him on the road."[48] The messenger belonged to the same caste as the patients: good. He had been breathing heavily on arrival, his garments were not too clean, and he had spoken facing south: bad, bad, bad. He wore a couple of ornaments: good. Here came a cow: good. Elephants were trumpeting in the distance: good. A bird whose name ended with a masculine termination was seen on the right: bad. A horse: good. In front of a farmhouse were corn husks, straw, and sesamum: all three bad. A eunuch and a cripple: both bad. They were talking about something being "cut": good in general, but not in relation to wounds. The sound of chanting Vedic verses: good. A dog running right to left: good . . .[49]

Patients Nos. 1 and 2: Arrow Wounds

When the vaidya reached the house, one of the wounded men was outside, under a tree. He lay on his back, as if pinned down by the feathered arrow-shaft rising vertically from his left shoulder. Bright red blood trickled from the wound, which was considered good; "black blood" was thought to mean poisoned arrows.[50]

The very first worry for the vaidya, before he could make any helpful move, was to find out whether his patient had been hit in a deadly spot or *marma*, because the Hindu surgeon, like his Greek and to some extent his Egyptian counterparts, would not take on a definitely fatal case.[51] The marmas being safe, the next step for any arrow casualty was to find out whether it was an *anuloma* situation or a *pratiloma* one (Ayurvedic medicine bristles with technical terms). Arrows that had to be pushed through, continuing their path, and therefore moving in the direction "from hair to root," were called anuloma arrows (lit. "along the hair root"); those that could be pulled back were called pratiloma ("against the hair root").[52] The vaidya tried a gentle tug on the shaft; it did not budge. Next, he tried the gentlest of the forward or anuloma methods: he held a small magnet next to the skin over the buried arrowhead[53] (most arrowheads were made of iron or steel) and waited. Again nothing happened.

So it was a tossup between applying more drastic anuloma methods, like striking the feathered end with a hammer,[54] or trying to yank out the arrow, pratiloma style. The ruse of shielding the barbs and easing the arrowhead

वैद्य

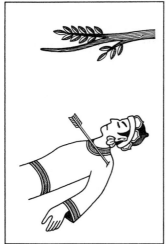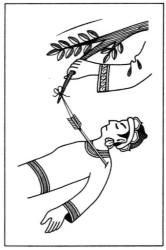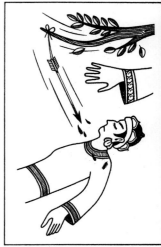

7.8 Sushruta's quick way of removing an arrow that cannot be easily pulled back out.

back out was apparently not yet known.[55] Speed was therefore essential. One possibility was to tie the shaft to the bridle of a horse and make the horse jerk its head.[56] But since the patient was lying under a tree, there was a simpler solution.[57] The vaidya strained down a branch, had it tied to the shaft, and let go (Fig. 7.8). Success came so fast that the extraction was scarcely painful.

Then, reaching for one of his earthen pots, the vaidya plastered the wound with a generous scoop of honey-butter paste and bandaged it "with a clean piece of linen."[58] The honey-butter paste was a favorite of Ayurvedic surgery.[59] It was essentially the same as the salve of the Smith papyrus, except that the fatty ingredient was a kind of oil (clarified butter or *ghee*) and that it was sometimes mixed with another wound-drug. Ghee, the commonest source of fat, was made like butter except that sour instead of fresh milk was used. It had the great advantage of keeping longer than ordinary butter; for use as a drug, it was even allowed to age beyond one hundred years.[60] There was practically no disease for which ghee was not rubbed on, swallowed, or offered to the gods. And a man who made sure to see his face reflected in ghee every day was sure to live a long life.[61]

The second wounded patient was more difficult to handle, because the broken arrow shaft was buried deeply in the thigh and the stump was out of sight. The vaidya began to search the wound with his blunt probe, the *eshani*. It was shaped much like the Greek wound probe, the spathomele, except that the blunt end was likened not to a small apple, or to an olive stone, but to the head of an earthworm:[62] tradition required that the working ends of surgical instruments be shaped like suitable animal heads.[63] The eshani, however, caused the patient too much pain. The vaidya, having expected this, had taken along three softer probes, the bamboo shoots.[64] But they, too, could not find a path in the swollen tissues. What was the direction of the buried shaft?

In this predicament, Sushruta suggested several tricks. The most elaborate was to load the patient into a carriage "with a broken or lopped-off wheel"[65] and drag it up and down a bumpy road. The sharp pain caused by

वैद्य

the jolting would indicate the position of the shaft.[66] Or one could plaster the skin with clarified butter, clay, or sandal paste.[67] The embedded arrow "is then exactly located at the spot where, owing to the heat of the affected part, the clarified butter, or earth, or sandal paste would be found to have melted, or dried up."[68] This is comparable to the clay method used by the Hippocratics to detect the center of an inflamed area.

But while the surgeon was studying the problem, the patient unknowingly provided the solution. His hand kept stroking and pressing a very painful spot on the back of the thigh. That was enough, for "the part which the patient repeatedly handles, or constantly presses with his own hand . . . and is marked by a sort of excruciating pain, or which he involuntarily withdraws from, or constantly guards against . . . should be regarded as clearly indicative of the exact location of the embedded Shalya."[69] So the arrow had been traveling from front to back.

The mouth of the wound was cautiously enlarged with a sharp knife,[70] and promptly the broken shaft appeared. The surgeon tried to seize it first with one of his most powerful forceps, the *sinha-mukha*, or "lion-mouth" (Fig. 7.9).[71] When that failed, he tried his trusty "heron-mouth" forceps (Fig. 7.10), because he knew that when other forceps failed, the long-jawed *kanka-mukha* often did the job.[72] It is no wonder that the same implement was reinvented a couple of thousand years later for the same purpose, and with very nearly the same name, as the French *bec de corbin* (Fig. 7.11). One tug, and out came the shalya. By great good luck, it was not a barbed arrow.[73] Its tip, shaped like a ferocious animal head,[74] seemed to express dismay.

Honey-butter, then a bandage in the shape of an 8 called a *svastika* ("cross"), and it was all over. The vaidya made sure that the knot of the bandage was not tied just above the wound, a preoccupation that the Hippocratics may have shared.[75]

Next came elaborate instructions for the attendants. The bedsteads had to be turned to face east: "The reason for the head being turned towards the East is that the patient may easily make obeisance to the (demons and) celestial spirits, who inhabit that quarter of the sky. Thus the patient shall lie in comfortable posture, attended upon by his sweet-talking friends and relations."[76] Afterward, "rites of benediction and divine peace should be done unto him. Wherefore? Because the monsters and demons of mighty prowess, who are the attendants of the gods Pashupati, Kuvera and Kumára, roam about in quest of prey, and visit the bedside of an ulcer-patient out of their fondness for flesh and blood, being attracted thereto by the smell of the secreted and morbid matter in the ulcer. These evil spirits come to take away the life of a patient in a case which is doomed to terminate fatally, while in a successful case their advent is due to the desire of extorting sacrificial oblations from him."[77]

In practice, subduing the demons meant burning incense sticks and making sacrifices of food.[78] Once subdued, the evil spirits tended to "spare the life of a self-controlled patient."[79] Therefore, the patient had to impress them with his light-heartedness and determination by keeping a weapon at

वैद्य

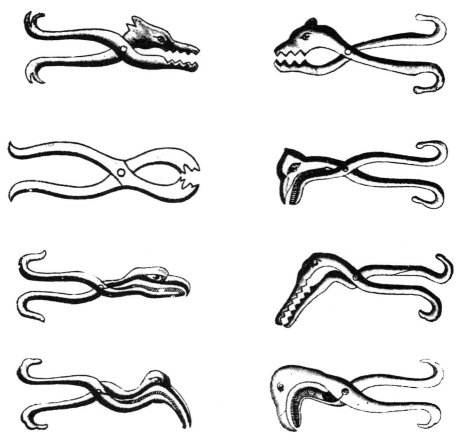

7.9 Hindu surgical instruments were named and fashioned after animals. *Left to right, from top:* The jackal-, cat-, lion-, bluejay-, hawk-, crocodile-, curlew-, and kite-mouth forceps. They were usually made of iron.

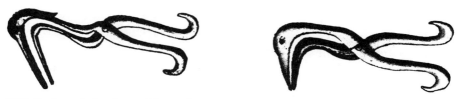

7.10 Sushruta's *kanka-mukha* and *kaka-mukha* forceps ("heron-mouth" and "crow-mouth"), for removing deep-seated foreign bodies.

Bec de corbin dentelé.

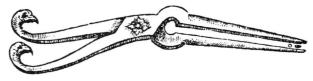

7.11 Ambroise Paré's *bec de corbin dentelé*, rediscovered in the 1500s under the stimulus of gunshot wounds.

his bedside, as well as by keeping flowers, garlands, fried paddy (rice in the husk), and lamps burning day and night, while his friends and relations contributed to the cure "with fond and loving topics to drive away the feeling of sleepiness with the prospect of a speedy cure."[80] Sleep during the day was considered dangerous.[81]

The whole room would have to be fumigated for ten days, morning and evening, with mustard, special leaves, clarified butter, and salt, all rolled into a kind of incense stick.[82] Morning and evening, the physician and some Brahman would perform rites of benediction as laid down in the four Vedas.[83] "Demons, that get abroad in the night, fly from the presence of an ulcer-patient protected as above, as herds of deer fly from the forest where lions are found."[84]

The diet would be boiled rice with clarified butter and some cooked meat,[85] but no cakes, treacle candy, meat of animals connected with water, milk, curd, or whey.[86] It is not very different from the Hippocratic diet, especially the prohibition of milk products. Another surprising parallel is the recommendation of barley powder in boiled water as "food and drink."[87]

To make the patient more comfortable, his wounded limb would be soothed with fumes "of pain-killing substances."[88] Because it was summer, the dressing would be changed every other day; in other seasons it would have been changed every third day.[89] However, in case of excruciating pain, the physician could rush in earlier, "as to a house in flames," and apply a warm salve of clarified butter boiled with *yashtimadhu*, "liquorice," which was thought to bring certain relief.[90] Whether liquorice really has any soothing effect I do not know, but it was also a favorite Chinese drug.[91]

The vaidya had now done all he could. But on departing, he chanted a couple of verses of the Ayurveda, reminding the bystanders that the success of medical treatment rested on four pillars: the physician and the drugs, but also the nursing and the patient.[92]

These two cases illustrate the great role that religion played in Indian medicine. Charaka's words leave no doubt:

Medicines are of three kinds . . .
First, Mantras [*magic formulas*] and religious acts;
Second, dieting and drugs;
Third, the subjugation of the mind by withdrawing it from every kind of injurious or harmful act.[93]

वैद्य

Religion is first, surgery last: Charaka gives it the fourth place (in this case, however, Sushruta disagrees: he has surgery at the top of the list[94]). Again, in Charaka's summary of the 152 most important principles of *medicine*, one is that "the atheist is the foremost of all persons to be avoided."[95]

A Parenthesis: How the Vaidya Saw the Body

When he removed an arrow, the vaidya could not visualize the damage that had been wrought inside. Dissecting the dead, in theory at least, was not permissible: mere contact with a corpse was a contaminating act. The vaidya's anatomy was therefore very poor. He had learned it—if at all—by Sushruta's method, which required a great deal of motivation: take a dead body, lay it in a still and solitary pool, enclose it in a cage (to keep it from drifting away or being eaten by fish), cover it with grass, and leave it there for a week. At that time "it will be thoroughly decomposed" and it will be possible to "slowly scrape off the decomposed skin etc. with a whisk made of grass-roots . . . or a strip of split bamboo, and carefully observe with his own eyes all the various different organs."[96] There is no touching, just poking with a little stick. Result: the taboo was successfully overcome, but anatomy was lost in the process. The proof is Hindu anatomy, which is almost nonexistent: all the blood vessels were supposed to come from the navel, no word existed for the lungs, and there was a bone in the penis.[97]

As to physiology, it hinged on the notion that the 700 vessels carried, in varying proportions, three basic *doshas* or "principles,"—plus blood: *vayu, pitta, kapha*—plus *rakta*.[98] The three doshas were very capricious, became easily deranged, and caused disease. The most dangerous was *vayu* or *vata*, "wind" (*vayu, vata,* and *wind* have in fact the same root); *pitta* has been translated as "bile," *kapha* (which may have the same root as *cough*[99]) has great similarities with "phlegm." *Rakta*, the blood, became upset everytime one of the three doshas was upset: it follows that venesection to draw out "bad blood" was as common as in Greece.

This theory, the mainstay of the vaidya's thinking,[100] overlaps in many ways with the Greek theory of the four humors. Despite differences in detail, the similarities are striking. How these similarities came about—whether by coincidence or exchange, and if by the latter, in which direction—is not known; but some sort of capillary, subhistorical, two-way exchange with the Greek world is most likely.[101]

Uniquely Hindu, instead, is the manner in which the Ayurvedic surgeons dealt with their ignorance in matters anatomical. They made up for it empirically—to some extent at least—thanks to centuries of experience with piercing weapons. This experience had taught them that wounds at certain precise points, which they called *marmas*, were critical or deadly (the word *marma* may well have the same root as *mortal*). Some marmas were said to cause paralysis; others hemorrhage, which was dreaded because Ayurvedic surgeons, just like the Hippocratics, did not know how to tie off a bleeding vessel. Thus, for example, the Hindu practitioner knew nothing about a nerve bundle running behind the knee, but he knew that "an injury to, or piercing of, the *Janu-Marma* situated at the union of the thigh and the knee, results in lameness of the patient."[102]

Each marma had its own name, and there were 107 in all.[103] Some do not really qualify as deadly, such as the eleven marmas on each hand (Fig. 7.12). Others correspond to definite anatomical danger points. The two *kukundara* marmas, for instance, are located on either side of the spinal column, slightly below the waist; a penetrating wound there led to "loss of feeling and motion in the lower limbs."[104] The famous paraplegic Mesopotamian lioness (Fig.

वैद्य

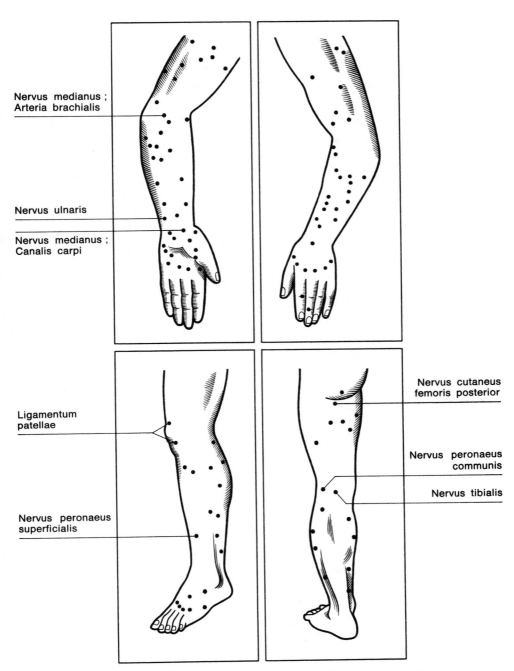

7.12 Vital points or *marmas* of the limbs, according to Hindu anatomy. Some correspond to major arteries, nerves, or tendons.

2.10) had been hit at just that place, but what the Akkadians had expressed solely as art, the Hindus had worked into a system.

Certain marmas were said to be fatal as soon as the weapon was extracted; others within one day, or two to four weeks.[105] A wound on the edge of a marma was expected either to cause death after some delay, or sometimes merely to cause a deformity.[106] Death was not always inevitable even with direct wounds. If a weapon stuck in the marmas of the temple, for instance, immediate death ensued if the weapon was pulled out, but if it was left in place and allowed to drop out on its own by suppuration, the patient could survive.[107] The meaning of "*deadly* point" should not be taken too literally, for the Hindus liked to embellish their truths with a glimmer of legend. Death by wounds in some marmas was explained as the result of excessive hemorrhage, but Sushruta also thought that the breath of life could escape out of the wounded marma in the form of vayu or vata, the bodily wind.[108]

For sheer antiquity, the doctrine of the marmas beats anything known of Greek medicine. It is already mentioned in the *Rig Veda*, which dates from about 1500–1200 B.C.[109] Vritra the demon, for instance, who fancied himself invulnerable, dammed up the river waters—but the warlike Indra killed him by piercing his marma.[110] Today, the idea survives not only in Ayurvedic medicine but also in Indian parlance: thus of someone who fell unconscious from a blow one might say, "he must have been hit in a marma." And some of the vital points have found a practical application in wrestling.[111]

Such was the practical anatomy of the Hindus, learned from studying wounds in the living rather than from dissecting the dead.

Sushruta's paragraph on human dissection has a puzzling appendix: "*Memorable Verses.* The Self, the occult or invisible Lord of the body cannot be detected except with the psychic eye or with that of the mind. He, who has observed the internal mechanism of the human body . . . is alone qualified in the science of Ayurveda and has a rightful claim to the art of healing."[112] Sushruta is using a favorite expression of the Greeks, the eye of the mind,[113] but it is a strange place to use it, right after discussing a very practical and messy job. Perhaps he is hinting that putrefied bodies had little to teach, and that human anatomy really had to be discovered by *thinking*. So it was, in a way, because the doctrine of the marmas was anatomy by dint of memory and correlation. Sometimes a very fine correlation: there is a marma that anticipated one of Galen's discoveries, and went beyond it, as we shall see in the last chapter.

Patient No. 3: A Snake Bite

वैद्य

Strolling back home, the self-satisfied vaidya in his white garment was the living image of Sushruta's perfect physician: he wore shoes, carried a stick and an umbrella, and walked "with a mild and benignant look, as a friend of all created beings, ready to help all."[114] And he pondered about the two wounded men. They certainly looked curable, but Sushruta warned that diseases affecting certain kinds of people "are apt to run into an incurable type, though appearing in a common or curable form at the outset."[115] Here is the list of such dangerous patients: "A Brahmana well versed in the Vedas, or a king, or a woman, or an infant, or an old man, or a timid person, or a man in the royal service, or a cunning man, or a man who pretends to possess a knowledge of the science of medicine, or a man who conceals his disease, or a man of an excessively irascible temperament, or a man who has no control

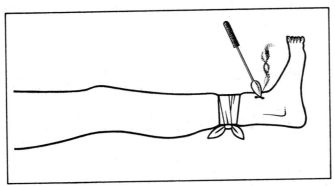

7.13 Sushruta's first aid for snake bite (besides sucking the wound): ligature and cautery.

over his senses, or a man in extremely indigent circumstances of life or without anyone to take care of him."[116] Sushruta had given much thought to his list of alibis.

Suddenly, as the vaidya came across the farm where he had seen the three bad omens, his well-trained ears detected signs of commotion. He speeded up and walked into the house. The family was clustered around a child, perhaps three years old, who had just been bitten in the left foot by a snake. The father glanced up and uttered one word—*darvi-kara*, "hooded cobra." Thanks to a smattering of Ayurvedic medicine, he had already applied the *arishta*, a strip of cloth tied four fingers above the ankle, very tight (Fig. 7.13).[117] He was now sprinkling cold water over the child's face, to counteract "the heat of the poison."[118]

The vaidya took over, acting "as fast as a man grabs a metal tool that has dropped in deep water."[119] It was good that the ligature had been applied: "Arishtas—says Charaka—are to poison what embankment is to the water"[120]—a marvellous statement, especially from people who did not know about the circulation. However, no ligature could be effective unless consecrated by the proper mantras, the sacred formulas. The vaidya had learned them as part of his training, during a special period of "self-control and cleanliness in body and spirit," while foregoing sexual intercourse, animal diet, honey, etc. . . . and lying on a mattress of *Kusha* grass." He chanted one over the arishta while the mother prepared an offering of clarified butter to burn on the family shrine:[121]

वैद्य

> I have gone about the race of snakes
>   as the sun about the sky
> As night about living creatures
>   other than the swan
> Thereby do I ward off your poison[122]

Then the vaidya rose, asked that someone fetch a clod of fresh earth, and turned to reassure the terrified child. The bite, he pointed out, was of the shallow variety known as *radita*, which meant that there was very little poison in the wound.[123] Whatever poison there was, the ligature would prevent it from climbing up into the rest of the body,[124] and maybe the poison was of poor quality anyway. The cobra could very well have been an old and miserable one, or a baby, or a member of the lower castes—because snakes, too, had castes; only the lustrous and sweetly smelling were Brahmans[125] (Fig. 7.14). Or it could have just cast off its skin, or been "attacked and discomfited by a mongoose,"[126] or simply been very frightened. All these kinds of cobras had a weak poison.[127] It would have done the patient a lot of good to be able to bite back into that wicked cobra, but it was just as good to bite into the clod of earth.[128] That was something he could do for himself. As for the doctor, he would take care of that little bit of poison in the wound; it really had to be taken out, even if it hurt.

The vaidya stuffed his mouth with a piece of linen and began sucking at the sore.[129] The gesture is still recommended in modern medical books, but it probably required more courage in ancient India, because the power of poison was overestimated. The flesh of an animal killed by a poisoned arrow or by a snake was thought to become venomous throughout and to remain so for about an hour after death.[130]

Next, with a dramatic gesture, while the parents held the boy, the surgeon plunged his blade between the marks of the two fangs, for he had learned that, "even as a tree does not grow when its roots are cut asunder, poison does not grow if an incision be made on the puncture."[131] Then he took a forceps, picked a blazing coal from the cooking fire, and quickly pressed it onto the wound. There was a scream, but the child felt a gush of relief when he saw the red coal fly out the door, toward the bushes where he had been bitten.[132]

Not much else could be done for the time being, as the child was too young for bloodletting, "the best treatment" for snakebite in an adult.[133] An apprentice would come along later with a special *agada*, an antipoison plaster.[134] In the meantime, a good agada-drink would be water blackened with the earth of an anthill;[135] and, if the mother had any in her herb garden,[136] a decoction of *sarpagandha* root. The last should have helped, for sarpagandha is none other than *Rauwolfia serpentina*, the source of reserpine, the potent drug that first earned the name of *tranquilizer* in the mid-1950s.[137] Perhaps this root was used against snake bite because it looks like a snake (hence its name *serpentina*).[138]

The mother then came with a gift of candy—fresh, succulent treacle— but the vaidya declined, for he was not allowed "to take anything but cooked rice from the hands of a woman."[139] He collected his fee and took his leave, recommending more sacrifices and prayer.

वैद्य

Everybody was prepared for the worst, for it was only too well-known that the bite of a "young" hooded cobra could be "as fatal as personified death."[140] In the vaidya's mental textbook the clinical picture of snake poisoning was carefully codified, like everything else, and subdivided into seven[141] or eight[142] stages. There was a treatment for each stage: emetics (*vamya*),[143] purges, collyria, antipoison snuffs (*nasya*),[144] even "brain purgatives" if the poison should rise as high as the head.[145] If consciousness began

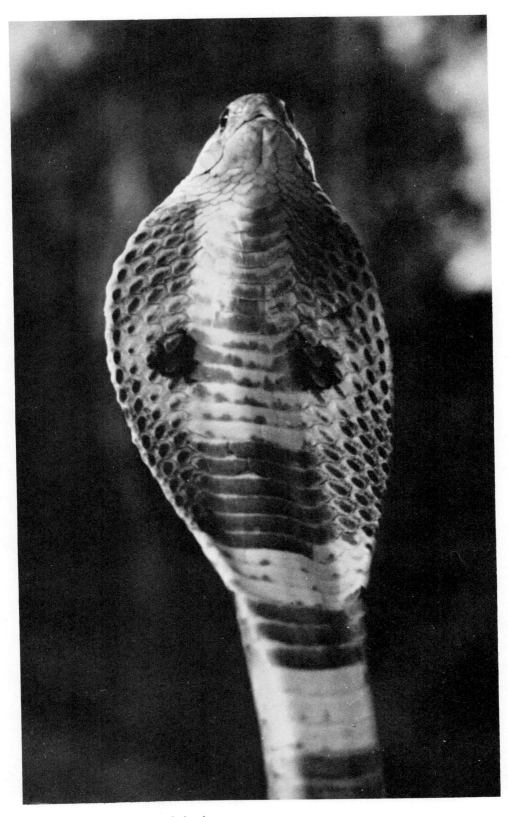

7.14 A *darvi-kara*—the hooded cobra.

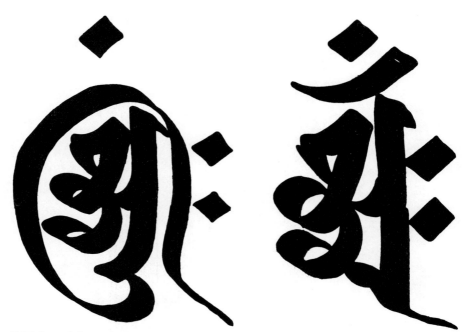

7.15 Sacred formulas or *mantras*. A mantra could be a short prayer, a word, even a single letter; eventually their spiritual value could be expressed by pure calligraphy. These two represent sacred syllables. By a Japanese Buddhist monk, twelfth century A.D.

to fade, it could still be revived with the noise of drums, perhaps smeared with antipoison plasters.[146] The vaidya would not give up until the symptoms had become overwhelming. By that time the patient, being in "an insane state like that of a drunkard,"[147] would no longer realize that he was being abandoned.

But despite it all the vaidya continued to believe that the mantras *never* failed: "The Mantras, full of occult energy and perfect truth and divine communion, never fail to eliminate the poison from the system, and hold their own even in cases of deadliest poisons" (Fig. 7.15).[148] And there is a good chance that the mantras did work. The local treatment was of a nature to help. In India, moreover, well over half of those who have been bitten by poisonous snakes escape without any symptoms of poisoning.[149] Many recover from cobra bites even without any effective treatment, perhaps because the snakes inject little venom when biting defensively.[150]

वैद्य

It was a tired man who walked back into his herb garden. The vaidya had just enough energy for the last chore of the day, testing the rain water by boiling Shali rice in his home. If the rice changed color, the clouds had been formed by vapors arising from the sea. If it did not, "the rain-cloud [had been] charged with vapors evaporated from the bosom of the Ganges."[151] That was the most wholesome water.

Outside, his eye caught one of the apprentices about to cull some medicinal herbs. Before doing so, he faced north.[152] The teaching had not been in vain.

Afterthoughts on the Arishta, the Hindu Ligature

Treatments that really treat are so rare in ancient medicine that the arishta deserves special mention. If it is true that Sushruta described the state of the art in the last centuries B.C., this is the first mention of a tourniquet in clinical practice.[153]

Note that this is not quite the same as the *hemostatic* tourniquet—a ligature tight enough to stop bleeding, already hinted in the Hippocratic books. Snake poison is reabsorbed and spread throughout the body by the veins as well as by the lymphatic vessels surrounding the bite; in both kinds of vessels, the pressure is so low that even a fairly loose ligature will close them (and therefore protect the bitten patient), even though blood continues to flow into the limb, beyond the ligature, through the arteries. To close the arteries, a much tighter ligature is required. However, the tourniquet for poisoned wounds does aim at stopping blood flow (although in the veins alone), and it is interesting that it was born as a response to snake bite, long before the circulation of the blood was recognized.

Much of India was covered with jungle. Poisonous snakes were everywhere, as they still are, for today they bring death to from 10,000 to 15,000 Indians every year.[154] The prevalence of snake bite in ancient India is proven by the lengthy chapters in Sushruta and Charaka, as well as by the dozens of antisnake charms in the much older *Atharva Veda*.[155]

Besides the tourniquet, another and perhaps even older response to the cobras had been to turn them into gods. The ancient snake-gods were called *nagas*, a word that may have the same root as *snake*.[156] One feels the presence of the nagas, as well as of real snakes, throughout Hindu art and literature (Fig. 7.16).

Alexander the Great was not prepared for the cobras. His men returned from India with terrifying tales. One was about a sacred snake living in a cave; it was 70 cubits long and had eyes the size of the large round Macedonian shields.[157] Snake bites became such a menace that Alexander felt obliged to hire Hindu physicians, who were kept on duty full time, and anyone bitten had to report immediately to the royal tent.[158]

None of the ancient historians who report these episodes mentions the ligature. Even Sushruta and Charaka deal with it in only a few lines, just enough to say that it is essential. Their descriptions of snake-bite poisoning show how the idea of the arishta developed. A bite in the foot causes symptoms in the head and neck.[159] Therefore, animal poison acts upward, with the inevitable corollary that plant poison acts downward.[160] If a poison rises from the foot, then a tie at the ankle comes about quite naturally.

वैद्य

Historically, the Hindus may have been the first to apply such ligatures, but the same idea was born, perhaps independently, in another snake-infested part of the world. In our days, the Mano tribe of Liberia has such trouble with snakes that it maintains a secret Snake-Bite Society;[161] and the Mano apply real tourniquets of bark. One, in fact, was applied to an American physician who had been bitten on a finger—after he had already applied two tourni-

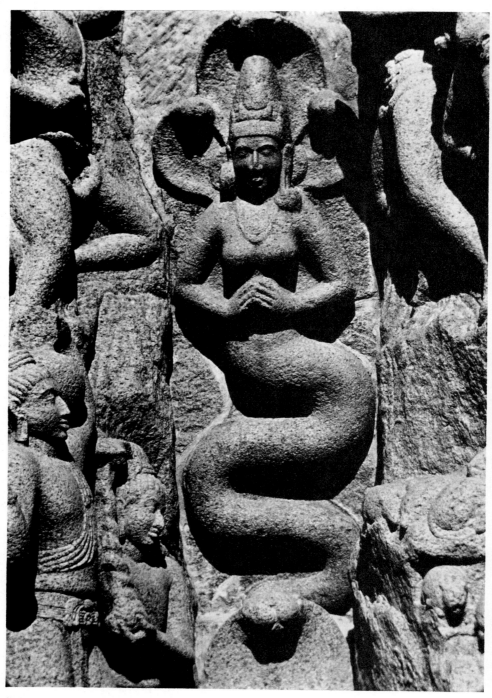

7.16 A statue to Nagini, the snake goddess: one of India's ways to cope with snakes.

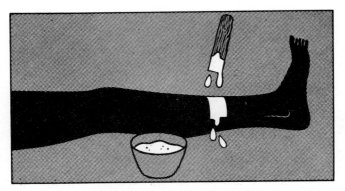

7.17 An early step in the development of the ligature for snake bite: the Manos in Liberia sometimes paint a white ring around the limb.

quets of his own. He reported that the Mano tourniquet was just tight enough to stop the return of venous blood, and therefore should have been at least partially effective. But the Mano practice is to apply ties on both wrist and ankle, regardless of the place where the victim was bitten, and even if the bite was not in a limb. Furthermore, at night, "to stop the poison from reaching the heart" before dawn, a ring of white clay is painted around the limb (Fig. 7.17). To the Mano, the tourniquet also symbolizes "binding the patient" until he has paid his fee,[162] a clear indication that many do recover. So Liberia offers a good example of a discovery in its embryonic stage, half rational, half magic, but already evolved enough to help—sometimes.[163]

In what is left of his books, Hippocrates never mentions snake bite. Surely he was aware of the problem. But his methods cannot have been too effective if Alexander's army doctors had to be replaced by Hindus.

Patient No. 4: A Problem of Earrings

The next morning, a nurse appeared, dragging by the hand a reluctant little boy. He was stark naked, except for an amulet of tiger claws around his neck,[164] and he was to have his ears pierced. It was none too early, said the nurse, for he had just recovered from a case of *shita-putaná*, one of the nine dreaded diseases of infants, which was due to the influence of the *Grahas*, the malignant stars.[165] The parents knew full well, of course, that pierced ears were not only for looks but also for protection against "the evil influences of malignant stars and spirits."[166] However, they had been obliged to delay the operation until the proper month of the year (the sixth or seventh) and until the right lunar and astral combinations.[167] Daily life was full of Beings, good and bad, that could not be neglected—like the Grahas. There was, for example, a *yaksha*—a particular kind of ghost—in each and every tree (Fig. 7.18).[168]

Piercing the earlobes was a standard operation:

The child should be placed on the lap of its nurse, and benedictions should be pronounced over it. Then having soothed it and lured it with toys and playthings,

वैद्य

285

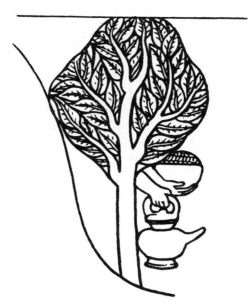

7.18 A *yaksha* in a tree: just one kind of ghost among the crowd of *a-mánusha* (non-humans) that haunted everyday life in India.

the physician should draw down with his left hand the lobules of its ears with a view to detect, with the help of the reflected sunlight, (the closed up) apertures that are naturally found to exist in those localities [*sic!*]. Then he should pierce them straight through with a needle held in his right hand, or with an awl (*Ará*), or with a thick needle where the appendages would be found to be too thick. The lobule of the right ear should be first pierced and then the left in the case of a male child, while the contrary should be the procedure in the case of a female. Plugs of cotton-lint should be then inserted into the holes of the pricked ear-lobules, which should be lubricated or rubbed with any unboiled oil. A copious bleeding attended with pain would indicate that the needle has passed through a place other than the natural (and closed up) fissure described above; whereas the absence of any serious after-effect would give rise to the presumption that the piercing has been done through the right spot.[169]

Over a sobbing child, the nurse was told what to do next:[170] "If all goes well, you will bring the child to me every third day; each time I will remove the lint, lubricate the hole with oil, and stretch it with a thicker plug. When the bodily humors in the ear will have settled down, I will then begin to expand the hole with rods of wood, or with lead weights." Perforating the lobes had been just a beginning: the real purpose was to stretch them into wide rings, flabby yet strong enough to carry heavy ornaments. In the famous paintings of the Ajanta caves[171] there is a fifth- or sixth-century lady who shows this very well (Plate 7.1). Some of her descendants need not envy her (Fig. 7.19). The custom also remains alive outside of India (Fig. 7.20).[172]

Why pierced or stretched ear lobes were supposed to protect, I do not know.[173] Buddha's heads show both features prominently (Fig. 7.4). In any event, the piercing carried a sizable risk, possibly including tetanus. Here is Sushruta's warning:

वैद्य

286

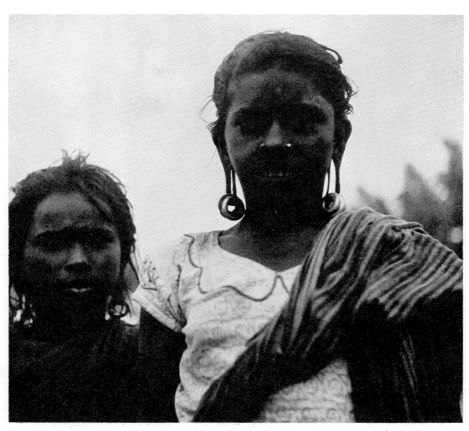

7.19 Stretched earlobes still exist in modern India.

Any of the local veins incidentally injured by an ignorant, bungling surgeon, may be attended with symptoms which will be described under the heads of Káliká, Marmariká, and Lohitiká.

Káliká is marked by fever and a burning pain in the affected part and swelling. *Marmariká* gives rise to pain and knotty formations about the affected region, accompanied by (the characteristic inflammatory) fever; while in the last named type (Lohitiká) symptoms such as, Manyá-Stambha (numbness of the tendons forming the nape of the neck), Apatának (a type of tetanus), Shirograha (headache) and Karna-shula (earache) exhibit themselves, and they should be duly treated with medicinal remedies laid down under their respective heads.[174]

The hole being stuffed with crude lint, some such infection was bound to occur. In cases of "extreme pain and swelling," Sushruta's advice was to remove the lint immediately, anoint the infected part with a paste of honey and clarified butter enriched with barley and four herbs,[175] wait for it to heal, then start all over again.

But woe to the surgeon who ran into this complication. The blame could be pinned on him, either for putting the hole "in the wrong place," or for making it "with a blunt, crooked or stunted needle," or for plugging it with an "inordinately large lint."[176] Sushruta was saying, in effect, that surgical infection is the surgeon's fault. Basically he was right, though for the wrong

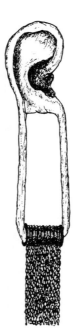

7.20 A stretched earlobe from East Africa. It was observed on a Masai man about 1900. The earring weight was made of copper wire.

reasons. An intriguing parallel occurs in a Chinese classic, the *Nei Ching*, where an abscess appearing at the site of acupuncture means that the acupuncturist is at fault, for having struck the wrong place.

Patient No. 5: A Torn Earlobe

The story of this patient is another landmark: the birth of plastic and reconstructive surgery. One reason that it happened first in India may be that the Greeks went to war with efficient helmets, whereas the Hindus probably wore none and were therefore especially liable to have ears and noses lopped off in battle.[177] They also ran the risk of judicial mutilation, for according to the ancient laws of Manu, every conceivable part of the body was liable to be amputated as a punishment, including the anus of any citizen who might break wind against the king.[178] If challenge breeds competence, plastic surgery was bound to be born here. Native enthusiasts even speak of whole heads being sewn back into place.[179]

वैद्य

Yet I believe that the principal stimulus for plastic surgery came from a very different, more peaceful, more commonplace event: torn earlobes. They were a major issue.[180] Sushruta gives ten pages to piercing earlobes and pertinent complications, but only two pages to repairing noses (how the nose was lost he does not say).

Now witness the facts in the vaidya's home. A very upset man stalks in, identified as a Brahman by the tuft of hair bunched together on top of his head. He asks for some perfumed water, fearing that he may have caught a filthy glimpse of a *chandāla*, an outcast of the lowest kind. The emergency is met; for it is wise to please the priestly caste without delay. As the stern gentleman washes his eyes clean of the awful sight,[181] the surgeon realizes why he has really come. The Brahman is wearing only one, heavy earring; the other earlobe has been torn open, probably as the result of an accident, and has now shrunk to a little, stumpy scar. This is a very familiar sight, and a safe one too, for it allows the surgeon to show off his art at its best. Said Sushruta, the ways to repair an injured earlobe are "innumerable."[182]

There is of course an established list of deformities related to torn or distorted earlobes. Each one requires a certain kind of treatment, with its own precise name (Fig. 7.21). The lobe of the Brahman has shriveled to almost nothing, so that it can be repaired only by making a new one out of the skin nearby. This too can be done—although nobody in the world knows how, except the vaidyas.

But there is a hitch. The patient would have to gather strength with a light meal[183] and drink some wine to decrease the pain.[184] Yet neither is feasible, because the traumatic experience of having seen a chandāla requires a Brahman to abstain from food and liquor for the rest of the day.[185] So he will have to return tomorrow, with friends and relatives to assist him.[186]

And there will be, of course, no fee for this operation. Brahmans tend to live off the other castes; the surgeon being a member of the Kshatriya caste, mainly comprising nobles and warriors, it is wholly in his interest to offer this gift to the Brahman. It will help his *karma*, or as we might say, his own investment in the next world, particularly the number of his reincarnations.[187]

The historic operation is described by Sushruta in two sentences, in which lies the beginning of that *shastra* or "science" now known as reconstructive surgery:

A surgeon well-versed in the knowledge of surgery should slice off a patch of living flesh from the cheek of a person devoid of ear-lobes in a manner so as to have one of its ends attached to its former seat [*cheek*]. Then the part, where the artificial ear-lobe is to be made, should be slightly scarified [*with a knife*] and the living flesh, full of blood and sliced off as previously directed, should be adhesioned to it.[188]

The details of the operation are not clear. Its Sanskrit name is *ganda-karna*, literally "cheek-ear." The cheek, if it meant then what it now means, is an unlikely place to carve out the flap. It would make more sense to lift the flesh from behind the ear, as in one of the modern methods (Fig. 7.22).[189] However, the principle is clear: Sushruta is using the classical technique of the pedicle flap, whereby an area of skin is outlined with a cut in the shape of a long *U*, then dissected free so that it can be moved about as a kind of tongue. Its free end can then be sewn onto any raw part within reach. Eventually the two surfaces grow together and exchange blood; at this point, if necessary, the base of the *U* can be cut free.

To prepare for the operation, the first duty of the surgeon was to collect the necessary items: "Surgical appliances and instruments . . . cotton, lint, thread, leaves, tow, honey, clarified butter . . . medicated plasters . . . fan, cold water, hot water . . . and moreover he shall secure the services of

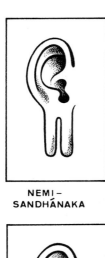

NEMI–
SANDHÁNAKA

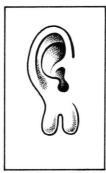

UTPALA–
BHEDYAKA

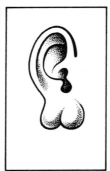

VALLURAKA

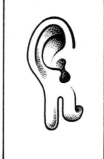

ÁSANGIMA

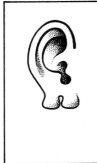

ÁHÁRYAYA

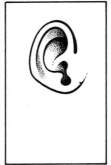

NIRVEDHIMA

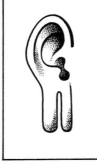

VYÁYOJIMA

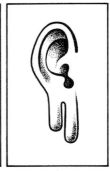

KAPÁTA–
SANDHIKA

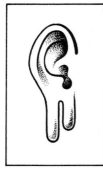

ARDHA–
KAPÁTA–
SANDHIKA

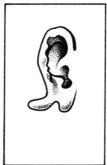

SAMKHIPTAM

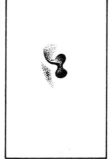

HINA–KARNA

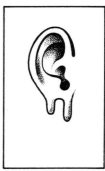

VILLAKARNA

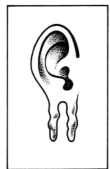

YASTHI
KARNA

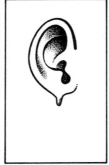

KÁKUSTHAKAPÁLI

7.21 The many problems caused by
Indian earrings were classified into
an elaborate system.

devoted and strong-nerved attendants."[190] He required three kinds of wound wash, to be used as we would use disinfectants. He chose among them on the spur of the moment, depending on the particular humor that seemed to be deranged. Unaccountably, he would also need a powder made of ground-up baked pottery, to dust on at the end.

The operation itself took place as follows:

> Then the hair of the patient, whether male or female, should be gathered and tied up in a knot, and the patient should be given a light food (so as to keep up his strength without hampering his digestion); after which his friends and relations should be asked to hold him firm. Then having ascertained the particular nature of adhesion to be effected in the case, the surgeon should examine the local blood by incising, excising, scarifying or puncturing the affected lobes as found necessary, and determine whether the same is pure or vitiated. Then having washed the blood with Dhányámla [*fermented rice gruel*] and tepid water, if found vitiated through the action of the deranged Váyu, or with milk and cold water in the event of the same being contaminated by the deranged Pitta, or with Surámanda ["*transparent surface-part of wine*"] and warm water in the case of its being vitiated by the action of the disordered Kapha, the surgeon shall bring about the adhesion by again scarifying the affected parts of the ear, so as not to leave the adhesioned parts elevated (raised), unequal and short. Of course the adhesion should be effected with the blood being still left in the parts that had been scraped. Then having anointed them with honey and clarified butter, they should be covered with cotton and linen, and tied with strings of thread, neither too loose nor too tight, and dusted over with powders of baked clay. Then directions should be given as regards the diet and nursing of the patient, who may be as well treated with the regimen laid down in the chapter on Dvi-vraniyam.[191]

And so it came to pass that, through the habit of stretching their earlobes, the Indians became masters in a branch of surgery that Europe ignored for another two thousand years. When the operation finally caught on, it was for a purpose much less common in India, but more applicable in Europe: making new noses.[192] In the ancient Indian operation, the new nose was built from a flap of skin folded down from the forehead. The flap itself was ingeniously drawn on the pattern of a leaf, with a stalk and two wings

7.22 A modern operation for making a new earlobe. Sushruta's *ganda-karna* or "cheek-ear" method must have been similar.

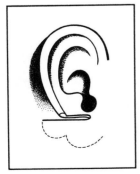 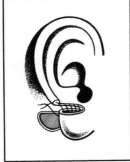 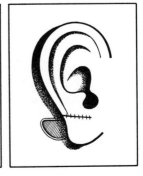

वैद्य

291

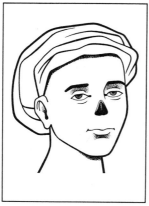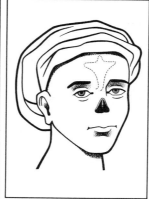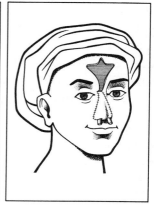

7.23 Reconstruction of the nose as described by Sushruta. A pedicle flap is brought down from the forehead and molded over two short tubes inserted in place of the nostrils. In 1794, the *Gentleman's Magazine* published a portrait of an Indian bullock-driver successfully operated on in this manner. The little tubes are still used in modern plastic surgery.

that gave the right contour when molded into nostrils (Fig. 7.23). The modern operation is essentially the same (Fig. 7.24); and the nostrils are still molded over two little tubes, as recommended by Sushruta.[193]

As to repairing earlobes, today's plastic surgeons still learn the technique, for the need persists. Sometimes the earring is torn out by its own weight; sometimes in the course of an argument.[194]

Another Parenthesis: Indian Infirmaries?

Sushruta never says where his patients are treated, but Charaka describes what appears to be, in that context, the ideal hospital. Here is most of the text:

In the first place a mansion must be constructed under the supervision of an engineer well-conversant with the science of building mansions and houses. It should be spacious and roomy. The element of strength should not be wanting in it. Every part of it should not be exposed to strong winds or breezes. One portion at least should be open to the currents of wind . . .

It should not be exposed to smoke, or the Sun, or dust, or injurious sound and touch and taste and form and scent. It should be furnished with staircases, with pestles and mortars, privies, . . . and cook-rooms.

After this should be secured a body of attendants of good behaviour, distinguished for purity or cleanliness of habits, attached to the person for whose service they are engaged, possessed of cleverness and skill, endued with kindness, skilled in every kind of service that a patient may require . . . competent to cook food and curries, clever in bathing or washing a patient . . . or raising the patient or assisting him in walking or moving about, well-skilled in making or cleaning beds, patient and skillful in waiting upon one that is ailing, and never unwilling to do any act that they may be commanded to do. A number of men should also be secured that are skilled in vocal and instrumental music, in hymning encomiums and eulogies,

वैद्य

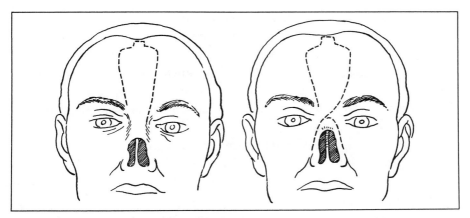

7.24 Two types of **modern operation** for rebuilding the nose with forehead flaps, essentially Sushruta's method and his leaf design. There still is a problem at the tip of the leaf: how to twist it by 180 degrees without choking the vessels.

conversant with and skilled in reciting verses and pleasant discourses and narratives and stories and legendary histories . . . fully conversant with all the requirements of time and place, and possessed of such politeness as to become agreeable companions. The mansion should also be stored with an adequate supply of partridge, hare, spotted deer, black antelope, black-tailed deer, etc. . . .

A cow also should be kept, yielding copious milk, of a quiet disposition, healthy, having all her calves living . . . So also should be kept little vessels or cups, larger vessels for washing the hands and face, water-vessels or jars, small jars or pitchers, dishes, metallic or earthen jars, cauldrons or pans . . . hollow vessels for covering articles, wooden or metallic ladles, mats . . . deer-skins and sheep-skins, rags, cloths made of cotton and wool, strings and cords, beds and seats, vessels called Bhringaras full of water and flatter vessels for holding spittle and evacuations, all placed ready for use, good beds placed upon bedsteads and overlaid with white sheets and containing pillows, for use when sleep is needed, beds and carpets for lying down or sitting upon . . . and diverse kinds of instruments, domestic and surgical. Smoking tubes, enemas . . . brushes and brooms, balances and weights, measuring vessels and baskets, Ghee, oil, fat, marrow, honey, treacle, salt, fuel, water, honey-wines, sour gruels of different varieties, different kinds of wines, whey, butter-milk, sour gruel of paddy or rice, and the different varieties of animal urine [*as drugs!*] should also be kept ready . . .

So also . . . emetics and purgatives, and articles that are both emetics and purgatives, those that are astringent, that increase the appetite, promote digestion, cool the system, and destroy the wind [*the most dangerous of the three doshas*] should be kept ready . . . Other things, again, that may conduce to the ease, comfort, and happiness of the patient, should similarly be kept ready.[195]

Truth or fairy tale? I believe truth, lapsing into fairy tale. That was the style of Sushruta or Charaka, who quite often describe something that is, then glide into what should be, or might be, to end in purely verbal fireworks. They are especially prone to do so when they enumerate, as in the text above. In the long list of patients who should not be treated (sometimes for good reasons), Charaka goes so far as to say that one should never treat, *even in wish*, people whose image reflected in a mirror is upside down or headless.[196] In listing patients who might need enemas, he goes from people to cows (still understandable) to camels, thence to a grand finale of fragrant enemas for snakes.[197] This is pushing snake worship too far. In listing the possible complications of enemas, he describes the ultimate possibility: the enema may reach high enough to come out of the throat, in which case the thing to do is of course to press on the neck.[198] All this does not mean that enemas were not given; it simply means that literature and fantasy had their share also in medicine.

So Charaka's infirmary surely existed, though probably only as an infirmary that rich people could afford as part of their household,[199] somewhat like the *valetudinaria* of Roman estates. Real Indian hospitals were not long in coming, however. Between 399 and 414 A.D., India was visited by Fa-hsien, a Chinese pilgrim and Buddhist monk, who was seeking the sources of the original faith.[200] With such a motivation, it was possible to brave the Headache Mountains and their eternal snows. "As far as the eye can reach, the route is marked out by the bleached bones of men who have perished in the attempt . . . scarcely one person in ten thousand survives . . . the wind, and the rain, and the snow, and the driving sand and gravel."[201] Crossing the Indus on a bridge of ropes, Fa-hsien reached Pataliputra. He marveled at the ruins of Ashoka's palace, which had been built, he says, with the help of Genii. Then he adds: "The respective nobles and landowners of this country have founded hospitals within the city, to which the poor of all countries, the destitute, cripples, and the diseased, may repair (for shelter). They receive every kind of requisite help gratuitously. Physicians inspect their diseases, and according to their cases order them food and drink, medicine or decoctions, everything in fact that may contribute to their ease. When cured they depart at their own convenience." Fa-hsien must have realized that this, too, was part of Buddha's heritage.[202]

Patient No. 6: An Internal Abscess

To be precise, this young man had more of a problem than just an abscess: he suffered from empyema—pus in his chest—just like Patient No. 3 whom we met at the Athenian clinic. For a couple of weeks, his horizon had been restricted to the bamboo frame of his bed.[203] The red, hot swelling on the side of his chest meant that pus, collected in that pleural cavity, was trying to find its way out. The vaidya was called to the bedside. Pneumonia was not in his books, nor was auscultation of the chest, so he merely studied the lump. It was rounded, painful. Because it reminded him of an anthill, it had to be an *antara-vidradhi* or "internal abscess."[204] One may disagree with this terminology, but for practical purposes it was correct.

A nice, ripe abscess is a temptation for any surgeon, but the vaidya faced a difficult question: could it be cut open without touching a marma? "In a case of surgical operation, the situation and dimension of each local Marma should be first taken into account and the incision should be made in a way so as not to affect that particular Marma, inasmuch as an incision, even

वैद्य

Color Plates

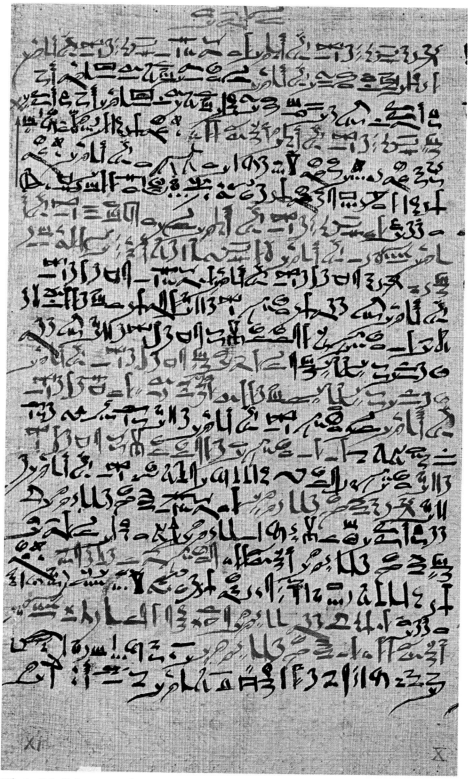

Plate 3.1 Column XI of the Smith papyrus, written about 1650 B.C. A red asterisk (arrow) shows where the scribe had left out the words "Thou shouldst say concerning him." He added them neatly at the top of the page.

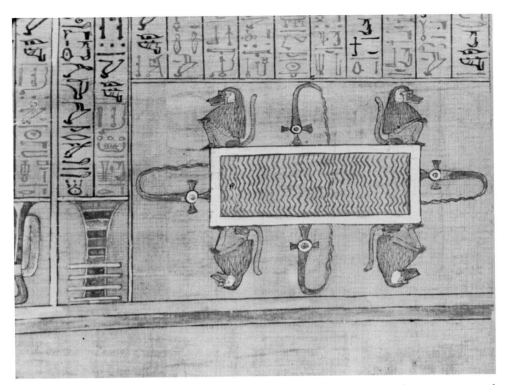

Plate 3.2 The hieroglyph for "hot" was clearly a brazier. Here it appears four times around the hellish Lake of Flames, as illustrated in a papyrus containing the *Book of the Dead*. The jagged lines ∿∿∿ stood conventionally for "water." From the papyrus of Ani, c. 1250 B.C.

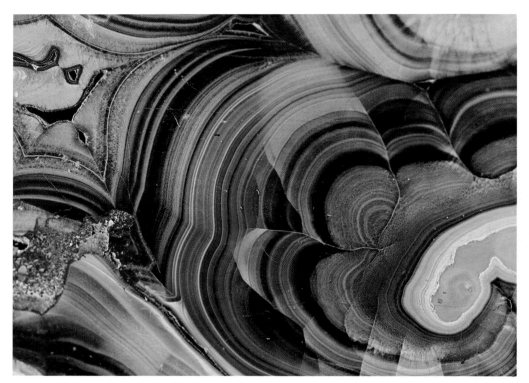

Plate 3.3 Malachite, the beautiful copper ore that was powdered to obtain green pigment for paint, eye shadow, and wound salves. Enlarged about 2x.

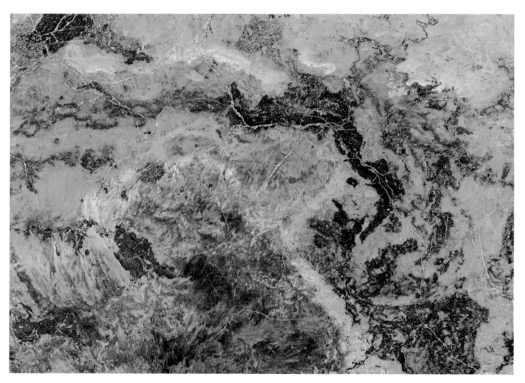

Plate 3.4 Chrysocolla, from a Greek word meaning "gold glue," is another lovely copper ore that was ground for pigment, used in paint, gold solder, and medicine. Enlarged about 2x.

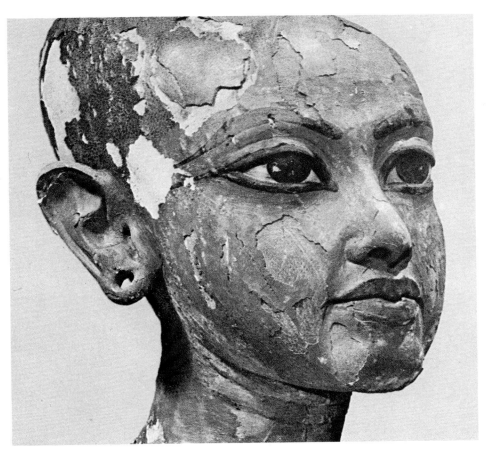

Plate 3.5 Typical Egyptian eye makeup with blue-green copper pigment (in this instance the precise variety is not known). Head found in Tutankhamun's tomb, c.1350 B.C.

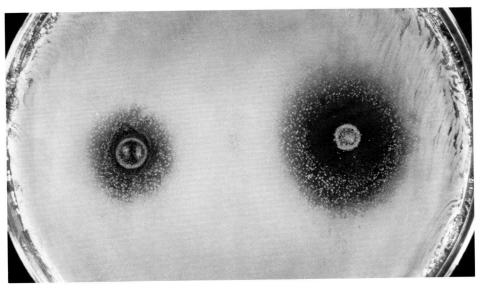

Plate 3.6 Effect of powdered malachite (right) and chrysocolla (left) on bacterial growth. Here the culture medium was sewn with harmless bacteria (*Sarcina lutea*); some powder was put into each of the two little wells and allowed to stand for eight hours at 4°C. Then the plate was incubated at 37°C. Bacterial growth (yellow background) failed to occur in a dark ring around each well; malachite was more effective.

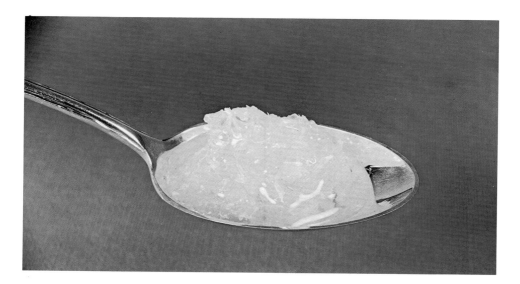

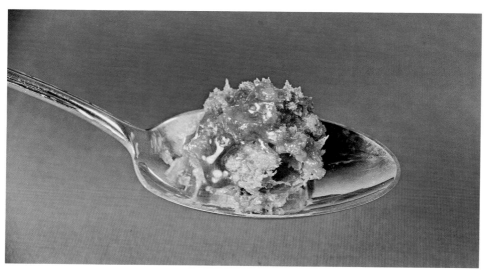

Plate 3.7 *Above:* A spoonful of honey in the comb. *Below:* Ancient honey, which lay underground in Paestum for about 2500 years. The color, consistency, and stickiness of the ancient honey were close to normal (the taste has yet to be tried).

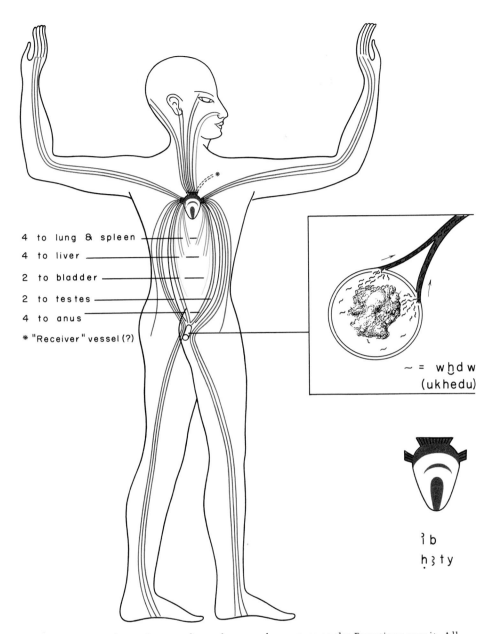

4 to lung & spleen
4 to liver
2 to bladder
2 to testes
4 to anus
* "Receiver" vessel (?)

~ = wḥdw
(ukhedu)

î b
ḥ₃ty

Plate 3.8 An informed guess about the vascular system as the Egyptians saw it. All vessels came from the heart, but they had a second assembly center around the anus. Some vessels carried blood (red), others mucus (green), urine (yellow), semen (black), water, and air (blue). Air entered the nose, passed through the heart, and went to the anus. *Upper insert:* A cross section through the anus, showing that the vessels opening to it could become flooded with excrement and carry elsewhere the dangerous *ukhedu*. Hence the central role of the anus in Egyptian medicine. *Lower insert:* The heart, which could speak through the vessels (a reference to the pulse?). Mysteriously, it had two names, *ib* and *ḥaty*; both could be abbreviated to ♡ .

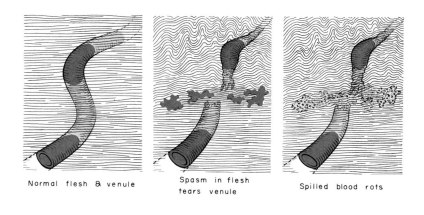

Normal flesh & venule

Spasm in flesh
tears venule

Spilled blood rots

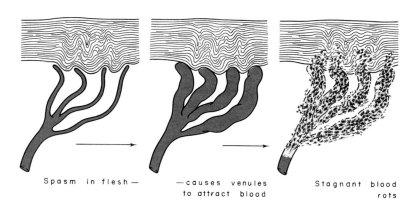

Spasm in flesh—

—causes venules
to attract blood

Stagnant blood
rots

Plate 4.1 The mechanics of disease as seen with the Greek "eye of
the mind." The basic theme is that spilled blood decays. In one case
(above) the trouble starts with a "spasm in the flesh," which makes the
venules burst. In another case (below) a spasm in the flesh "attracts"
too much blood in the venules, with the same result.

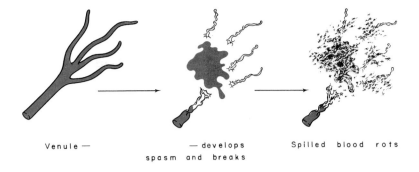

Venule —   — develops   Spilled blood rots
                    spasm and breaks

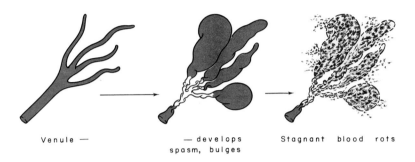

Venule —   — develops   Stagnant blood rots
                    spasm, bulges

Plate 4.2 "Spasms in venules." A spastic venule can either tear itself apart and spill out its content (above) or trap the blood into a pocket, whence it seeps out and decays (below).

Plate 4.3 Basic procedures of Hippocratic wound care. Whether the sutures were continuous, in separate stitches, or of both kinds, is not known. One obscure passage suggests that both kinds of stitches *may* have been used on the ends of the bandages. It is often claimed that Hippocrates wisely recommended applying poultices *around* the wound, but this was not always the case.

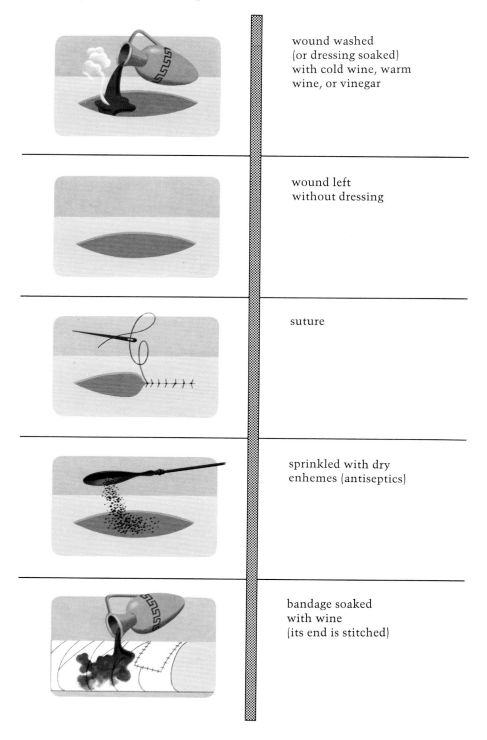

wound washed
(or dressing soaked)
with cold wine, warm
wine, or vinegar

wound left
without dressing

suture

sprinkled with dry
enhemes (antiseptics)

bandage soaked
with wine
(its end is stitched)

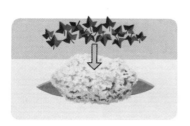

sponge, soaked in
oil and wine,
covered with leaves

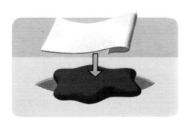

wool, soaked in
oil and wine

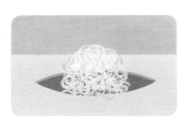

poultice on wound,
then linen pad
soaked in vinegar

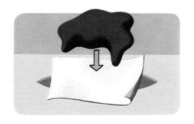

linen pad soaked in oil
and wine on wound,
then poultice

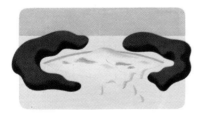

poultice around wound
(recommended for suppuration)

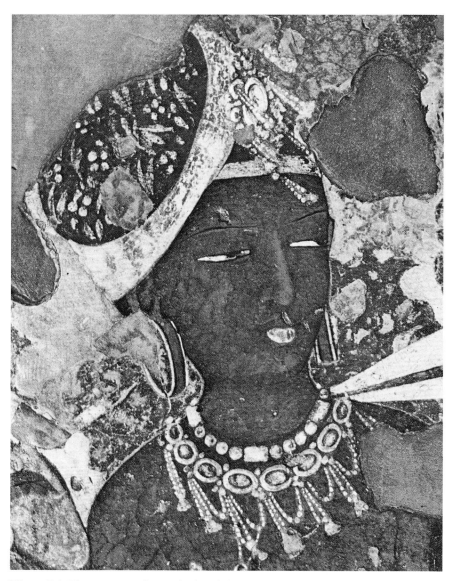

Plate 7.1 The purpose of stretched earlobes in ancient India, as shown by an *apsaras*, a celestial nymph. From a painting in the Ajanta caves, fifth-sixth century A.D.

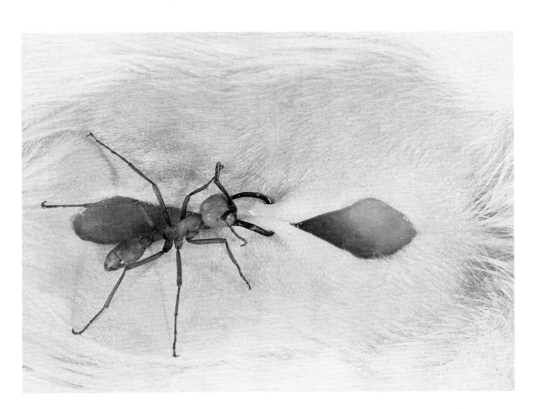

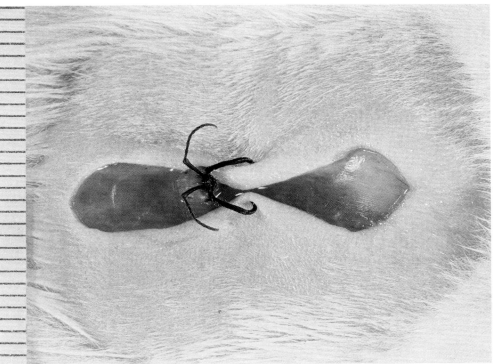

Plate 7.2 The jaws of *Eciton burchelli* holding together the edges of a wound (top), in an experiment with a dead ant on a dead rat. In the second step of the clamping process (bottom), the body of the ant is twisted off. Scale in mm.

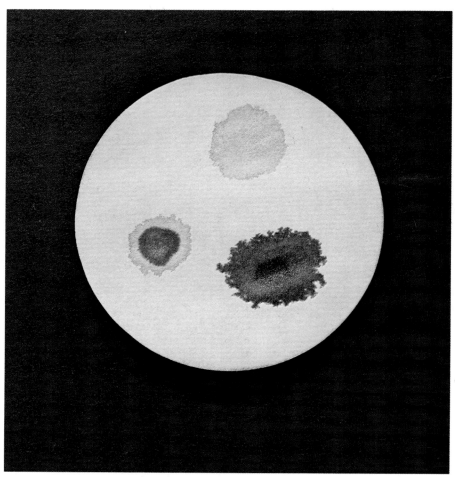

Plate 9.1 Chemical reaction described by Pliny to detect the adulteration of green copper acetate with green ferrous sulphate. A disk of filter paper—used here in place of papyrus—was impregnated with tannic acid (oak gall) and dried. *Top:* Effect of a drop of water. *Left:* 10 percent copper acetate. *Right:* 20 percent ferrous sulphate.

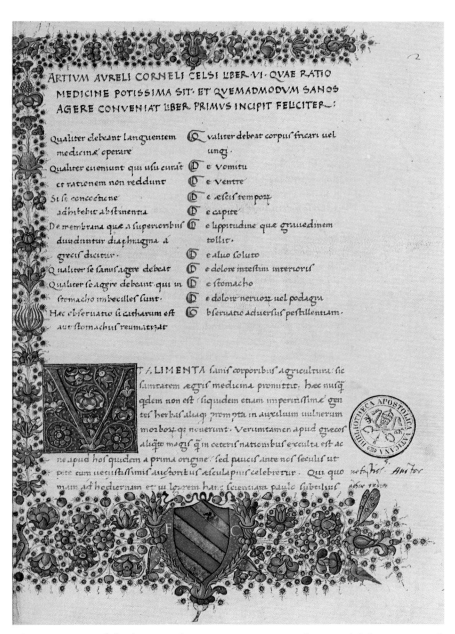

Plate 9.2 One of the fourteenth-century manuscript editions of Celsus, prepared from the ancient codices that had just been rediscovered.

extending or affecting in the least, the edge or the side of the Marma, may prove fatal."[205]

While studying how to incise without touching a marma, the vaidya asked cryptically: "Are you in the habit of taking strong wine?"[206] The patient did not quite know how to answer, because drink, he did, although he was not supposed to do so. The Brahmans, who were in charge of public mores, frowned upon fermented drinks. Yet there were dozens of such drinks—made from fruit juice, coconut juice, rice, barley, palm sap, and sugar cane; peppered, spiced, and perfumed; with a price for all pockets, up to grape wine, which was the most expensive.[207] Unlike most patients, the young man finally confessed, and he was rewarded, because the surgeon was on his side. Sushruta had no objection to fermented drinks and had written lavishly about their curative properties.[208] Better yet, if a patient was accustomed to liquor, he "should be provided with a meal before a surgical operation, or strong wine given to him . . . The effect of a good meal . . . will be to keep up the strength of the patient and to guard against his swooning during the operation, while the effect of wine will be to make him unconscious of the pain.[209] *The rule as regards the feeding and anaesthetising (wine giving) of the patient should be strictly adhered to.*"[210]

So the young man drank his way into a legitimate haze, feeling doubly good about it. It is hard to understand, incidentally, why the wine-loving Greeks did not mention wine in relation to surgery, except for external use. Maybe they left tipsiness to private initiative.[211]

A servant appeared, loaded down with bags and equipment.[212] The operating room was to be the great outdoors,[213] so the patient was directed to sit on the ground, facing east, while the servant tied his hands and feet.[214] The surgeon tested his steel blade by cutting a human hair.[215] Then, with "courage, light handedness, non-shaking, non-sweating, sharp instruments, self confidence and self command,"[216] and facing west, he cut the skin and helped the pus to flow out, while the servant dashed cold water on the face and eyes of the patient.[217] Afterward the wound was washed with an "astringent" decoction of herbs and wiped thoroughly dry with clean linen. A plug of lint, soaked in a herb preparation, was "plastered over with the paste of sesamum, honey and clarified butter . . . and . . . inserted deep into the wound."[218] Then came another plaster, spread on against the direction of the hair (*pratiloma*), to make it penetrate better;[219] followed by a thick layer of tow, "such as the leaves and bark of the Indian fig-tree;" and finally a wrapping of linen.

वैद्य

The patient could now relax, while the vaidya recited the appropriate mantras. The servant produced a long, light, flexible tube and began to set up the *nadi-sveda* (Fig. 7.25). This was an important operation. The word *nadi* is Sanskrit for "tube," and *sveda* has the same root as "sweat." The operation was in effect a sort of steam bath, with the double purpose of chasing away the pain as well as the malignant spirits.

The tube itself was a masterpiece of ingenuity. It was fashioned of woven

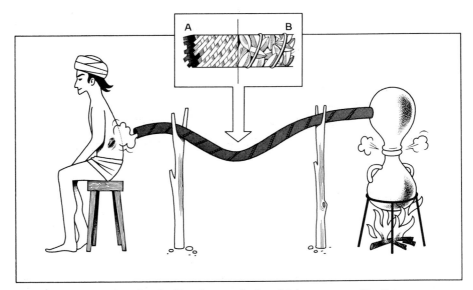

7.25 The *nadi-sveda*, a kind of local steam bath, which was part of Indian postoperative care. The pipe was made of woven grass (A), wrapped in leaves (B). The vapor was supposedly "made delightful" by bends in the pipe.

grass[220] and was made airtight with a wrapping of leaves.[221] The vapor, which came from a boiling soup of milk and urine,[222] was collected in an inverted pot, with an opening for the tube in its side. The critical feature was the shape of the tube: it had to have "three bends or turns in its body to resemble the trunk of an elephant."[223] "The reasons for the bending tube," explains the translator, "are to make the fomentation delightful, in consequence of the vapor not passing in a straight course,"[224] and to "break the strength of the vapor." The idea could only spring from the mind of a smoker. In fact, Charaka deals at length with the right length and shape of smoking pipes, the favorite materials for them being the same as for enema tubes. Smoke does no harm, he maintains, "if inhaled through a pipe made of three limbs."[225] Thus, the nadi-sveda blew gentle puffs at the wound as the vaidya chanted on. The patient listened, and his mind floated away, away from pain.

वैद्य

The wound would have to be dressed again every other day. There was no question of trying to sew it up "as long as the least bit of morbid matter, or pus remains inside it"[226] (three cheers for Sushruta). Then it would be essential to take measures against a relapse. As the patient certainly realized, an internal abscess meant that the three doshas or basic principles of his body were extremely "deranged, through eating heavy, incompatible and incongenial articles of food or of dry, putrid and decomposed substances, or by excessive coition and fatiguing physical exercise, or by voluntary repression of any natural urging of the body."[227] Hence, a list of "cures" which called for exceptional stamina: the unabridged version runs to sixty items.[228] Following are a few that could be prescribed for this patient:

> No sex, no meat, no exercise, no emotions of grief or fright, or ecstasies
> of joy.[229]

Fasting, again to bring under control the enraged doshas.[230]

Vomiting would also help, as by taking a stomachful of barley gruel, then ejecting it by sniffing a medicated flower.[231]

Sneezing too, since the wound was fairly high up in the body, by means of *nasya* or nose drugs,[232] such as pepper mixed with cow's urine or the watery exudation of cow dung.[233]

Purging,[234] plus added purification with "light agents," such as the urine of cows, buffaloes, goats, sheep, mules, horses, or camels[235]—there were six hundred purgatives in all.[236]

Enemas, with the urine group of drugs,[237] although enemas were best for sores in the lower part of the body.[238] Sushruta's directions for using the bladder-and-pipe contraption are the most detailed of antiquity, including lubrication of the tip with clarified butter.[239]

And venesection: "Venesection . . . *properly performed is half the treatment in surgery*, like the application of enematic measures in the therapeutics"![240]

On the whole, then, the young man's treatments would have been about the same as in Greece—the local techniques fair, the general ones dreadful. The Indian operation was less aggressive, no drain being left in the wound and no oil injected into the chest, and psychotherapy was more highly developed.

Patient No. 7: A Broken Nose

A *vaishya* or "workingman" came in next, holding a bloody rag over his face. It covered the result of a tavern brawl,[241] a fractured nose. Nothing serious; the sunken bone was raised with the help of a rod, just as in Greece. But the Indian technique was a touch more elegant. Instead of stuffing a leather plug into each nostril, the vaidya inserted two short pipes of bamboo cane.[242] He probably borrowed the idea from his plastic operation for making a new nose, in which the nostrils were molded around two little tubes. Again, concern for the patient.

His nose was bandaged, and sprinkled with the inevitable clarified butter.[243] The bonus was a lotus stem for sucking milk, if chewing was painful.[224]

वैद्य

Patient No. 8: An Instant Ulcer

It had been a bad fall from horseback: a fellow Kshatriya of the warrior caste was brought in with a wound in his leg, bleeding profusely. Such a wound was called a *sadyovrana*. *Vrana* was a general name for "sore," including wounds as well as ulcers, like the Greek *hélkos* (Fig. 7.26);[245] *sa-dyás* stood literally for "same-day"; *sadyovrana* therefore meant "same-day sore," "recent sore," or in the words of the translator of Sushruta, "instant ulcer."[246]

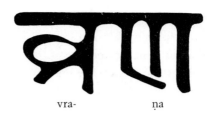

vra-　　　ṇa

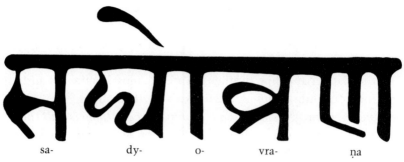

sa-　　dy-　　o-　　vra-　　ṇa

7.26 Two Sanskrit words for wound: *vraṇa*, for any type of wound (including sores and ulcers); and *sadyovraṇa*, literally "same-day wound," for fresh wounds. In modern Russian the word for wound is *rana*, a close relative.

The trouble was that the vaidya knew very little about stopping hemorrhage. One way was to sew up the wound as fast as possible and bind it,[247] but he rightly decided against that method, because it was unclean—again a fine decision.[248] He tried pouring on some warm clarified butter; he gave some to swallow, and even a squirt by enema;[249] but the blood kept pouring. A poultice of rice and beans did no better. Eventually he took a bag of sand, put it over the wound, and sang over it the hemostatic charm of the *Atharva Veda* which went with that specific maneuver:[250]

> About you hath gone
> 　　a great gravelly sandbank
> Stop and be quiet
> I pray

It worked. The Kshatriya was then bandaged and asked to return every third day.[251]

But he disobeyed, stayed at home, and tried to treat himself. A month later, when he reappeared, the dressing gave off a typical smell of putrid meat. This was duly noticed, for the sense of smell played an important part in all medical examinations.[252] A smell of dog, horse, or putrid meat, for example, was unfavorable; a smell of lotus "or any celestial flower" announced death. Note that the deadly smells are those that are clearly impossible: the same odd correlation occurs in other lists of symptoms.

Now the vaidya, besides his general policy of not accepting fatal cases, had an absolute rule: not to "take in hand the treatment of an ulcer-patient" without first examining the ulcer to determine whether it was curable.[253]

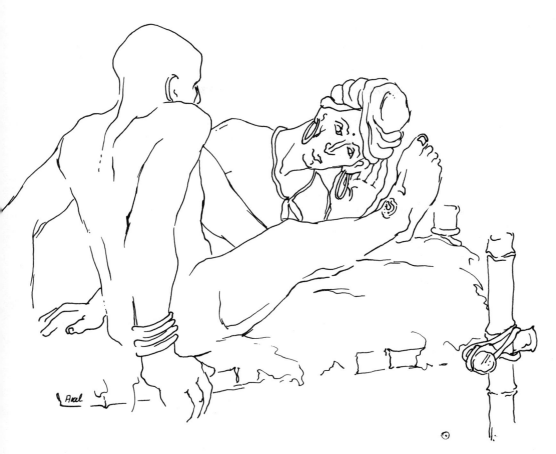

7.27 Auscultation of an ulcer, Indian style. Most diseases were caused by deranged *vayu* or *vata*, the "inner wind"; hence, in the words of Sushruta, "a distinctly audible sound or report is heard in . . . ulcers which are found charged with wind."

Sushruta's warning was probably suggested by hopeless cancerous sores. Considered incurable, for instance, was "an ulcer cropping up like a fleshy tumor . . . with its edges raised like the genitals of a mare."[254] Highly suspicious, and rightly so, were also those ulcers entirely devoid of pain.[255]

Removing the homemade dressing, the surgeon found that the sore was filthy, but acceptable; it was merely creeping with maggots.[256] "Worms due to flies," he said,[257] causing no great worry. These were only one in a list of twenty kinds of vermin that were a daily concern.[258] Maggots could be enticed out of the ulcer with a little piece of flesh, or smothered with a paste of herbs and cow urine; but the quickest way to take care of them was with an alkaline wash.[259] Afterward the ulcer looked better, though not yet clean enough to look "like the back of the tongue."[260] The vaidya leaned over to sniff the cleaned-out ulcer at close quarters. Now the smell was just fishy, and therefore "normal" for an ulcer.[261] But what about the sound?

He listened carefully, his ear to the ulcer. There was a definite sound of blowing, he said. The ulcer was charged with vayu, wind, that troublesome dosha (Fig. 7.27).[262]

वैद्य

Standard treatment for a sore such as this was a good scraping with a linen pad and rock salt. The raised edges were scarified with a steel blade, much as in Greece, except for the final ointment of honey and clarified butter.[263] The dressing was a pad of selected leaves, again as in Greece (Pl. 4.3), but here we are told why: the "rationale . . . is that the leaves tied by an intelligent physician . . . serve to generate heat or cold and retain the liniment or medicated oil in their seat of application."[264] Since the patient could afford it, the leaves were bound on with a bandage of expensive, imported *Chinapatta*: Chinese cloth.[265]

The prognosis was fairly good, because the outline of the sore did not resemble any of the shapes that were regarded as fatal: the barb of a spear, a banner, a chariot, a horse, an elephant, a cow, an ox, a temple, or a palace.[266] The Kshatriya went home.

Two days later he was back again with a flare-up of inflammation, fever, a throbbing foot, and a throbbing headache; the surgeon's suggestion, to drain blood out of the temples, made good sense to him. It happened to be an acceptable time of the year (the rainy season) and an acceptable day, without rumblings from a thundercloud.[267] So, with the courage of a soldier, the patient followed orders: he sat on a stool, faced east, drew up his legs, rested his elbows on the knees, closed his fists, thumb inside, and rested his neck on them, one fist on either side of the neck. At that point, an apprentice wrapped a band of cloth around his neck, passing it over the fists, and held it rather tight so that he was practically handcuffed, while his fists were also pressing against the jugular veins. The temporal veins bulged, recalling to the vaidya the lotus stems on which he had practiced venesection (Fig. 7.28). He chose a point far removed from all the marmas, told the patient to hold his breath, keep his mouth open—and before he slit the vein "to the depth of a barley corn,"[268] he paused a moment, thinking of the twenty things that could go wrong with venesection: *durviddhá,* "bad incision"; *atividdhá,* "excessive incision"; *kunchitá,* "crooked incision"; *pichchitá,* "thrashed incision"; *kuttitá,* "lacerated incision"; *aprasrutá,* "non-bleeding incision"; *marma-viddhá,* "a deadly cut on a marma"; and then on to *atyudirná, parisushká, vepitá, shastrahatá, apaviddhá . . .*[269] He recited a mental mantra, and plunged his lancet.

Few indeed are the medical emergencies in which bleeding may help, and then only as a palliative. As for the Kshatriya's ulcer, there was not a chance in the world that it was being helped.

वैद्य

Patient No. 9: A Thorn, and a Nonpatient

A professional hunter, who had just sold a cart load of venison at the market,[270] stopped his wagon at the door and walked in carrying a little girl in tears. A huge thorn was buried in her foot.

The vaidya shuddered: the thorn had sunk straight into a marma. His mental text was formal: "The Marma known as *Kshipra* . . . between the first

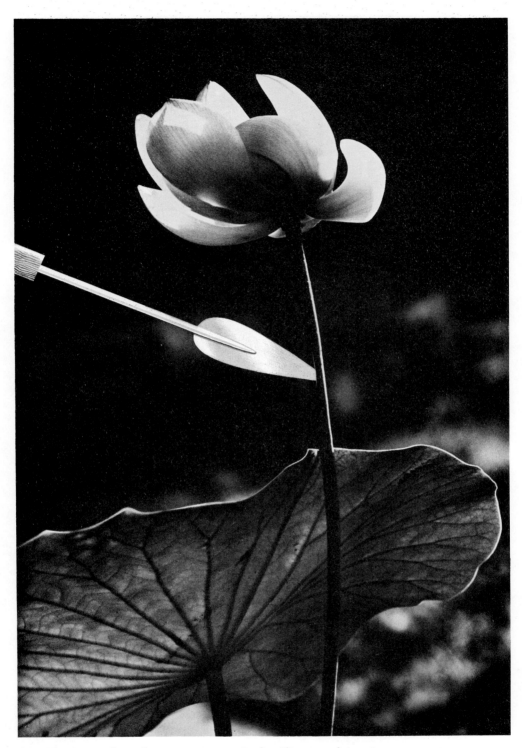

7.28 There were days when surgeons practiced swift cuts on lotus stems.

and second toes . . . being injured or pierced, brings on death from convulsions."[271] Sushruta had probably generalized from one or more cases of tetanus, after a piercing wound in the foot. His conclusions were equally formal: "in case of piercing or injury to any of these Marmas [in the hand or foot], the hand or leg should be immediately amputated at the wrist or at the ankle, respectively."[272]

The father listened to this injunction in disbelief. Cut off the whole foot because of a thorn? That tender little foot? No, he would take the responsibility. There would be no amputation. It is very unlikely, in fact, that all such formal injunctions were taken literally. This one should perhaps be seen as an alibi for the surgeon. In any event, he finally gave in and set about the job of cutting out the thorn, in the deadly territory of a marma. It was the father's responsibility.

A steel blade, however, would not do. On children and on patients who "dreaded the knife," it was recommended to use cutting edges of "strips of bamboo skin [sic], crystals, bits of glass, and the rock known as Kuruvinda."[273] The bamboo blades recall the Egyptian and Roman reed knives—but the motivation is purely Indian. So the vaidya picked up a little bamboo blade: less effective, but more considerate. The thorn came out, in the beak of the heron-mouthed forceps. Cradled in her father's arms, the little girl stopped sobbing.

One of the father's arms appeared to be bandaged. "What happened there?" asked the surgeon.

"It was this morning. The hunting knife slipped while I was skinning a deer."

A fresh, clean cut: what a golden opportunity for a suture, with cotton, Chinese silk, hemp, linen, plaited horsehair, or any other thread that would fit the vaidya's special surgical needles.[274] But both men knew that this was impossible. An Ayurvedic surgeon was not allowed to treat a professional hunter, a professional fowler, or a habitual sinner.[275] All in all, it had been a frustrating visit.

Two aspects of this episode call for comment. First, the surgeon's ethics throughout were not very consistent: he refused to treat a hunter, and yet he was allowed to extract information from him about medicinal herbs of the forest.[276] Second, in his readiness to amputate he was more aggressive than the Hippocratics— though only in the case of injured marmas. The rather confused philosophy here is expressed by Sushruta as follows: by a wound in the marma "a man . . . meets doom like a tree whose roots have been severed"; whereas if the limb is actually cut off, it "does not necessarily prove fatal, like lopping off the branches of a tree."[277] Sushruta somehow believed that there was less hemorrhage by amputation than by injury to a marma: "The vessels become contracted in the case of [amputation of hand or foot], and hence the incidental bleeding is comparatively scantier."[278]

वैद्य

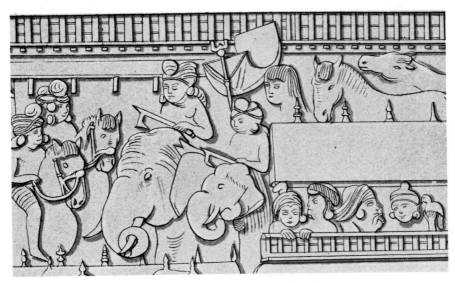

7.29 Indian elephant drivers. Buddhist bas-relief, perhaps first century A.D.

Patient No. 10: Enemas for the Elephant, Too

The poor old man could hardly walk. He had been an elephant driver as far back as he could remember (Fig. 7.29), lately also in the service of the king, but nothing like this had ever happened. His bottom, thighs, and groins were covered with eruptions—red, hot, painful boils, some as open sores. And he shook with fever.

This was a serious problem. The elephant had probably been poisoned, so as to poison the king. There was no limit to the treachery that a king had to expect. Poison could be placed in his turban, his garlands, his food, his bath, his cosmetics.[279] Even in his women. Sometimes a woman, slowly habituated to poison, was presented to a king: with a single embrace he could die "almost instantaneously."[280] So in this case it was necessary to treat the driver as well as the elephant.[281] Had the elephant been restless, the vaidya asked, or red-eyed? Had the driver noticed that flies died after eating the elephant's food, or that shadows were not reflected in his drinking water?[282] If so, it might be necessary to give the elephant a good healthy enema. There was a method laid out, all in verse.[283] As to the driver, his sores would be treated with clarified butter and herbs, and left unbandaged.[284]

Now for the fever. The surgeon had memorized over forty pages about fever,[285] and he feared it. Fever, begotten by the wrathful fire of Rudra,[286] the god of destruction, "is a dangerous disease. It affects . . . appetite and the strength as well as the complexion of the body and is virtually the sum-total of all the other diseases. It is therefore called *the lord of all bodily diseases*. It is common to all created beings (men and animals), affects the whole of the organism (including also the mind), is extremely hard to cure and is present in all cases at the time of the death of all creatures. Hence it is rightly called the destroyer of created beings."[287] Elsewhere this thought is carried further:

fever is the lord of ailments because it is *perhaps an indispensable condition under which a creature can come into being or can depart from this life.*[288]

With all this, fever had no satisfactory treatment. Fasting was still the favorite cure[289] and of course also purging, or drinks of diluted barley gruel,[290] the same as the Hippocratics. Then there was also another famous therapy for the chills of fever: "Damsels young, beautiful and skilled in the sport of love, with faces glowing like the full moon of autumn and darting forth beams of love from their languid blue-lotus-like eyes, with eye-brows moving in the ardour of desire . . . clad in thin transparent garment, fumigated and scented . . . should be asked to take the patient into a firm embrace like a forest-creeper entwining itself around a sylvan tree, and the girls should be told to keep off as soon as the patient would feel himself heated" (Fig. 7.30).[291]

No, this was not for the old elephant driver. Maybe he could do with a lukewarm plaster of herbs in cow's urine and curd-cream.[292] And Sushruta never says how he would treat the chills of fever—in a woman!

The Ant Saga

Sushruta's pages on gored bellies are too vivid to represent theory alone. When the intestines spill out of a wound, he explains, to coax the slippery loops back into place, try to make your patient vomit by gently rubbing his throat with a finger, or lift him up into the air and shake him like a bag; and if in the meantime the intestines have dried up, wash them first with milk and lubricate them with clarified butter.[293] His advice in cases of intestinal perforation: "According to others . . . large black ants should be applied even to the perforated intestines [?] . . . and their bodies should be separated from their heads after they had firmly bitten the perforated parts with their claws [*jaws*]. After that the intestines with the heads of the ants attached to them should be gently pushed back into the cavity and reinstated in their original situation therein."[294]

Sutures with ant heads are often mentioned in connection with primitive medicine.[295] I had always dismissed them as probable nonsense, for I could not see how severed ant-heads could keep clinging to the skin. However, since Sushruta mentions the technique, albeit at secondhand, I decided to look into the matter. In a classic on entomology, Wheeler's *Ants*, I found this precise statement: "The huge heads of the soldiers of the South American leaf-cutting ants (*Atta cephalotes*) [Fig. 7.31] have been employed by the native surgeons in closing wounds. After the two edges of the wound have been brought together and have been grasped by the mandibles, the ant's head is severed from its body and left as a ligature."[296] William Beebe confirmed that Guiana Indians suture their wounds with the jaws of giant *Atta* "maxims," the largest workers. He added that a whole year after returning from the jungle, he found the jaws of two Attas clamped onto his own boots, "with a mechanical vise-like grip, wholly independent of life or death."[297]

वैद्य

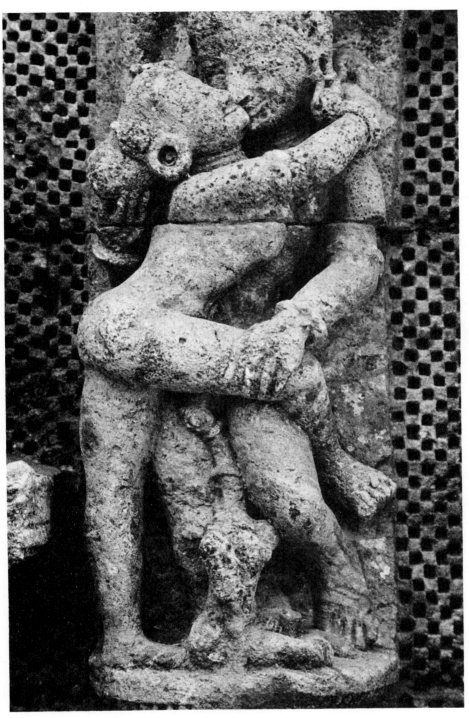

7.30 Indian treatment for the chills of fever (in adult males).

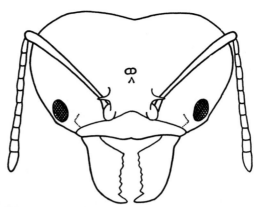

7.31 The jaws of *Atta cephalotes* were made for chopping leaves. They can cause 6mm wounds but are not suitable as wound clamps. Their actual size is about like that of one of the eyes in this drawing.

Outside the Brazilian jungle, *Atta cephalotes* is hard to find. However, I secured a couple of pickled specimens and tried to use them. Complete failure. The jaws worked like scissors—as they should, being the jaws of the leaf-cutting ant—and could not possibly be used as clamps. Both Wheeler and Beebe were no longer there to argue the point, so I was ready to return to my original skepticism.

However, I kept writing letters, and the trail finally led to Prof. Neal A. Weber of Swarthmore College. He replied:

You have a good opportunity in your book to lay at rest the myth that leaf-cutting ants were used to suture wounds in South America. The ants that were used were soldiers of *Eciton burchelli* (Westwood) and *Eciton hamatum* (Fabricius). These have a wide distribution in both middle and South America. My experience frequently here is that, when I am attacked by these soldiers, their fish-hooked shape mandibles engage so firmly in the skin or clothing that the heads remain when I try to brush off the ants. I am enclosing an old photo of my leather gloves with these soldiers impaled by their mandibles after death. In addition to the shape of the mandibles, the adductor mandibular muscles are stronger than the abductor and tend to keep the mandibles closed.

Through Prof. Weber I had the good fortune of finding another entomologist who had been personally sutured by ants, that is, bitten so effectively that his clothes had become sutured to his skin: the late Dr. T. C. Schneirla of the American Museum of Natural History. I quote from his letter:

वैद्य

It is most likely that the major worker of *Eciton burchelli*, the largest swarm-raiding army ant in the New World, would be used in suturing wounds, the smaller *Labidus praedator* or (next in order of probability) the majors of other *Eciton* species . . . In Africa and most of Asia, the leading probability would be the major worker of one of the driver ant (*Dorylus*) species. There are still other possibilities. In any case, use of the major workers of *Eciton* species in suturing wounds is definite, as it is a real problem to get the fish-hook-shaped and very sharp mandibles of these insects out of your skin once they have been firmly implanted. In most cases, I have removed them by inserting a pair of tweezers and spreading the points to forcibly extricate the hooked tips. Sometimes the rather brittle tips break off in the wound . . . There is no question that the mandibles remain firmly implanted after the body

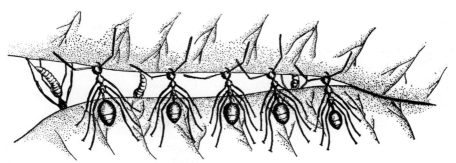

7.32 The oldest silk suture: a brigade of *Oecophylla smaragdina* building a nest. Workers in front draw together the edges of two leaves, while workers in back bind them with silk spun by larvae.

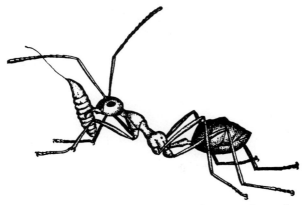

7.33 An *Oecophylla smaragdina* worker holding a larva, used as a shuttle for weaving leaves together.

has been snipped off from the head. The mandibles are held firmly in the wound by virtue of their being sharply pointed and recurved so that the edges catch firmly on each side of the suture as would a pair of opposed fishhooks . . . To sum up, I think there is nothing mythical about the story of suturing wounds with these ants, as unavoidably I have been subjected to this operation countless times.

This letter was followed by six stupendous ants, looking more like miniature horses, fixed in alcohol. I did not feel like subjecting a live rat to the test of *Eciton* jaws, but on a dead one they worked beautifully (Plate 7.2).

Indian ants may still be at work. Recently an entomologist was exploring the jungle of southern Bhutan, at the foot of the Himalayas and not far from Ashoka's ancient capital, when a Bhutanese guide pointed out to him a nest of ants that were used, he said, for closing wounds.[298] The species was *Oecophylla smaragdina*, which performs some marvelous sutures of its own. When it is time to build a nest, a battery of workers line up along the edge of a green leaf, facing outward. Then they rise, snap their jaws into the edge of a leaf above, and pull down (Fig. 7.32). Last, a worker comes along, holding in its jaws one of the family larvae, in which the silk glands happen to be extremely well developed; and using the larva as a shuttle, it sews the two leaves together (Fig. 7.33).[299] This feat is surely the oldest suture on earth.[300]

वैद्य

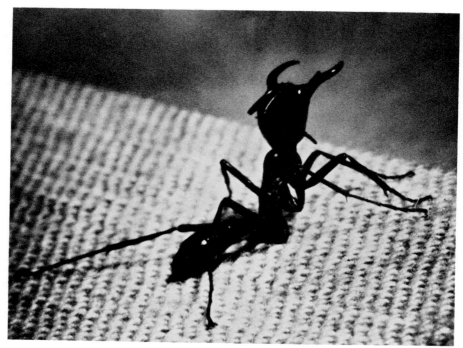

7.34 Ready to clamp: a sentinel of *Dorylus*, the African army ant, photographed in the Congolese jungle. It has climbed onto a piece of cloth dropped at the edge of the advancing army and taken its typical posture. Length up to 13mm.

I have ceased to doubt about the ancient Hindu sutures; in fact, I am beginning to suspect that the ancient Hindus may have borrowed the idea from *Oecophylla smaragdina*. In Africa, where the practice still exists, the fearful sight of driver ants on a swarm raid should be enough to suggest clamping even to the unprepared mind: the streaming black river is flanked by motionless, ferocious-looking sentinels, ready to clamp onto anything in sight (Fig. 7.34).

Hippocrates has nothing to say about ants; maybe he did not have the right kind.[301] This practical use of ant mandibles, however, recalls Raymond Dart's theory, whereby mammalian jaws may have been among the first tools of man-apes, three or four million years ago; especially antelope jaws, which can be used for cutting as well as sawing.[302] And did not Samson slay one thousand men with the jawbone of an ass?[303] Jaws, after all, are natural tools.

For use as wound clamps, even those of the beetle have been tried. One traveler returning from Algeria in 1845 claimed to have seen wounds clamped with *Scarites pyracmon*.[304] I did procure a specimen (Fig. 7.35), but so far, no insect clamp that I have seen comes anywhere near the mandibles of *Eciton* (Fig. 7.36).

वैद्य

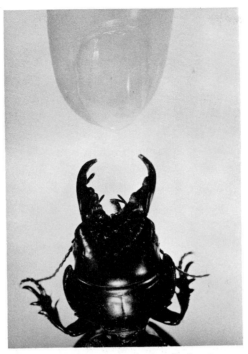

7.35 Another candidate as a wound clamp, the beetle *Scarites pyracmon*, common in all Mediterranean countries. The finger is for scale.

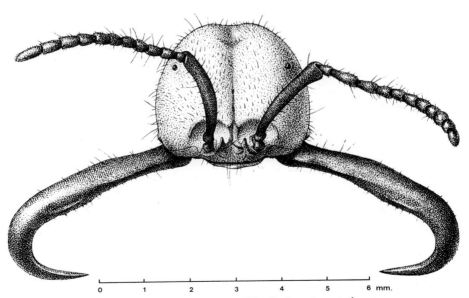

7.36 Head and jaws of an *Eciton* soldier, possibly the best insect-clamp.

The Vaidya, the Iatrós, and the Yang I

At a summit meeting of a vaidya, a iatrós, and a yang i there would have been agreement on several basic points: on the importance of diet (but not on how to use it), on "draining out" some diseases (but not on how to do it—and the Chinese also "drained in") and more astonishingly, on a theoretical point so specialized that some sort of unconscious communication seems inevitable. This was the notion of "wind" as a cause of disease. In China, the internal *ch'i* was a "breath" not very different from meteorologic wind;[305] the *Nei Ching* reports that "winds contribute to the development of a hundred diseases."[306] In India, vayu, the bodily wind, was an inner equivalent of external and even cosmic winds;[307] it caused, says Charaka, 80 of the 140 diseases.[308] In Greece, there is a whole Hippocratic treatise *On Winds*,[309] which closes with the statement that "winds are, in all diseases, the principal agents."

Among neighbors, similarities were even greater. Sushruta's and Charaka's endless lists of five elements, six tastes, eight properties, five salts, four oils, and eight urines, not to mention the six triples followed by eight triples that had to be kept in mind in order to drink wine properly,[310] have a distinct flavor of Chinese numerology. Nor can it be an accident that the two neighboring cultures created similar doctrines of vital points, the marmas and the points of acupuncture.[311] Sushruta, after all, used Chinese silk for sutures and Chinese cloth for bandages.

The Indian exercises in experimental surgery have no parallel. The nearest approach was in Persia, where a believer in Zoroastrian religion had to practice first, not on a lotus stem, but in the flesh of a nonbeliever. Such is the rule as laid out in the sacred books of the *Zend-Avesta*:[312]

> O Maker of the material world, thou Holy One! If a worshipper of Mazda [God] want to practice the art of healing, on whom shall he first prove his skill? on worshippers of Mazda or on worshippers of the Daêvas [demons]?
> Ahura Mazda answered: On worshippers of the Daêvas shall he first prove himself, rather than on worshippers of Mazda. If he treat with a knife a worshipper of the Daêvas and he die; if he treat with the knife a second worshipper of the Daêvas and he die; if he treat with the knife for the third time a worshipper of the Daêvas and he die, he is unfit to practise the art of healing for ever and ever . . .
> If he shall ever attend any worshipper of Mazda, if he shall ever treat with the knife any worshipper of Mazda, and wound him with the knife, he shall pay for it the same penalty as is paid for wilful injury [possibly amputation of six fingers].
> If he treat with the knife a worshipper of the Daêvas and he recover; if he treat with the knife a second worshipper of the Daêvas and he recover; if for the third time he treat with the knife a worshipper of the Daêvas and he recover; then he is fit to practise the art of healing for ever and ever.[313]

The apprentice surgeon is thus graded, as in the Chinese system, by counting successes and failures. The infidels were of course Indians, Greeks, or Romans living in Iran.

वैद्य

If a Greek physician had been confronted with the medical practice in Pataliputra around 400 B.C.—assuming that this period for the writings of Sushruta is right—he would probably have been shocked, primarily by the use of religion as a part of medicine. He himself had split away from religion and from the psychotherapy it afforded, leaving both to the temples of Asklepios. The vaidya, instead, practiced the whole gamut. To him, religious acts were medicine of the first order. Nowhere as in India did religion mingle so thoroughly with private and public behavior.[314]

To the iatrós, the ethical standards of India would look familiar,[315] but not identical. The caste barriers would appear unreasonable, as also the outright recommendation not to treat the very poor.[316] Perhaps the concern with the patient's feelings would also look overplayed.

Technically, the iatrós would marvel at the Indian plastic surgery, especially at rhinoplasty or reconstruction of the nose, although his own clientele had few such problems with ears and noses. He would be equally aghast at the daring feat of "couching the cataract," an operation that destroyed many blind eyes, but restored partial eyesight to a large number of otherwise hopeless patients.[317] He would probably admire the courage of Hindu surgeons in amputating limbs, and their ability to stop the bleeding with hot oil. He would feel somewhat dizzy at the number of drugs, about six hundred of them or twice his own list,[318] and would wonder at the rare use of inorganic drugs.[319]

At the conceptual level, the Greek would surely recognize that vayu, pitta, kapha, and rakta behaved very much like wind, bile, phlegm, and blood. On one point, however, he would definitely recoil: the Indian passion for names, for splitting hairs, for classifying.[320] That was entirely against his grain. To him, in practice, the Greek four humors were an excuse to make all diseases more or less alike. In India, it was the other way around. Sores, for instance, had special names according to the particular humor supposed to be affected; thus there were fifteen *groups* of sores, but then varieties were "practically innumerable":

वैद्य

> *vataja,*
> *pittaja,*
> *kaphaja,*
> *raktaja,*
> *vata-pittaja,*
> *kapha-vataja,*
> *kapha-pittaja,*
> *vata-raktaja,*
> *vata-pitta-raktaja,*
> *kapha-pitta-raktaja,*
> *vata-pitta-kapha-raktaja,*

and so forth, each one with its own special clinical picture.[321] Nothing could be farther removed from the Greek sense of synthesis.

And what could the vaidya have learned from the Greek?

Despite much thought, I still cannot see any major lesson that the Greek could have given in exchange. For all of his mantras and endless superstitions, the vaidya, particularly in his surgery, helped more people and saved more lives.

There is something unnerving about the ancient vaidya, because he cannot be placed exactly in time. Was it 400 B.C.? 200 B.C.? 200 A.D.? But the answer is not especially relevant, because the vaidya—unlike the asu, the swnw, and the iatrós—never disappeared. Ayurvedic medicine is still the medicine of millions.[322]

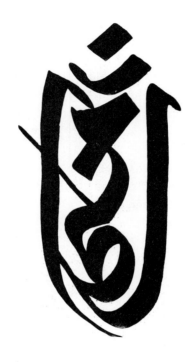

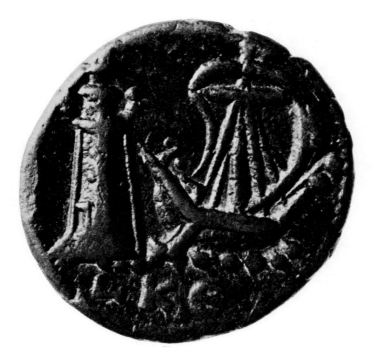

8   Alexandria the Great

Back to the Mediterranean, about 250 B.C. Here is the lighthouse of Alexandria, one of the seven wonders of the world: perfect symbol of that city, whose glory came and went like a flash, unique in the history of antiquity.

The very birth of Alexandria is something of a fairy tale. Imagine a crown prince who is also a private pupil of Aristotle, a Macedonian lad of twenty-two who sees himself as a descendant of Hercules, and fired with an ambition that will one day lead him to stab a friend in anger.[1] Imagine him taking off at the head of an army, crossing the sea, conquering all the land from Asia Minor to Egypt, then heading east into the vague territories of India—and founding a string of at least seventeen Alexandrias as he goes.[2] He will burn out on his path, like a falling star, but one of his cities will pick up the flame: Alexandria of Egypt.

As Plutarch tells the story, after the conquest of Egypt (it was 332 B.C.), Alexander's engineers dutifully mapped out, somewhere, the site for a new city.[3] But then the king had a dream in which a grand old man appeared to him, reciting verses about an island named Pharos. Alexander was a scholar worthy of his former tutor (he even slept with Aristotle's edition of the *Iliad*, and a dagger, under the pillow):[4] he recognized the old man as Homer and took the hint. True to style, he tore off to visit Pharos a few hundred yards offshore, west of the Nile Delta. The island itself was too small for settlement, and the coast just opposite was a dismal strip of wasteland, later called the

8.1 Rough map of ancient Alexandria: a poor harbor, were it not for the Heptasta-dium, a jetty (now silted up on both sides). Lake Mareotis was a huge tidal pool from the Nile floods. Rhakotis was a settlement of Egyptian fishermen and pirates, preexisting on the site of Alexandria; it left no known trace.

Taenia, running between swampy Lake Mareotis and the sea (Fig. 8.1): a flat, unsafe, unlikely place for a city.[5] But for Alexander there would be no other. Chalk to mark the boundaries was not on hand, so his men had to use flour. Birds ate up the flour; Alexander brushed aside the bad omen. The city shot up, and Alexander marched off to the East, never to return alive. Pharos was connected to the mainland by a jetty, the Heptastadium, which made two large harbors out of nature's small one. Within a matter of years this desolate strip of land was a bustling city and the hub of the Mediterranean world.

After the death of Alexander, one of his generals, Ptolemy, took over Egypt and finally declared himself king and Pharaoh, with residence in Alexandria. When he retired fifty years later, this genial Macedonian soldier had something to show for his reign, having founded the great lighthouse, the Mouseion or House of Muses (we call it Museum), and the library. The best of Greece was now happening in Egypt.

Near Egypt, I should say. By pedigree, Alexandria had little to do with the people of the pyramids, and its citizens were primarily Greeks: so the prevalent name in antiquity was "Alexandria near Egypt," *Alexandrea ad Aegyptum*.[6]

The Museum, though not the first nor the last of its kind, certainly became the prototype.[7] It was a fabulous, state-supported institution, where scholars from all branches of knowledge, set aside in majestic surroundings, were paid to think, search, read, and write. Strabo tells us that it included "a promenade, a place with seats for conferences, and a great hall where the scholars had their meals in common."[8] In fact and in principle, the House of Muses sounds very much like the Rockefeller Institute of the twentieth

314

century, except that its members did not pay for their meals in the common hall; they did not even have to pay taxes. The results, measured in science and scholarship, were phenomenal: within two or three generations the Museum could boast of such achievements as a figure for the diameter of the earth, accurate to better than 1 percent,[9] and a membership list with names like Euclid, and maybe even Archimedes.

Maybe: a historical drama in five letters. The astonishing truth is that *there is very little we can say with certainty* about the Museum, beyond a few superlatives. There is no ancient book about it. We have a long list of Alexandrian firsts—the valve, the pump, the screw[10]—and whole new fields, like hydraulics and pneumatics, but we cannot say how much of it all happened at the Museum—except for the medical events.

One of the few definite statements that can be made about the Museum is that is was *almost* unique. Almost, because six thousand miles away, unbeknown to the Mediterranean world, another state academy was born in the very same years, in the never-never land of China. It was the Academy of the Gate of Chi, founded in 318 B.C. in the state of Chhi.[11] It welcomed scholars from all other states as well as Chhi, and provided them with quarters and maintenance. But that was rather an academy of philosophers, much like the Athenian academies of the same period or the later Chinese Imperial Academy, which was called the Han-Lin Yuan or *"Forest of Pencils"*;[12] whereas the Alexandrian Museum cultivated the humanities as well as the sciences.

In both of these fields, the Museum could not have become what it was without the library. Run by bibliomaniacs in the homeland of papyrus, the library bought, copied, or pirated all the literature available. The library of Aristotle, and probably also that of the Hippocratic school, landed here; indeed, it seems that this is how we have come to inherit the Hippocratic Collection. Travelers were required to declare their books and, if necessary, to surrender them until copied; they got back only the cheaper certified copy.[13] A by-product of this huge enterprise is the very structure of this printed line, for it was the library staff who invented punctuation.[14] When the library was first threatened by fire under the last Ptolemy—Cleopatra—in 47 B.C., it may have contained 700,000 volumes.[15]

Pearls in the Rubbish

All this ancient history may sound as remote as Noah's ark; but something snaps—and everything comes alive—if you manage to peek through the secret window of the papyrologists. These elusive people belong to a breed as rare as any of the 120 mammalian species now threatened with extinction. They are known to be delightful company if you can only find one and coax him or her into conversation (for they live two thousand years ago, and do not advertise in the present). You may then be entertained for hours about the lives, deeds, quarrels, even the wounds of Greco-Egyptians as if they were next-door neighbors. You will also discover that papyrologists study Egypt and papyri, but *not* Egyptian papyri, and that they specialize in broken pottery. Here are the facts.

The Greeks imported into Egypt their habit of using bits of broken pots, óstraka, as ordinary writing material. These were cheap, handy, and long-lasting, so that the family archives might be a jarful of óstraka: bills, tax receipts, letters, and daily budget, often dated to the day. Sometimes the same kind of message was written on the more costly papyrus, which later might be treated as waste paper, ending up in the cartonnage casing of mummies (a sort of papier mâché)[16] or simply on rubbish heaps.

The climate of Egypt preserved all these scribblings until the papyrologists came along, armed with saintly patience and devices such as a *Konträr-index*, a dictionary in which words are spelled backward, to help find suitable heads for decapitated words. Thanks to their unsung labors, the Greco-Egyptian trash of shards and papyrus scraps yielded precious facts and gossip such as we do not have for practically any other ancient people, and most of which is now buried once again, alas, in highly specialized publications, often without translation, sometimes with footnotes in Latin.[17]

These texts now number in the tens of thousands, ranging from 311 B.C. (the oldest known) to about 750 A.D.: this is the period during which Greek was one of the vernacular languages of Egypt, and in fact the message is usually written in Greek, more rarely in Latin.[18] In most cases it consists of a few lines scribbled in black ink. Here is a handful of the topics, mostly from the index of a *Papyrological Primer*.[19] Note the prevalence of legal documents:

> Protest against an appointment
> Contract with a castanets dancing girl
> Circumcision of a priest's child
> Statement of taxes
> Prayer
> Minutes of a session held by the Chief of Police
> Loan of money upon mortgage
> Action to state forgery in a document
> Contract with a stenographer
> Letter to an unfaithful manager
> Account of taxes on sacrifices[20] and wool
> Sale of a slave
> Sale of a handmill
> Notification of a surprise attack
> Preparations for an official visit

Since the Greeks did not have surnames, in many of these legal documents the individuals are identified by their given name plus any identifying scar (*oulé*):

> Cháretos, one-scar-small-finger-right-hand. . .
> Máron, eldest son of Onnóphreus, aged 40, with a scar on his forehead, made an agreement with his brother Onnóphreus, born of the same father, aged 18, with no marks.[21]

There seems to have been enough trauma to ensure accurate identification. Otherwise, the individual was labeled *ásemos*, "not marked."[22]

Some of the texts refer to doctors and disease. From the second century B.C. there is this short letter, apparently from mother to son:

I heard that you are learning Egyptian, and I was very happy, for you as well as for myself; because now, arriving in the city, you will tutor the sons of Phal . . . the enema-doctor, and make money towards old age.[23]

The "enema-doctor," *iatroklýstes*, must have been a specialist of intestinal diseases, a latterday Shepherd of the Anus.[24] One piece of pottery bears a crudely spelled statement sworn before a judge by two brothers, who deny having beaten up the third brother (Fig. 8.2). The tone is somewhat as follows: "The wound that you have we aint done it and we dont know who did it."[25]

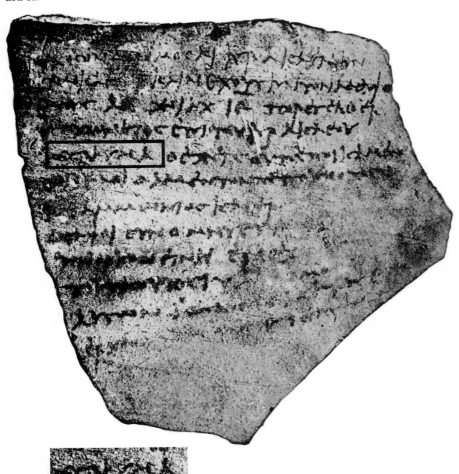

8.2 A legal document, crudely written on an *óstrakon* (shard), presumably before a judge: "The wound that you have we ain't done it. . ." The detail of the boxed area shows how the word *trauma* (wound) is deciphered. Second century B.C.

τραυμα

Hear also this pitiful tale, which gives a rare glimpse of medicolegal practices. It is the morning of the seventh day of Athyr (November), 182 A.D.; Leonidas writes from Senepta to the police chief of Oxyrhynchus:

> Yesterday evening, during a local festivity, as the castanets dancers were performing as required . . . the 8-year old slave boy Epaphrodeitos, wanting to see the dancers, leaned over too far from the roof and fell to his death.[26]

Leonidas then requests the police to send someone. Miraculously, another bit of papyrus turned up showing that the chief of police took care of the matter the very same day: he sent one of his men, accompanied by a state physician (*demósios iatrós*), to examine the body and draw up a written report.[27]

The following was written in 237 B.C., on a small bit of papyrus recovered from the wrappings of a mummy:

> The 17th year [*of Ptolemy III*], on the 2nd day of Phaophi. We have had measured out to us by Stratius 5 artábes of rice-wheat as the physician-tax, and 9 artábes of rice-wheat as the police-tax. Total 14 artábes of rice-wheat. Farewell.[28]

This is a tax receipt. It concerns the *iatrikón* (Fig. 8.3), a tax that went to support public physicians[29] such as the one we just met in Oxyrhynchus. Since one *artábe* came close to 40 litres,[30] to carry his 14 artábes Stratius must have gone to the office of the tax collector with a cart; so imagine the problem of the tax collector who then had to cart the rice-wheat to the iatrós. To avoid this trouble, the iatrikón was sometimes paid by the citizen directly to the physician. Witness this receipt from the wrappings of a different mummy dated 231 B.C:

> [*Name lost*] . . . Cyrenean, of Zoilus's troop, private, to Eucarpus, physician, greeting.
> It has been ordered that I shall pay you 10 artábes of rice-wheat, or 4 drachmae, as the iatrikón for the 38th year.[31]

Physicians too had their burdens. Another tax receipt says that "Petronius the physician has paid his camel tax."[32]

Alexandrian Patents

The Alexandrians developed, almost from the start around 300 B.C., a real passion for gadgets such as is not found again until modern times. One can appreciate it by leafing through Heron's astonishing book entitled *Pneumatics*. Heron of Alexandria came rather late (he lived in the first century A.D.) but many of his gadgets are borrowed from the third century B.C.: fountains with singing birds, revolving model theaters, a constant volume dispenser for liquids (Fig. 8.4), and most amazing of all, a kind of steam engine (Fig. 8.5).[33] More complicated schemes could make a toy bird drink "while its neck is being severed in two";[34] a priest could perform miracles,

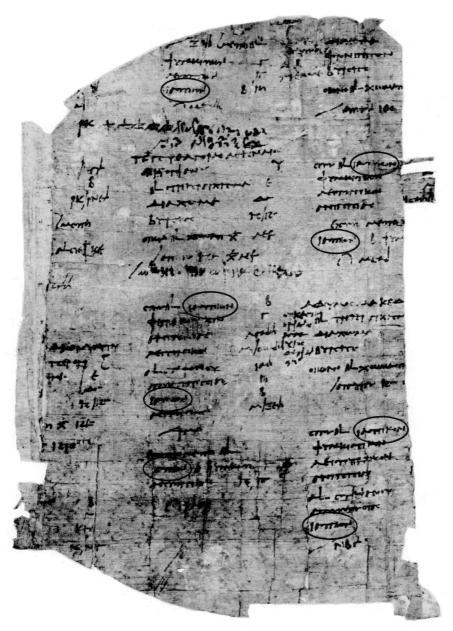

8.3 A list of taxes paid by orphans, on a Greco-Egyptian papyrus of the third century B.C. The physician tax, *iatrikón* (ιατρικον, circled), figures eight times in the amount of β, which means 2: in this case, two measures of wheat.

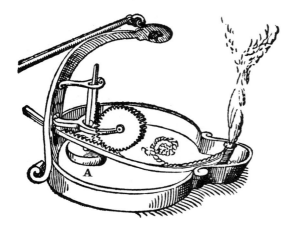

8.4 Examples of Alexandrian tricks and gadgets as described by Heron. *Left:* An oil lamp with an automatic feed for the wick. The float (A) rests on oil. *Below right:* A fountain with whistling birds. *Below left:* A constant volume dispenser, the *dikaiómeter*, which may or may not have worked.

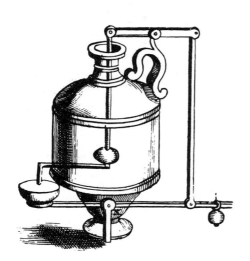

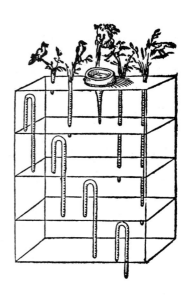

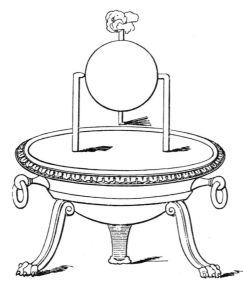

8.5 A steam turbine. The cauldron stands over a flame (not shown); it is full of water and covered with a flat lid, in which two vertical tubes are fitted. At the top, the tubes are bent toward each other to function as pivots for the hollow sphere. Steam rises through the right tube into the sphere and escapes through two smaller L-shaped tubes, causing the sphere to rotate.

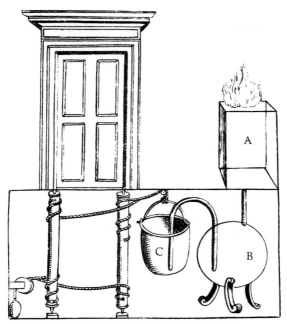

8.6 A gadget to promote religion. The priest lights a fire on *A*; the heated air expands and is driven down into the sphere *B*, which is full of water. The water escapes into the bucket *C*, which drops and causes the door of the temple to open, as if by a miracle.

8.7 A coin-in-the-slot machine, for dispensing holy water.

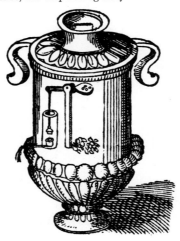

like the hilarious one illustrated (Fig. 8.6), while collecting five-drachma pieces on the side; and the world's first coin-in-the-slot machine dispensed tiny squirts of holy water (Fig. 8.7). The lighthouse itself carried its load of trickery: the 23-foot statue of Ptolemy I on its top could veer into the wind, which was not as simple as it sounds;[35] the bronze tritons may have been steam-driven foghorns;[36] and a radar system of sorts, based on mirrors, projected a view of the horizon to people stationed in the tower one hundred feet below (Fig. 8.8).

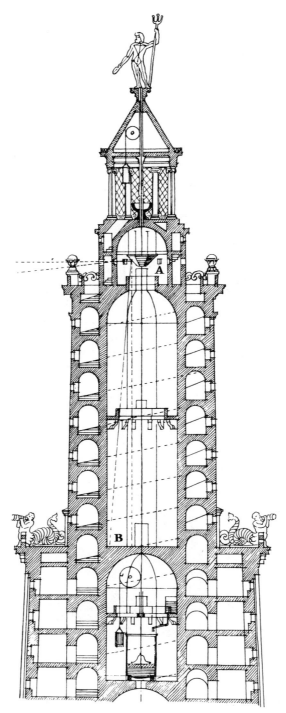

8.8 Gadgetry on top of the lighthouse of
Alexandria. The 23-foot statue revolved as
a weathervane. The upper section of the
tower contained an optical system (A) for
viewing the horizon from a platform one
hundred feet below (B). The tritons may
have been foghorns.

It is usually stated that all this Alexandrian machinery never outgrew the stage of toys for grownups. I must claim an exception for the syringe. Oddly enough, the syringe steps into medical history as an aid for the treatment of wounds. Here is how it happened.

From Barbers to Pistons

The syringe—in fact the very concept of piston and cylinder— was born in a barbershop, at the hands of a Greek, in Alexandria of Egypt about 280 B.C.[37] (Fig. 8.9). The story, as told by a Roman architect, Vitruvius, 250 years later, is a good example of the Alexandrian love for tricky gadgets:

Now Ktesibios was the son of a barber and was born at Alexandria. He was marked out by his talent and great industry, and had the name of being especially fond of mechanical contrivances. On one occasion he wanted to hang the mirror in his father's shop, in such a way that when it was pulled down and pulled up again, a hidden cord drew down the weight; and he made use of the following expedient.

He fixed a wooden channel under a beam of the ceiling, and inserted pulleys there. Along the channel he took the cord into a corner where he fixed upright tubes. In these he had a lead weight let down by the cord. Thus when the weight ran down into the narrow tubes[38] and compressed the air, the large amount of air was condensed as it ran violently down through the mouth of the tube and was forced into the open; meeting with an obstacle, the air was produced as a clear sound. Ktesibios, therefore, when he observed that the air being drawn along and forced out gave rise to wind-pressure and vocal sounds, was the first to use these principles and make hydraulic machines. He also described the use of water-power in making automata and many other curiosities, and among them the construction of water-clocks.[39]

"Curiosities" indeed: this barber's son went on to invent nothing less than the valve, and because of the valve, the pump (Figs. 8.10-8.11). Ktesibios is acknowledged as one of the greatest engineers of antiquity. It is also true, as Vitruvius remarked, that he applied his basic discoveries to a colorful family of machines, toys, water clocks and automata. Though all his works are lost, they survive in the compilations of Philon of Byzantium (perhaps a generation later) and of Heron.[40]

One of these applications he called the water-flute. It was actually an organ that used water as a pressure regulator. The word *hydraulics*, born in the chatter of a barbershop, still echoes the song of this old *hydr-áulis*, "water-flute" (Fig. 8.12).

Another application was the syringe. Its precise birth record is lost, but it first appears in Heron's *Pneumatics*, with no reference (Fig. 8.13). Heron, who otherwise had no particular bent for things medical, may have lifted it from an Alexandrian medical text.[41] The instrument, he notes, is also good for injecting liquids; but the primary use is for sucking pus out of wounds, hence the Greek name *pyúlkos* latinized as *pyulcus*, the "pus-puller."[42] A

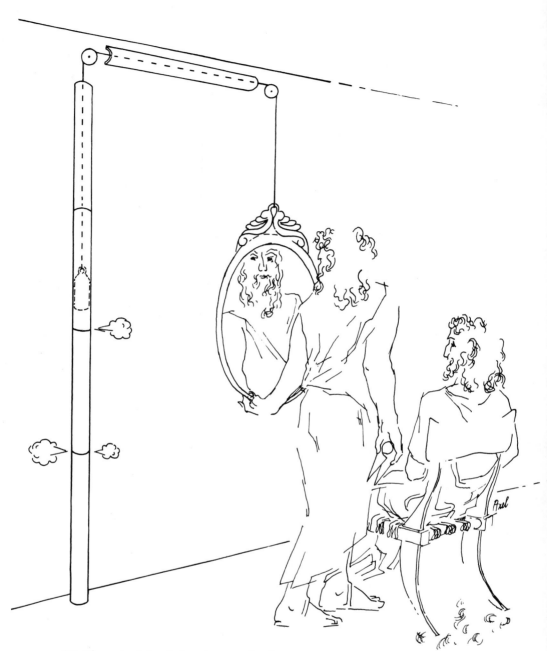

8.9 The principle of the piston and cylinder, as discovered by Ktesibios in the barbershop of his father. The original purpose of the gadgetry was to set up a mirror of adjustable height, with concealed cables and concealed weights. Whistles caused by the dropping weights suggested that compressed air could be exploited mechanically.

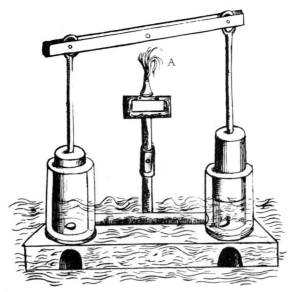

8.10 The valve and the pump, also invented by Ktesibios, as applied to a fire extinguisher in Heron's description. The water spouts at *A*.

8.11 Scheme of the Ktesibios pump, as described about 50 B.C. by Vitruvius. The points *F* are fixed.

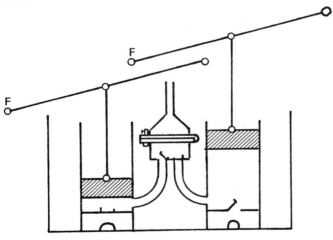

humanitarian toy, to be sure, but to a gadgeteer it is the principle that counts, not the application. In a book on warfare, Heron proposes the syringe as a flamethrower (Fig. 8.14).[43]

The subsequent fate of the syringe, that contrivance of the Greek colony, could be considered a revenge of the ancient Egyptian gods. The flamethrowing feature, so far as I know, never caught on; and the pus-pulling was never a great help, though Ambroise Paré still refers to the pyulcus as the "matter-drawer."[44] Forgotten by warfare and neglected by surgery, this great instrument spent its next two thousand years aiming at a target highly reminiscent of ancient Egypt: the anus.[45]

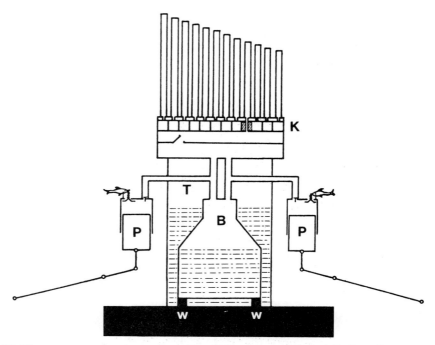

8.12 The organ, another invention of Ktesibios. Its name *hydraulis*, literally "water-flute," gave *hydraulics*. The tank (T) is half full of water, which flows freely into the mouth of the bell (B), raised on wooden blocks (W). Pistons (P) pump air into *B*, which displaces some of the water; this reservoir of compressed air supplies the pipes above the keyboard (K) with a relatively constant flow of wind.

8.13 The piston-and-cylinder principle was put to use in the syringe, described by Heron as *pyúlkos* or "pus-puller," to be used on wounds.

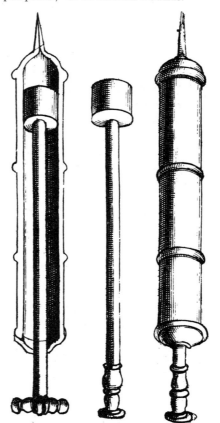

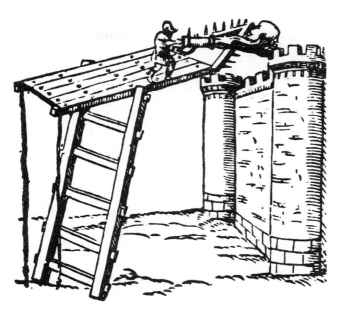

8.14 The syringe as a flamethrower, in Heron's book on war machines.

Alexandrian Medicine

In the hot climate of Alexandria some parts of the Museum must have spread quite a scent: the major field of medical research was anatomy, which included dissection of animals, human corpses—and even live men, growled Celsus three centuries later.[46] Let us hope that Celsus was wrong; but anyway, this was real, full-time, professional research, as new as the new world that had produced it.

It all happened so fast that the two top anatomists, Herophilos and Erasistratos, were just twenty or thirty years younger than the city itself.[47] To place them in time with respect to Hippocrates: if we assume that they started working roughly around 270 B.C., the great Master had died 110 years earlier. They were well aware of him. In fact, it is said that Erasistratos was the one who collected the Hippocratic books during his travels;[48] and Herophilos, whose teacher actually came from the school of Cos, wrote the first commentaries to the Hippocratic works.[49] Thus, both Alexandrian anatomists were free to inherit the knowledge as well as the handicaps of the Hippocratics. Unfortunately all their books have been lost, but later authors credited Herophilos with discovering and naming such unlikely organs as the prostate and the duodenum, as well as an oblong, hidden structure of the brain, which he named *calamus scriptorius* because it reminded him of the Greek writing pen.[50] As for his contemporary, Erasistratos, by a stroke of luck Galen found him particularly irritating: he took the trouble to write two books against Erasistratos, and vilified him on at least sixty separate occasions, while making concessions on about twelve others.[51] In the process we learn something about the man.

The personality of Erasistratos emerges as that of a surgeon-scientist, whose hand and whose beliefs were firm enough to slit open a belly and apply drugs directly onto the liver.[52] Despite Galen's wrath, there are some views of Erasistratos that will last as long as medicine. I like to think of him at work in his laboratory at the Museum, in front of a large balance, performing his famous "metabolic" experiment: he put a bird in a pot, kept weighing it together with its excrement, and found a progressive loss of weight. This he took to mean that there was an emanation "perceptible only to the mind"— *lógoi theoretén*.[53] The experiment is usually extolled as the world's first measure of basal metabolism; in fact, nobody could deny its three novel features: identifying a subtle metabolic problem, asking a question that is technically answerable, and using quantitative means to arrive at the answer. In the last respect Erasistratos was measuring up to his neighbors in the math department, where the chief was Euclid. At a more down-to-earth level, however, I find it difficult to repress a heretical thought: perhaps all that Erasistratos was really finding is that bird droppings, in a hot climate, tend to dry up!

With these two giants, Alexandrian medical science soared to its zenith; then, oddly enough, it petered out. Although Alexandrian training remained fashionable for almost a millennium, and even Galen studied there, the famous names remained those of old. Alexandrian physicians spent their time splitting hairs and acquired the reputation of being, on the whole, a frivolous bunch.[54] But once again, all this is essentially hearsay, for not a single medical work of the Alexandrians has come down to us—not one, not a page of Erasistratos—only short, scattered quotations. We are somewhat in the position of trying to understand the shape, life, and history of a beautiful frigate by studying its reflection in the sea.

Among the outsiders who saved something of Alexandrian medicine by quoting or discussing parts of it, the most important is a Roman: Cornelius Celsus, who wrote in the first century A.D. In fact, after the Hippocratic books, his *De medicina* is the first complete medical work. In between there is nothing but debris.

The first impression on reading Celsus, after Hippocrates, is that something major has happened to surgery. Hippocratic scalpels had never gone beyond what is today called minor surgery: mostly a matter of removing hemorrhoids or nasal polyps, draining pus, and slitting veins. The closest that Hippocrates ever came to amputation was watching people's legs falling off bit by bit from gangrene. But the operations listed by Celsus could figure in the daily schedule of a modern surgical ward: removal of goiters (I shudder at the thought), operations for hernia or stones in the bladder, amputation of limbs. What has happened?

The answer is in the preface to *De medicina:* after Hippocrates there had been the Alexandrian boom.[55] And the Alexandrian physicians had discovered a major technical trick, the most important step in the treatment of wounds until the advent of asepsis: the ligature of blood vessels. Celsus takes this technique for granted.

The name of the genius who first tied a bleeding artery has not been preserved. Perhaps it was Erasistratos, or at least one of his pupils (although it is strange that Galen should not have mentioned it), for Erasistratos was deeply interested in the body's plumbing system, from the heart to its finest roots. This brings us to examine his concept of tissues, which has a lot to do with plumbing problems.

Tissues and Their Plumbing System

A severed artery bleeds, because the heart pumps out the blood: it sounds so simple, yet few biological events drew as many pages of nonsense. By the time the Alexandrian virtuosi of dissection started to look into it, the muddle was perhaps at its peak.[56]

Hippocrates had had no means of recognizing the heart as a pump, because there was no such item in his world, and no such word in his vocabulary. However, an unknown anatomist, perhaps a Greek from Sicily, whose treatise *Perí kardíes* or *On the Heart* is now in the Hippocratic Collection, dissected the mammalian heart (some think also the human) with unusual skill; and though he saw it as containing two cavities only, he discovered in it two interesting sets of "membranes" (*hyménes*), the sigmoid valves at the root of the aorta and the pulmonary artery (Fig. 8.15). He marveled at them:

> The last topic to discuss, concerning the heart, are the hidden membranes, a structure most worthy of attention . . . There are two aortae [*the aorta and pulmonary artery*]; at the entrance of each are arranged three membranes, rounded at their extremities, in the shape of a half-circle; and when they come together, it is marvelous to see how they close the orifices, at the border of the aortae. And if someone who knows the ancient ritual [*probably the technique of the augurs at sacrifices*] takes the heart after death, and [*the membranes*] are spread out and made to lean against each other, water poured in will not penetrate into the heart, nor will air blow in; and this especially on the left; for that side has been constructed more precisely, as it should be, since the intelligence of man lies in the left cavity.[57]

What the writer is saying is that these marvelous membranes, the valves, are useful, because they keep blood and its impurities *out* of the heart; think what a mess would happen, especially in the left heart, if blood were to pour in and mix with the intelligence that is held in there! This was in fact a brilliant suggestion: what else could he think, having discovered one-way valves in an organ through which, as far as he knew, nothing was flowing? The only solution was to interpret them as static safety devices. I note with due humility that his novel experiment is now routine in modern pathology: that is, the act of pouring water into the stumps of the aorta and pulmonary artery, to check whether the valves close properly (Fig. 8.15). The ancient author actually went further, for no modern pathologist ever blows into these severed vessels.

This short but important treatise *On the Heart* was probably written in Sicily, a few years before Erasistratos broached the same subject, perhaps

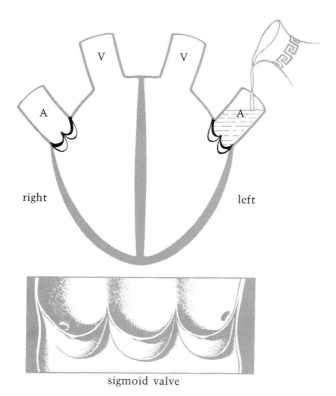

sigmoid valve

8.15 About 280 B.C. the heart was understood in this manner by an unknown Hippocratic anatomist. The scheme (top) shows the heart from the front in cross section. The four stumps represent the beginnings of the four main vessels—arteries (A) and veins (V)—which were then known. The heart was also known to consist of two sides, right and left, separated by a vertical septum, but the horizontal separation of each side into atrium and ventricle was not known. The right side of the heart was thought to hold blood (without pumping it); the left side contained intelligence. At the root of the large arteries, the anatomist discovered the three pockets forming the sigmoid valve (also shown below as it appears when the arteries are slit open). He tested this valve by pouring water into the stump.

around 280 B.C.[58] Another author who came after Hippocrates, and before Erasistratos, was Aristotle. For him, too, the heart was the seat of intelligence. He mistook its four cavities for three, and failed to notice the valves altogether.[59] With heart physiology in this state, the meaning of the pulse could not be understood. It was thought that every artery had the innate capacity to beat, like the heart, and that the real problem was to find out whether the active beat was inward, or outward.[60]

Finally, just half a century after the death of Hippocrates, the ultimate bit of vascular nonsense swept out of Cos: the great news that veins contain blood, arteries air ("pneuma").[61] This fascinating mistake found easy access into Alexandria, because it originated with the teacher of Herophilos, Praxagoras of Cos (c.350–300 B.C.). It enjoyed a career of five hundred years. How could anybody believe that arteries contain air? The excuse traditionally offered is that, after death, most of the blood goes to swell the large veins, which leaves very little blood in the large arteries.[62] Still, there is a long way

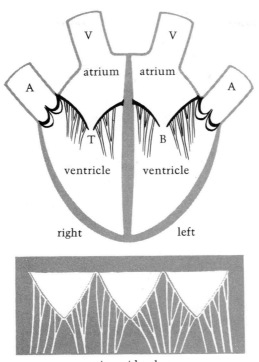

tricuspid valve

8.16 About 270 B.C. an Alexandrian physician, Erasistratos, realized that the heart is a pump. He discovered that each side of the heart is divided into two parts, upper and lower (atrium and ventricle), separated by the bicuspid (B) and tricuspid (T) valves (top). These valves are made, respectively, of two and three roughly triangular flaps, anchored to the inner surface of the heart by cords (bottom). In the scheme of the heart they are shown in profile. When the heart contracts, they are pressed together and prevent the blood from returning to the upper chamber. Thus, Erasistratos realized that the heart received blood from the veins and pumped it out into the arteries.

between "very little blood" and plain "air." Some years ago a Swedish pathologist attempted to bridge that gap. He measured the blood pressure in the carotid and femoral arteries, after death, and found negative values. Thereupon he opened the chest and severed the large vessels emerging from the heart: arterial pressure rose to zero, because the large arteries—due to their negative pressure—had drawn in some air.[63] Thus, it is indeed *possible* to find air in large arteries in dissecting a dead body; but I do regret having to admit that even the great Alexandrians fell into that trap—and went along with the myth that living arteries convey air.

Despite all these handicaps, when Erasistratos came to dissect the heart, he found in it two new sets of membranes: flat triangles that reminded him of *cuspids*, "spear points." He named them *bicuspid* and *tricuspid*,[64] and even understood that they were flaps of one-way, inlet valves, which opened and closed with the heartbeat (Fig. 8.16). It was Galen who preserved this gem of a discovery, "a golden fragment among the miserable ruins of Alexandrian

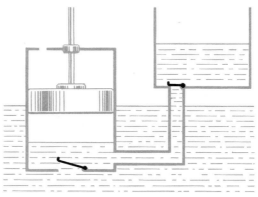

8.17 About 270 B.C. an engineer, Ktesibios of Alexandria, invented the valve and the pump.

medicine."[65] This is how Galen sums up the function of all the heart valves according to Erasistratos:

> The use of these membranes . . . is to perform for the heart contrary functions, alternating at successive intervals . . . Those attached to the vessels that bring in material [*bicuspid and tricuspid*], when pressed from without inward, yield to the influx of materials, and falling into the cavities of the heart, throw open its orifices and leave an unobstructed passage . . . The membranes attached . . . to the vessels of exit [*sigmoid valves*] act in the contrary way.

Erasistratos also knew, and understood, the aortic and pulmonary outlet-valves. Perhaps he had read about them in *On the Heart*; perhaps he had re-discovered them. Anyway, he was able to jump ahead of the anonymous pioneer and conclude that the four sets of "membranes" were flap valves belonging to a one-way pump. But then he also enjoyed the decisive advantage of working in the very birthplace of hydraulics. I envision that the brainstorm of Erasistratos—realizing that the heart is a pump—may have been helped by lunchtime discussions with a colleague from the physics department who had just invented the flap valve and the force pump: Ktesibios (Fig. 8.17).[66] Although the dates of these various steps are not quite certain, it is obvious that biology and physics interwove in the discovery of the valve and pump concepts (Figs. 8.15–8.17).

If ever a discovery came too early, it was this one of the heart as a pump. Veins and arteries were seen as sets of independent, dead-end canals; blood and air were supposed to slowly seep toward the periphery, where they were used up. So there was no real need for a busy, powerful, one-way pump; in fact it was an embarrassment. Galen inherited this difficulty and twisted the facts to fit an improved scheme that was horribly wrong.[67] The heart as a pump made no sense, really, until Harvey in 1628.

Branching out of the heart, the veins and arteries were thought to form two separate trees, whose branches intertwined and became thinner and thinner until they faded out of sight. And here Erasistratos made two everlasting contributions, using what we have called the Greek "microscope," a compound of genius and wishful thinking. First:

> All living parts are a tissue of vein, artery and nerve, and each part is nourished by the vein contained in it: namely, the simple vein apprehensible by reason [*lógoi theoretés* again].[68]

This is the original concept of *tissues*, which I have attempted to render in Fig. 8.18. It was referred to as the *triplokía* ("trinity" or "three-ply"). There is still more to it. Some tissues, notes Erasistratos, like the brain, fat, and liver, are different, because a deposit of nutriment is "poured-in-between" the tissue, *par-en-chyma* (Fig. 8.19).[69] The word *parenchyma* still means the cells that fill the spaces between the vessels and fibers of the connective tissue; and fat cells are, without any stretch of the imagination, a deposit of nutriment.

Now for a wound. Even Erasistratos could not escape the blatant truth that when an artery is severed, blood escapes, not air. But he stuck to his guns and invented this far-fetched explanation: the wall of the arteries is a tissue like all others, and it therefore includes the endings of innumerable little veins. When the artery is severed, its "pneuma" escapes and leaves a vacuum, so the little veins will instantly bleed into the artery to fill the void (an extenuating circumstance for the author: he was echoing the current Alexandrian jargon about pneumatics and the effects of a vacuum).[70] Yet notice that this *tour de force* obliged Erasistratos to postulate a fundamental truth, the communication between arteries and veins. He may have drawn the idea from the Hippocratic book *On Joints*,[71] and it was the beginning of a major discovery. But he carried it no further.

Practical Applications: Alexandrian Tourniquets

So much for the mechanics of the tissues; now see how they could explain illness. Erasistratos borrowed one of the favorite Hippocratic themes, the *plethora*, an "overabundance of blood,"[72] and built it up. Most diseases, he said, came about because the tissues receive more blood than they can use. Within his scheme of the triplokía, this meant that the tips of the little veins, when overloaded with blood, would bulge dangerously close to the tips of the arteries, filled with air: one more step and the two would form *synanastomoses*, "end to end connections," and the veins would spill blood into the arteries (Fig. 8.20).[73] In the case of a wound, for example, if the skin all around became red, hot and inflamed, the reason was simple: the arteries had lost all their pneuma and become flooded with blood. This concept was used to explain not only what we call now acute inflammation, but practically any disease.

Absurd, of course, but how much more absurd it would have seemed to postulate that the outside world was crawling with untold billions of tiny, invisible creatures, and that *they* were the cause of inflammation. If a part of

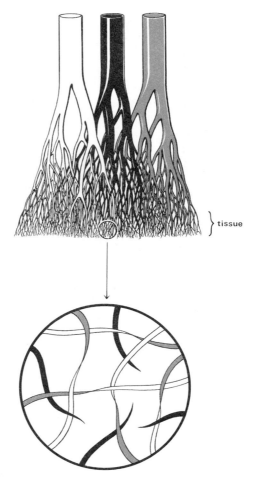

} tissue

8.18 The mental picture of tissues as first conceived by Erasistratos must have been something like this. Since the eye could perceive three sets of branching structures—veins, arteries, nerves (top)—all tissues had to be composed ultimately of the finest branches of these structures (bottom).

8.19 In some tissues, Erasistratos thought, nutriment (*parenchyma*) was "poured in" between the branches: another remarkable extrapolation.

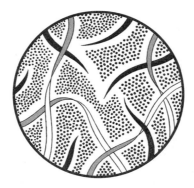

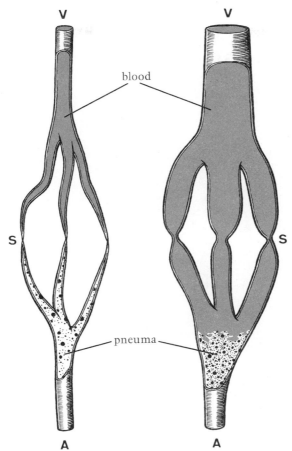

8.20 The mechanism of inflammation—and of most diseases—according to Erasistratos. *Left:* Normal veins contained blood, arteries air (*pneuma*). Their endings were dangerously close, being connected through extremely fine channels called *synanastomoses* (S). *Right:* An excess of blood (*plethora*) in the veins would force blood through these channels into the arteries. Nonsense, but it contained a good guess, that there are indeed connections between arteries and veins.

the body is sick, the likeliest cause (the gods have been ruled out) must be something within. So for Erasistratos it was an error of place (*parémptosis*): blood in the wrong place.[74] This concept had the further advantage of offering one and the same mechanism for the majority of diseases, and therefore one type of treatment.

Given a predicament like plethora, the logical treatment might have been bleeding; but Erasistratos was loathe to get rid of good blood, especially since he did not believe in the four humors and their faulty mixtures. He preferred cutting off the supply at the roots by starvation. And his authority surely contributed to the starving of thousands of wounded, up to the days of—pardon the shock—Napoleon. Behold, however, this other and more imaginative treatment of plethora: why not try to "blood-starve" the congested part, by trapping some of the blood supply in other parts of the body—until the sick tissues had used up their plethora? This was done by putting ligatures at the roots of the limbs, not too tightly. The limbs would

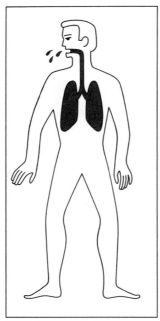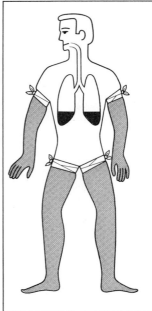

8.21 The treatment for patients who spat blood, according to Erasistratos. It was inferred that these patients suffered from too much blood in the lungs; hence, ties were placed on the limbs, to hold blood there. In some cases it could have worked.

become congested, and hold the blood within them, out of mischief (Fig. 8.21).

Do not mistake these ligatures for hemostatic tourniquets: in the case of a wounded limb they would be applied to all the limbs *except* the wounded one.[75] And here we miss, incidentally, an important piece of theory. I wonder how Erasistratos explained that a ligature at the root of a limb would cause congestion. It does, of course; but in his view, the blood flowed—very slowly—from the heart to the periphery, so his ligatures should have prevented the blood from flowing into the limb, rather than holding it there.

Anyway, a wounded patient would be forced to lie with tight, uncomfortable bands around his arms and thighs, and starve. As a treatment for wounds, these ligatures made no sense: they did subtract a certain amount of blood from the circulation, but never enough to stop the gush from a severed artery (somewhat as opening three faucets in a house would scarcely affect a leak in the main). However, the Erasistratean ligatures were especially recommended for plethora of the lungs: that is, for patients who spat up blood. Now, if the bleeding was due to pulmonary tuberculosis, there is no chance that the ligatures could work: by holding blood in the limbs it is impossible to lower arterial pressure to the point of stopping an arterial hemorrhage.[76] If, instead, the plethora of the lung meant the bloody froth that suffocates a patient in acute cardiac failure, the ligatures should have worked. They still work, and in a spectacular way. By retaining blood in the limbs, they do just what Erasistratos had in mind: they keep blood away from the lung. When the left side of the heart fails suddenly, it can no longer clear the lungs of the blood that the right ventricle, still vigorous, pumps into them; the lungs become congested, and there is danger of sudden edema. One emergency procedure (besides drugs) is to cut down the supply of venous blood flowing into the right ventricle. This is done "by *venostasis,* which consists in applying tourniquets to three limbs. Every few minutes a tourniquet is placed on the fourth extremity and one of the others is released."[77] If the technique saved a few in ancient times, it was worth the discomfort of the others.

So much for Alexandrian insight. I should not close this chapter without attempting to analyze that curious Alexandrian failure, at first sight so very unlikely. There was Erasistratos, a born experimenter, with enough genius to recognize the heart as a pump, and to postulate connections (albeit "abnormal") between arteries and veins; yet he failed to recognize the circulation of the blood. He apparently never thought of filling a good Alexandrian syringe with ink, injecting it into the veins, and seeing if it came back through the arteries.

But think of the body's plumbing as he saw it. Arteries and veins formed two separate systems, one for blood, the other for air. There was no reason to look for a circulation between the two, when it was *obvious* that the two had to remain separate, because blood, spilled into the arteries, caused inflammation. If I may use a twentieth century comparison, Erasistratos visualized the arterial and venous systems about as separate as we see the water and gasoline ducts in our cars. There would be no purpose in trying to force one to mix with the other.

In practice, from the point of view of a wounded patient, none of the fancy new Alexandrian theories would have helped (even though they did help, by accident, some patients in cardiac failure). The trend against bleeding was good, but was probably canceled by the emphasis on starvation; and Galen reversed that trend anyway. The one great gift of Alexandrian medicine—the anonymous gift that made it possible for surgery to rise as a separate profession—was the ligature of bleeding vessels.

The flamboyant outburst of science and scholarship was already losing monentum after a century; its last great contribution was the Ptolemaic system.[78] In 295 A.D., during a revolt, the Museum was destroyed. Its head-quarters were provisionally transferred to the nearby temple of Serapis, but in 391 the temple was sacked by a Christian mob, the library was burned, and the shell converted to a church. A few years later the last scholar—a woman, Hypatia—was seized by the Christians, dragged into a church, and lynched.[79] Whatever the Arabs burned in 642, if indeed they did,[80] could only have been a ghost.

Today, ancient Alexandria is almost out of sight; it has sunk below sea level, and the new city sits over it so tightly that archeological exploration is nearly hopeless.

Nothing is left of the Museum.

In 1847, in the garden of the Prussian consulate, a block of stone turned up. It was square, with a deep hollow, and one of its sides read: THREE TOMES OF DIOSKOURIDES. If this was a stone box for papyrus scrolls, it is all that is left to mark the site of the Museum and its library.[81]

As to the lighthouse, on 8 August 1303, an earthquake shook the island and the great tower collapsed.[82] But its light kept shining. On the opposite shore of the Mediterranean, in Greek, Italian, Spanish, and French, the word for "beacon" is the name of the tiny island facing Alexandria:

pharos
faro
faro
phare

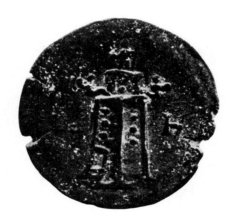

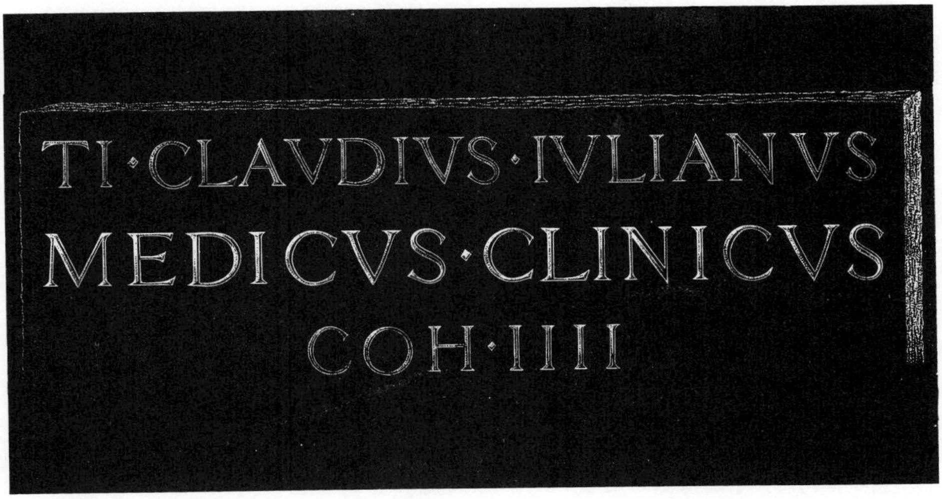

TI·CLAVDIVS·IVLIANVS
MEDICVS·CLINICVS
COH·IIII

9   The Medicus

Hippocrates passed away; Alexandria sprang up; Greek medicine discovered the laboratory. And all this time the Romans had no physicians at all.

Ignorance? Pliny has a six-word explanation: *non rem antiqui damnabant, sed artem;* "it was not medicine itself that the forefathers condemned, but medicine as a profession . . . chiefly because they refused to pay fees to profiteers in order to save their own lives."[1] So for six hundred years the frugal Romans carried on with folk remedies. Surely there was no reason to pay for *those*. To put crushed cabbage on a wound, as Cato recommended,[2] there was no need for an expert.

Then the plague struck; it was 293 B.C. The elders, if they were well informed, must have debated several alternatives: whether to follow tradition and just purify the air with the smoke of bonfires,[3] or try to import an Egyptian specialist (a *medicus*, "physician," assuming that the word appeared in Rome before the profession)—or perhaps one of those Greek iatrói. Finally the Sibylline books were consulted; their advice was to summon Asklepios from his shrine in Epidauros. A trireme was dispatched; it brought back Asklepios in the form of a snake (Fig. 9.1), the snake settled on the Island of the Tiber, and the plague abated.[4]

Quite a while later, in 219 B.C.,[5] the first Greek physician drifted over from the Peloponnesus. His name was Archágathus, and his start was brilliant. "Citizen rights were given him, and a surgery at the crossway of Acilius was bought with public money for his own use. They say that he was

MEDICVS

339

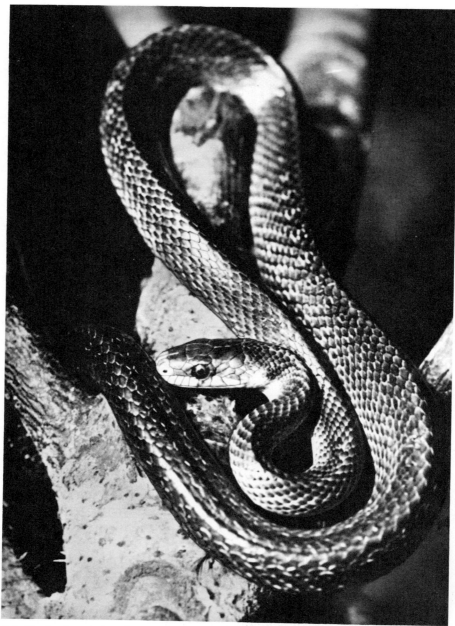

9.1 *Elaphe longissima longissima,* the first Greek healer that Rome imported, a century after the death of Hippocrates.

MEDICVS

a wound specialist [*vulnerarius*] and that his arrival at first was wonderfully popular, but presently from his savage use of the knife and cautery he was nicknamed the executioner [*carnifex*] and his profession, with all physicians, became objects of loathing."[6] Cato the Censor raged: the Greeks, he wrote to his son Marcus about 200 B.C., "are a quite worthless people, and an intractable one, and you must consider my words prophetic: when that race gives us its literature it will corrupt all things, and even all the more if it sends hither its physicians. They have conspired together to murder all foreigners with their physic, but this very thing they do for a fee, to gain credit and destroy us easily . . . I have forbidden you to have dealings with physicians."[7]

Cato died just in time to be spared the inevitable: another iatrós, much wiser, took aristocratic Rome by storm with the irresistible therapeutic slogan "swiftly safely and sweetly" (*cito tuto jucunde*). That was Asclepiades (124–50 B.C.). He prescribed few medicines, among them wine and music, and went so far as to oppose venesection.[8] Native Romans could not possibly compete with these people—who had nine rational ways to reset a shoulder, to mention only one problem—when the best the Romans could do to the same end was to bind on two pieces of a green reed and sing over them the gibberish of Cato the Censor:[9]

> Huat haut haut
> Istasis tarsis
> Ardannabou dannaustra

There was no choice, to use Pliny's sarcasm, but to be "swept along on the puffs of the clever brains of Greece."[10]

The Setting: Roman Life As Seen by Pliny

When Vesuvius buried Pompeii in 79 A.D., Rome was at its height. Most of the facts discussed in this chapter belong to that period. To understand them best, we need a human portrait, one showing a Roman of the first century, with his thoughts, his background, his prejudices, and all that he took for granted. For this role I have chosen Pliny the Elder: for he lived from 23 to 79 A.D., and though by no means an average citizen, he was almost the caricature of a Roman.[11] He started his career as a public officer in Germany, by serving in the cavalry, then returned to Rome and studied law. Under Nero at first he kept quiet, but eventually he resumed public life and went to Spain as a procurator. All this time he was writing books, on subjects from history to grammar to the use of the javelin. When Vespasian took over, he again returned to Rome and was admitted to the intimate circle of the emperor, an old-time army acquaintance.

At age fifty-two, feeling that digests (*thesauroi*) were more needed than new books,[12] Pliny set out to write his only extant work, the *Historia naturalis* or *Natural History*. He compiled it at record speed in two years, setting an all-time example of compulsive, obsessive data-collecting, writing only during the night, having books read to him literally every spare moment—on vacation, even in the street, not *in* the bath but certainly while being rubbed down and dried, at table—and scolding friends for interrupting without good reason ("your interruption has cost us ten lines!").[13] As his readers droned on, he occasionally misheard the Greek or Latin words, so that the notes he was jotting down were sometimes garbled.[14] What he chose to record was not too critical, and was often colored by his love of the marvelous. But in his thirty-seven books he finally assembled (he says, and he

MEDICVS

is probably right) 20,000 facts from about 2000 volumes by 100 selected authors,[15]—a gigantic enterprise for his day.

For 1600 years the *Natural History* was revered as a pillar of human knowledge. Nowadays, Pliny's reputation outside his native Como is low, for he is unjustly remembered for the poorest of his 20,000 facts; yet if he had not undertaken that ghastly two-year marathon, we would be denied a major source of information about antiquity. And we have it by mere chance. Barely two years after dedicating his finished work to a friend,[16] Pliny had become involved with the navy. On August 24 of the year 79, at age fifty-six, while he was in command of the fleet off the bay of Naples, a great mushroom-cloud rose from Mount Vesuvius.[17] It was unthinkable for Pliny to stand by and watch. He moved in with his quadriremes, braving the waves, the rising sea-bottom, and the hail of stones and ashes; he landed, and died on the shore the next day, in a cloud of poisonous fumes.[18] His nephew, Pliny the Younger, left a touching portrait of him in his letters to Tacitus and to another friend.[19]

I will now let Pliny speak for himself, out of the pages of his *Natural History*. To this effect I have chosen about one hundred passages that I considered typical or relevant, and I have grouped them by topic. Pliny's own words are italicized, the rest is my shortened version.

On the World and Physics

The Greeks call the world *cosmos*, "ornament," and the Romans *mundus*, "elegant," *because of its perfect finish and grace.*[20]

The world is a sphere that rotates with undescribable velocity. [Pliny may have seen the Alexandrian toy model of the earth as a sphere (Fig. 9.2)].[21]

Light travels faster than sound.[22]

Certainly it is found that every liquid becomes smaller when frozen [surprisingly wrong].[23]

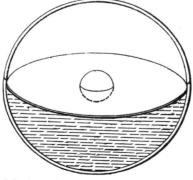

9.2 An Alexandrian model, described by Heron, to represent the earth as a sphere in the center of the universe: a ball floating on water, inside a glass globe. The globe is half full, and the ball is held in place by a perforated bronze plate. First century A.D.

On God and the Afterlife

What is this mad idea that life is renewed by death?[24]

I deem it a mark of human weakness to seek to discover the shape and form of God. Whoever God is—provided there is a God—and wherever he is, he consists wholly of sense, sight and hearing, wholly of soul, wholly of mind, wholly of himself.[25]

On Mankind

Snakes do not bite snakes, *whereas to man, I vow, most of his evils come from his fellow-men.*[26]

Man enters the world *wailing and weeping, and none other among all the animals is more prone to tears.*[27]

A foreigner scarcely counts as a human being for someone of another race.[28]

People will even give their name to a new variety of fruit, as if it were an outstanding achievement.[29]

Man is the only animal for whom mating for the first time is followed by repugnance.[30]

Nature appears to have created everything for the sake of man.[31]

Our civilization depends largely on paper.[32]

On the Good Old Days

It was not this way in bygone generations: there was no need to keep watch on domestics.[33]

In the past, *a certain barrenness of fortune made it necessary to exercise the gifts of the mind . . . but later generations have been positively handicapped by the expansion of the world and by abundance.*[34]

Craftsmanship of working in metals has quite disappeared; for this . . . like everything else, has now begun to be practiced for the sake of gain.[35]

The skill of casting in bronze has perished.[36]

Nobody knows any more what wine he is drinking. *Our commercial honesty has sunk so low that only the names of the vintages are sold, the wines are adulterated as soon as they are poured into the vats.*[37]

What an absurd idea to pay more money for an object [of crystalware], just because it is more breakable.[38]

What a difference from the old days, when Cato the Censor suggested that even the Forum be paved with sharp stones, to prevent loitering.[39]

Amber is now so expensive that *a human figurine, no matter how small, costs more than several human beings [slaves] alive and in good health.*[40]

Who could be blamed for complaining nowadays? *The cost of living has been raised by luxuries and extravagance.*[41]

On Women and Cosmetics

The reason why women are kissed by men is to know whether they have been at the wine—says Cato.[42]

Women have in their womb an animal called a mole, and it moves about.[43]

By the lowest reckoning India, China and the Arabian peninsula take from our empire 100 million sesterces every year: that is the sum which our luxuries and our women cost us. What fraction of these imports, I ask you, now goes to the gods or to the powers of the lower world?[44]

I find that a woman's breast-band tied around the head relieves headache.— Over and above this there is no limit to a woman's power.[45]

Perfume was probably invented by the Persians to quench the smell of dirt.[46]

The highest recommendation for perfume is that when a woman passes by, her scent may attract the attention even of persons occupied in something else (and it costs 400 denarii per pound!).[47]

Almond oil . . . smoothes the skin, improves the complexion.[48]

Perfume is the most superfluous of luxuries: it dies in the very hour when it is used.[49]

On Food and Wine

To gain weight, drink during meals. [Modern medicine gives the same advice in reverse: to avoid gaining weight, avoid drinking during meals. The rationale: dry food, being more difficult to swallow, allows one to eat less.][50]

A civilized life is impossible without salt.[51]

To think that the only pleasing quality of pepper is that it stings—and we go all the way to India to get it.[52]

Who discovered that great boon—the liver of stuffed geese [pâté de foie gras]?[53]

The pith at the top of the palm-tree is called "the brain," and it has a sweet taste [palm heart].[54]

Arabia produces a brittle kind of honey that collects in reeds [cane sugar]. It is used only in medicines.[55]

Butter is used by barbarian tribes, where it distinguishes the rich from the poor.[56]

Sergius Orata invented oyster ponds; he also invented shower baths and sold them to outfit country houses [about 90 B.C].[57]

Oysters are served on snow; thus luxury has wedded the tops of the mountains to the bottom of the sea.[58]

MEDICVS

Refrigerated drinks were invented by Nero. He boiled water and then put the container in snow. In this way one gets the coolness without the injurious qualities of the snow. [Little did Pliny know that the Chinese had been doing that for centuries!][59]

Artificial colors are now added to wine. So many poisons are employed to force wine to suit our taste—and we are surprised that it is not wholesome! [Pliny was right, although unaware of the most dangerous poison in Roman wine: lead.][60]

There is no topic more difficult to handle than wine . . . It is hard to say whether wine does good to more people than it harms . . . Medical opinion is very divided.[61]

On Geography and Peoples

Italy is much longer than it is broad, and bends toward the left at its top; it is 1020 Roman miles long [actually about 650 miles as the crow flies, along the backbone, the Roman mile being about 95 yards shorter than the modern English mile].[62]

One is ashamed to borrow an account of Italy from the Greeks.[63]

The Egyptian Sphinx is 243 feet long [almost exact: the Sphinx is 73.5m long, so Pliny's figure is about 1.5m short].[64]

The danger of lighthouses, such as are now burning in several places, is that their uninterrupted light can be mistaken for a star.[65]

The first international agreement was the adoption of the Ionian alphabet.[66]

The ambassadors from Ceylon were amazed at Roman honesty.[67]

The pirates of Germany navigate on boats made of a single tree hollowed out.[68]

I am of the opinion that the Assyrians always had writing, but others . . . hold that it was invented in Egypt [we are still not sure].[69]

Nowadays immense crowds go on voyages, but their object is profit, not learning.[70]

On Natural History, Biology, and Chemistry

How do bees multiply, since they can never be seen having intercourse?[71]

Dust in wool and clothes breeds moths.[72]

Many people have said that insects do not breathe.[73]

Fish run away from the bodies of dead fish. [This was the basis of a shark repellent developed in Woods Hole, Mass., during World War II.][74]

It is known from antiquity that amber is a form of resin.[75]

Glossopetrae [tongue stones] are said to fall from the sky; this is probably false.[85] [Sure enough, they are fossilized shark teeth (Fig. 9.3)][76]

To detect adulterations of copper acetate, smear it on a sheet of papyrus steeped in an infusion of plant gall. It should leave a black mark if genuine. [Although Pliny has it backward, this is still the world's first reactive paper (Plate 9.1).][77]

Going into the cellar, where the wine vats are, can be fatal. A good test is to let down a lamp; if it goes out, it means danger.[78]

On Superstition and Magic

MEDICVS

Does foreknowledge really exist, or is it a matter of chance like most things?[79]

Have words and incantations any effect? This is a most important question, and one never settled.[80]

When somebody sneezes, why do we say "good health"?[81]

We certainly still have formulas to charm away hail, various diseases, and burns, some actually tested by experience, but I am very shy of quoting them, because of the widely different feelings they arouse. Wherefore everyone must form his own opinion about them as he pleases.[82]

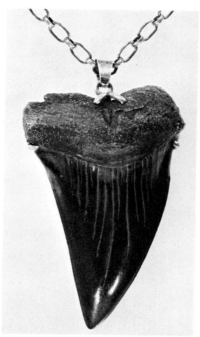

9.3 The source of an ancient drug: fossilized shark teeth, which were called "tongue stones" (*glossopetrae*). Ground up, they were said to be very effective, both internally and externally, until the 1600s. Actual size.

Magic is detestable, vain and idle . . . though it has what I might call shadows of truth. [Pliny has a personal grudge against the Magi, whom he calls liars, yet fears. Originally they were a tribe of the Medes (Persia), who became a priestly caste, not unlike the Levi among the Hebrews. Their religion seems to have been somewhat esoteric, so that the word *Magi* slowly passed from meaning "wise men of the East" to "magicians." By Pliny's time the word had gone halfway on its journey.][83]

Magic arose in Persia with Zoroaster. Its power comes from a seductive mixture of medicine, religion, and astrology, and thus *holds men's emotions in a three-fold bond.*[84]

Here are some lies of the Magi . . . to prevent a wound being painful they prescribe wearing as an amulet, tied on the person with a thread, a nail or other object that he has trodden on . . . To relieve headaches, they advise the rope used by a suicide tied around the temples.[85]

The Magi recommend the eggs of a horned owl. *Who could ever have looked at a horned owl's egg, when it is a portent to have seen the bird itself?*[86]

Even today Britain practices magic . . . It is beyond calculation how great a debt humanity owes to the Romans for sweeping away the monstrous rites in which to kill a man was the highest religious duty, or to eat man a passport to health.[87]

In quartan fevers [malaria] *ordinary medicines are practically useless, for which reason I shall include several of the magicians' remedies.*[88]

On Prodigious Events

There have been rains of milk, blood, flesh, iron, sponges, wool, and baked bricks.[89]

There are islands that float and drift with the wind.[90]

People in Pontus cannot sink—it is reported—even if weighted down with clothes.[91]

King Cyrus knew all his soldiers by name.[92]

There are fish that grunt, others that climb trees [true].[93]

Pigeons have carried important messages.[94]

There was a man who could see 123 miles.[95]

The champion for love-making was Messalina: she beat a prostitute with a score of 25 in 24 hours.[96]

In the School of Gladiators of Gaius only two men of 20,000 did not blink and were therefore unconquerable.[97]

One professor of logic died of shame because he could not solve a problem put to him in jest.[98]

Julius Caesar could dictate or listen to four secretaries; *seven if he was not otherwise occupied.*[99]

Truth Misinterpreted

Bees have a government.[100]

Whales have their mouth on their forehead.[101]

Species with more than four feet [insects] have no blood.[102]

In Persia there are trees that bear wool [cotton].[103]

All trees are of both sexes, say the experts [varieties mistaken for sexes].[104]

Lime has a remarkable quality: once it has been burnt, its heat is increased by water.[105]

The human race is becoming smaller; in Crete there are remains of colossal men [probably fossils of prehistoric animals].[106]

Glass globes full of water become so hot when facing the sun that they can set clothes on fire.[107]

Naphtha has a close affinity with fire, which leaps to it at once when it sees it in any direction.[108]

Some Nonsense

Nails grow after death.[109]

Certain animals stop growing if they drink wine, it is said.[110]

Mixing several sorts of wine is bad.[111]

Sexual intercourse cures dullness of vision.[112]

Poisonous mushrooms are neutralized by cooking with vinegar.[113]

Haircuts are best just after the full moon—so as not to go bald, says Varro.[114]

On Doctors and Disease

New diseases, unknown in past years, have come to Italy and to Europe.[115]

The variety of diseases is unlimited. There was a poet who had fever only on his birthdays.[116]

Hippocrates is the prince of medicine [*princeps medicinae;* quite a concession by Pliny to a Greek] . . . *He founded that branch of medicine called "clinical"* [generous but debatable].[117]

Nature distributed medicines everywhere; *even the very desert was made a drug store.*[118]

For bruises, your hearth should be your medicine chest [quoted from Varro].[119]

For a tiny sore a medicine is imported from the Red Sea, though genuine remedies form the daily dinner of even the very poorest. But if remedies were sought in the kitchen garden . . . none of the arts would become cheaper than medicine.[120]

Physicians acquire their knowledge from our dangers, making experiments at the cost of our lives.[121]

Physicians make enormous amounts of money, up to 600,000 sesterces a year [roughly 100 times the minimum living wage].[122]

Heaven knows, the medical profession is the only one in which anybody professing to be a physician is at once trusted [there being no recognized medical diplomas], *although nowhere else is an untruth more dangerous. We pay however no attention to the danger, so great for each of us is the seductive sweetness of wishful thinking.*[123]

Our pleasures we enjoy ourselves, but our life we entrust to someone else [a physician], which *I personally hold to be the worst possible disgrace.*[124]

On Barbarians, Greeks, and Romans

There is a marvellous neatness in the titles of Greek books: but when you get inside them, good heavens, what a void![125]

There are foreign people who live like savages and then have the courage to complain when they are taken over by the Romans. Fortune ought to spare them as a punishment.[126]

The outstanding race in the whole world is undoubtedly the Roman.[127]

On Death

I do not indeed hold that life ought to be so prized that by any and every means it should be prolonged. You holding this view, whoever you are, will none the less die . . . Of all the blessings given to man by nature none is greater than a timely death.[128]

MEDICVS *Folk Remedies—and a Lost Pearl*

In his monumental collection of folk remedies, Pliny does not specify which ones were those of the forefathers; but here are a few that might qualify:[129]

"To commence with admitted medical aids, that is, wools and eggs" . . . wool is applied with honey to old sores. Wounds it heals if dipped in wine, or vinegar, or cold water and oil, and then squeezed out.

White of egg cools inflamed eyes and closes wounds.

Earth worms have a great reputation for uniting fresh wounds; they are used in honey or vinegar . . . also pounded cypress leaves.

A slice of veal will prevent wounds from swelling . . . and to make them close fast, use leaves and bark of the elm . . . or of the vine.

Pig dung, fresh or dried and powdered, is good for wounds made by iron.

Pellets of goat dung kneaded in vinegar and warmed are good for ulcers on the shins.

For poisoned arrows use dog's blood, for snake bite, a mouse cut in two.

For a painful wound, any pebble right side up—or a potsherd applied just as it was taken up—those applying it must not look back, and make sure that the sun does not behold them.

For chafings caused by foot wear, ash of an old shoe.

For sores of a whipping, fresh sheep skin.

And all wounds will heal faster if bound up with the very difficult Hercules knot [probably true; for a knot with invisible ends reduced the patient's chances of being treated].

Once in a while, one of Pliny's simples scores a bull's eye. Fern, for instance, is recommended for intestinal worms; it is a very effective drug.[130] Still other treasures may be lost in the thicket of Pliny's 20,000 data—perhaps even a drug that would be good on wounds.

In fact, I did find a lost treasure, when looking among the styptics. There were the famous cobwebs, still used in Italy.[131] There was the rennet again, as in Greece—kid rennet, hare rennet, deer rennet—[132] and this time it is obvious that its purpose is to "coagulate" or "bind," because it is used also to stay the diarrhea of infants, by applying it to the mother's breasts.[133] But then, reading on, I could scarcely believe my eyes. Pliny talks of a plant that "some call *ephedron* . . . The Greeks hold various views about this plant . . . assuring us that so wonderful is its nature, its mere touch stanches a patient's bleeding . . . its juice kept in the nostrils checks hemorrhage . . . and taken in sweet wine it cures cough."[134] One cannot help but be startled by the association of a plant named "ephedron" with stopping hemorrhage and curing cough: for these are the two main effects of a powerful drug called *ephedrine*. A surgical incision in skin injected with ephedrine is almost bloodless; and a spell of asthmatic cough can be relieved almost as if by miracle. Coincidence? The data are repeated elsewhere with a description of the plant: "*Ephedra* . . . has no leaves, but numerous, rush-like, jointed tufts . . . (Fig. 9.4). For cough, asthma and colic it is given pounded in dark-red, dry wine." MEDICVS

By Hercules, this is an accurate description of both the plant *Ephedra* and its product, ephedrine, the precious drug supposedly discovered only by the Chinese. I quote from a modern textbook of pharmacology: "Ephedrine . . . was used in China for over 5000 years before being introduced into Western medicine in 1924."[135] In fact, the introduction of ephedrine from China is a classic episode in the recent history of medicine. Between 1922 and 1924, a young American physician, Carl Frederic Schmidt, worked at the

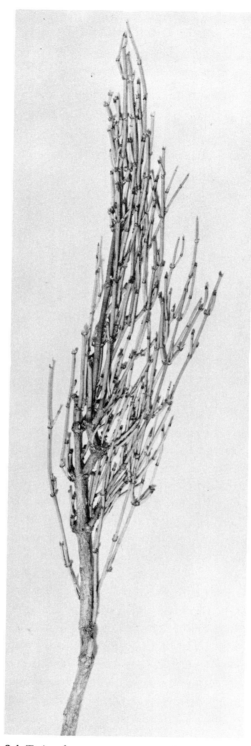

9.4 Twig of a contemporary *Ephedra nebrodensis Tin.*, gathered in Sardinia. Note the typical segmented branches, with no leaves, as described by Pliny. Actual size.

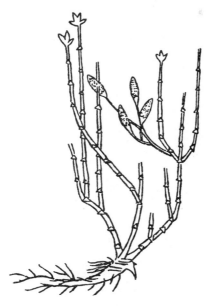

黃　麻

9.5 *Ma huang:* this is *Ephedra* as it was known to the Chinese, perhaps as far back as 2000 B.C.

9.6 Chemical formulas of ephedrine and adrenaline.

epinephrine (adrenaline)

$$HO—\bigcirc—CH—CH—NH$$
$$\quad\quad\quad\;|\quad\;|\quad\;|$$
$$\quad\quad\quad OH\;\;H\;\;CH_3$$

ephedrine

$$\bigcirc—CH—CH—NH$$
$$\quad\quad\;|\quad\quad|\quad\quad|$$
$$\quad\;OH\;\;CH_3\;CH_3$$

Peking Union Medical College, testing some of the most popular Chinese traditional herbs, in the hope of discovering some new active principle. Of the five drugs that were selected out of nearly two thousand, only one gave significant results: an extract of *Ephedra*, locally known as *ma huang* (Fig. 9.5). When injected intravenously in dogs, it caused a spectacular increase in blood pressure. Thus began the modern career of ephedrine.[136]

Ephedrine (Fig. 9.6) has essentially the same effects as adrenaline, a hormone produced by the adrenal glands, but with two advantages: it can be given by mouth (as Pliny gives it), and its effects, though weaker, last longer. Its classical uses are for asthma, allergic cough, and hemorrhage; Pliny has all three.

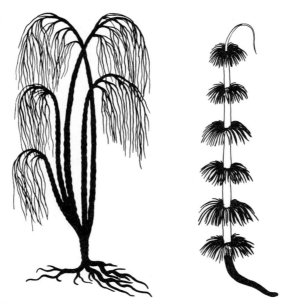

9.7 *Ephedra* (left) in a drawing of 512 A.D., labeled "Two Species of Ippouris." It would have been difficult to recognize *Ephedra* here, because the distorted name *Ephudron* is given as the last of fifteen possible synonyms, and *Ephedra* is associated with a similar but unrelated plant, *Equisetum arvense* (right). These drawings may well derive from originals drawn at the time of Dioscorides.

Could it be that Pliny somehow inherited the notion of *Ephedra* from China? It is extremely unlikely. His immediate source could have been Dioscorides, who has essentially the same information (Fig. 9.7).[137] There is no record of anyone from China going to Rome in antiquity.[138] The Romans knew little about China, except that there were "people called Seres . . . famous for the woollen substance obtained from their forests."[139] If the use of ephedrine had come from China, it should have increased in Europe as contacts increased; but in fact, it was completely forgotten. In ancient India, Sushruta and Charaka do not mention it.[140] There are many *Ephedrae* in Europe, including an *Ephedra helvetica*; among the Italian varieties, some from Sardinia were even studied in 1940 for possible industrial exploitation.[141] So we are probably dealing with an independent Mediterranean discovery, not related to ma huang.

The most obvious lesson here is that treasures are buried in ancient books. Dr. Schmidt retrieved this one by sifting through the two thousand drugs of China. One might say that he could also have sifted through the one thousand drugs of Pliny. But the story of ephedrine is loaded with irony: Dr. Schmidt might almost have ordered his precious drug from a catalog. As he and his Chinese collaborator, K. K. Chen, were wondering what to call their newly discovered substance, they found out that a crystalline substance extracted from ma huang had already been prepared in 1885; it had been called ephedrine in 1887, and even synthesized. Thereafter it had become a victim of its own progress. Because ephedrine had become available in large amounts, it had also become possible to prepare potent solutions and to inject huge doses into experimental animals. The animals dropped dead, whereupon ephedrine was branded as highly toxic, and forgotten. Asthmatics went on coughing and wheezing—and all the while it lay written in the books of Pliny and Dioscorides that a gentler, impure decoction of *Ephedra* would have brought them instant relief.

The Star Witness: Cornelius Celsus

Aside from the usual flurry of minor historical tidbits, up to the first century A.D. there are only two major sources on wound care in Rome, both from the height of the empire: first Celsus, then Pliny.[142] Celsus is a special case. If this were a play, all the spotlights would be on; Cornelius Celsus would stride out in the glare and hold forth in impeccable, soul-stirring Latin, for his style has few equals in the drab world of medical literature. Practically all we know about him is that he lived under Tiberius (14–37 A.D.) and wrote in his mother tongue a vast treatise covering agriculture, warfare, rhetoric, medicine, and possibly more.[143] The medical section was entitled *De medicina*, "On Medicine," in eight books. Writing extensively on medicine, *in Latin*, was almost an act of courage: Pliny—who took the same risk in his *Natural History*—felt quite sore about the fact that "if medical treatises are written in a language other than Greek they have no prestige even among unlearned men ignorant of Greek; and if any should understand them they have less faith in [them]."[144]

Celsus was the second of three Roman authors—after Varro, and before Pliny—who wrote encyclopedias about fifty years apart. Of Varro, a few books survived; Pliny's *Natural History* sailed through the ages almost unscathed; Celsus very nearly shipwrecked. Shortly after his time, one stuffy grammarian acknowledges him only as a man of "average intellect."[145] The conscientious Pliny quotes him twenty-four times, mostly on matters nonmedical,[146] but then makes an interesting slip. As he sets about writing on medicine in Latin, half a century after Celsus, he says that "no one hitherto has treated the subject in Latin."[147] Apparently *De medicina* had made no great splash, even with Pliny (perhaps *because* it was written in Latin). Then the curtain dropped.

For thirteen centuries the manuscripts of Celsus were almost as good as buried. Someone cared enough to copy the eight books on medicine before they crumbled to dust; but all the others disappeared for good. The very name of Celsus recurs only four times in known documents of the Middle Ages.[148] Finally, as the new wind of the Renaissance sent Italian scholars rummaging for Greek and Latin codices, two copies of Celsus were unearthed: one in 1426 (promptly recopied and lost again) and one the year after, already five hundred years old, in the Basilica of Saint Ambrose in Milan (Plate 9.2).[149] For the discoverers the find was almost too good to be true: Greek medicine in perfect Latin dress! As soon as Gutenberg made it possible, Celsus rolled off the press, first among all medical authors (1478), and the only complete medical text that came down from antiquity: the Smith papyrus stops at the waist; the Hippocratic books are a jumble; *De medicina* is a gem with all facets intact.

MEDICVS

353

Celsus on Human Vivisection

The substance of *De medicina* is Hippocratic (which also means that its surgery is far superior to its internal medicine), but enriched by Alexandrian progress, and almost surely by Indian imports.[150]

In his opening chapter Celsus discusses human experimentation. In principle, he asks, is it useful to use wounds as windows, to study what is going on inside the body? His answer:

> For when pain occurs internally, neither is it possible for one to learn what hurts the patient, unless he has acquainted himself with the position of each organ or intestine; nor can a diseased portion of the body be treated by one who does not know what that portion is. *When a man's viscera are exposed in a wound, he who is ignorant of the colour of a part in health may be unable to recognize which part is intact, and which part damaged; thus he cannot even relieve the damaged part.*[151]

In other words, knowledge of anatomy is essential.

Celsus draws this conviction not from the Hippocratic books but from the later studies at the Alexandrian Museum:

> They hold that Herophilos and Erasistratos did this in the best way by far, when they laid open men whilst alive—criminals received out of prison from the kings—and whilst these were still breathing, observed parts which beforehand nature had concealed, their position, colour, shape, size, arrangement, hardness, softness, smoothness, relation, processes and depressions of each, and whether any part is inserted into or is received into another.[152]

This gruesome story did not fail to draw thunder from two Fathers of the Church, Tertullian and St. Augustine, which led George Sarton to draw the obvious conclusion: "Celsus had been able to tell the story without disapproval because pagan ruthlessness had not yet been assuaged by Christian tenderness."[153]

Shock must have prevented all three eminent scholars from reading further,[154] because in the next breath Celsus goes on to blast human vivisection. Others believe, he says, that people's entrails are exposed often enough by accident:

> For sometimes a gladiator in the arena, or a soldier in battle, or a traveller who has been set upon by robbers, is so wounded that some or other interior part is exposed in one man or another. Thus, they say, an observant practitioner learns to recognize site, position, arrangement, shape, and such like, not when slaughtering, but whilst striving for health; and he learns in the course of a work of mercy, what others would come to know by means of dire cruelty.[155]

And here is the opinion of Celsus himself:

> I believe that medicine should be rational . . . But to open the bodies of men still alive is as cruel as it is needless [*et crudele et supervacuum*]. To open the dead is necessary to those who learn, who must know the positions and relations, which the corpse shows better than does a living and wounded man. As for all the rest that can

be learned only from the living, actual practice will demonstrate it in the course of treating the wounded, in a somewhat slower, but much milder way.[156]

This "opening the dead" was wishful thinking, for Rome was not ready to follow Alexandria in breaking the taboo.[157] But using wounds to study anatomy was true Roman reality. A century and a half later Galen, who raised it almost to an art, called it *vulneraria speculatio*, "the contemplation of wounds."[158]

The Celsian Surgeon and Some of His Tools

Surgeons will relish these lines. After diet and drugs,

The third part of the Art of Medicine is that which cures by the hand . . . It does not omit medicaments and regulated diets, but does most by hand. The effects of this treatment are more obvious than any other kind; inasmuch as in diseases since luck helps much, and the same things are often salutary, often of no use at all, it may be doubted whether recovery has been due to medicine, or a sound body, or good luck . . . But in that part of medicine which cures by hand, it is obvious that all improvement comes chiefly from this, even if it be assisted somewhat in other ways . . .

Now a surgeon (*chirurgus*) should be youthful or at any rate nearer youth than age; with a strong and steady hand which never trembles, and ready to use the left hand as well as the right; with vision sharp and clear, and spirit undaunted; filled with pity, so that he wishes to cure his patient, yet is not moved by his cries, to go too fast, or cut less than is necessary; but he does everything just as if the cries of pain cause him no emotion.[159]

Celsian surgery is clear and practical, free of Greek-style aesthetic frills.[160] Yet many and perhaps most of the surgeons liable to read his lines were Greeks.[161] Pliny says that even the Romans who practiced medicine soon became "deserters to the Greeks."[162] Why not, after all: they practiced an art that was mostly Greek, and I suspect that even many of their instruments came from overseas. Look at the monument to the otherwise unrecorded practitioner Publius Aelius Pius Curtianus *medicus bene meritus* (Fig. 9.8). His name is as Roman as could be, but his folding surgical kit is astonishingly similar to a Greek model (Fig. 9.9).

Greek or homemade, the instruments of the Roman surgeon were many and specialized. The richest collection is that of Pompeii, with hundreds of specimens.[163] Its scalpels are identical to those represented on sculptures (Fig. 9.10). Folding kits like that of Curtianus were not preserved; but kits of another kind, cylinders now known as *thecae vulnerariae*, "wound boxes," are fairly common. The remains of one whole collection came to light in a dramatic setting. Among the Pompeians who were smothered by the ashes and fell to their death in the streets, some carrying their worldly possessions, one man tried to flee with a case that was more precious to him than money; he finally collapsed over it, and it was found under his skeleton. In it were several cylinders of polished metal, each containing half a dozen instruments. Unfortunately no photographs were taken on the spot, but a similar kit is shown in Fig. 9.11.[164]

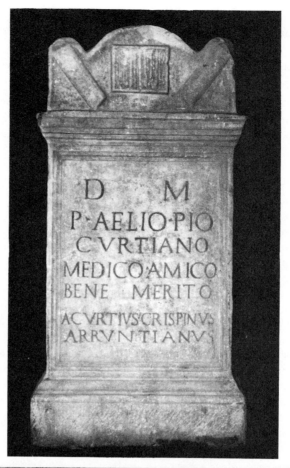

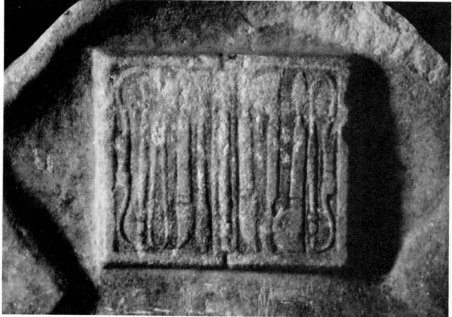

9.8 The Roman physician remembered in this monument had probably used a Greek-style instrument kit (shown in detail).

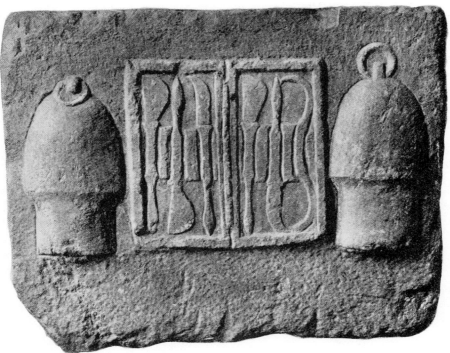

9.9 Instrument box of a Greek physician, and two cupping jars. Bas-relief found in Athens and dated 400 B.C.—100 A.D. About one-quarter original size.

9.10 Rusty surgical knives found at Pompeii. Unlike any modern scalpel, they were double-ended tools: Celsus says that the bronze handle (*manubríolum*) was used for blunt dissection in working around cysts or varicose veins. Apparently the surgeon did not mind holding the scalpel by the blade! About two-thirds original size.

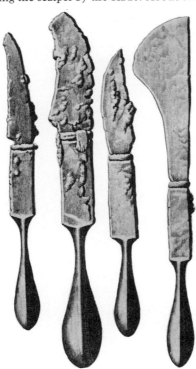

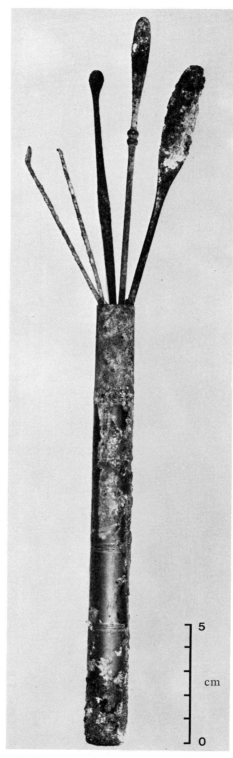

9.11 The commonest type of Roman medical kit: a pocket-sized cylindrical case. From Pompeii, first century A.D.

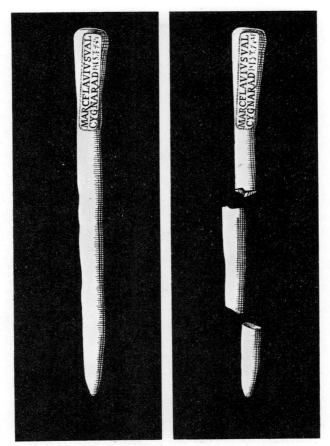

9.12 A guess at the shape and size of a collyrium stick, used as a probe (left) or in solution (right). One of the best varieties was the *cygnarium* (swan-white), made of starch and lead-white.

The two spoon-shaped probes emerging from the kit illustrated are made of bronze; they are typical examples of *spathoméle*, the simplest and most versatile tool of Greek medicine. Celsus mentions also another kind of probe, which—strangely enough—was soluble: a medicated stick, called *collyrium*. Collyria were made up of a glutinous paste rolled into long thin cones (Fig. 9.12). Nowadays their name sounds improper, because collyrium is the technical term for eyedrops. Actually, there is no mistake. The little sticks could be used as probes to explore wounds or fistulae, or they could be broken up and dissolved to make up a "medicated" solution. Eventually the second use prevailed, and the resulting solutions were used mainly for the eyes.[165]

Most famous of all the Pompeian instruments are the dilators, also because they are one of the earliest known applications of the screw (Fig. 9.13). Their use for dilating wounds, although not described, is certainly possible. For extracting barbed arrows, Celsus describes the Greek "spoon of Diokles."[166] In 1880, no original specimen having yet been found, H. Frölich (the German military surgeon who had studied Homer) proposed a model based on the description of Celsus (Fig. 9.14). His was a good guess, as proven by the specimen that was eventually discovered (Fig. 9.15).[167]

MEDICVS

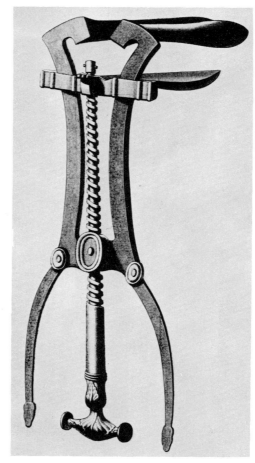

9.13 The *speculum* or dilator, a famous Pompeian medical instrument. Its prongs (top) are slowly spread by the powerful, square-threaded screw. About one-half actual size.

Celsus on Wounds and Ulcers

"There are still," writes Celsus, "some other things to be learnt about wounds and ulcerations in general, of which we will now speak . . . Blood comes out from a fresh wound or from one which is already healing . . . pus from an ulceration."[168]

MEDICVS Here is, at long last, the use of two separate terms, "wound" and "ulcer," a distinction that does not yet exist in the Hippocratic books (an ulcer is characterized by its poor tendency to heal, due to infection, mechanical irritation, poor circulation, or the like). Celsus even refers to ulcers *of the stomach*,[169] and Pliny goes so far as to say that an ulcerated stomach (*stomachum exulceratum*) is cured by drinking milk.[170] Knowing that human dissection in Rome was almost certainly nonexistent, one is left to wonder how it was realized that ulcers can develop also in the stomach. Perhaps they were seen only (and it can be done) with that tool that the Greeks and the Hindus liked to use, the "eye of the mind."[171]

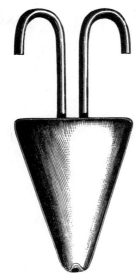

9.14 The spoon of Diokles for extracting barbed arrowheads, as drawn in 1880 from the description of Celsus, before an actual specimen had been found. The perspective is somewhat misleading: visualize the object not as a solid cone, but as a hollow spoon.

9.15 The spoon of Diokles (left, about one-half actual size) and how it worked (right). From a bronze specimen.

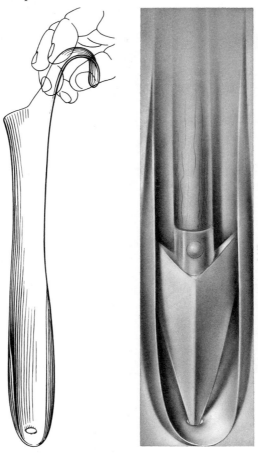

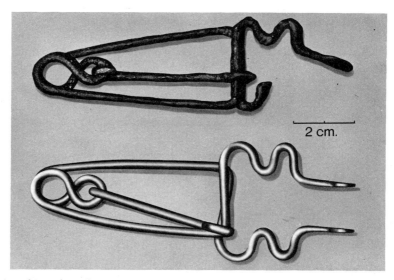

9.16 An object found in a Roman camp (above), which has been reconstructed (below) and interpreted as a "vein clamp." From Saalburg, Germany, second–third century A.D.

Celsus on Hemorrhage

This is how Celsus describes the basic problems of a wounded patient: "When a man has been wounded who can be saved, there are in the first place two things to be kept in mind: that he should not die from hemorrhage or inflammation."[172] Perfect: even Hippocrates is not as clear on this point. For "inflammation," of course, read "infection." Now see how Celsus deals with each problem. First, the bleeding:

If we are afraid of haemorrhage which can be judged both from the position and size of the wound and from the force of the flowing blood, the wound is to be filled with dry lint, and over that a sponge applied, squeezed out of cold water, and pressed down by the hand. If the bleeding is not checked thus, the lint must be changed several times, and if it is not effective when dry, it is to be soaked in vinegar.[173]

All this is essentially Hippocratic. Pliny adds wisely that "old sponges do not close wounds."[174] Celsus continues:

Vinegar is powerful in suppressing a flow of blood; and some, therefore, pour it into wounds. But then there is an underlying fear of another kind, that if too much diseased matter is forcibly retained in the wound it will afterwards cause great inflammation [*namely, if you suppress a healthy outflow of blood, the retained blood will become pus: Hippocrates again*]. It is on this account that no use is made, either of corrosives or of caustics, owing to the crust they induce, although most of these medicaments suppress bleeding; but if for once recourse is had to them, choose those which have a milder action. But if even these are powerless against the profuse bleeding, [*and now comes something quite new*] THE VEINS THAT ARE POURING OUT BLOOD ARE TO BE SEIZED, AND ROUND THE WOUNDED SPOT THEY ARE TO BE TIED IN TWO PLACES, and cut across in between, so that each end may retract on itself, and yet have its orifice closed.[175]

MEDICVS

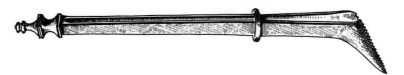

9.17 Forceps closed by a sliding ring, another Roman tool that could have been used to pinch bleeding vessels. This one is from Great Britain; one like it was found in Pompeii. Two-thirds actual size.

9.18 Pompeian forceps, which could very well be the one that Celsus had in mind when he wrote: "The veins, that are pouring out blood, should be seized." The detail (right) shows its serrated edge, as in the modern hemostatic forceps. About one-half actual size.

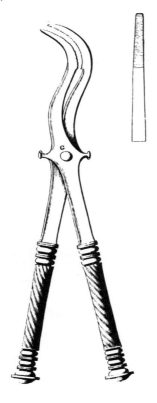

Surgery has finally learned its lesson from plumbing, probably thanks to the Alexandrian scientists. This is what allows Celsus to explain, for the first time, how to amputate a leg, on which occasion he even omits to mention the blood vessels, taking it for granted that they will be tied off.[176]

Presumably this was done with a special forceps. The difficulty here is to identify the right gadget among the many possible ones that have come to light. One of the candidates looks more like a clasp for the daily mail (Fig. 9.16). Whatever it is, I doubt it could be used as a hemostat. Much more likely is that variety of forceps which is closed by a sliding ring (Fig. 9.17). Another possibility is the well-known Pompeian instrument (Fig. 9.18) which looks like the *bec de corbin* that Ambroise Paré invented 1500 years later "to stanch the bleeding when the member is taken off" (Fig. 9.19).[177] But the

MEDICVS

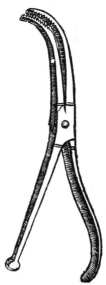

9.19 A "new kind" of forceps devised by Ambroise Paré in the 1500s: "The Crows-beak fit to draw the Vessels forth of the flesh, wherein they lie hid, that so they may be tied or bound fast." Under the name of *bec de corbin* (crow's beak) Paré grouped several types of curved forceps; this one was for seizing vessels.

9.20 Gallo-Roman surgical forceps, which locks automatically when closed (below), like the modern hemostatic forceps. First–third century A.D.

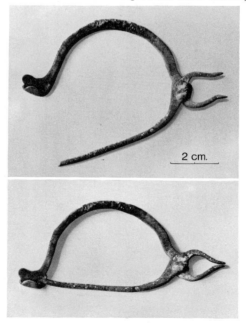

2 cm.

prize find belonged to one of the so-called Gallo-Roman "oculists"[178] and operates on the principle of the modern surgical hemostat (Fig. 9.20).

When circumstances did not allow for tying the bleeding *vena*, Celsus says that "it can be burnt with a red-hot iron." Or else, "apply a [suction] cup to a distant part, in order to divert thither the course [*cursus*] of the blood." There were good reasons to give this method last: it could not possibly work.

Note that Celsus always speaks of bleeding *venae;* he still has in mind that arteries contain air.[179]

Bleeding and inflammation in a wound, in the mind of a modern surgeon, are about as unrelated as leak and a fire on board, in the mind of a skipper; but the Greeks, obsessed with the notion that blood is attracted around the wound and causes inflammation, felt that bleeding *protected* the wound against inflammation. If one remembers this, the following passage of Celsus becomes understandable:

> Against bleeding there is help in the foregoing measures; but against inflammation it lies simply in the bleeding itself. Inflammation is to be feared when a bone is injured or sinew or cartilage or muscle, or whenever there is little outflow of blood compared to the wound. Therefore, in such cases, it will not be desirable to suppress the bleeding early, but to let blood flow as long as it is safe; so that if there seems too little bleeding, blood should be let from the arm as well, at any rate when the patient is young and robust and used to exercise, and much more so when a drinking bout has preceded the wound [*back to the awful practice of bleeding the wounded*].
>
> Now, when bleeding has been suppressed if excessive, or encouraged when not enough has escaped of itself, then by far the best thing is for the wound to become agglutinated.[180]

In other words: once the wound has bled, let it heal (rather than keeping it open to let the bad humors drain out). This wiser choice is stated much more emphatically than in the Hippocratic books.

Celsus on Closing Wounds

To close a wound, "there are two treatments. For if the wound is in a soft part, it should be stitched up, and particularly when the cut is in the tip of the ear or the point of the nose or forehead or cheek or eyelid or lip or the skin over the throat or abdomen."[181] Stitching has become much more commonplace. As in Greece, it is recommended mostly for the face. For very fine work, as on the eyelids, Celsus recommends the hair of a woman[182]—a method that has only just died away: the last Deaconess sister to provide her hair for corneal sutures still works at the University Eye Clinic in Geneva (her hair is no longer requested, but I understand that it served the purpose quite well[183]).

Celsus continues:

> But if the wound is in the flesh, and gapes, and its margins are not easily drawn together, then stitching is unsuitable; fibulae (the Greeks call them *anctéres*) are then to be inserted, which draw together the margins to some extent and so render the subsequent scar less broad.[184]

Closing wounds with metal pins, *fibulae,* must have been introduced sometime during the four hundred years since Hippocrates—a rather late development, since the method is used among primitive peoples. The very fact that Celsus feels compelled to quote the technical name of *ancteres* points to a

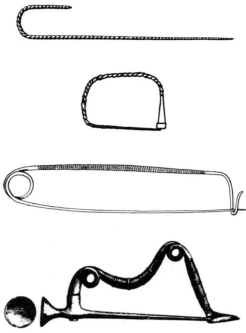

9.21 Stages in the evolution from pin to safety pin (from top). All these shapes were called *fibulae* in Latin. Greek and Mycenaean specimens.

9.22 The simplest fibulae were nothing but small skewers. For surgical sutures they were used essentially as shown here; the tips were snipped off for safety. From a French manual of 1858.

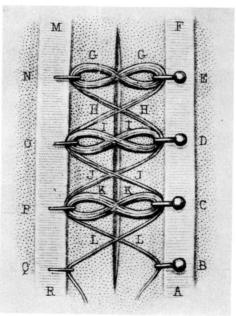

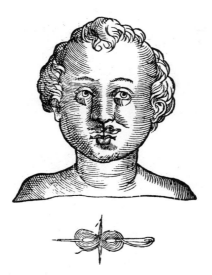

9.23 The same principle as used by Ambroise Paré in 1564 to close a harelip. Here a threaded needle serves as fibula (see detail).

Greek or Alexandrian import, and a useful one too. Fibulae as clothespins must be as old as clothes.[185] In classical Greece and Rome they had evolved to complex safety pins, but these seem to have stayed out of surgery except for fixing the ends of a bandage (Fig. 9.21). Those used for sutures were the simplest, being essentially small skewers (Fig. 9.22), and lasted until recently for the correction of harelip, another facial operation (Fig. 9.23).

Now from the above it can be gathered also whether flesh which is hanging free at one part and attached at another,—if it is still capable of juncture,—demands suture or fibula. But neither of these should be inserted until the interior of the wound has been cleansed, lest some blood-clot be left in it. For blood clot turns into pus [*Celsus really knows his Hippocrates*] and excites inflammation, and prevents agglutination of the wound. Not even lint which has been inserted to arrest bleeding should be left in, for this also inflames the wound [*tweezers handy for picking out foreign bodies came in a variety of shapes; Fig. 9.24*]. The suture or fibula should take up, not only skin but also some of the underlying flesh, where there is any . . . Neither procedure needs any force . . . Generally . . . fibulae leave the wound wider open, a suture joins the margins together, but these should not be brought actually into contact throughout the whole length of the wound, in order that there may be an outlet for any humour collecting within [*this is surgical drainage in its simplest form, already hinted in the Egyptian papyri; the Hippocratic idea of a tin tube apparently failed to catch on*]. If any wound admits of neither of these[*suture or fibula*] it should none the less be cleaned. Hence, upon every wound there is to be applied, first a sponge squeezed out of vinegar; or out of wine if the patient cannot bear the strength of vinegar.[186]

MEDICVS

Vinegar is very painful indeed. The closing comment is beautifully chosen: *"And a wound can be treated without foreign and far-fetched and complicated medicaments."*

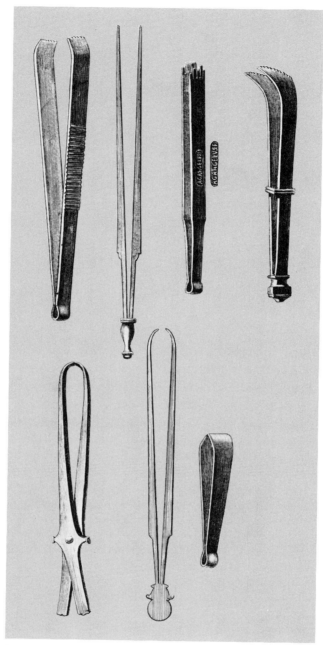

9.24 Various kinds of tweezers found at Pompeii and Herculaneum. One is marked AGATH[AN]GELUS F[ECIT], "made by Agathangelus"—a Greek name.

To judge from the number of ancient wound-plasters, few were those who appreciated this great truth; it should have been engraved in marble, in the verses of Ovid:

> Curando fieri quaedam majora videmus
> vulnera, quae melius non tetigisse fuerit

> We see wounds grow larger by being treated,
> Which would have done better untouched.[187]

Roman Antiseptic Wound-Dressings

The text just quoted continues, for the sake of those who prefer aggressive treatments: "But if any one has not confidence in this treatment, a medicament should be put on, which has no suet in its composition, chosen from those which I have stated to be suitable for bleeding wounds [*the Greek enhemes*] and especially, if it is a flesh wound, the composition called barbarum."[188]

Here is the formula for barbarum, in metric equivalents:[189]

Copper acetate (*scraped verdigris*)	48 gm		oil	250 cc
Lead oxide (*litharge*)	80 "			
Alum	4 "	Mix with		
Dried pitch	4 "		vinegar	250 cc
Dried pine resin	4 "			

Mixed in my laboratory, these ingredients gave a murky, brownish lotion. No need for tests to recognize it as an antiseptic.

This is no accident: Celsus prescribes antiseptics with unmistakable purpose. For wounds he has a list of thirty-four plasters and ointments, all but five of which contain heavy doses of lead and copper salts, and those five, according to Celsus, are especially meant to produce pus.[190] Alum, mercury, and antimony sulphides are also used; the main excipients are resins, pitch, bitumen, wax, oil, and vinegar; and the doses of antiseptic salts are generous indeed, up to ½ or ⅔ of the mixture. An example:

Lead acetate (*cerussa*)	
Lead oxide (*litharge*)	
Antimony sulphide (*stibium*)	equal parts[191]
Wax	
Suet	

With this we reach the height of antiseptic treatment in antiquity—though not without danger, because antiseptics like mercury and lead salts are also anti-people; and Celsus knew it. He gives an "antidote" for poisoning with *cerussa*, lead acetate.[192] And Pliny says of cinnabar (mercuric sulphide) and red-lead (lead carbonate) that, as they are "admitted to be poisons, all the current instructions on employment for medicinal purposes are in my opinion decidedly risky."[193]

Although the amount of lead absorbed through a wound may have been relatively small, the hazard of saturnism was great for the Romans, because they took in lead from several other sources.[194] If they could afford running water, they drank the lead of their plumbing; they definitely sipped it with their wine. A current wine preservative was made with must, which Columella recommends to boil in leaden vessels, because "brazen vessels throw off copper-rust and spoil the flavor."[195] Pliny agrees.[196] More danger came from cosmetics: ladies smeared lead-white on their faces and dusted it onto their hair.[197]

The use of metallic compounds—including rust—on wounds was featured in the myth, popular in Pliny's days, of Achilles treating the wound of Telephos with scrapings from the tip of his lance, "whether he did it with a bronze or an iron spearhead"[198] (Fig. 9.25). Copper acetate (verdigris) was not as dangerous as the lead salts; it gave its green color to several wound-drugs recommended by Celsus and Pliny. An intriguing explanation for this use of copper is offered in Pliny's *Natural History:* "Copper ores and mines supply medicaments in a variety of ways; inasmuch as in their neighbourhood all kinds of ulcers are healed with the greatest rapidity."[199] I wish I knew whether this had any basis in fact. The text continues, "yet the most beneficial is *cadmea,*" which is silicate and carbonate of zinc. Zinc happens to be one of the latest fashions in wound treatment,[200] but it seems that the beneficial effect, if any, is quite small.[201]

For myself, I would probably choose the antiseptic dressing that Celsus recommends for cleansing old sores: *tincta in melle linamenta.*[202] Readers not familiar with Latin will be proud to recognize this wound dressing if I translate it into Egyptian hieroglyphs:

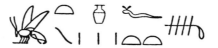

byt and *ftt,* honey and lint, here reappearing a couple of thousand years later![203]

In content as well as in form, there has been progress since Hippocrates; but the road is still long. In the crystal bowl of Celsian Latin you will be served an occasional piece of dung. The thirty-four caustics of Celsus include not only quicklime, cantharides, salt, and pepper, but also salamander ash and dung of lizard, pigeon, wood-pigeon, swallow, and sheep.[204] His drugs for "closing a wound" include myrrh, white wine, and vinegar, but also eggwhite, pounded snails, and cobwebs.[205] And pain may call for poppy-tears,[206] but for headache the opium is soaked in bread—and worn like a hat.[207]

Birth of the Four Cardinal Signs

Thus far, on the subject of inflamed wounds, I have been discussing the practice of Celsus; tradition requires that I also mention his theory about inflammation—or rather his single line about it. Words for "inflammation" had existed ever since the Akkadian ⟨glyph⟩ *ummu* and the Egyptian ⟨glyph⟩ *shememet,* but nobody had ever bothered, it seems, to define its clinical symptoms. History assigned that role to Celsus.

The famous Celsian passage actually applies only to that variety of inflammation—perhaps the commonest—which is technically known as "acute" and which a layman might consider "typical" (good examples being a boil or an infected wound). Perhaps Celsus lifted his definition from some other work; perhaps he drew it out of his own pen. One thing is sure: on the day that he wrote it he was being assisted by Fortuna, the blindfolded goddess. For

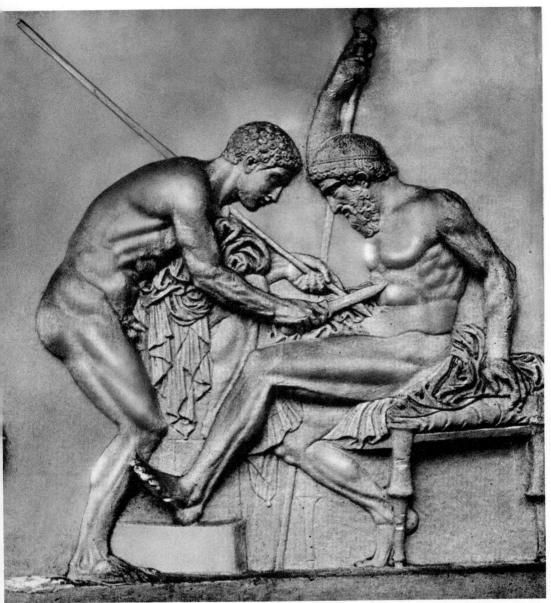

9.25 Achilles treats the war-wound of Telephos with scrapings off his lance. Both "iron rust" and "bronze rust" were supposed to be good for cleansing sores. Telephos was a Mysian wounded in the thigh by Achilles on his way to Troy. The oracle predicted that the wound would not heal except by the lance of Achilles; hence the reconciliation. Rust was recommended for sores much as was verdigris. Pliny agrees but finds it strange that iron should be good for wounds, since "it is with iron that wounds are chiefly made." Pliny could actually have seen this bas-relief, which was buried in Herculaneum in 79 A.D.

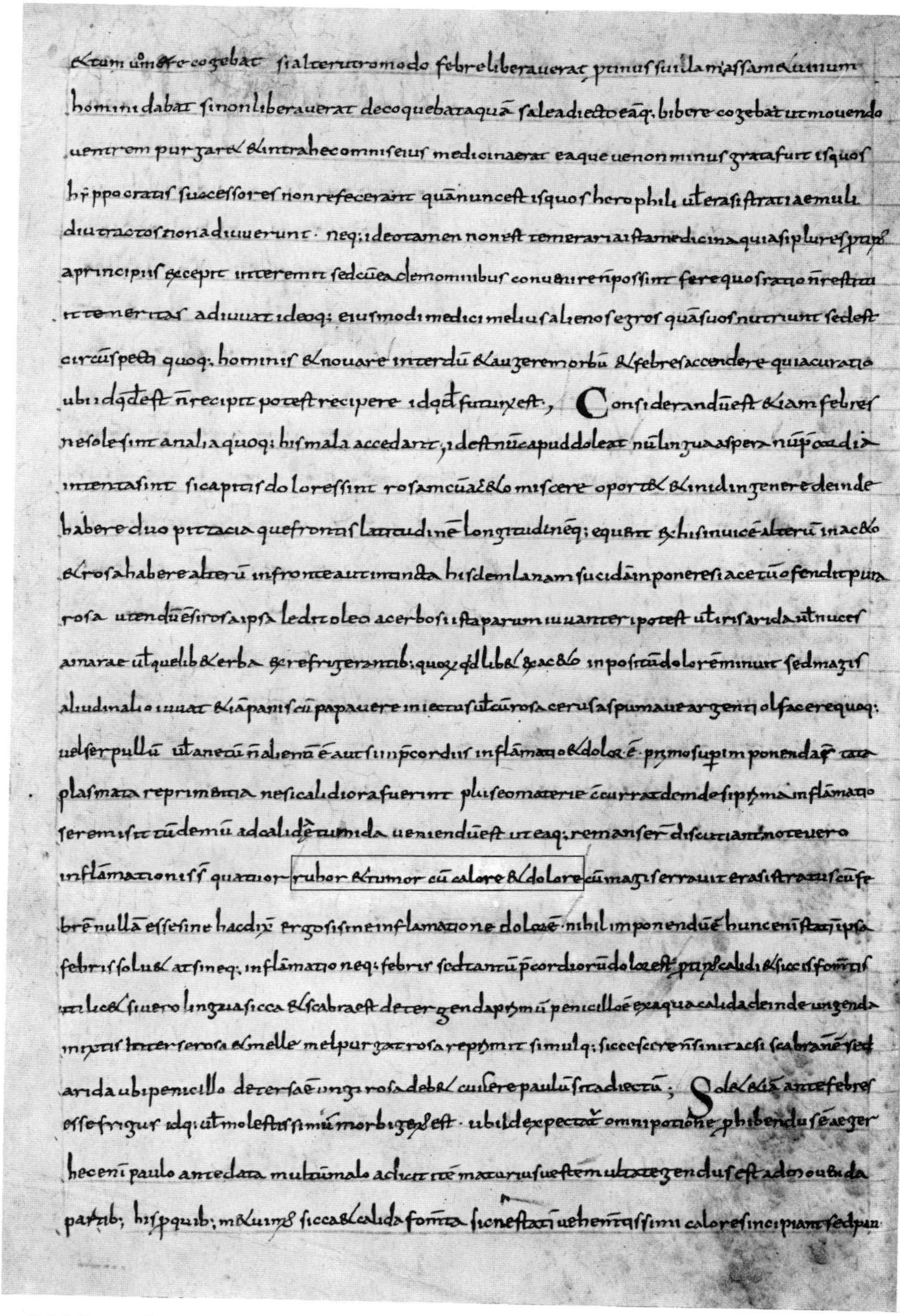

9.26 In tenth century handwriting, the page of *De medicina* that mentions the four cardinal signs of inflammation (box).

he buried it in a paragraph that I find singularly obscure, I daresay un-Celsian (Fig. 9.26):

> But if there is inflammation and pain in the chest, the first thing is to apply to it repressing plasters, lest more diseased matter should gather there, if hotter ones were

applied; next, when the primary inflammation has subsided, and not before, we must go on to hot and moist plasters, in order to disperse what remains of the matter. Now the signs of an inflammation are four: redness and swelling with heat and pain. Over this Erasistratus greatly erred, when he said that no fever occurred apart from inflammation. Therefore if there is pain without inflammation, nothing is to be put on: for the actual fever at once will dissolve the pain. But if there is neither inflammation nor fever, but just pain in the chest, it is allowable to use hot and dry foments from the first.[208]

"Redness and swelling with heat and pain:" if there is one item of information common to all medical students alive (at least in the so-called West), it is that the signs of acute inflammation are four: *rubor et tumor cum calore et dolore* (Fig. 9.27). Deservedly so, for it would be difficult to improve on these four "cardinal signs," which evoke so succinctly the clinical picture.

Notice that Celsus, despite pages and pages on inflamed wounds, slips in his great definition in a context that nowadays seems entirely irrelevant: he is discussing a disease that causes pain *inside the chest*, presumably pleuritis. No modern medical writer would dream of using this as an example of disease that causes a visible inflammation of the skin. But things were different before the advent of antibiotics: pus that had accumulated in the pleural cavity could "come to a head" through the skin (hence the Greek operation for empyema). This is the course of events that Celsus must have in mind when he mentions "repressing plasters" to prevent matter from "gathering" in the skin, in cases of chest pain.

Whatever Celsus had in mind, posterity swept away the fog, rescued the line, and raised it to the status of a medical slogan. Quite a success for Celsus the encyclopedist, who may have been no more a physician than he was a beekeeper, a general, or a grammarian.

I would propose for second prize another beautiful Celsian definition. Granted that *rubor, tumor, calor, dolor* are the signs of acute inflammation, what is the meaning of *acute*? Medical students today learn that it implies a quick pace; the Oxford dictionary says "coming sharply to a crisis" (be it a good or bad crisis). When Celsus says *acutus*, he means exactly the same. He

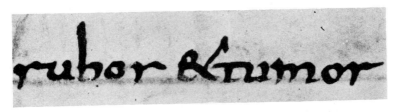
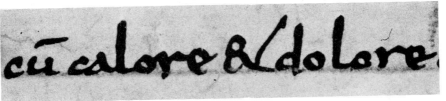

9.27 Detail: RUBOR ET TUMOR CUM CALORE ET DOLORE, "redness and swelling with heat and pain."

explains the condition with classic elegance but in more concrete terms: acute diseases are those that *cito vel tollunt hominem, vel ipsi cito finiuntur*—"either finish the man quickly, or finish quickly themselves."[209]

Rome's Debt to Indian Medicine

Historical clichés do make life easier, at least for the historian. One of them is to brush off Roman medicine, Celsus and all, as a product of Greek thought. I will submit that this is grossly unfair, at least to the Hindus.

Consider that while Celsus was buying up new scrolls of papyrus for his *De medicina,* or maybe a couple of generations later while Pliny was gazing at the mushroom cloud of Vesuvius, Charaka in India was revising the ancient medical treatise of Agnivesa. Buddha's message had already rung for six hundred years; India had long since shrugged off the Persian and then the short-lived Greek rule; the great Mauryan Empire had come and gone, leaving Ashoka but a memory; and waves of invaders had since poured into the plains through the same old gaps in the northwest. But in the meantime, communication with the Mediterranean world had grown to an established trade. All over the Indian peninsula, local merchants—following the ancient Indian custom of burying treasure[210]—were looking for places to hoard their Roman gold and silver coins (Fig. 9.28). No longer was there anything unusual about the gentleman in Virapatnam who treated his guests to Tuscan wine (bits of his amphorae are there to prove it[211]), or about the Pompeian gentleman who drilled a hole in the head of a little Indian statue, perhaps to make a handle for his wife's mirror (Fig. 9.29).[212] Pliny himself shows how close India had become when he describes it as a huge country, covering "one third of the entire surface of the earth," and extremely populous, the Indians being "almost the only race that has never migrated from its own territory." Its people were known to be "divided into many classes . . . there is a fifth class of persons devoted to wisdom, which is held in high honour . . . and almost elevated into a religion."[213] India was also teaming with marvels, most of them legendary, like the people of the umbrella-foot tribe, who in hot weather lay down on their backs, enjoying the shade of their huge feet; or the Imavi Mountains (the Himalayas), inhabited by people unable to breathe in another climate.[214] But some marvels were true, like the wool that grew on trees (cotton), or the fish that crawled out of the rivers (*Anabas scandens* does exactly that).[215]

The average Roman had more contact with India than does the average Italian nowadays with, say, Canada or Peru. The use of Indian pepper had become commonplace; there had even been attempts to import and grow the pepper plant.[216] For reasons that I do not know, segments of huge Indian bamboo canes were a common sight in Roman temples.[217] Painters used an Indian black and the beautiful purple *indigo*.[218] Wealthy Romans bought Indian pearls.[219] When they spiced their warm wine with expensive *malabathrum* they were actually using two Sanskrit words, *tamala pâtra,* "cinnamon leaves."[220] Some may have ploughed through Strabo's *Geography* far

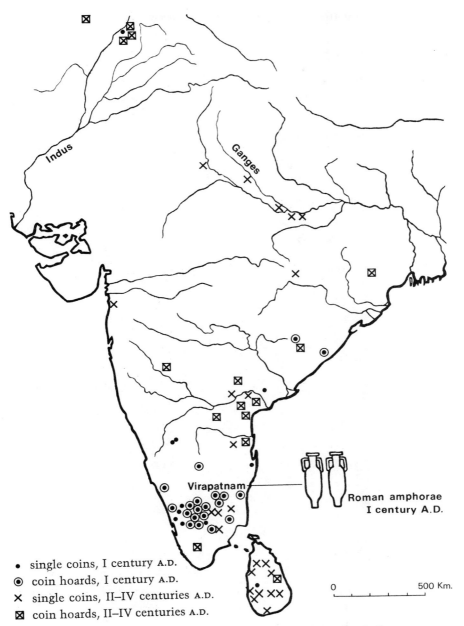

Roman amphorae
I century A.D.

0 ⸺ 500 Km.

9.28 Distribution of ancient Roman coins and amphorae found in India.

enough to reach Book 15 on India; for the adventurous who could afford to go there in person, using the newly discovered monsoons, it was advisable to have a party of archers on board, on account of the pirates.[221] Yet the trip had become common enough to warrant publication of a sort of guidebook, called *The Tour of the Indian Ocean,* written by an old salt who had obviously been there.[222]

Under these conditions, it would be strange indeed if no Indian medicine had found its way to Rome. In fact, so many *medicamenta* came from India that Pliny complains about it. Arabia and India, he writes, are

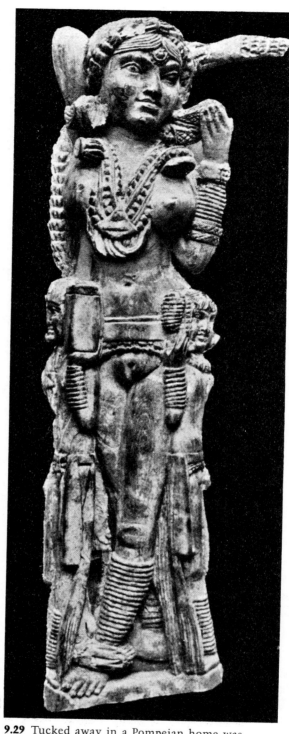

9.29 Tucked away in a Pompeian home was Lakshmi, Indian goddess of beauty and happiness. Carved ivory, height 25cm.

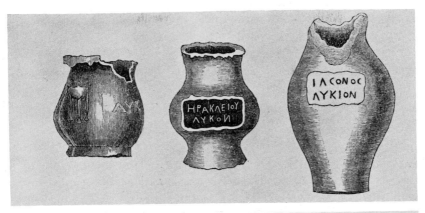

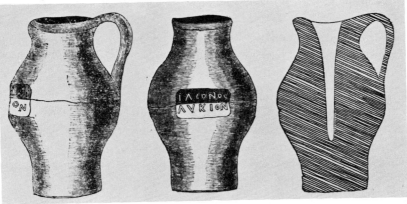

9.30 Tiny pots of eye salve, labeled LYKION (misspelled at top); this is their actual size. The best lycium came from India and was very costly; hence the small capacity of the pots (bottom right). Probably from Taranto, Southern Italy.

supposed to be storehouses of remedies, and nobody looks into his own kitchen garden.[223] The reputation of these drugs was high, for even Pliny had to admit that only one commodity imported from India, myrrh, was of worse quality than that of other countries.[224] Perhaps the most popular Indian drug was *lycium*, a plant extract used especially for eye troubles.

The only medical vases of Greco-Roman times that have come down to us with a label are tiny containers of the precious *lýkion* (Fig. 9.30). There was also a Greek variety, but the best was by far the Indian.[225]

When a drug is imported, it is not only the substance but also the idea that travels. Lycium was an Indian eye medicine, and as such, it was still in use in the 1800s.[226] So here is a definite example of Indian medical practice in Celsian Rome. Of course, not all that came from India was worth the trip; lycium itself may have been perfectly dreadful for the eyes. The point I am making here is that Indian imports existed. For variety, I will now propose an example of a different sort—one that looks to me like typical imported Indian nonsense.

In the year 19 A.D. Germanicus, legate of Emperor Tiberius, came down in Antioch (Syria) with a mysterious illness. He was sure that he was being slowly poisoned by his enemy Piso, legate to Syria, and he may have been right. When he died, his body was burned on the pyre, as was customary; but those who came to collect the remains found that the heart lay "intact between the bones." Suetonius, who records the event, comments: "it is said that this organ cannot be consumed by fire, when it is soaked with poison."[227] Now the tale of poisoned hearts not burning in fire is mentioned by Sushruta.[228] Most likely the Syrians knew this bit of Indian lore and passed it on to their Roman bosses, who took it seriously enough to discuss it in the trial that followed. Piso seems to have defended himself by submitting the notion (on what evidence is not reported) that *all* sick hearts resist fire, not only those that have been poisoned.[229] Once again, nonsense—but it serves to show how Indian medical ideas, good or bad, could travel across the Roman Empire.

As regards surgery, Celsus does not acknowledge any debt to the land of Buddha; we have to read between the lines. In looking among the surgical novelties since Hippocrates—significant, useful novelties—I find at least three that smack of India.

The first is the operation for cataract. "Couching the cataract" is the established term for the procedure described by Celsus. *Couching* comes from the French *coucher*, "to lay down." The purpose of this operation is to push down and out of the way the crystalline lens in the eye when it has become opaque (Fig. 9.31). This is accomplished with a needle, a lancet, or even a thorn, stabbed sideways into the edge of the cornea; the pain is reported as minimal.[230] If infection does not occur, some vision is restored—even excellent vision if the patient happens to be also extremely shortsighted.[231] It is a bold and tricky operation, which appears suddenly in Celsus.[232] Charaka remarks that there are ninety-six diseases of the eye, but he refrains from discussing them because "full descriptions are laid down in treatises of

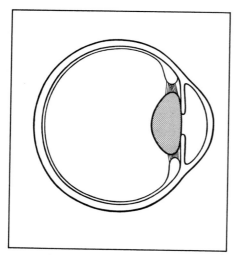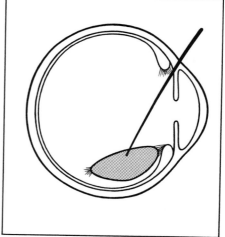

9.31 Steps in the operation for "couching" the cataract. When the crystalline lens in the eye becomes clouded (left), the lens is tilted over with the aid of a needle inserted behind the iris (right), like a lid on a horizontal hinge, or is sometimes pushed down completely free. This was most likely an Indian invention.

surgery, together with the methods of treatment."[233] We just have to turn to the classic Hindu treatise of surgery, Sushruta's, and there are the promised descriptions; the chapter on eye diseases is at least four times as long as in *De medicina*, and the operation for cataract is given in much the same terms, including the advice to pierce the right eye with the left hand, and vice versa.[234] Of course, the priority for the discovery of cataract-couching rests, as usual, on the hazy dates of Indian history; but if my tentative dates are right, this was an Indian, not an Alexandrian discovery. Until very recently it was a part of Indian folk medicine.[235]

Another surgical advance that recalls India is plastic surgery. Of this, too, there is no hint in the Hippocratic books. The main example of plastic surgery in Celsus is a simple pattern of incisions suitable for repairing a large gap in the skin.[236] The basic idea is to carve out two pedicle flaps pointing toward each other, and then to draw them together (Fig. 9.32). This is nowhere nearly as imaginative as the Indian pedicle flap, twisted down from the forehead to make a new nose. It rather looks as if the lesson of Sushruta had not quite come through.

Oddly enough, Celsus also mentions two ways to handle perforated earlobes.[237] If "a man, for instance" wants to get rid of the holes, it is enough to cauterize their edges; thereafter it is easy to make them grow together. "But if the hole is enlarged, as is usually the case with those who have worn heavy ear-rings, the part of the lobule that is in excess should be incised, and the edges above should be made raw with a scalpel. Then the wound is sewn up and covered with a drug that will promote healing." The description is not too clear; I see it as in Fig. 9.33. But again it does not equal Sushruta's reconstruction of a lost earlobe.

On this subject, I was quite surprised to find men in Rome who would perforate and stretch their earlobes. It sounded so unlikely for a people of warriors. However, in searching for documents about perforated ears in antiquity,[238] and in ancient men, I came across this passage in the Old Testament:

THE LORD SAID TO MOSES, Say this to the Israelites . . . These are the laws you shall set before them:
When you buy a Hebrew slave, he shall be your slave for six years, but in the seventh year he shall go free and pay nothing . . .
But if the slave should say, "I love my master, my wife, and my children; I will not go free," then his master shall bring him to God: he shall bring him to the door or the door-post, and his master shall pierce his ear with an awl, and the man shall be his slave for life.[239]

Now going back to the passage of Celsus about the man with perforated ears to whom the holes suddenly "become offensive" (*offendunt*), I believe I can piece together a human drama: not the story of a vain young man who wants to keep pace with fashion, but that of a slave become a freedman, who wants to erase the physical traces of his past.

Surgical operations of this kind were not unknown in Rome during the

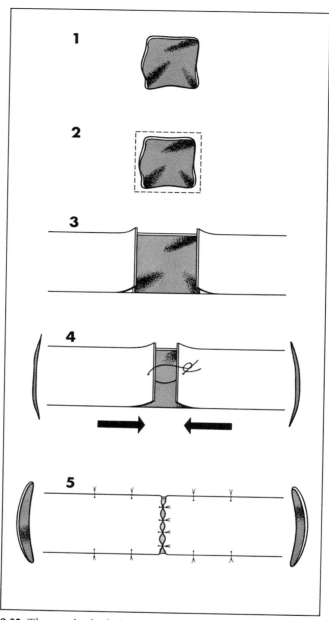

9.32 The method of plastic surgery described by Celsus for covering a large gap in the skin. (1) A skin lesion that needs to be remedied, such as a sore which refuses to heal. (2) The edge of the sore is cut out so as to leave a regular square. (3) The upper and lower cuts are prolonged horizontally, so as to define two flaps, which are dissected free and lifted. (4) The flaps are drawn together; if stretching is excessive, a curved cut is made at the root of each flap. (5) Flaps are sewn in final position.

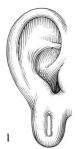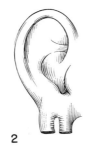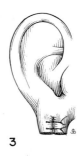

9.33 The method described by Celsus for closing up a hole in an earlobe, for people who "change their mind." This is real plastic surgery, although not as advanced as that of the Indians (Fig. 7.22). (1) An earlobe with a large hole. (2) The lobe is cut shorter and the stumps are scraped raw. (3) They are sewed together.

first century A.D. Martial mentions a certain Cinna, a barber, who was an expert in removing brand-marks from ex-slaves, a practice already mentioned in Hammurabi's Code eighteen centuries earlier (p. 43, law 226).[240] Plastic surgery and psychology are allies of old.

The third surgical novelty in Celsus—not mentioned in the Hippocratic books, but treated extensively in both Hindu classics—is the treatment for snake bite. Celsus says:

> The ancients had very various methods . . . for each kind of snake . . . but in all it is the same measures which are most efficacious. Therefore first the limb is to be constricted above this kind of wound, but not too tightly, lest it become numbed; next, the poison is to be drawn out. A cup does this best. But it is not amiss beforehand to make incisions with a scalpel around the wound, in order that more of the vitiated blood may be extracted. If there is no cup at hand . . . a man must be got to suck the wound. I declare there is no particular science in those people who are called Psylli, but a boldness confirmed by experience. For serpent's poison, like certain hunter's poisons, such as the Gauls in particular use, does no harm when swallowed, but only in a wound . . . Anyone, therefore, who follows the example of the Psylli and sucks out the wound, will himself be safe, and will promote the safety of the patient. He must see to it, however, beforehand that he has no sore place on his gums or palate or other parts of the mouth.[241]

The Psylli were an African people with a reputation as snake charmers.[242] Celsus quotes them in relation to the sucking technique, but he does not indicate where he learned about the ligature. Certainly not from Hippocrates; I suspect from India, where snake bite was a daily concern.[243]

Celsus mentions India only in passing, as a source of nard.[244] He probably did not realize that some of his *medicina* was Indian.

Roman Army Hospitals

It is high time to visit the Roman army and see how it dealt with casualties. In the heroic days of the forefathers, when regular doctors were not yet around (let alone hospitals), Rome had a very practical way of dealing with wounded soldiers. Livy tells that in 480 B.C., after a victory over the Etruscans, the consul Manlius, remembering "that policy which he had adopted in the

beginnings of his consulship, of winning the affections of the plebs . . .
billeted the wounded soldiers on the patricians, to be cared for. To the Fabii
[*a prominent family*] he assigned the largest number, nor did they anywhere
receive greater attention." Livy points out that this was a good political investment: "For this the Fabii now began to enjoy the favour of the people, nor was
this end achieved by aught but a demeanour wholesome for the State."[245]
After another battle, even enemies were "quartered among the citizens . . .
until their wounds were healed."[246]

This manner of dealing with mass casualties was revived in the time of
Celsus, when a major catastrophe hit the town of Fidenae, five miles from
Rome—major enough to recall the emperor from his retreat in Capri. It was
27 A.D. when one Attilius, determined to become popular cheaply and on a
large scale, offered the city a gladiatorial contest in a rickety amphitheater
that he had built for the purpose, on unsafe ground. The structure collapsed,
and over 20,000 people were killed or injured.[247] Tacitus sets the figure at
50,000. Wealthy homes, he says, opened their doors to the wounded, and
Rome was a sorry sight, recalling the old days when citizens, in the aftermath
of battle, used to care for the wounded.[248]

The method worked as long as battles remained close to home; when the
frontiers expanded, sending the wounded back to Rome became unthinkable.
They had to be kept at the camp. But sharing quarters with the casualties
could be too much to bear even for the tough Roman legionaries.[249] After a
battle with the Samnites in 294 B.C., "the soldiers were dispirited; all night
long they had been kept awake by the groans of the wounded and the dying.
Had the enemy attacked the camp before daylight, their fear would have been
so great as to cause them to desert their ranks; as it was, they were . . . as good
as beaten."

Eventually, Roman generals afield were obliged to provide special quarters for the sick and wounded, the *valetudinaria*. Remains of at least twenty-
five have been found; they are all strung out along the frontier, from Scotland
to Palestine (Fig. 9.34), another proof that they were born of a military need,
as "islands of hope" at the limits of the empire.[250] *Limes*, "the limit," was the
actual name of the frontier; life at the outposts there, weeks and months from
home, must have been an exercise in loneliness (Fig. 9.35).

MEDICVS

Most of the known valetudinaria sprang up during the first and second
centuries A.D. The larger ones, typical of the legionary fortresses, were all
built on the same plan (Fig. 9.36), possibly derived from an earlier layout of
tents along the sides of a rectangle.[251] This standard plan identifies the
hospital at a glance on the map of a Roman camp (Fig. 9.37). In its simpler
version the plan corresponds to a single row of small rooms around the sides
of the rectangular court; in the more complex version, illustrated here, the
buildings are deep enough to have a central corridor running all the way
around the quadrangle, with small rooms on either side. Auxiliary forts had
smaller hospitals, built of timber. They were rectangular, with a corridor
running from one end to the other, and small cubicles on both sides,
resembling one wing of the larger legionary hospitals.[252]

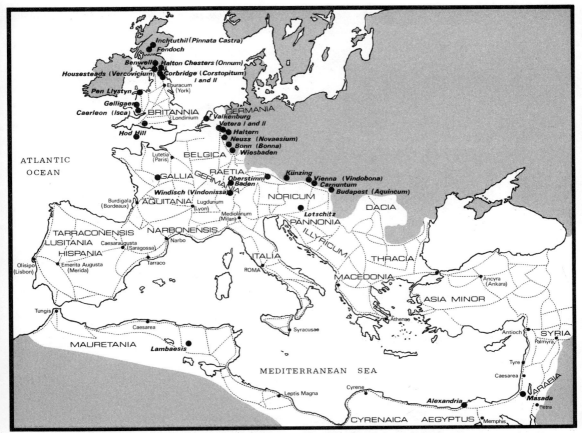

9.34 Roman military hospitals (large dots) were scattered along the borders of the empire, especially along the Rhine, the Danube, and the frontier with Scotland. None were found in Italy.

The Roman legion that was fighting the *barbari* of Scotland around 85 A.D. built a timber hospital of the larger kind at Inchtuthil (Fig. 9.37). Here the central corridor and the two flanking rows of small wards were built as separate units, each with a gabled roof (Fig. 9.38). There were sixty-four wards, one per *centuria* (company), and each could accommodate four or at most five men (Fig. 9.39), which means that the commanders were prepared for a casualty rate of 2.5 to 10 percent.[253] This camp was evacuated in haste (a hoard of almost a million precious new iron nails had to be left behind) and its buildings were dismantled. All that is left of the hospital is a large number of faint traces of holes in the ground.[254] However, the design formed by these holes is a true monument to those who planned it, being a fine example of functional architecture, rational for the patients as well as for the hospital staff.

MEDICVS

It could be argued that the small size of the wards—in depth—was a matter of structural necessity rather than of hygienic thinking, having been determined by the length of the roof's timbers. Perhaps so; but the partitions were definitely a matter of choice. Evidently the architects disliked the notion of long, narrow wards (such as those that became prevalent in much

383

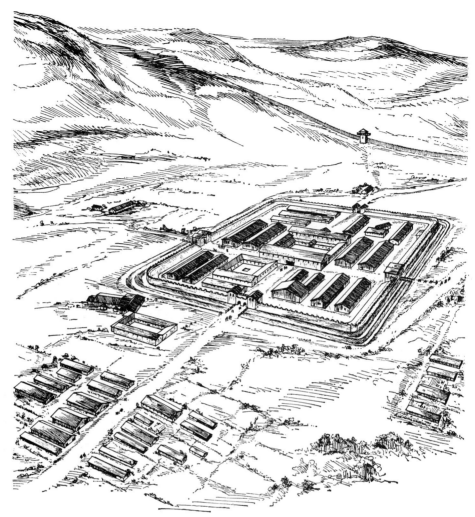

9.35 Artist's view of the Roman camp at Saalburg along the northern frontier, with the border stockade in the distance. Army hospitals were a must in this loneliness.

later days), so they cut them up lengthwise, which added to the cost, but also helped morale, fought cold and draughts, and (incidentally?) decreased the spread of infection.

MEDICVS

Medical instruments were found in several of these hospitals and actually helped to identify them as such.[255] The valetudinarium of Baden, Switzerland, yielded 120 probes and a pot of ointment: animal fat mixed with a lead salt.[256] At Novaesium (now Neuss on the Rhine) two accidents, millennia apart, added up to a wonderful stroke of luck. First, sometime during the first century A.D., fire destroyed a part of the local Roman army hospital. The roof collapsed, and that section was abandoned. Then in 1962 plans were made to lay a canal through that area, and bulldozers cut a trench two meters deep through part of the known valetudinarium. However unkindly one may look on this enterprise, near the bottom of the ditch

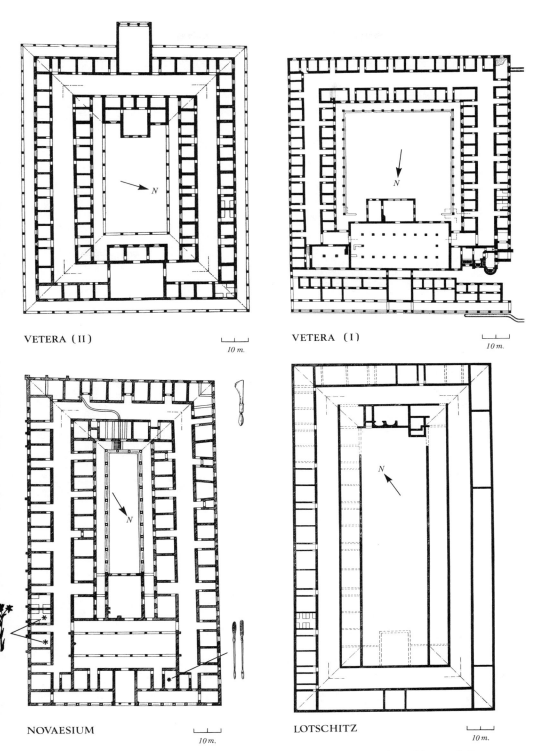

VETERA (II)

10 m.

VETERA (I)

10 m.

NOVAESIUM

10 m.

LOTSCHITZ

10 m.

9.36 Plans of four typical stone-built Roman army hospitals. Sets of partitions subdivide each wing into small wards (in the Lotschitz hospital the subdivision appears to be incomplete, but little is left of that building). Instruments and herbs were found in different parts of the Novaesium hospital, where shown.

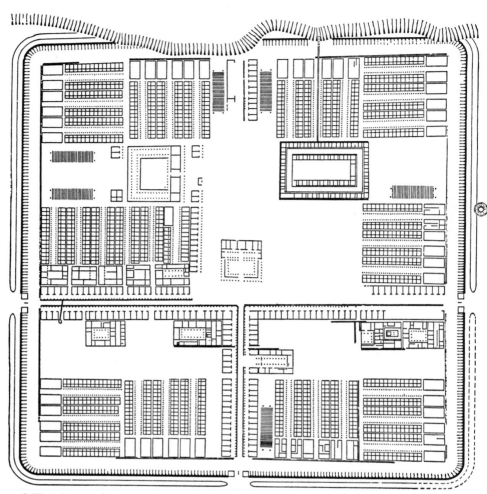

9.37 A Roman legionary fortress in Scotland, at Inchtuthil. The plan of the hospital building stands out clearly (top right).

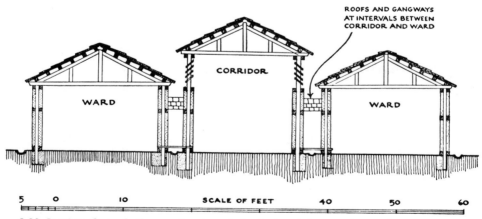

9.38 Section through the north wing of the Inchtuthil army hospital, a wooden structure.

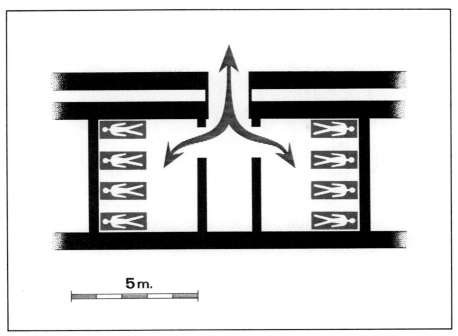

9.39 Functional scheme of the wards at the Inchtuthil hospital. Note the small rooms and rational circulation.

workers came upon a layer of carbonized material mixed with debris of roof tiles; in it were also broken pots, containing carbonized lentils and peas. Nearby was some carbonized wood—and a very black layer of fibrous material a few centimeters thick. The material was collected, dubbed "carbonized hay," and sent to be examined. Then the pipe was laid down and the ditch closed for good.[257]

The "hay," loosened in water and examined under the microscope, turned out to be something much more valuable: a stack of selected herbs, including unmistakable medicinal herbs.[258] There were, for instance, thirty-nine seeds of henbane, *Hyoscyamus niger* (Fig. 9.40). Celsus recommends them as a sedative: "some induce sleep by draughts of decoction of poppy and hyoscyamus."[259] Henbane seeds contain scopolamine, which is still used as a preanesthetic medication, inducing drowsiness and amnesia. In high doses, however, it is dangerous, recalling its close relative atropine, which received its name from Atropos, the goddess of fate who cuts the thread of life.[260]

The bulk of the material was made up of carbonized centaury, *Centaurium umbellatum Gilib.* (Fig. 9.41). For centaury, I must use the words of Pliny: "Centaury is said to have been the treatment given to Chiron [*the Centaur*] when an arrow fell on his foot as he was handling the arms of Hercules, who was his guest; for which reason some call it Chironion . . . Its power to cure wounds is so strong that even pieces of meat, they say, coalesce if they are boiled with it."[261] I did not try this experiment but cannot help wondering at the fame of centaury (Fig. 9.42). The herb is practically forgotten except as a source of "bitters:" perhaps this very taste was the cause

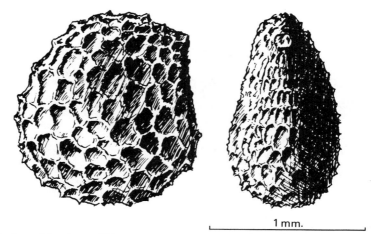

9.40 Grains of henbane (*Hyoscyamus niger*) found in the Roman hospital at Novaesium. Though dangerous, they were better than nothing for the relief of pain.

9.41 Centaury (*Centaurium umbellatum Gilib.*) was highly esteemed as a healer of wounds. This specimen was among the remains of one or two hundred centaury flowers found in a room of the Novaesium hospital.

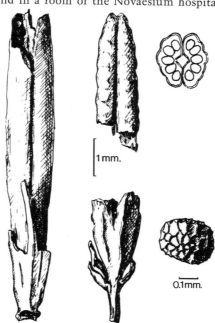

of its ancient popularity, for bitterness was somehow connected with healing properties, in Greek as well as Indian medicine.[262]

No other find like this one has ever been made in Europe, for humidity usually destroys such remains. The herbs of Novaesium were preserved because the part of the hospital where they were stored burned down; the herbs were heated, without burning, then left to carbonize in the rubble.

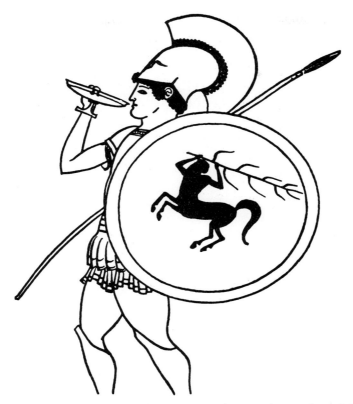

9.42 Centaury took its name from the Centaur Chiron, who taught Achilles the art of healing with herbs. Here is Chiron on the shield of Achilles. Greek amphora, c.490 B.C.

Another unique discovery was made at the Roman camp of Corbridge in Northumberland, a couple of miles south of Hadrian's Wall. Inside a wooden chest, buried under a room of the valetudinarium, was a peculiar kind of treasure: bundles of iron spearheads, several tools, several hundred nails, a block and tackle, keys, pieces of scrap metal, bronze fastenings, and other objects, often broken. Some were wrapped in cloth or leather. What could have been on the mind of those who buried this chest, why did they choose the hospital, and why did they wrap up bits of scrap metal? I am much inclined to accept the suggestion of R. W. Davies, whose arguments begin, once again, with Pliny. According to the *Natural History*, iron rust as well as verdigris are good for wounds: "Rust of iron is obtained by scraping it off old nails with an iron tool dipped in water. The effect of rust is to unite wounds and dry them and staunch them . . . For recent wounds it is useful diluted with wine and kneaded with myrrh . . . Scale of iron, obtained from a sharp edge or point . . . has an effect extremely like that of rust only more active . . . Its chief recommendation is its use in a wet plaster for cleaning wounds and fistulas."[263] So the purpose of the old chest may have been to make rust and verdigris for the hospital pharmacy.[264] As to the real effect of rust on wounds, infected or not, I have no data.

Roman Army Doctors

For lack of documents, the story of the Roman army and navy surgeons cannot be written; but it is safe to state that under the empire there was a regular medical corps.[265] At least eighty-five army physicians are recorded, mainly because they died and earned an epitaph.[266] Some of their names are Greek; the majority are Latin.

Of their lives little is known. A rare exception is Marcus, who was stationed at Alexandria about 270 A.D. One day, after a local skirmish, he took a piece of papyrus and wrote a letter to his parents, in Greek. Here is part of it:

Marcus to Antonia, Sarapion, and Cassianos[*grandfather?*], my parents, many greetings. I make obeisance toward you before the gods in the local temple, because nobody can go to make obeisance up the river, on account of the battle that has taken place between the Anoteritae [?] and the soldiers. Fifteen soldiers of the *singulares* have died, not to count the legionaries, the *evocati*, and those exhausted.

Now I am writing you to send me as fast as possible the short woollen coat that you are making, so that I may have it here. The palm trees should be watered three times, as is proper at this season . . .

And as in every letter, I write you to shake the dust off my medical books, shake it off and remove them from the window, where I left them on my departure.[267]

Most famous of the eighty-five army physicians was Dioscorides, a native of Cilicia (now Turkey), who followed Nero's army and wrote in Greek the most celebrated herbal of antiquity.

A tacit tribute to the army's foreign medics[268] may be engraved on the famous bas-relief of the Trajan Column in Rome, showing how the wounded were treated on the spot (Fig. 9.43).[269] The five men involved in the first-aid scene are all shod with *caligae*, the sandals of the Roman regulars; but there are two kinds of uniform. The two men at the left wear the armor of Roman citizens, as praetorian legionaries. The three others are dressed as auxiliaries, with the typical scarf and leather jacket; they are non-Romans. In the context of the action, this seems to suggest that blood was shed by Romans (2) as well as by foreigners (5), but that the art of healing was only in foreign hands (4, perhaps also 3).

The Romans did not develop an inferiority complex about Greek medicine, as far as I can tell. Hear Pliny: "Medicine alone of the Greek arts we serious Romans have not yet practiced; in spite of its great profits only a very few of our citizens have touched upon it."[270] The reason, in his words: *Romana gravitas.* Pliny's view of professional medicine must have been low indeed to make him say that the Romans were too serious to join it.

Civilian Infirmaries

Back in the Eternal City there were no hospitals at all; or more precisely, there are no remains, and no records, of any army hospital in Rome. As for civilians—what might have happened, for instance, to a citizen who had been run over by a cart?[271] Anybody who could afford it would surely be taken to

MEDICVS

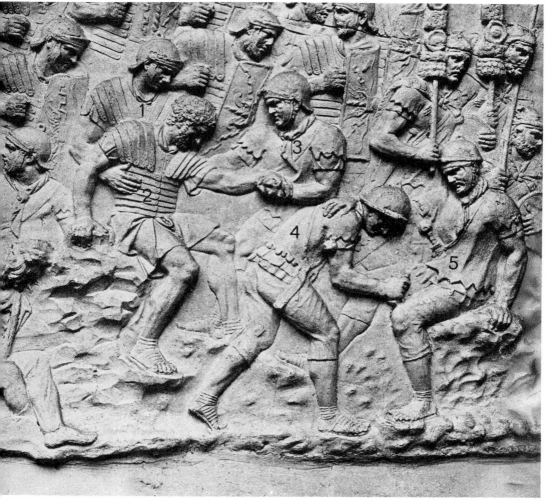

9.43 First aid in the Roman army. This bas-relief from Trajan's column may indicate that medical care was in the hands of non-Romans (see text).

a private physician.[272] Beyond this, the evidence is skimpy. It is possible that an artisan might be taken to the physician of his guild.[273] A slave from a country estate would probably be taken to the infirmary in that household. If badly mangled, he might be patched up and sold, or abandoned on the island of the Tiber, site of the ancient temple of Aesculapius, where Claudius decreed that if they recovered, they must be freed.[274]

Some of these patients may have been taken over by the public physicians. The Romans had found this institution at work in Greece as well as in Gaul.[275] They had tried it out themselves under the republic, when they hired Archagathus, the wound specialist, and paid for his *taberna*, "workshop," as Pliny calls it, out of public funds. The trouble is that after him there are no further records of Roman public physicians until the decree of Antoninus Pius (137–161 A.D.).

The text of this decree suggests that this good emperor was worried about public physicians because of some current abuse regarding the exemptions

MEDICVS

391

and privileges that came with the office: "The smallest cities may have five tax-exempt [*immunes*] physicians, three sophists and as many grammarians; larger cities may have seven physicians, and four teachers of the above-named branches; the largest cities may have ten physicians, five rhetoricians and as many grammarians. Beyond these numbers, even the largest cities may not confer tax-exemption [*immunitas*] . . . It is not permissible to exceed these numbers . . . for any reason; but it is possible to decrease them."[276] Later these public physicians came to be known, in the Roman Empire, by the Latinized Greek name of *archiatri*, from *archiatrós*, meaning "court physician," "official physician," or more generally, "responsible practitioner."[277] There is little doubt that one of their major duties was the medical care of the poor,[278] but to see this mentioned in the law—and then most emphatically— we have to wait for a Christian emperor, Theodosius, in 368 A.D.[279]

In stating the duty of caring for the poor, this decree rises to the tone of a sermon: "There shall be as many Archiatri [*in Rome*] as there are regions in the city, over and above the two of the Porticus assigned to the Gymnasium and to the Virgin Vestals [*a Christian bow to the waning pagan institution*]. May these physicians, knowing that their annual moneys will come from the people's money, prefer to serve with honesty the poor, rather than the rich with disgrace. We shall tolerate that they accept the fees that those in good health may offer for their services, but not the fees that those in danger may promise for being saved."[280] Ultimately, these public physicians must have become a very popular institution, considering that *archiater* gave the German word for "doctor," *Arzt*.[281]

It is also unclear where these public physicians took care of the citizens. Of archiatric hospitals there is no trace. In the first century A.D., Celsus has a passing comment about "large valetudinaria" (whether public or private, he does not say), but from the context I guess that he himself would never be taken to one of those places. He brings up the matter of large infirmaries only incidentally, in a startling passage in which he discusses the importance of theory versus practice; or rather of medicine as an art, as opposed to empirical healing gestures. And he concludes (hear this) that *there are three kinds of doctors who cannot bother with theory*: "those who treat cattle and horses, since it is impossible to learn from dumb animals particulars of their complaints . . . so also do foreigners, as they are ignorant of reasoning subtleties . . . again those who take charge of large valetudinaria, because they cannot pay full attention to individuals"![282]

MEDICVS

Within a few years of these lines, Columella was writing his treatise on farming (*De re rustica*), which tells that infirmaries, again called valetudinaria, were a regular part of large country estates. It is implied, however, that they were for slaves only, perhaps even being run by slaves with medical skills (*servi medici*), and that they were nothing more than rooms set aside for the sick.[283] Visualize them from Columella's own words, in the chapter dealing with the duties of the bailiff's wife: "Then too she will have to see that the kitchen and the cowsheds and also the mangers are cleaned, and she will have to open the sick-wards [*valetudinaria*] from time to time, even if they contain no patients, and keep them free from dirt, so that, when necessary, the sick may find them in an orderly and healthy condition."[284] Should the farmer's wife find a slave "even pretending to be ill, she must without delay conduct him to the valetudinarium; for, if he is worn out by his work, it is better that he should rest for a day or two under observation than that he come to some real harm by being forced to overwork himself."[285]

To sum up these few data on civilian infirmaries, their general context is cattle, cowsheds, and slaves. Here the question arises whether there was any parallel institution for wealthier citizens. The fairest answer is that we do not know. There are two oft-quoted passages by Seneca, from the first century A.D., in which valetudinaria are mentioned in passing, rather as figures of speech ("If I were to walk into a valetudinarium, or into the house of a rich . . ."[286]). Not much can be squeezed from such lines. Perhaps some medici had nursing facilities where they lived, but wealthy Romans were most likely treated in their own homes.[287]

So we are left with good military hospitals, good data on slave infirmaries, and next to nothing on private clinics for the rich. All this appears to fit a logical scheme, which suggests that the rich took care of themselves but made sure that proper care was given to the two groups on which their power depended, soldiers and slaves. If humanitarian considerations were involved, they probably remained in the background; private infirmaries were—like army hospitals—part of good business administration.[288]

The Romans, who insisted on manslaughter as part of their weekly amusement,[289] could not be expected to produce highly philanthropic laws. However, the public physicians were a beginning. From Greece to Rome, to distant China, antiquity recognized—in token form at least—the right of the citizen to medical care.[290]

"Medicina"

The greatest Roman innovation in medicine was perhaps the military hospital. Architecturally, it was almost ideal. Yet after the empire it was forgotten—so thoroughly forgotten that many of today's physicians trained in wards where patients were lined up by the dozen, in two rows. The reason, I assume, has to do with the motivation of the Roman hospital: it was a product of army efficiency. When the army and its efficiency collapsed, the beautiful hospitals went with it.

A different motivation had to arise, either from the law—giving all men equal rights—or from religion. In Rome, the religious motivation came first, as it did in India, where Buddhism had a 500-year headstart over Christianity. About 350 A.D. a wealthy Roman lady, Fabiola, embraced the Christian faith and founded with her own money a home for the sick. Her *nosokoméion*, "sick-tending-place," may not have included medical care as known today, but it reflected a concern for human beings that in the Western world was entirely new, and which ultimately found expression in real hospital care. Saint Jerome tells that Fabiola went herself to pick up in the streets, and carry

MEDICVS

393

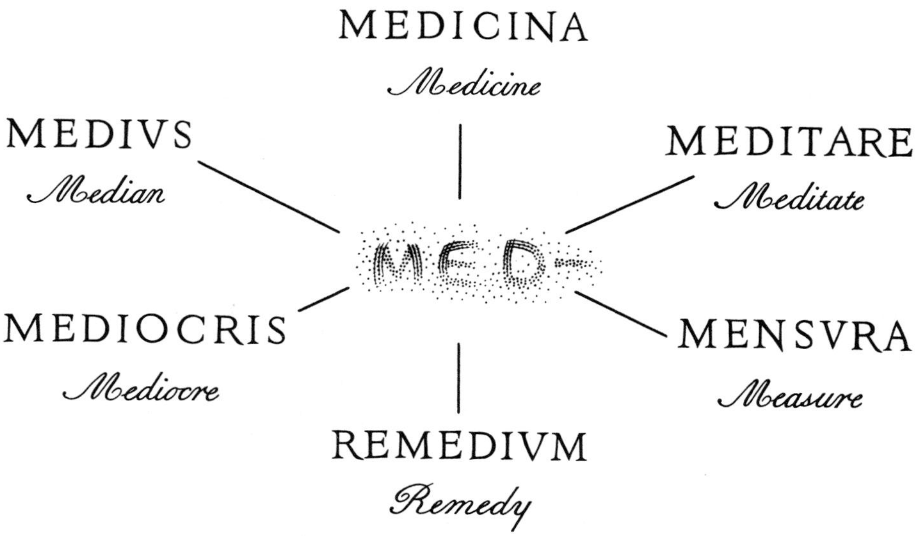

MEDICINA
Medicine

MEDIVS   MEDITARE
Median   *Meditate*

MED

MEDIOCRIS   MENSVRA
Mediocre   *Measure*

REMEDIVM
Remedy

9.44 Greek gave us *clinic* and *surgery* (*cheirurgía*), but Latin gave us *medicina*, from the Indo-European root *med-*. Here are some of its relatives. The root *med-* seems to imply the general connotation of "thoughtful action to establish order."

away on her shoulders, wretched beings with "leprous arms, swollen bellies, shrunken thighs, dropsical legs . . . their flesh gnawed and rotten and squirming with little worms . . . How often did she not wash the pus of festering wounds that others could not bear to see?"[291]

So Christ took over the work of Asklepios. If the Christian poorhouses and hospitals of the Middle Ages have precedents, they are not the valetudinaria of the Roman army, but the homely public Roman infirmaries and the special buildings attached to the temples of Asklepios, where the worshippers could live.[292]

It is certainly true that Roman medicine was basically Greek; but Europe's center of gravity had also shifted from Greece to Rome. As the Roman Empire came to embrace practically all of the Western world, the art of healing grew, blending the knowledge of three continents. Hence its name in most European languages (except Greek) was taken from the language of the conquerors: *medicina* (Fig. 9.44).[293]

And the last flash of Greek medicine came from Rome: Galen.

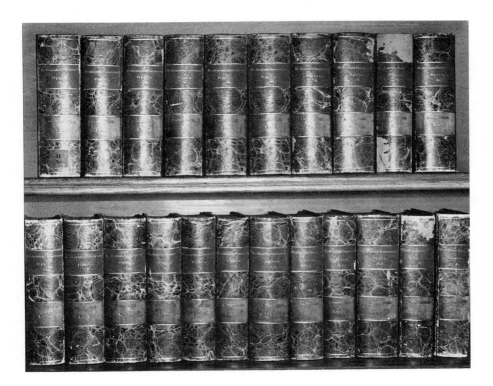

10 Galen—and into the Night

Galen's fame rests on a self-made monument of two and a half million words: twenty-two volumes in the only edition available, a forbidding sight—as illustrated above.[1] All this amounts to two-thirds of what he wrote; the rest is lost.[2]

The next most wondrous fact about Galen is that, today, he is scarcely read at all. There are many reasons for not reading Galen. A simple one is that very few of his works have been translated from the original Greek, except into Arabic, or Latin for the really ignorant.[3] Even in the few that are available in English, the general style is so consistently boring that the sparks of genius tend to be lost in the smoke. To make matters worse, Galen was a very pompous gentleman, and he also wrote that way. A genius he was, of course, or he would not have dominated medicine for nearly fifteen centuries. But the critics of the Renaissance toppled him so effectively that a lasting revival never took place. He is still in disgrace, "doubtless from the extravagant homage formerly paid to him." Somebody even took the trouble of counting his anatomical mistakes.[4] But if Galen's writings could be condensed into two or three books, those books would be full of pearls.

Galen was born in 130 A.D. in Pergamon, on the coast of Asia Minor (Fig. 4.1). His father, a wise and wealthy architect, provided him with the best possible education and independent means for the rest of his life; his mother impressed him especially with her vicious character, of which we shall have more to say. Pergamon had fallen to the Romans almost three centuries before Galen's birth. It was a beautiful and intellectual city, famous for its Asklepieion, which drew crowds of pilgrims, and for its library, second only to that of Alexandria. In fact, it was through the influence of the library in Pergamon that parchment (*charta pergamena*) was developed. Pliny explains how it happened: "When, owing to the rivalry between King Ptolemy and King Eumenes [*of Pergamon*] about their libraries, Ptolemy suppressed the export of paper [*papyrus*], parchment was invented at Pergamum; and afterwards the employment of the material, on which the immortality of human beings depends, spread indiscriminately."[5]

Galen's father owned a small farm, where he liked to retire to perform his favorite experiments: anticipating Pasteur's *Etudes sur le vin*, he studied the aging of wine as affected by the heat of the fireplace.[6] Little Galen watched other children play,[7] but wasted no time himself. At the age of thirteen he had already written three books. By twenty he had completed four years of medical study at the school of the Asklepieion, but to him this background was not enough. The best of science was still concentrated in Alexandria, so he went there and stayed several years, studying especially anatomy. When he returned home, he was an accomplished dissector and could boast of twelve years of training. This would be a lot even now, and was surely unique at that time: two Roman epitaphs remember "physicians" who died at the age of seventeen; and a certain Thessalus offered in Rome a medical course of six months![8]

Although his home remained Pergamon, Galen spent twenty-four years in Rome, where he rose to the position of court physician to none other than Marcus Aurelius. In Rome he lived as a haughty Greek; some say that he never even bothered to learn much Latin.[9] He wrote, lectured, gave public demonstrations, and found time for private practice, often ending in verbal fights with his colleagues. Toward the end of his life, when he returned to Pergamon, he had written so many works (perhaps five or six hundred) that he felt the need to write two more books about his own writings. He died in 200 A.D.

Galen had no brothers or sisters, never married, left no pupils, and does not mention any friends.[10] His one and only idol was Hippocrates. The Hippocratic Collection had already gathered five hundred years of dust; he revived it, adopted it as if he were its new messiah—which he surely was—and wrote much about it that is now extremely valuable. Indeed, his comments on the Hippocratic books are usually much longer than the books themselves.[11]

Yet, while his medicine was essentially Hippocratic, Galen had also been to the Alexandrian school; thus, for all his faults, his scientific horizon reached at least one order of magnitude beyond that of Hippocrates: *he practiced dissection and experiment* (Fig. 10.1). Whereas Hippocrates had studied disease essentially as a naturalist, Galen dared modify nature as a scientist. His thirst to understand *The Use of the Parts* (the title of one of

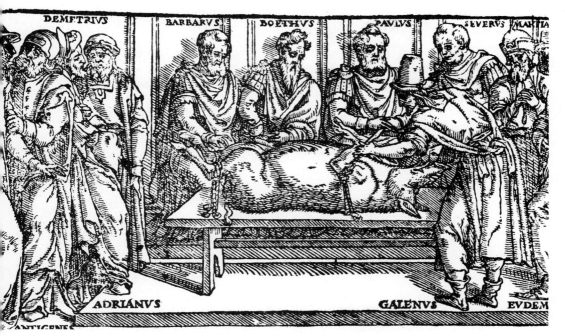

10.1 Galen's systematic experiments on animals were a great advance over Hippocrates. Here Galen is vivisecting a pig, presumably to demonstrate his famous "nerve of the voice." Boethus was a scholarly Roman ex-consul who once paid for a stenographer to record the proceedings of such a demonstration. From a 1609 edition of Galen.

his books) led him to perform experiments on a scale totally unheard of. He opened live arteries and determined that they contained blood, not air (not so easy when everybody maintains the contrary); he tied the ureters of living animals—cruel, but technically a tour de force—to show that urine comes from the kidneys; he severed spinal cords at different levels and described the kinds of paralysis that ensued.[12]

And yet, after this dazzling start, Galen abandoned truth for theory, and dug his own grave as a scientist. In retrospect, the step was a short one, irrational but understandable: anatomy became revelation. It became the tangible proof of an infinitely wise Creator. With this perspective, Galen slipped from dissection into philosophy, to create a system in which every organ, function, and disease made perfect, ultimate sense. So deep was his conviction that he could speak of a nerve as of a religious experience. The following excerpt is an excellent self-portrait, taken from the book *On the Usefulness of the Parts of the Body:*

> I want you now to pay me closer attention than if you were being initiated into the mysteries of Eleusis or Samothrace or some other sacred rite and were wholly absorbed in the acts and words of the hierophants [*priests*]. You should consider that this mystery is in no way inferior to those and no less able to show forth the wisdom, foresight, and power of the Creator of animals, and in particular you should realize that I was the very first to discover this mystery which I now practise . . . Ac-

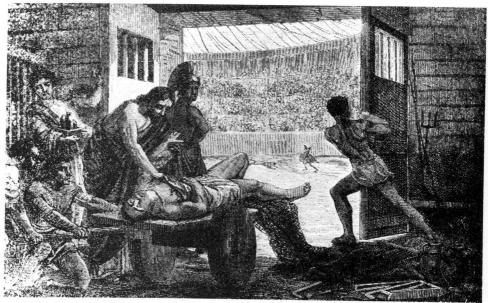

10.2 Galen treating a wounded gladiator in the amphitheater at Pergamon, as visualized by Jan Verhas about 1870. It is likely that Galen had better working quarters than the animal den.

cordingly, even if you have not done so before, fix your mind now on holier things, make yourself a listener worthy of what is to be said, and follow closely my discourse as it explains the wonderful mysteries of Nature.[13]

No pagan was ever more pious. This is the language that allowed Galen to be worshipped, century after century, by Christians, Muslims, and Jews.

Galen's prime interests were science and internal medicine, not surgery. In fact, he never wrote a book on surgery. However, he tended a vast number of wounds during three years as a surgeon to the gladiators (Fig. 10.2), and he left some interesting notes on that experience.[14]

Galen and the Gladiators

Pergamon was a Greek city, and as such, it had nothing to do with gladiators. But when the Romans came, the conquerors could not do without their favorite show. On Greek soil, however, the first reaction was horror, and some Greek cities went as far as forbidding gladiatorial games altogether.[15] The Romans solved the problem by a technique of immunization: they organized combats anyway, but stopped them—at first—as soon as blood appeared. Gradually, the public became accustomed. By the time Galen was twenty-eight, Pergamon had full gladiatorial games and needed a surgeon (Fig. 10.3). This is what Galen has to say about his appointment:

On my return from Alexandria to my native land, while still a young man in my twenty-eighth year, I had the good fortune to work out a successful dressing for wounded nerves and tendons. I demonstrated this to physician friends not only in Pergamon, but in neighboring cities so that they might confirm my findings by exper-

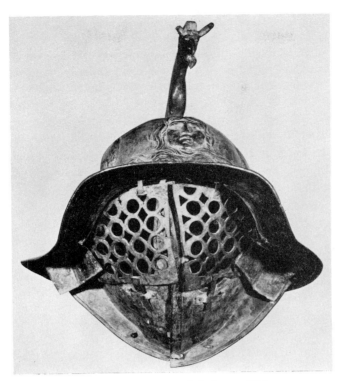

10.3 Galen's patients, the gladiators, wore such helmets. This one was worn in Pompei until 79 A.D.

iment. This treatment coming, I know not how, to the knowledge of the Pontifex of our city [*president of the games*] he entrusted me with the care of the gladiators while still a young man, for I was arriving at my twenty-ninth year . . .

Since many died in previous years [*and*] not one of those treated by me died, the succeeding pontifex appointed me likewise.[16]

The "successful dressing" is more precisely a sauce. It may have been an improvement over local practice, but surely not over the Hippocratic school:

Though previous gladiatorial physicians bathed the wound in hot water and put on a dressing of wheat flour moderately cooked in a mixture of oil and water, I omitted the water entirely and made the dressing of flour cooked in oil and poured an additional small amount of oil over it. The result was excellent, for not one of my cases died, though fatalities were numerous previously.[17]

In Galen's dressings I would not detect the mark of a genius. He seriously believed in dove's dung, on which he has a whole chapter,[18] and was quite happy to pour his favorite fluid, writing ink, onto live flesh.[19] If this was real ink made from the soot of torches, the net effect of the soot was probably that of all foreign materials: favoring infection (although it could be argued that the small amount of tar present in the soot could act as a short-lived antiseptic).[20] If, instead, it was the so-called shoemaker's blacking, made of tannin and iron salts, that was an old wound-drug and perhaps slightly more acceptable as an antiseptic.[21] Luckily there was always wine, the trustiest friend of all wounded Greeks:

As I have previously explained, it is necessary to keep the wound continually moist, because if the dressings dry out, the ulcer becomes inflamed. This is true especially in summer, at which time when the pontifices of Pergamum were celebrating the appointed gladiatorial games, I cured the most seriously injured by covering the wounds by a cloth wet with astringent wine kept moist both day and night by a superimposed sponge.[22]

Technically, as a wound surgeon, Galen could do better than Hippocrates, because he knew more about stopping hemorrhage, and he sutured muscles. Both these methods were already current. On wound healing in general he had nothing new to offer.[23] Fortunately he did recall the sane old Hippocratic principle that pus is not essential to normal healing:

Those who believe that inflammation necessarily follows a wound show great ignorance, since it is possible for anyone to see even large ones reach the stage of being practically healed in two to four days without inflammation, in connection with the countless fighting in a single day in the arena.[24]

Here is a typical case history:

I found one of the gladiators called *horsemen* with a transverse division of the tendon on the anterior inferior surface of the thigh, the lower part being separated from the upper, and without hesitation I brought them together by sutures. I knew that the fleshy parts of muscles had been sutured before, but I had never seen my teachers suture tendons. In fact in wounds of this kind some physicians only stitch together the skin edges, others put the sutures only through the anterior part of the muscle, and the posterior part fails to unite. When the muscular injury is longitudinal, proper bandaging alone will bring the parts together, but when transverse they must be held by sutures or they will remain permanently separated. When the edges of the ruptured tendon were ragged, I trimmed them. Some unskilled surgeons, imitating my work, tear away the membrane covering the muscle, not knowing that this should be included in the stitches.[25]

All this makes good surgical sense, especially the comments on wounds in muscles. When a muscle is split lengthwise, it behaves as if it consisted of two separate muscles, and the damage is not great; the two parts will grow together again even if left unsutured. If, instead, the muscle is cut transversely, the two stumps will pull away from each other, leaving a broad gap; if they are not drawn together by stitches, the muscle becomes useless. It is worth adding that Galen worked this out correctly, despite his total misunderstanding of muscular contraction. In fact, he did not realize that muscles are themselves able to contract; he believed that the pull exerted by the muscle-tendon apparatus was due to a shortening of the tendon—and he interpreted the bulge of a muscle, during contraction, as a passive slackening.[26]

Since Galen's forte was anatomy and dissection, he took his tenure at the games as a prolonged lesson in human anatomy. Like Sushruta, he describes the difficulty of pushing back the intestines when they have slipped out of the belly (how right he is).[27] In one case it was the omentum that had come out; he cut it off and the gladiator survived.[28] Many gladiators were wounded

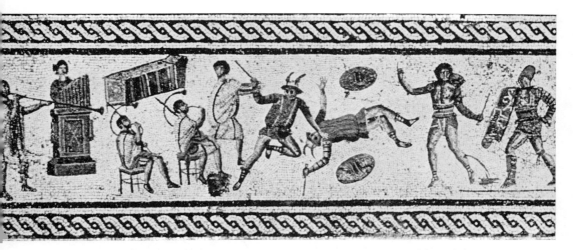

10.4 Gladiator fights were accompanied by music. The woman (second from left) is playing a water-organ (Fig. 8.12). Beside her is a casket, ready for the next casualty; another casket is at far right (not shown). From a Libyan mosaic, third century A.D.

in the heart. Galen noticed that they died faster if the wound reached into the left cavity. If the wound did not poke through, they could survive a whole day and a night thereafter, then they died "of inflammation. And assuredly, all these maintain their mental faculties as long as they survive, and this phenomenon confirms the ancient principle that the intelligence of the soul does not reside in the heart."[29]

All this official butchering seems to have left Galen relatively cold. He actually despised athletic professions,[30] and he describes the gladiators' wounds as if they had happened to nonpeople. Dr. J. Walsh of Philadelphia, who between 1934 and 1937 wrote a series of essays on Galen, tries to explain the indifference to cruelty that seems to have prevailed in Galen's days:

> We see in our football games the player carried off the field injured or possibly dead, without the spectators knowing or even caring much which, occupied as they are with the irritation produced by the delay. Later they may read of his death in the newspaper with sympathy, particularly if he was a good player, but with little or no sense of horror.
>
> In the year 1935 there were in the United States 30 deaths due to football casualties and about 13,000 players injured. During the same year there were 36,400 deaths due to motor cars and about 1 percent of the population, or 1,250,000, injured . . . Our humaneness does not particularly stand out.[31]

While still regretting Galen's lack of sympathy, I will add that he too had undergone a certain degree of immunization. For thirty-five months he stood by as men whom he personally knew slaughtered each other to the sound of music (Fig. 10.4). Gory details of the proceedings, in full color, are preserved in many mosaics, especially in North Africa. Roman citizens may have been trained to enjoy the show since their early days. On the floor of a Roman villa in Carthage (now Tunis) one can see eight children having fun spearing cats, hares, and the like.[32] And when they grew up to become regular spectators, they behaved accordingly.[33] Sometimes one of them would step forth and

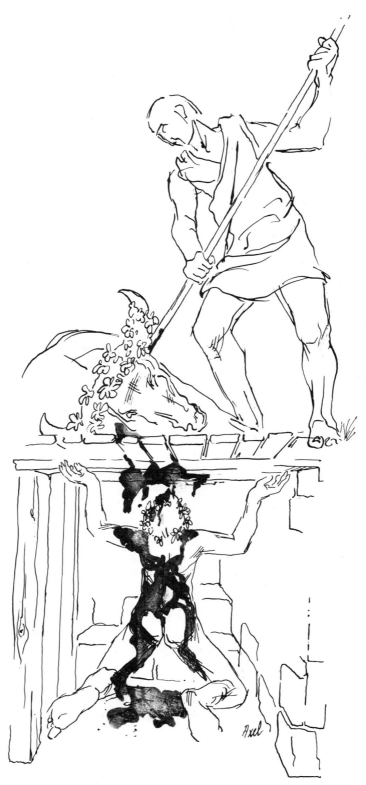

10.5 The *taurobolium,* symbolic rebirth through a blood-bath. This ritual came to Rome from the East and was current in Galen's days.

snatch a piece of liver from a gladiator lying gutted in the dust: gladiator liver, taken nine times, was a cure for epilepsy.[34] Another might come to drink blood from the wounds, for the same purpose.[35]

The ultimate in blood cure, in great vogue at that time, was a ceremony called *taurobolium*. Once in a while in Rome, Galen's peace may have been disturbed by the sound of flutes and a cheering crowd: a leading senator, drenched in blood from head to foot, was returning home after having been "taurobolized." This was a rebirth ceremony connected with the cult of Cybele. The man who wished to be spiritually reborn descended a few steps into a pit covered with stout planks, loosely joined and pierced with many holes. Then above him, a priest sacrificed a bull; the blood trickled down into the pit, to the sound of flutes, and the man soaked up as much of it as he could. Then he walked out at the other end of the pit, as out of a grave, happily reborn (Fig. 10.5).[36]

Galen and Hemorrhage: Still No Tourniquet

A trusty gladiatorial surgeon should have stood by holding a strip of cloth, ready to use as a tourniquet; but Galen did not.[37] His first aid in case of hemorrhage was essentially to raise the injured part, put a finger into the wound, find the gaping vessels, and compress them "gently, without causing pain."[38] Whether the patients were live apes or gladiators, this was his first device. He added, "very useful is also an assistant who co-operates with you, and in the manner described compresses for you the places in which you are in need of it."[39] Ten fingers could go a long way.

If this did not work, "what is also helpful is a hook with which you grasp the part from which the outflowing blood is coming, and twist it around" (Fig. 10.6).[40] Today, twisting a bleeder is standard technique. It is not quite clear to me, however, whether Galen transfixed the bleeding vessel with the hook, or whether he just "fished" in a pool of blood, hooked up whatever he could, and twisted.

The last step was to tie the vessels, by then already an ancient method. Sometimes Galen tied arteries with Chinese silk ("many rich ladies have it in Roman territories, especially in the large cities"[41]). It was high time for silk to appear in surgery: the Old Silk Road had been open for almost three hundred years, and Galen's master, Marcus Aurelius, had been the first to send a mission of merchants to China.[42]

To stop bleeding, Galen relied heavily on locally applied "styptics." The best of these mixtures, he says, was made as follows: frankincense, one part; aloes, one part; mix with eggwhite to the consistency of honey, and add a pinch of clippings from the fur of a hare.[43] He used it "perfectly safely" on a wound exposing the meninges!

And this is all—which means that even Galen, for all of his science, failed to appreciate the possibilities of the tourniquet for stopping hemorrhage. He must have known of its current use in a different context (for cases of snake bite); and he may even have heard of its sporadic use against bleeding, as we shall presently see.

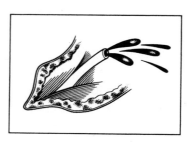

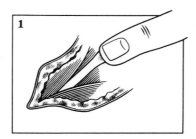

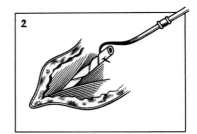

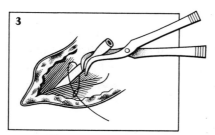

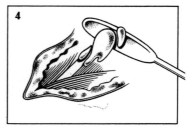

10.6 A severed vessel (*top*) and four of Galen's ways to stop the bleeding: (1) press the vessel with a finger; (2) twist it with a hook; (3) seize it with a forceps, then tie it; (4) apply styptics—or rather, drugs that were *supposed* to be styptics.

I find this failure hard to understand, but one can try to rationalize. First, Galen's crude method of squeezing with the fingers may have worked well enough, especially since he did not worry about the wound being infected. Second, he was preoccupied with the wound itself and did not realize the danger of blood loss as a cause of death, by what is now called hemorrhagic shock. Third, he may have had the wrong mental image of what the tourniquet really does.

I found this "wrong image" forcefully expressed in the homely booklet of Scribonius Largus, presumably written in Rome some 150 years earlier.[44] The passage is precious, because it shows how surgeons could reason about bleeding before they had learned about the circulation of the blood; it shows how the "obvious" is entirely dependent on the point of view; and it reveals incidentally that some form of tourniquet was in use in first century Rome, perhaps as a passing fad.[45] Somewhat shortened, the text reads:

> One should sponge the wound with water or vinegar and prevent the limb from being constricted [*by a tourniquet*], which most doctors do, not realizing that by compressing the muscles they force more blood out of the wound . . . In the same way, if you tie a rope around a skin bag and tighten it, if that bag has a leak, it will of course squirt out its contents (Fig. 10.7).[46]

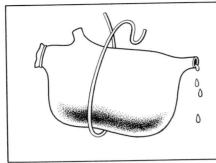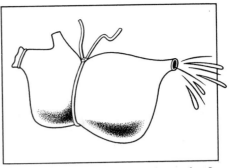

10.7 An argument against the tourniquet, from Scribonius Largus early in the first century A.D. In his view the tourniquet should make the bleeding worse.

Scribonius finds this so exasperatingly obvious that his language lapses into invective. Referring to those doctors who, in his view, are making hemorrhage worse by applying tourniquets, he concludes: *Et, o bone deus . . .*—"And, good Lord, these are the same physicians who always give the fault to the medicines!"

Wounds As Windows

One of Galen's concessions to modesty was to admit that he never dissected ants, gnats, fleas, "and other minuscule creatures."[47] The list of animals that he did dissect remains difficult to match: apes, horses, asses, mules, cows, camels, sheep, lions, wolves, dogs, lynxes, stags, bears, weasels, mice, snakes, a variety of fish and birds, and several elephants.[48] Human bodies he did not dissect, except cadavers "in which all that overlies the bones is decayed and the bones alone remain."[49] He always had at hand "a large number of specially prepared bones of apes." The best way to obtain these, he says, is to bury the ape for four months in moist soil.[50] Surely his laboratory was decorated with skeletons and choice dissected specimens (Fig. 10.8).

Some of Galen's visitors must have cringed at heartrending animal cries. Galen was passionately interested in the functions of the body; and to understand them, he dissected live animals strapped on a board. His favorite animal for dissection was the barbary ape: *Macaca sylvanus*, the only European ape, a little tailless creature that still lives around Gibraltar (Fig. 10.9). But for vivisection, he recommends, use pigs or goats: "leave live apes alone."[51] They were human enough to be a nuisance, even to him.

It was in this manner that Galen worked out the functions of the nerves and the spinal cord:

But if you cut the marrow [*spinal cord*] behind the first thoracic rib, then that damages the hand of the ape [*so it was an ape anyway!*]. And should the cut follow a line behind the second thoracic rib, then that does not damage the arm, except that the skin of the axillary cavity . . . and . . . upper arm . . . become deprived of sensibility.[52]

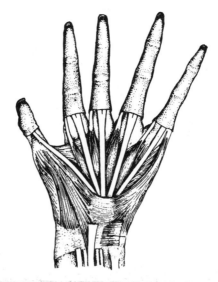

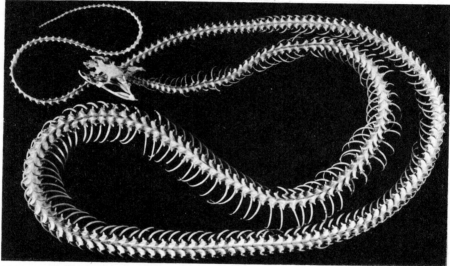

10.8 Galen, who was proud of his dissections on a variety of animals, may have displayed specimens such as these: the hand of an ape (top), the skeleton of a snake.

More inventive yet was his method to detect the function of the optic nerves:

When you have divided the frontal bone . . . you will be met by two nerves that go to the eye. If you divide the larger of the two, then the visual sense of the animal will be impaired . . . But that the animal can no longer see . . . you can only appraise by deduction, from the fact that you find that it does not blink with its eye at anything which you bring near it, pretending to be about to stab home with it.[53]

Galen put to use even the squeals. To study the brain, "you must procure either a pig or a goat, in order to combine two requirements. In the first place, you avoid seeing the unpleasant expression of the ape when it is being vivisected. The other reason is that the animal on which the dissection takes place should cry out with a really loud voice, a thing one does not find with

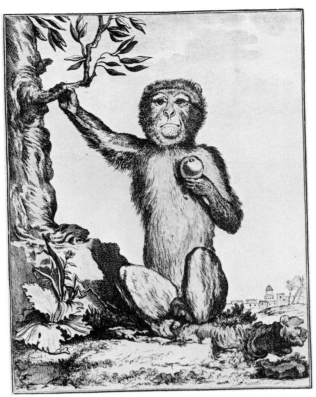

10.9 The barbary ape (*Macaca sylvanus*), Galen's favorite subject for dissection—though not for vivisection.

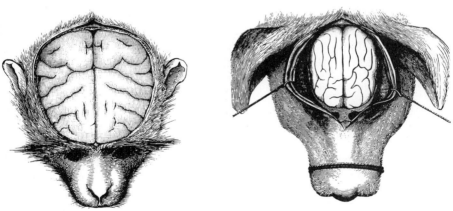

10.10 Opened heads of a monkey and a dog, from a French manual on vivisection of 1882. Galen, too, dissected the brain; he also exposed it in living animals.

apes."[54] The text goes on to recommend that all cuts should be performed swiftly, without pity or compassion (Fig. 10.10).

Galen's pitiless approach allowed him to make his most important discovery. He was vivisecting a pig. To find out whether the nerves in the region of the neck had any effect on respiration, he was cutting them one by one. The pig squealed helplessly, despite a slave who tried to muzzle it. Suddenly, as Galen cut one of the two nerves now known as "recurrent" or

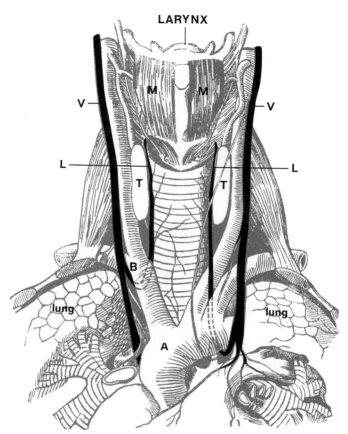

LARYNX

10.11 Two U-shaped cords (black) occur on either side of the neck. Each one is formed by the vagus nerve (V), running downward, and by one of its branches, Galen's recurrent laryngeal nerve (L), returning upward. Galen was intrigued by the peculiar course of the laryngeal nerves along this route: instead of taking the shortest path from the brain to the muscle (M) in the larynx, they travel within the vagus down into the chest, turn around a large artery, and come back up to the larynx—(A) aorta, (B) a branch of the aorta, (T) thyroid.

"inferior laryngeal nerves" (there is one on each side), the squealing stopped. The experiment was repeated on dogs, goats, and other animals. The result was always the same: *the recurrent laryngeal was the nerve of the voice*.[55] This was a revolutionary experiment, for it proved beyond doubt that the brain was in charge. According to the ancient theory of Aristotle, mental faculties resided in the heart; that theory was now finished for good.[56]

Galen's scalpel, and Galen's pen, became busier than ever. Knowing his connections with the arena, where wild animals were killed by the thousands, it is not altogether unexpected to read that the nerve of the voice is easily demonstrated in the lion.[57] Whether the lion's roar could also be dampened is left to the reader's imagination; but Galen had several opportunities to see his nerve sectioned, and his theory confirmed, on live people. One of them was a child who had a large goiter removed by another physician (whereby we learn, incidentally, that this operation—already mentioned by Celsus—was being performed routinely). The operation was successful, but the child remained mute: both nerves had been cut.[58]

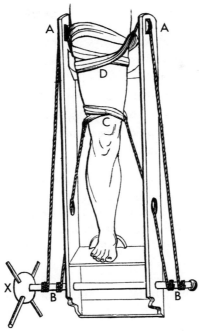

10.12 The *glossocomion*, for reducing fractures. For a fracture between points *C* and *D*, if the wheel *X* is turned clockwise, *C* and *D* will be drawn apart. In other words, the rope can pull *down* on *C* because it loops around the bar *BB*. In the same way, says Galen, the recurrent laryngeal nerve has to loop down and up around an artery in order to pull at the laryngeal muscles (a blunder, but the analogy made sense in the context of Galen's physiology).

Then Galen went one step too far. He felt compelled to prove that these laryngeal nerves, like all other parts of the body, were laid out in the best possible way; yet here was a very peculiar arrangement to explain. Why would a nerve, coming down from the brain and aiming for the larynx, descend first into the chest, curl around a large artery, and then return upward to the larynx? (Fig. 10.11).

It is all too easy to say, now, that the reason is purely accidental, being due to displacements of organs that take place during embryonic development. Galen's physiology was so primitive that it ignored even muscular contraction; and surely it had no place for accident. So Galen worked out the problem as follows. He pointed out that the muscle, in which the laryngeal nerve ends, runs vertically (Fig. 10.11). Thus, the pull "of its tendons"—in Galen's way of thinking—has to occur vertically. The nerve that causes the pull must therefore line up with the direction of the muscle; so it makes "perfect sense" that it should first run down to the chest, use a large, strong artery as a pulley, and return upward vertically.

To give a practical example of his pulley theory, Galen used the comparison of the *glossocomion*, a machine worked by a crank, vertical ropes, and pulleys, used in his day for reducing fractures of the femur and tibia (Fig. 10.12). Placed side by side, the two situations illustrate well the seduction of analogy. Although hopelessly wrong, Galen had achieved his ultimate purpose: to demonstrate that the use of the parts was, in his words, "a hymn of glory to the Divine Creator of Man."[59]

Galen's Nerve and the Hindus

The recurrent laryngeal is now known as *Galen's nerve.* Galen missed no opportunity to repeat that he was the first to discover its function. I wonder what he might have said if a visitor from India had told him that his famous symptom—loss of the voice—had been observed by the Hindus several centuries before, together with another symptom that he never even suspected. A visiting vaidya could have recited the passage from Sushruta's chapter concerning vital points or marmas:

Now we shall describe the marmas which are situated in the regions above the clavicles . . . There are four Dhamani [*"ducts," nerves as well as arteries*] . . . on either side of the wind-pipe.[60] Two of them are known as *Nila,* and the other two as *Manya.* One Nilá and one Manya are situated on either side of the larynx. An injury to any of them produces dumbness, and change of voice (hoarseness), and also the loss of the faculty of taste.[61]

Galen could pinch his animals to make them squeal; he could threaten them to make them blink; but he could not ask them about taste. The Hindus, on their part, would not vivisect pigs; but they took lessons as they came from war casualties. Translated into anatomical terms, the symptoms they describe for an injury of the two marmas in the neck mean that an arrow, or any pointed weapon, plunging into the neck could sever one of three nerves on that side (Fig. 10.13): the glossopharyngeal, abolishing the

10.13 The hoarse voice, described by Galen after cutting the recurrent laryngeal nerve, had been observed centuries before by Sushruta in India after an injury to one of the vital points or *marmas* in the neck. (1) vagus nerve, (2) Galen's recurrent laryngeal nerve, (3) glossopharyngeal nerve.

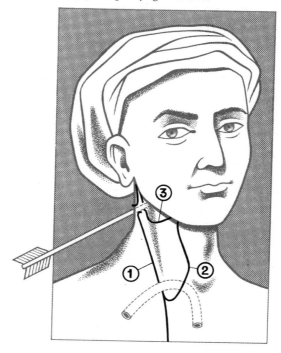

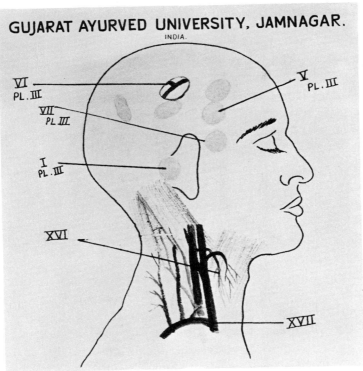

10.14 Drawing of the marmas in the neck, from a contemporary Ayurvedic medical school. The number XVI corresponds to Sushruta's *Neela-Manya* marma, which, when hit, causes hoarseness and loss of the sense of taste. The modern topographic correlations are somewhat fanciful, but the marma, anatomically and functionally true, is still there: it preceded Galen's nerve by several centuries.

sense of taste on that side; Galen's recurrent laryngeal nerve, resulting in a hoarse voice; or the main trunk of the vagus nerve, again resulting in a hoarse voice (because this nerve also carries the fibers that branch off further down to become Galen's nerve; the symptoms, however, would be more complex than those resulting from a pure injury of Galen's nerve). If struck by a pointed weapon coming from the side, as illustrated, the victim might come away with a hoarse voice *and* a loss of the sense of taste, but still without a fatal injury to the major vessels that run close by.

Yet Galen could not have read Charaka or Sushruta, for they had never been written: they were just learned by heart in Sanskrit. And no visiting vaidya seems to have come within Galen's orbit.

Since Sushruta's medicine is still alive as Ayurveda, I wrote to India to have the last word on the topic of marmas in the neck. The Gujarat Ayurved University was kind enough to send me lists and charts of marmas, which show a clearcut effort to line up with modern anatomy and its Greco-Latin terminology. In one plate, on the side of the neck, appeared the same vital point described by Sushruta, where wounds cause loss of voice and taste; its name was unchanged, Neela-Manya marma (Fig. 10.14). The names of the deep anatomical structures—which explain the symptoms—were given in modern terms, including the glossopharyngeal nerve, which transmits the sense of taste. Oddly enough, Galen's nerve was omitted![62]

Galen on Inflammation: The True Story

To medical students today, the name of Galen should bring up at least two associations: Galen's nerve and *functio laesa* or "disturbed function," the fifth sign of inflammation. The discussion of Galen's nerve has shown that it was not Galen's alone. The story of Galen's fifth sign is even more heretical: Galen had practically nothing to do with it.

The notion of the fifth sign, as taught in pathology courses, can be summarized as follows. Celsus described the four cardinal signs of inflammation, REDNESS, SWELLING, HEAT, and PAIN; then came Galen, who supposedly added the missing fifth sign, DISTURBED FUNCTION, meaning that an inflamed part does not work as well as it should. I too have contributed to spreading this bit of lore. The concept of a fifth sign is definitely catchy. It is the adventure of a square becoming a pentagon. It sounds like progress. Everybody remembers it. How could a teacher forget it?

Eventually I decided to check the sources, and spent nights leafing through dusty Latin editions of Galen. There were pages and pages on *inflammatio*; but not the slightest hint about the discovery of a fifth sign. Nor was there any trace of the basic four signs, though they had been announced to the world by Celsus some 150 years earlier. Finally I realized that my search was pointless: Galen wore down many a Roman quill, consumed gallons of Roman ink, but took no notice of anything Roman, let alone of a Roman like Celsus, who had chosen to write about medicine in Latin.

The truth is, therefore, that Galen never added a fifth sign. He does mention "disturbed function" here and there—it would be difficult to write about medicine without using these two words—but never specifically as a symptom of inflammation. He never even mentions Celsus. Unnerving as this may sound, I hope the retraction reaches at least some of my former students.

The story of how the fifth sign actually originated furnishes first-rate material to anyone interested in the birth and survival of medical legends. It was another great man, Rudolf Virchow, who first spelled out the functio laesa as a fifth sign. I found the reference by sheer accident, staring out of a page in that epoch-making book called *Cellularpathologie*, "Cellular Pathology," a collection of lectures published in 1858, which was instantly accepted as the cornerstone of modern pathology:

> Nobody would expect a muscle which is inflamed, to perform its function normally . . . Nobody would expect an inflamed gland-cell could secrete normally.
> Now there can be no doubt . . . that —a point upon which all the more recent schools at least are agreed—to the four characteristic symptoms [*of inflammation*] *lesion of function* (functio laesa) must be added.[63]

It "must" be added, says Virchow, and it was. His wording shows that the fifth symptom was already in the air; but his authority had the effect of transforming a vague notion into general law. The impact of statements issued by Virchow, their metamorphosis into law, is a unique phenomenon in the history of pathology. After publication of the *Cellular Pathology*, Virchow's fame became so overwhelming that anything he wrote or said spread throughout the medical world and became absorbed as diffuse, nonspecific medical knowledge. Thus, within six years of 1858, the author of a pathology *Handbuch* quoted the fifth sign, functio laesa, as general knowledge (and gave it no father). Then the fifth sign carried on with varying success until a mutation occurred in 1919: the author of another *Handbuch*, presumably recalling that the functio laesa had sprung up somewhere in the great and nebulous past, skipped from Prussia to Pergamon—and assigned the fatherhood to Galen.[64]

So this is the true story of the fifth sign. But it may come too late to straighten out the textbooks. A brilliant journalist once tried to recall a hoax of his own, perpetrated through the newspapers; he never succeeded: it had become too true in the process.[65] And nobody will ever undo the myth of Galileo dropping cannonballs from the Leaning Tower of Pisa.[66]

Galen on Bites and Poisons: The Theriac Saga

I do not wish to sound destructive, but another undeserved gem in Galen's crown is "Galenic" drugs. A course in Galenic pharmacy is still given at the University of Geneva; it deals with drugs extractable from plants; yet the word *Galenic* cannot be traced back to any particular kind of drug discovered by Galen (*Galenic* has become a loose term, says George Sarton, "the semantic variations of which are difficult to follow.")[67]

Although he did not push back the frontiers of pharmacology, Galen contributed a great deal to the success of the dreadful concoctions called theriacs, creating his own brand which somehow rose to the rank of Top Drug.[68] Its incredible career deserves to be mentioned here, because it betrays the ancient fear of bites and poisons.

Today we can no longer appreciate the ancient concern with being bitten.[69] There was a *Book of Bites* in Egypt. The herbal of Dioscorides, from the first century A.D., mentions bites 329 times.[70] After his chapter on wounds, where a modern treatise might proceed to discuss burns, Celsus continues: "I have spoken of those wounds that are mostly inflicted by weapons. My next task is to speak of those that are caused by the bite, at times of a man, at times of an ape, often of a dog, not infrequently of wild animals or of snakes. For almost every bite has in it poison of some sort."[71]

Note the mention of human bites, and the fear of poison in every bite. Galen informs us that when his mother lost her temper with her servants, she used to bite them.[72] According to Pliny, "the bite of a human being is considered to be a most serious one."[73] Human teeth, he explains "contain some sort of virus [*poison*], for they dim the brightness of a mirror when bared in front of it, and also kill the fledglings of pigeons."[74] The wounds they leave are conveniently treated with ear wax, if possible from the ear of the bitten.[75]

Ear wax apart, Pliny was right: human bites are still a very serious injury, indeed worse then dog bites. Hear this from a modern textbook of surgery:

"The dog bite is considered to be a cleaner wound than the human bite . . . The human bite is a serious injury because of the tremendous number of organisms present within the mouth . . . The secondary infection as a result of the human bite is usually mixed, but the spirochete and the fusiform bacillus are frequently found, and these are thought to be responsible for the gangrenous character of the lesion . . . The patient should be kept under close observation following the human bite, since amputation of fingers, hand and arms may be necessary because of the rapid spread of cellulitis and gangrene."[76]

To return to antiquity, most bites were those of wild animals—in Greek *thería*—especially when Greek and Roman armies began to roam the world. Books appeared, called *theriaká*,[77] about dangerous beasts: snakes, angry mammals, rabid dogs. To cope with this threat, there grew up a special kind of drug, the *theriacs*, which had to differ from drugs for ordinary wounds because most bite-wounds, as Celsus explains in the passage above, were thought to be poisoned. Though worthless as antidotes, except perhaps psychologically, theriacs gave enough comfort to become very popular. By 50 A.D. the Roman traveler relied on his theriac as we now do on vaccination: "For your protection," writes Scribonius Largus, "also whenever you go to the country, I shall set down the making of theriac, a medicament for the bites and strokes of serpents" and scorpions.[78]

What happened thereafter to theriacs is almost incredible. At first they were used against bites, considered poisonous; then they began to be used against poisons in general; and finally they were used against anything. They became all-purpose drugs, mushrooming into one of history's best examples of the power of wishful thinking. They were always surrounded by an aura of legend, related to the gruesome tale of their "scientific" beginnings at the court of a Persian king: Mithridates, king of Pontus (132–63 B.C.).

Mithridates and the Drugs of Fear

It was actually poison, rather than bites, that worried this high-strung monarch. On the world scene he was one of Rome's fiercest enemies, famous also for his terrifying war-chariots, equipped with rotating scythes. A savage tyrant, but also one who passed from history to legend for his knowledge of twenty-two languages and his passion for things medical,[79] he studied poisons on a scale perhaps never matched. His guinea pigs were "criminals," whom he had poisoned or bitten by venomous beasts. Then he tested the effect of antidotes on them, and eventually compounded the best ones into a single drug for his own use. He had, in fact, good reasons to fear that someone might want to poison him. During the fifty-seven years of his thunderous reign he survived by killing four of his sons. In the end, defeated by Pompey and cornered by his fifth son, he had to take his own life; and tradition has it that being immune to all poisons, he was obliged to seek death by the sword.[80]

Pompey was careful to retrieve all of the books and notes that he could find in Mithridates' quarters, and Roman experts began to produce Mithridatic antidotes. They, too, had good reasons for being interested in antidotes: poisoning was becoming part of life. Just a century later Nero employed a professional poisoner from Gaul, named Locusta.[81] Meanwhile the *praegustatores* or "foretasters" grew into a guild with its own officials. In this serene environment the call for new and better "antidotes" was inevitably great.

It was then that Nero's physician, Andromachus, delivered his inspirational masterpiece. He started out with a traditional "antidote" called *Mithridatium*, already effective because of its name and fame. Then he raised its level of complexity by bringing the number of compounds to sixty-four, enriched it with chunks of viper flesh, and multiplied the opium content by five. The new theriac truly deserved its name of *galene*, meaning "tranquility" (unrelated to the name of Galen). It was, in effect, an addicting tranquilizer (Fig. 10.15).[82]

From then on galene became the theriac par excellence, known simply as theriac, and there never was a more successful drug.[83] Galen wrote a whole book about it, called *Theriaké*. He accepted the addition of viper flesh as perfectly sound: was it not logical that the antidote, *theriaké*, should contain the *therion*, the beast itself?[84] He personally prepared it for three emperors. Production was a major enterprise, lasting a couple of months. The final product was supposed to mature for years, but Marcus Aurelius liked it fresh and possibly became an opium addict in the process.[85] Those who could afford it gulped down a bean-sized lump of theriac for practically everything from the Black Death to nothing at all, as a preventive. It also went into plasters. When applied over bites, according to Galen, "it drew out the poison like a cupping-glass."[86] Once he tried it over an abscess, because the patient's father was reluctant to allow an operation: "it divided the overlying tissues more quickly than a scalpel."[87]

Skip 1300 years, and the creation of Nero's doctor has become an object of major international trade, being taken to China as a gift to the emperor. The chinese called it *tê-ya-ka* (Fig. 10.16), and it seems that they were not overly enthused.[88] As to the Indians, I found no record of their buying theriac (though they surely did); but they had brands of their own. Charaka mentions an antidote called *Mahagandhahasti* with sixty ingredients, almost the same as its European analog.[89] Sushruta has a similar one with eighty-five ingredients.[90]

Theriac survived even the onslaught of the Renaissance, though there was much discussion about the brand of vipers and whether heads and tails should be included. In several European cities the making of theriac became an official ceremony, preceded by public display of the vipers and the sixty-three other ingredients. A visitor to Venice in 1646 came away with his supply of prized "Venice treacle," but also stayed for the "extraordinary ceremony thereof . . . for 'tis extremely pompous and worth seeing."[91] Theriac became almost synonymous with medicine.

Theriac died, but ever so slowly. The German official pharmacopoeia still included it in 1872, vipers and all; the French in 1884. By then you could order your *Theriaca Andromachi* by telephone (Fig. 10.17).

Theriaca Andromachi senioris.

℞ Throchiscorum Stiliticorum ℥ xij ,
    Viperinorum ,

Magmatis Hedycroi ,   Therebinthinæ Chiæ , ana ℥ j ß ,
Piperis longi ,   Radicum Gentianæ ,
Opÿ Thebaici , ana ℥ vj ,   Acori Veri ,
Rosarum rubrarum ,   Meu Athamantici ,
Iridis ,   Valerianæ majoris ,
Succi Glycyrrhizæ ,   Nardi Celticæ ,
Seminis Buniadis ,   Amomi racemosi ,
Scordij ,   Chamæpytheos ,
Opobalsami ,   Comæ Hyperici ,
Cinnamomi ,   Seminis Ameos ,
Agarici, ana ℥ iij ,   Thlaspeos ,
Costi ,   Anisi ,
Nardi Indicæ ,   Fœniculi ,
Dictamni Cretici ,   Siseleos Massiliensis ,
Rhapontici ,   Cardamomi minoris ,
Radicis Pentaphylli ,   Malabathri
    Zinziberis ,   Comæ Polij montani ,
Prassÿ albi ,   Chamædryos ,
Stœchadis Arabicæ ,   Carpobalsami ,
Schænanthi ,   Succi Hypocistidos ,
Seminis Petroselini Macedonici , Acaciæ Veræ ,
Calaminthæ montanæ ,   Gummi Arabici ,
Cassiæligneæ ,   Styracis Calamitæ ,
Croci ,   Terræ Lemniæ ,
Piperis albi ,   Chalcitidis ,
    Nigri ,   Sagapeni ana ℥ j ,
Mirræ Trogloditidis ,   Radicum Aristolochiæ tenuis ,
Thuris masculi ,   Comæ Centaurij minoris ,
    Seminis Dauci Cretici ,
    Opopanacis ,
    Galbani ,
    Bituminis Iudaïci ,
    Castorei ana ℥ ß ,
    Mellis optimi despumati ℔ xxviij.
    Vini generosi quantùm satis.

10.15 The drugs that went into *galene*, the classical theriac, according to a French *Pharmacopée Royale* of 1676. The drawing is a modern addition; it underscores the two most important ingredients: viper flesh, on which the myth of theriac was based, and opium, perhaps the only component that was medically—and commercially—effective.

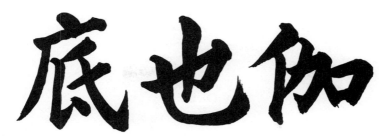

10.16 Theriac went as far as China, where it became *tê-ya-ka* (now *ti-yeh-chia*).

After Galen

After Galen, the history of the wound grinds to a halt for at least one thousand years. Europe sank into the Dark Ages; Indian surgery declined; even in China, where science advanced, surgery made no progress.[92] Only the number of wounds did not decline; for the wound remained, as I fear it always will, a basic means of human communication.

And wounds continued to become sores. For all of his greatness as an experimenter, Galen had left no message, and no surgical dressing, that really helped. His wound biology had moved not one step beyond that of Hippocrates. It could scarcely have been otherwise, for he had totally endorsed the hopeless theory of the four humors, and even built further upon it. Under his influence, during the Middle Ages the theory acquired still new layers, of no advantage to medicine (Fig. 10.18); it simply became an effort to fit man into the universe by a scheme of fours, the same as the Chinese were trying to do by a scheme of fives.

10.17 The theriac contained in this pot may have been on sale one hundred years ago.

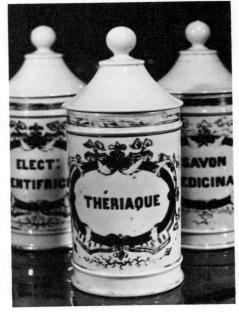

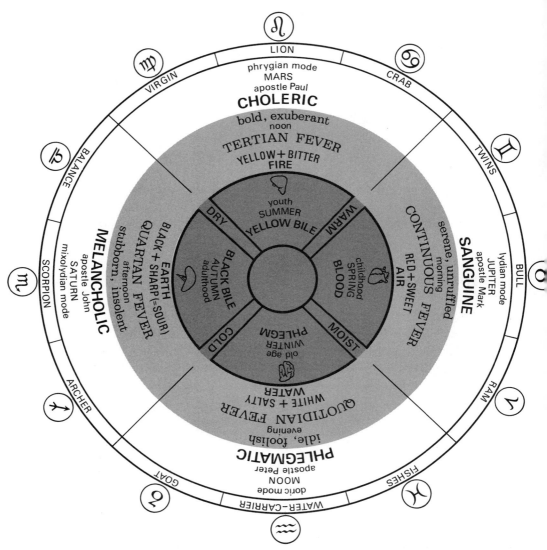

10.18 The Hippocratic scheme of the four humors (dark gray ring) and its growth through the ages. Galen added some correlations (light gray ring); others accrued in the Middle Ages (white ring), in an attempt to fit man's microcosmos with the universe. This scheme of fours recalls the Chinese fivefold scheme (Fig. 6.20).

Galen's handling of the wounded patient, as of the sick in general, remained as bad as ever. Even his diets were unhealthy. In this respect he was again following in the footsteps of Hippocrates, whose strong interest in diet, usually hailed as a great advance, was actually a road to vitamin deficiency. The Hippocratics found fault with most vegetables, and fruits were considered even worse. The prejudice against fruit is also echoed by Pliny: spring apples are harmful, pears are indigestible even to the healthy, plums and cherries are bad for the stomach, walnuts poison the brain.[93] The prevalence of bladder stones in children, a condition now almost unknown, was probably due to lack of vitamin A. The risk of vitamin lack was probably greater for the rich, for only they could afford the optimal Greek diet—mainly meat.[94]

Besides the drugs, which were generally useless or dangerous, Galen's treatment rested again on that indefensible Hippocratic triad: STARVING, PURGING, BLEEDING. Galen became, most unfortunately, the apostle of the bloodthirsty school. There was in Rome at that time a group of physicians who followed the conservative line of Erasistratos, opposed to bleeding. They infuriated Galen to such a degree that he wrote the book *On Venesection Against Erasistratos*, besides a pamphlet, *On Venesection*.[95] How could anybody be so thick-headed as not to understand that *ulcers called for bleeding?* Here is a case he gave to prove the point:

After a man had an ulcer on his thigh for a long time, the veins lying above it which were varicose, were excised. Immediately the ulcer healed. Yet the incision by means of which the veins were removed did not get well. Later in the year, one of my preceptors at Pergamum, Stratonicus, a disciple of Sabinus Hippocrates, opened a vein at the elbow, and when he saw the escaping blood thick and black he repeated the venesection for four days. In addition he purged the black humor by medicaments, prescribed a nourishing diet, and thus healed the ulcer.[96]

The conservatives lost the battle. Venesection for ulcers was so easy to rationalize: injury attracted blood (everybody could see that); blood stagnated around the injury and decayed (everybody could see the decay too); so blood had to be drained out before it decayed. The Hippocratic books had spelled out the theory; the Alexandrians had reinforced it; Galen, who gave it the final touches, thereby became responsible for rivers of blood—and for cemeteries prematurely full.

Bleeding for wounds and ulcers alone would have been bad enough; but remember that interesting Hippocratic remark to the effect that *every* disease may be considered as a wound of some sort. Galen followed this trend, bled for practically every disease—and *even bled for bleeding.*

This paradox became standard practice; three centuries later we find it recommended by Caelius Aurelianus, an eminent compiler (Fig. 10.19):

10.19 The Hippocratic principle of curing hemorrhage by bleeding, as recommended by Caelius Aurelianus in the fifth century A.D.

CAP. XIII. *Hæmorrhagiæ curatio.* 415
enim de *fchemate* jacendi, atque *phlebotomia*, & 183
ligatione, & conftrictivis, vel frigidis *cataplafmati-*
bus, & *aceto* bibendo, varia difceptatione pugnatum
eft. De *fchemate* inquam jacendi: fiquidem alii fu-
pinos jubent ægrotantes jacere, vel fuper eas partes,
quæ non patiuntur. *Afclepiades* z confequenter ap- z inconfe-
probat fupra partes quæ patiuntur, effe locandos æ- quenter
grotantes: fiquidem cum fcriberet neceffarias effe
curationes, adprehenfa caufa, fic fuerit elocutus,
etiam fanguine, inquit, fluentes ita effe locandos. *a*Si- *a* At quidem

under the heading *Haemorrhagiae curatio,* "Treatment for Bleeding," he lists *phlebotomia,* "venesection"! The hemorrhage here meant by Caelius Aurelianus is from the lungs (presumably in tuberculosis), but the reasoning applied to any form of bleeding. The paragraph concludes that not everyone who bleeds should be bled, but those who are not "are deprived of a great help."[97] Medicine never produced a greater absurdity.

All this was, in essence, a revival of Hippocrates. Centuries passed. The Roman Empire broke up. The flame of Greek medicine flickered, but never died out. Three times at least it was revived. The first revival occurred in Persia, between the fifth and tenth centuries; the second took place in Europe when the printing press first made the texts more easily available; the third came in the early 1800s, as a reaction to despair. It happened in Paris, where medicine seemed to have run aground. Operations that had been routine at the time of Hippocrates could no longer be performed, because the patients died of infection. As for drugs, it was more and more obvious that they were worthless.[98] In this gloomy state of affairs a learned physician, Emile Littré, decided that it was time to return to the original sources and make them available to everyone, even to those who could not read Greek or Latin. So he gave twenty-two years of his life to translate all the works of Hippocrates. When he finally came to the last page of the tenth volume, in 1861, it was just too late: Claude Bernard, Virchow, Pasteur had broken the impasse—and the new word was to look forward. Hippocrates and Galen had stepped out of medicine and into history.

To end, I must pay tribute to the earliest and most important revival of Greek medicine: its reappearance in oriental dress, during the Middle Ages, in one of the most interesting and least known detours of history—the Nestorian epic.[99] In the year 431 A.D., a church crisis ended dramatically at the Council of Ephesos when Nestorios, the tough patriarch of Constantinople, was excommunicated for heresy. He maintained that the divine and human persons were not entirely merged in the person of Christ, and especially that Mary should not be called *Theotókos,* "Mother of God," as was then customary. Nestorios was exiled, and died—probably in Egypt—in 451. His followers, the first Nestorians, were forced to flee. Their first refuge was among the erudite monks of Edessa, in upper Mesopotamia (Fig. 10.20). But the long hand of the church reached them even there and caused them to scatter as far as India and China. One group found permanent asylum in Persia, thanks to its tolerant king. They settled in his capital, Jundi Shapur, an ancient and beautiful city not far from Susa, with a university and a hospital that functioned also as a medical school. Happily transplanted, the Nestorians flourished. Partly through their influence, partly through its fortunate circumstances, the University of Jundi Shapur became one of the leading intellectual centers of the time. Its geographical setting allowed it to become a unique meeting point of cultures—Persian, Greek, Alexandrian, Jewish, Hindu, and Chinese—and its tolerant atmosphere allowed scholars of different creeds to work together in peace, as nowhere else in the world. When the city fell to

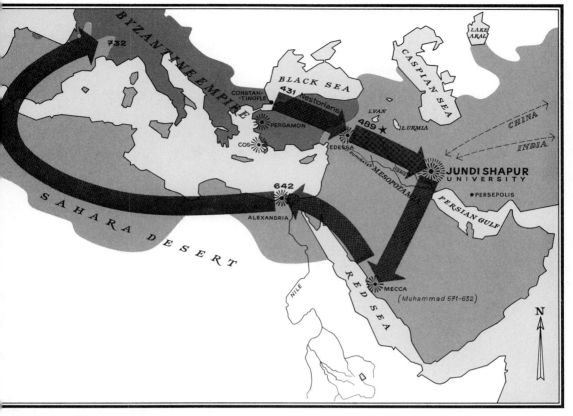

10.20 The route of Hippocratic medicine as it returned to Europe through the Nestorians, via the University of Jundi Shapur, and then the Muslims.

the Arabs in 636, the university was not disturbed; in fact, the conquerors adopted it and made of its medical school their principal training center.[100] Two of the Prophet's physicians were graduates of Jundi Shapur. All the while, the Nestorians were performing a huge bibliographic task: translating Greek books into Syriac, the language of the university. Hippocrates and Galen were among their first translations. Then Muslims worked at Arabic translations of the Syriac. Eventually a large body of Greek literature became available in Syriac and Arabic.

Toward the end of the tenth century Baghdad, having become the capital of the caliphate, began to drain away the talents of Jundi Shapur. The end came fast. Today, nothing is left of that glorious city except for a few vague trenches in the ground.

The adventure of the Nestorians explains why some Greek works have come down to us ultimately as Latin versions from an Arabic text translated from the Syriac. A new book of Galen, in Arabic, was discovered in Constantinople as late as 1931.[101] The Nestorian experience also explains why the great Arabic physicians—Rhazes, Avicenna, Albucasis—not only revered the Greek masters, but spoke their same words, and tempered them with Hindu medicine.

It is not known whether the Nestorians of Jundi Shapur and their colleagues made any original discoveries in the field of medicine. But this is irrelevant, for they were foremost among that crowd of unknown, unsung scholars who, during the so-called Dark Ages, cared to transmit the knowledge of antiquity. Without their labors, some of our roots would have withered—and much of the story that I have shared with you in this book could not have been told.

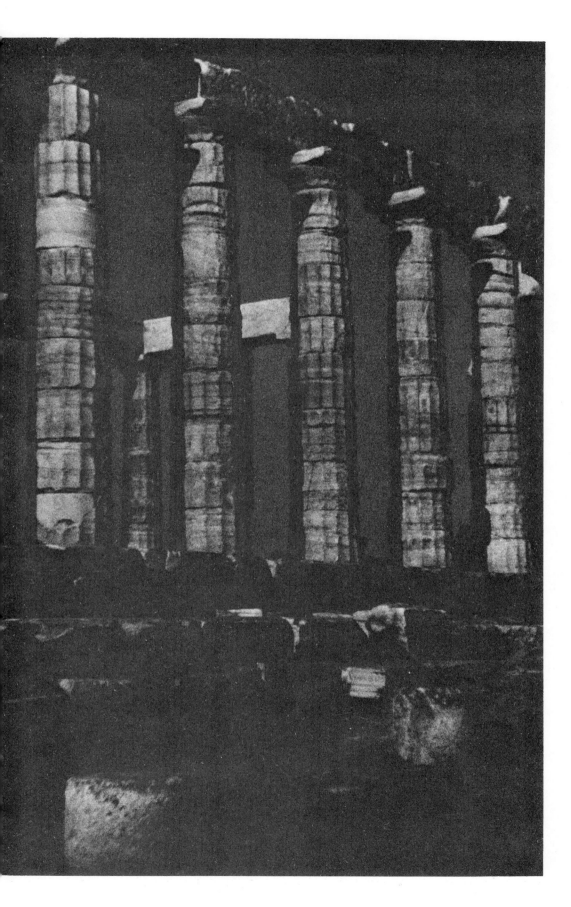

Bibliography

1. Prelude

Ackerknecht, E. H., 1946: Contradictions in Primitive Surgery. Bull. Hist. Med. *20*, 184–187.

———, 1967: Primitive Surgery. Ch. 51 in Brothwell and Sandison 1967 (pp. 635–650; see ref.).

———, 1971: *Medicine and Ethnology: Selected Essays.* Bern, Huber.

Ardrey, R., 1967: *African Genesis.* New York, Dell.

Barghoorn, E. S., 1971: The Oldest Fossils. Scientific American *224*, 30–42.

Bartels, M., 1893: *Die Medicin der Naturvölker.* Leipzig, Grieben.

Bössneck, J., 1971: Mosaik der Geschichte der Tierchirurgie. In H. Schebitz, *Allgemeine Chirurgie für Tierärzte.* Hamburg, Parey-Verlag.

Bourne, G. H., ed., 1969 and 1970: *The Chimpanzee.* Basel, Karger (vols. I and II).

Bradley, W. H., 1963: Unmineralized Fossil Bacteria. Science *141*, 919–921.

———, 1968: Unmineralized Fossil Bacteria: A Retraction. Science *160*, 437.

Brain, C. K., 1967(a): Hottentot Food Remains and Their Bearing on the Interpretation of Fossil Bone Assemblages. Scient. Papers Namib Desert Res. Stn. No. 32, 1–11.

———, 1967(b): Bone Weathering and the Problem of Bone Pseudotools. South Afr. J. of Sci. *63*, 97–99.

———, 1969: The Contribution of Namib Desert Hottentots to an Understanding of Australopithecine Bone Accumulations. Scient. Papers Namib Desert Res. Stn. No. 39, 13–22.

Breuil, H., 1920: Les roches peintes de Minateda. L'Anthropologie *XXX*, 1–50.

Brothwell, D., and Sandison, A. D., 1967: *Diseases in Antiquity.* Springfield, Ill., C. C. Thomas. [A comprehensive, extremely useful volume.]

Cartailhac, E., 1889: *La France préhistorique d'après les sépultures et les monuments.* Paris, Alcan.

Clark, G., 1965: *World Prehistory: An Outline.* Cambridge, Cambridge Univ. Press.

Clement, A. J., 1956: Caries in the South African Ape-Man: Some Examples of Undoubted Pathological Anthenticity Believed to be 800,000 Years Old. Brit. Dent. J. (London) *101*, 4–7.

Cloud, P. E., Jr., 1965: Significance of the Gunflint (Precambrian) Microflora. Science *148*, 27–35.

Cloud, P. E., Jr., and Hagen, H., 1965: Electron Microscopy of the Gunflint Microflora: Preliminary Results. Proc. Nat. Acad. Sci. *54*, 1–8.

Courville, C. B., 1967: Cranial Injuries in Prehistoric Man. Ch. 48 in Brothwell and Sandison 1967 (pp. 606–622; see ref.).

Daland, J., 1936: Depressed Fracture and Trephining of the Skull by the Incas of Peru. Ann. Med. Hist. *7*, 550–558.

Dart, R. A., 1925: *Australopithecus africanus:* The Man-Ape of South Africa. Nature (London) *115*, 195–199.

————, 1949: The Predatory Implemental Technique of Australopithecus. Am. J. Physical Anthropol. *7*, 1–38.

————, 1953: The Predatory Transition from Ape to Man. Internat. Anthropological and Linguistic Review *1*, 201–219.

————, 1955: Cultural Status of the South African Man-Apes. Ann. Report, Smithsonian Inst., 317–338.

————, 1957: The Osteodontokeratic Culture of Australopithecus Prometheus. Transvaal Museum Memoir No. 10.

————, 1958(a): The Gradual Appraisal and Acceptance of Australopithecus. In *Evolution and Hominisation,* G. Kurth, ed. Stuttgart, Fischer (2nd ed.; pp. 230–256).

————, 1958(b): The Minimal Bone-Breccia Content of Makapansgat and the Australopithecine Predatory Habit. Am. Anthropologist *60*, 923–931.

————, 1959(a): An Australopithecine Scoop from Herefordshire. Nature (London) *183*, 844.

————, 1959(b): Osteodontokeratic Ripping Tools and Pulp Scoops for Teething and Edentulous Australopithecines. J. Dental Assn. of South Africa *14*, 164–178.

Dart, R. A., and Craig, D., 1959: *Adventures with the Missing Link.* New York, Harper.

Dastugue, J., 1959: Un orifice crânien préhistorique. Bull. et Mém. Soc. Anthropol. de Paris *10*, 357–363.

Drew, I. M., Perkins, D., Jr., and Daly, P., 1971: Prehistoric Domestication of Animals: Effects on Bone Structure. Science *171*, 280–282.

Felkin, R. W., 1884: Notes on Labour in Central Africa. Edinb. Med. J. *29*, 922–930.

Fischer, H., 1864: Klinisches und Experimentelles zur Lehre der Trepanation. Arch. klin. Chir. *6*, 595–647.

Florey, H. W., 1970: *General Pathology.* London, Lloyd-Luke (4th ed.).

Frank, R. M., and Brendel, A., 1966: Ultrastructure of the Approximal Dental Plaque and the Underlying Normal and Carious Enamel. Arch. Oral Biol. *11*, 893–912.

Freeman, D., 1964: Human Aggression in Anthropological Perspective. In *On Aggression, a Symposium,* Carthy and Ebling, eds. London, Acad. Press (pp. 109–119).

Gabbiani, G., Hirschel, B. J., Ryan, G. B., Statkov, P. R., and Majno, G., 1972: Granulation Tissue as a Contractile Organ. A Study of Structure and Function. J. Exptl. Med. *135*, 719–734.

Gardner, R. G., 1963: *Dead Birds* (feature-length motion picture, produced by Film Study Center, Harvard University; Contemporary Films and Mutual Distributors).

Gardner, R. G., and Heider, K. G., 1968: *Gardens of War: Life and Death in the New Guinea Stone Age.* Introduction by Margaret Mead. New York, Random House.

Gilmore, C. W., 1912: The Mounted Skeletons of Camptosaurus in the United States National Museum. Proc. U.S. Nat. Museum *41*, 687–696.

Goodall, Jane, 1965: Chimpanzees of the Gombe Stream Reserve. In *Primate Behavior,* I. DeVore, ed. New York, Holt, Rinehart and Winston (pp. 425–473).

Gorjanović-Kramberger, K., 1906: *Der diluviale Mensch von Krapina in Kroatien. Ein Beitrag zur Paläoanthropologie.* Wiesbaden, Kreidel.

Guex, J., 1967: Contribution à l'étude des blessures chez les ammonites. Bull. des laboratoires de géologie, minéralogie, etc., Université de Lausanne, No. 165, 1–16 (also: Bull. Soc. vaudoise des Sci. nat. 69, No. 323, 1967).

Hare, R., 1967: The Antiquity of Diseases Caused by Bacteria and Viruses: A Review from a Bacteriologist's Point of View. Ch. 8 in Brothwell and Sandison 1967 (pp. 115–131; see ref.).

Hengen, O. P., 1967(a): Weitere wahrscheinliche Krankheiten im Tier-Mensch-Uebergangsfeld (Teil I). Folia Historica, Reihe A, No. 20, 25–27.

———, 1967(b): Uebrige pathologische Befunde and paläohygienische Umweltbedingungen der frühesten Hominiden. Folia Historica, Reihe A, No. 17, 21–24b.

———, 1969: Probleme und Ergebnisse der Paläomedizin, Selecta XI, 651–659.

Hilton-Simpson, M. W., 1922: *Arab Medicine and Surgery. A Study of the Healing Art in Algeria.* London, Oxford University Press.

Holloway, R. L., 1970: Australopithecine Endocast (Taung Specimen, 1924): A New Volume Determination. Science 168, 966–968.

Howell, F. C. and the Editors of Time-Life Books, 1970: *Early Man.* Life Nature Library. Time-Life International, Nederland.

Howells, W., 1962: *Ideas on Human Evolution: Selected Essays, 1949–1961.* Cambridge, Mass., Harvard University Press.

———, 1967: *Mankind in the Making: The Story of Human Evolution.* Garden City, N.Y., Doubleday.

———, 1973: *Evolution of the Genus Homo.* Reading, Mass., Addison-Wesley.

Jaeger, W., 1944: *Paideia.* New York, Oxford University Press (vol. III).

Janssens, P. A., 1957: Medical Views on Prehistoric Representations of Human Hands. Medical History 1, 318–322.

Jarcho, S., 1966: *Human Palaeopathology* (proc. of a Symposium on Human Palaeopath., Washington, D.C., Jan. 14, 1965). New Haven and London, Yale University Press.

Klindt-Jensen, O., 1957: *Denmark before the Vikings.* London, Thames and Hudson.

Kobayashi, K., 1967: Trend in the Length of Life Based on Human Skeletons from Prehistoric to Modern Times in Japan. J. of the Fac. of Science, University of Tokyo, Sect. 5 (Anthropol.) III, 107–160.

Koehler, W., 1927: *The Mentality of Apes.* Trans. E. Winter. New York, Harcourt, Brace & Co.

Kortlandt, A., and von Zon, J. C. J., 1969: The Present State of Research on the Dehumanization Hypothesis of African Ape Evolution. Proc. 2nd. Internat. Congress of Primatology III, 10–13.

Kurth, G., ed., 1968: *Evolution and Hominisation.* Stuttgart, Fischer (2nd ed.).

Lawick-Goodall, Jane van, 1971: *In the Shadow of Man.* London, Collins.

Lawrence, J. W. P., 1935: A Note on the Pathology of the Kanam Mandible. In Leakey, L. S. B., *The Stone Age Races of Kenya*, Oxford University Press, 1935 (Appendix A, p. 139).

Leakey, L. S. B., 1932: The Oldoway Human Skeleton. Nature (London) 129, 715 and 721–722.

———, 1961(a): Exploring 1,750,000 Years Into Man's Past. Nat. Geogr. Magazine 120, 564–589.

———, 1961(b): New Finds at Olduvai Gorge. Nature (London) 189, 649–650.

Leroi-Gourhan, A., 1958: Le symbolisme des grands signes dans l'art pariétal paléolithique. Bull. Soc. Préhist. Française 55, 384–398.

———, 1964: *Les religions de la préhistoire (paléolithique).* Paris, Presses Universitaires de France.

———, 1967: Les mains de Gargas. Essai pour une étude d'ensemble. Bull. Soc. Préhist. Française 64, 107–122.

———, 1968: Les signes pariétaux du Paléolithique supérieur franco-cantabrique. In *Simpósio Internacional de Arte Rupestre.* Barcelona (pp. 67–77).

———, 1971: *Préhistoire de l'art occidental.* Paris, Editions d'art Lucien Mazenod.

Levey, M., 1959: *Chemistry and Chemical Technology in Ancient Mesopotamia.* Amsterdam, London, New York, and Princeton, Elsevier.

Lindblom, G., 1920: *The Akamba in British East Africa.* Uppsala, Appelbergs (Arch. d'Etudes Orientales, J.-A. Lundell, ed., vol. 17).

Lisowski, F. P., 1967: Prehistoric and Early Historic Trepanation. Ch. 52 in Brothwell and Sandison 1967 (pp. 651-672; see ref.).

Lorenz, K., 1952: *King Solomon's Ring.* London, Methuen.

Lucas, A., and Harris, J. R., 1962: *Ancient Egyptian Materials and Industries.* London, Arnold (4th ed.). Abbr. LH.

MacCurdy, G. G., 1923: Human Skeletal Remains from the Highlands of Peru. Am. J. Physical Anthropol. 6, 217–329.

Majno, G., Gabbiani, G., Hirschel, B. J., Ryan, G. B., and Statkov, P. R., 1971: Contraction of Granulation Tissue in Vitro: Similarity to Smooth Muscle. Science 173, 548–550.

Malvesin-Fabre, G., Nougier, L. R., and Robert, R., 1954: *Gargas.* Toulouse, Privat.

Manouvrier, L., 1904: Incisions, cautérisations et trépanations crâniennes de l'époque néolithique. Bull. et Mém. Soc. Anthropol. Paris 5, 67–73.

Margetts, E. L., 1967: Trepanation of the Skull by the Medicine–men of Primitive Cultures, with Particular Reference to Present-day Native East African Practice. Ch. 53 in Brothwell and Sandison 1967 (pp. 673–701; see ref.).

McGrew, W. C., and Tutin, C. E. G., 1972: Chimpanzee Dentistry. J. of the American Dental Ass. 85, 1198–1203.

——, 1973: Chimpanzee Tool Use in Dental Grooming. Nature (London) 241, 477–478.

McKenzie, W., and Brothwell, D., 1967: Disease in the Ear Region. Ch. 38 in Brothwell and Sandison 1967 (pp. 464–473; see ref.).

Mennerich, G., 1968: *Römerzeitliche Tierknochen aus 3 Fundorten des Niederrheingebietes.* Doctoral thesis, Munich, Institut für Paläoanatomie, Domestikationsforschung und Geschichte der Tiermedizin.

Miles, W. R., 1963: Chimpanzee Behavior: Removal of Foreign Body from Companion's Eye. Proc. Nat. Acad. Sci. 49, 840–843.

Miller, M. G., 1913: Human Vertebra Transfixed by a Spearpoint of Antler. J. Acad. Nat. Sci., Philadelphia XVI, 477–480.

Moodie, R. L., 1923: *Paleopathology: An Introduction to the Study of Ancient Evidences of Disease.* Urbana, Illinois, University of Illinois Press.

——, 1926: Studies in Paleopathology, Second Series, I: A Prehistoric Surgical Bandage from Peru. Ann. Med. Hist. 8, 69–72.

——, 1927: Studies in Palaeopathology. XXI. Injuries to the Head Among the Pre-Columbian Peruvians. Ann. Med. Hist. 9, 277–307.

Morel, C., 1951: *La médecine et la chirurgie osseuses aux temps préhistoriques dans la région des Grands Causses.* Paris, La Nef (also: Doctoral Thesis, Montpellier, 1951).

Morel, C., and Baudouin, M., 1928: Un cas intéressant de pathologie préhistorique. Une pointe de silex dans une vertèbre néolithique. Le progrès médical No. 25, 142.

Morice, A. G., 1901: Dené Surgery. Trans. Canad. Inst. 1900–1901, 15–28.

Muniz, M. A., and McGee, W. G., 1897: Primitive Trephining in Peru. Bureau of American Ethnology, 16th Annual Report, 11–72.

Oakley, K. P., 1957: Tools Makyth Man. Antiquity 31, 199–209. Reprinted in Ann. Report Smithsonian Inst. 1958, 431–445; Howells, W., *Ideas on Human Evolution* 1962 (pp. 422–435; see ref.).

——, 1968: The Earliest Tool-Makers. In *Evolution and Hominisation*, G. Kurth, ed. Stuttgart, Fischer (2nd ed.; pp. 257–272).

Pales, L., 1930: *Paléopathologie et Pathologie Comparative.* Paris, Masson (also: Doctoral Thesis, Bordeaux, 1929).

Pliny [The Elder]: *Natural History.* Trans. H. Rackham, W. H. S. Jones and D. E. Eichholz. Loeb Classical Library, Cambridge, Mass., Harvard University Press, and London, Heinemann (1956-1966; 10 vols.). Abbr. PNH.

Protsch, R., and Berger, R., 1973: Earliest Radiocarbon Dates for Domesticated Animals. Science 179, 235–239.

Raff, R. A., and Mahler, H. R., 1972: The Non Symbiotic Origin of Bacteria. Science *177*, 575–582.

Robinson, J. T., 1959: A Bone Implement from Sterkfontein. Nature *184*, 583–585.

———, 1968: The Origin and Adaptive Radiation of the Australopithecines. In *Evolution and Hominisation*, G. Kurth, ed. Stuttgart, Fischer (2nd ed.; pp. 150–175).

Ross, R., 1969: Wound Healing. Scientific American *220*, 40–50.

Rouillon, A., and Baudouin, M., 1924: L'inclusion des silex taillés, révélée par la radiographie, dans les os préhistoriques. Le progrès médical No. 11, 170–173.

Schopf, J. W., Barghoorn, E. S., Maser, M. D., and Gordon, R. O., 1965: Electron Microscopy of Fossil Bacteria Two Billion Years Old. Science *149*, 1365–1367.

Schultz, A. H., 1939: Notes in Diseases and Healed Fractures of Wild Apes and their Bearing on the Antiquity of Pathological Conditions in Man. Bull. Hist. Med. 7, 571–582.

———, 1969: *The Life of Primates*. London, Wiendenfeld and Nicolson.

Simpson, G. G., 1967: *The Meaning of Evolution*. New Haven and London, Yale University Press.

Smithers, R. H. N., 1966: *The Mammals of Rhodesia, Zambia and Malawi*. London, Collins.

Solecki, R. S., 1957: Shanidar Cave. Scientific American *197*, 59–64.

———, 1960: Three Adult Neanderthal Skeletons from Shanidar cave, Northern Iraq. Smithsonian Inst., Ann. Report for 1959, 603–635.

———, 1963: Prehistory in Shanidar Valley, Northern Iraq. Science *139*, 179–193.

———, 1971: *Shanidar, the First Flower People*. New York, Knopf.

Sollas, W. J., 1911: *Ancient Hunters and their Modern Representatives*. London, Macmillan.

Stewart, T. D., 1959: The Restored Shanidar I Skull. Smithsonian Inst., Ann. Report for 1958, 473–480.

———, 1966: Some Problems in Human Palaeopathology. In *Human Palaeopathology*, S. Jarcho, ed. New Haven and London, Yale University Press (pp. 43–55).

———, 1969: Fossil Evidence of Human Violence. Transaction 6, 48–53.

Straus, W. L., Jr., and Cave, A. J. E., 1957: Pathology and the Posture of Neanderthal Man. Quart. Rev. Biol. *32*, 348–363.

Tasnádi-Kubacska, A., 1962: *Paläopathologie (Pathologie der vorzeitlichen Tiere)*. Jena, Fischer. [Very useful book with many interesting figures.]

Teleki, G., 1973: *The Predatory Behavior of Wild Chimpanzees*. Lewisburg, Bucknell University Press.

Tobias, P. V., 1962: A Re-Examination of the Kanam Mandible. Actes du IVe Congrès Panafricain de Préhistoire et de l'Etude du Quaternaire. Tervuren, Belgium, Annales du Musée Royal de l'Afrique Centrale, Série in-8⁰, Sciences Hum., No. 40.

———, 1964: The Olduvai Bed I Hominine with Special Reference to its Cranial Capacity. Nature *202*, 3–4.

Underwood, E. A., 1951: *Catalogue of an Exhibition Illustrating Prehistoric Man in Health and Sickness*. Wellcome Medical Historical Museum. London, Oxford University Press.

Vallois, H. V., 1937: La durée de la vie chez l'homme fossile. L'Anthropologie 47, 499–532.

Verbrugge, A. R., 1956: La main dans l'art préhistorique. L'Ethnographie, N. S. No. 51, 13–20.

———, 1965: Les mains mutilées. Congrès Préhist. de Monaco, XVI Session, 1959, 1–9.

———, 1969: *Le symbole de la main*. Author's possession, 41 R. St. Lazare, 60 Compiègne, France (2nd ed.).

———, 1970: *Corpus of the Hand Figurations in Primitive Australia*. Ophrys. Compiègne, France.

Virchow, R., 1886: Buschmänner. Ztschr. f. Ethn. *XVIII*, 221–239.

Weidenreich, F., 1939: The Duration of Life of Fossil Man in China and the Pathological Lesions Found in his Skeleton. Chinese Med. J. *55*, 34–44.

Wells, C., 1965: *Bones, Bodies and Disease.* New York and Washington, Praeger. [A most readable, well-illustrated account of disease in early man.]

Wells, L. H., 1958: A Reconsideration of Some Mandibular Profiles. South Afr. J. of Sci. *54,* 55–58. Reprinted in Howells, W., *Ideas on Human Evolution,* 1962 (pp. 460–465; see ref.).

Wolbach, S. B., 1954: The Glorious Past, the Doleful Present and the Uncertain Future of Pathology. Harvard Med. Alumni Bull., June 1954, 45–48.

Wolberg, D. L., 1970: The Hypothesized Osteodontokeratic Culture of the Australopithecinae: A Look at the Evidence and the Opinions. Current Anthrop. *11,* 23–38.

Wormington, H. M., 1957: *Ancient Man in North America.* Denver Mus. of Nat. Hist., Denver, Colorado (4th ed.).

Zeuner, F. E., 1963: *A History of Domesticated Animals.* London, Hutchinson. See also German translation, 1967, revised by J. Bössneck and T. Haltenroth, *Geschichte der Haustiere.* Munich, Basel, and Vienna, Bayerischer Landwirtschaftsverlag.

2. The Asu

For a general background on Mesopotamian civilization, Oppenheim's *Ancient Mesopotamia* is an excellent eye-opener, expressly written to communicate with non-Assyriologists. It includes a chapter on medicine (see also Meissner 1920; Saggs 1962; Mallowan 1965; Chiera 1966). Oppenheim belongs to the "pessimistic" school of Assyriologists who feel that very little is known about the people of Mesopotamia, hence the subtitle of this book, *Portrait of a Dead Civilization.* Its contents, however, will convince the reader that an awful lot is known; in fact, I was amused to find that in the French translation the subtitle is *Portrait of a Civilization* (Oppenheim 1970). Another book of absorbing interest, in which Akkadians *really* come alive, is Oppenheim's *Letters from Mesopotamia* (1967). Kramer's *History Begins at Sumer,* very much an example of the enthusiastic school, offers a gripping portrait of Sumerian life. On Mesopotamian medicine the papers of Labat, and his *Treatise of Prognoses,* are a must; Contenau's book on Assyrian and Babylonian medicine is useful, though old; so is Sigerist's chapter on Mesopotamian medicine (in which the translations would need to be revised, and the religious aspects of medicine are erroneously emphasized; see Biggs 1969 p. 95). Some of Thompson's pioneer studies have become so outdated as to be dangerous in the hands of a layman. Köcher's several volumes of medical texts in cuneiform may contain treasures, but Assyriologists have not yet come around to translating them. In general, the bulk of data on Mesopotamia is enormous, but that on medicine limited; one is forced to admit that it is inadequate for tracing a real, continuous history over three-thousand years. Without joining the pessimistic school, I believe one should always keep in mind Oppenheim's closing lines: "This material covers only a restricted area and period, permitting but an occasional insight into a perhaps unique situation whose relationship to the over-all picture can well be likened to an accumulation of irregular blotches and short lines meandering from nowhere to nowhere . . ." (Oppenheim 1964 p. 334).

Bibliography

Akkadisches Handwörterbuch. See von Soden.

The Assyrian Dictionary of the Oriental Institute of the University of Chicago. The Oriental Institute, Chicago, Ill., 1968. Abbr. CAD.

Bible, Dictionary. Abbr. DB. See Buttrick 1962.

————, *The New English Bible.* Oxford University Press and Cambridge University Press, 1970.

Biggs, R., 1969: Medicine in Ancient Mesopotamia. In *History of Science,* A. C. Crombie and M. A. Hoskin, eds. Cambridge, Heffer (vol. VIII, pp. 94–105).

Bishop, C. W., 1939: The Beginnings of Civilization in Eastern Asia. J. Am. Oriental Soc. *4,* 45–61.

Buttrick, G. A., and others, eds., 1962: *The Interpreter's Dictionary of the Bible*. New York and Nashville, Abingdon (4 vols.). Abbr. DB.

Cardascia, G., 1969: *Les lois assyriennes*. Paris, Ed. du cerf.

Ceram, C. W., 1967: *Gods, Graves and Scholars: The Story of Archaeology*. New York, Knopf.

Chiera, E., 1966: *They Wrote on Clay*. Phoenix Books. Chicago and London, University of Chicago Press.

Civil, M., 1960: Prescriptions médicales sumériennes. Revue d'Assyriol. *54*, 57–72.

———, 1961: Une nouvelle prescription médicale sumérienne. Revue d'Assyriol. *55*, 91–94.

———, 1969: The Sumerian Flood Story. In W. G. Lambert and A. R. Millard, *Atra-ḫasīs*. Oxford, Clarendon (pp. 138–145, 167–174).

Contenau, G., 1927: *Manuel d'archéologie orientale depuis les origines jusqu'à l'époque d'Alexandre*. Paris, Picard.

———, 1938: *La Médecine en Assyrie et en Babylonie*. Paris, Maloine.

———, 1940: Les débuts de l'écriture cunéiforme et les monuments figurés. Rev. des études sémitiques et Babyloniaca, 55–67.

———, 1947: *La magie chez les Assyriens et les Babyloniens*. Paris, Payot.

Denton, G. B., 1943: A New Interpretation of a Well-Known Assyrian Letter. J. of Near Eastern Studies *2*, 314–315.

Dictionary of the Bible. Abbr. DB. See Buttrick 1962.

Diringer, D., 1968: *The Alphabet: A Key to the History of Mankind*. London, Hutchinson (3rd ed.; 2 vols.).

Ebeling, E., 1932: *Arzt*. In E. Ebeling and B. Meissner, *Reallexikon der Assyriologie*. Berlin, de Gruyter.

Flückiger, F. A., and Hanbury, D., 1879: *Pharmacographia: A History of the Principal Drugs of Vegetable Origin Met with in Great Britain and British India*. London, Macmillan. Abbr. FH.

Forbes, R. J., 1965: Chemical, Culinary and Cosmetic Arts. Ch. 11 in *A History of Technology*, C. Singer, E. J. Holmyard, and A. R. Hall, eds.. Oxford, Clarendon (vol. I, pp 238–298).

Gelb, I. J., 1963: *A Study of Writing*. Chicago and London, University of Chicago Press.

Ghirshman, R., and Ghirshman, T., with Haeny, Jaquet, Vicari, Siebold, Sixtus, Weatherhead, Auberson, and Gasche, Architects, 1966: *Tchoga Zanbil*. I: La Ziggurat. Mémoires de la Délégation Archéol. en Iran, *XXXIX*. Paris, P. Geuthner.

Glotz, D., 1968: Mitteilungen über ein assyrisches Apothekeninventar. Arch. internat. d'hist. des sciences *21*, 95–114.

Harper, R. F., 1892–1914: *Assyrian and Babylonian Letters Belonging to the Kouyounjik Collections of the British Museum*. London, Luzac (14 vols.).

———, 1904: *The Code of Hammurabi King of Babylon about 2250* B.C. Chicago, University of Chicago Press, and London, Luzac.

Hastings, J., 1909: *The Dictionary of the Bible*. New York, Scribner.

Herodotus. Trans. A. D. Godley. Loeb Classical Library. Cambridge, Mass., Harvard University Press and London, Heinemann (1920–1925, repr. 1960–1966; 4 vols.).

Hole, F., 1966: Investigating the Origins of Mesopotamian Civilization. Science *153*, 605–611.

Hood, M. S. F., 1968: The Tartaria Tablets. Scientific American *210*, 30–37.

Humbert, P., 1964: Maladie et médecine dans l'Ancien Testament. Revue d'Hist. et de Philos. Relig. *44*, 1–29.

Ivánovics, G., and Horváth, S., 1947: Isolation and Properties of Raphanin, an Antibacterial Substance from Radish Seed. Proc. Soc. Exper. Biol. Med. *66*, 625–630.

Jacobsen, T., 1968: Mesopotamia. In H. Frankfort, H. A. Frankfort, J. A. Wilson, and T. Jacobsen, *Before philosophy*, Baltimore, Pelican Books, pp. 137–234.

Jastrow, M., Jr., 1917: Babylonian-Assyrian Medicine. Ann. Med. Hist. I, 231–257.

Jean, C.-F., 1950: Lettres diverses, transcrites et traduites. In *Arch. Royales de Mari*, A. Parrot and G. Dossin, eds. Paris, Impr. Nationale (vol. II).

Johns, C. H. W., 1904: *Babylonian and Assyrian Laws, Contracts and Letters.* New York, C. Scribner.

———, 1905: *The Oldest Code of Laws in the World: The Code of Laws Promulgated by Hammurabi, King of Babylon,* B.C. 2285–2242. Edinburgh, Clark.

Johnston, C., 1898: *The Epistolary Literature of the Assyrians and Babylonians.* Baltimore, Doctoral thesis, Johns Hopkins University.

Köcher, F., 1955: Keilschrifttexte zur assyrisch-babylonischen Drogen- und Pflanzenkunde. Deutsche Akad. der Wissensch. zu Berlin, Veröffentl. 28. Berlin, Akademie-Verlag.

———, 1963 and 1964: *Die babylonisch-assyrische Medizin in Texten und Untersuchungen.* Berlin, de Gruyter (vols. I-III). [All in cuneiform!]

Kramer, S. N., 1956: *History begins at Sumer.* The Falcon's Wing Press (paperback: Garden City, N.Y., Doubleday, 1959).

———, 1959: The World's Oldest Known Prescriptions. The CIBA Journal, No. 12, 1–7.

Kramer, S. N., and Levey, M., 1955: The Oldest Medical Text in Man's Recorded History: A Sumerian Physician's Prescription Book of 4000 Years Ago. The Illustrated London News, Feb. 26, pp. 370–371.

Labat, R., 1951: *Traité Akkadien de Diagnostics et Pronostics Médicaux. I: Transcription et Traduction.* Collect. de Trav. de l'Acad. Internat. d'Hist. des Sci., No. 7. Leiden, Brill.

———, 1952: *Manuel d'Epigraphie Akkadienne* (signes, syllabaire, idéogrammes). Paris, Impr. Nat. Abbr. MEA.

———, 1953: La médecine babylonienne. Conférences du Palais de la Découverte, Univ. de Paris, Série D, No. 20.

———, 1954: A propos de la chirurgie babylonienne. Journal Asiatique, 207–218.

———, 1957: Remèdes assyriens contre les affections de l'oreille, d'après un inédit du Louvre (AO. 6774). Riv. degli Studi Orientali 32, 109–122.

———, 1959: Le premier chapitre d'un précis médical assyrien. Revue d'Assyriol. 53, 1–18.

———, 1961: A propos de la fumigation dans la médecine assyrienne. Revue d'Assyriol. 55, 152–153.

———, 1962: Jours prescrits pour la confession des péchés. Revue d'Assyriol. 56, 1–8.

———, 1964(a): Fieber. In E. Ebeling and B. Meissner, *Reallexikon der Assyriologie.* Berlin, de Gruyter (p. 61).

———, 1964(b): Geschwulst, Geschwür, Hautkrankheiten. In E. Ebeling and B. Meissner, *Reallexikon der Assyriologie* (vol. III, p. 231-233).

———, 1966: La Mésopotamie. In *La science antique et médiévale.* I: La médecine. Paris, Presses Universitaires de France (pp. 89–103).

Laki, K., 1969: On the Origin of the Sexagesimal System. J. of the Washington Acad. of Sci. 59, 24–29.

Lambert, W. G., and Millard, A. R., 1969: *Atra-ḥasīs—The Babylonian Story of the Flood. With the Sumerian Flood Story by M. Civil.* Oxford, Clarendon.

Landsberger, B., 1959: *Materialien zum Sumerischen Lexikon.* Roma, Pontificium Institutum Bibl. (vol. VII).

Levey, M., 1955: Evidences of Ancient Distillation, Sublimation and Extraction in Ancient Mesopotamia. Centaurus 4, 22–33.

———, 1959: *Chemistry and Chemical Technology of Ancient Mesopotamia.* Amsterdam, London, New York, and Princeton, Elsevier.

———, 1961: Some Objective Factors of Babylonian Medicine in the Light of New Evidence. Bull. Hist. Med. 35, 61–70.

Levin, S. S., 1970: *Adam's Rib: Essays on Biblical Medicine.* Los Altos, Calif., Geron-X.

Limet, H., 1960: Le travail du métal au pays de Sumer au temps de la III Dynastie d'Ur. (Biblioth. de la Fac. de Philos. et Lettres de l'Univ. de Liège, Fascicule CLV). Paris, Soc. d'Ed. "Les Belles Lettres."

Littré, E., 1851: *Oeuvres complètes d'Hippocrate.* Paris, Baillière (vol. VII). Abbr. LTT.

Lods, A., 1925: Les idées des Israélites sur la maladie, ses causes et ses remèdes. Beihefte z. Ztschr. f. die Alttestam. Wissensch. 41, 181–193.

Maksymiuk, B., 1970: Occurrence and Nature of Antibacterial Substances in Plants Affecting *Bacillus thuringiensis* and Other Entomogenous Bacteria. J. of Invert. Path. *15*, 356–371.

Mallowan, M. E. L., 1964: Noah's Flood Reconsidered. Iraq *26*, 62–82.

———, 1965: *Early Mesopotamia and Iran*. New York, McGraw-Hill.

Meissner, B., 1920–1923: *Babylonien und Assyrien*. Heidelberg, Winters (2 vols.).

Mendenhall, G. E., 1954: Ancient Oriental and Biblical Law. Biblical Archaeologist *17*, 26–46.

Miller, J. I., 1969: *The Spice Trade of the Roman Empire* (29 B.C. to A.D. 641). Oxford, Clarendon Press.

Neugebauer, O., 1957: *The Exact Sciences in Antiquity*. Providence, R. I., Brown University Press.

Nickell, L. G., 1959: Antimicrobial Activity of Vascular Plants. Economic Botany *13*, 281-318. [A listing in table form; 174 refs.]

Oppenheim, A. L., 1962: Mesopotamian Medicine. Bull. Hist. Med. *36*, 97–108.

———, 1964: *Ancient Mesopotamia: Portrait of a Dead Civilization*. Chicago and London, University of Chicago Press (repr. 1965).

———, 1967: *Letters from Mesopotamia*. Chicago and London, University of Chicago Press.

———, 1970: *La Mésopotamie: portrait d'une civilisation*. Paris, Gallimard.

Osborn, E. M., 1943: On the Occurrence of Antibacterial Substances in Green Plants. Brit. J. Exper. Path. *24*, 227–231.

Parrot, A., 1949: *Ziggurats et tour de Babel*. Paris, Michel.

———, 1953: *Archéologie mésopotamienne. Technique et problèmes*. Paris, Michel.

———, 1968: *Sumer*. Paris, Gallimard (2nd ed.).

Pfeiffer, R. H., 1935: *State Letters of Assyria*. New Haven, American Oriental Society.

Piggott, S., 1968: The Beginnings of Wheeled Transport. Scientific American *219*, 82–90.

Preuss, J., 1894: Der Arzt in Bibel und Talmud. Arch. path. Anat. u. Physiol. *138*, 261–283.

———, 1923: *Biblisch-talmudische Medizin*. Beiträge zur Geschichte der Heilkunde und der Kultur überhaupt. Berlin, S. Karger.

Pritchard, J. B., 1950: *Ancient Near-Eastern Texts Relating to the Old Testament*. Princeton University Press (pp. 163–180: The Code of Hammurabi, trans. Theophile J. Meek).

Raikes, R. L., 1966: The Physical Evidence for Noah's Flood. Iraq *28*, 52–63.

Reallexikon der Assyriologie, 1964: Ebeling E. and Meissner B., Founders. Berlin, de Gruyter.

Ritter, Edith K., 1965: Magical-Expert (= $\bar{A}\check{S}IPU$) and Physician (= $AS\hat{U}$). Notes on two complementary professions in Babylonian medicine. Assyriological Studies, No. 16, The Oriental Inst. of the University of Chicago (Studies in Honor of B. Landsberger, etc.). Chicago, Ill., University of Chicago Press.

Röllig, W., 1970: *Das Bier im Alten Mesopotamien*. Berlin, Inst. f. Gärungsgewerbe u. Biotechnologie.

Rosengarten, F., Jr., 1969: *The Book of Spices*. Wynnewood, Pa., Livingston; Macrae and Smith, distr., Philadelphia.

Rowton, M. B., 1969: The Role of the Watercourses in the Growth of Mesopotamian Civilization. In *lišān mithurti* (Festschrift für W. F. von Soden; M. Dietrich and W. Röllig, eds.). Neukirchen, Verlag Butzon & Bercker Kevalaer (pp. 307–316).

Rutten, M., 1940: Notes de paléographie cunéiforme. Rev. des études sémitiques et Babyloniaca, 1–53.

Saggs, H. W. F., 1962: *The Greatness That Was Babylon*. New York, Hawthorn Books (repr. 1966).

Salonen, A., 1951: Die Landfahrzeuge des alten Mesopotamien. Ann. Acad. Scient. Fenn., Helsinki. Ser. B, 72 (3).

Santillana, G. de, and Dechend, H. von, 1969: *Hamlet's Mill: An Essay on Myth and the Frame of Time*. Boston, Gambit.

Singer, C., Holmyard, E. J., Hall, A. R., and Williams, T. I., 1965: *A History of Technology*. Oxford, Clarendon. (5 vols.).

Scheil, V., 1902: *Textes Elamites-Sémitiques*, Series 2. Mémoires de la Délégation en Perse. Paris, Leroux (vol. IV).

Soden, W. von, and Meissner, B., 1965: *Akkadisches Handwörterbuch*. Wiesbaden, Harrassowitz.

Thompson, R. C., 1907: Assyrian Prescriptions for Diseases of the Head. Am. J. of Semitic Languages and Lit. *24*, 1–6 and 323–353.

————, 1923: *Assyrian Medical Texts from the Originals in the British Museum*. London, Oxford University Press. [Includes only copies of the tablets, in cuneiform.] Abbr. AMT.

————, 1924(a): *The Assyrian Herbal*. London, Luzac.

————, 1924(b): Assyrian Medical Texts. Proc. Roy. Soc. Med. *17*, 1-34.

————, 1925(a): Assyrian Medical Texts. Proc. Roy. Soc. Med. *19*, 29–78.

————, 1925(b): *The Chemistry of the Ancient Assyrians*. London, Luzac.

————, 1930: Assyrian Prescriptions for Treating Bruises or Swellings. Am. J. of Semitic Languages and Lit. *47*, 1–25.

————, 1931: Assyrian Prescriptions for Ulcers or Similar Affections. J. Soc. Oriental Res. *15*, 53–59.

————, 1937: Assyrian Prescriptions for Diseases of the Head. Am. J. of Semitic Languages and Lit. *53*, 217–238.

Thorwald, J., 1962: *Histoire de la médecine dans l'antiquité*. Paris, Hachette.

Thureau-Dangin, F., 1921: Rituel et amulettes contre Labartu. Rev. Assyriol. et Archéol. Orientale *18*, 161–198. [Labartu is the outmoded reading of Lamashtu.]

Townend, R. R., 1938: An Assyrian Dental Diagnosis. Iraq *5*, 82–84.

Trease, G. E., and Evans, W. C., 1972: *Pharmacognosy*. London, Baillière Tindall (10th ed.).

Tschesche, R., 1971: Progress in the Chemistry of Higher Plant Constituents with Antibiotic Action. Pharma International, 17–23.

Vollenweider, M. L., 1967: *Catalogue raisonné des sceaux, cylindres et intailles*. Genève, Musée d'Art et d'Histoire (vol. I).

Waterman, L., 1930: *Royal Correspondence of the Assyrian Empire*. Ann Arbor, University of Michigan Press (Part II).

White, W., 1969: An Assyrian Physician's *Vade mecum*. Clio Medica *4*, 159–171.

Woolley, C. L., 1965: *Ur of the Chaldees*. New York, Norton.

3. The Swnw

The principal "medical" papyri are: *Kahun* veterinary and *Kahun* gynecological (c.1850 B.C., 3 fragmentary pages); *Smith* (c.1650 B.C., 17 pp.); *Ebers* (c.1550 B.C., 108 pp.); *Hearst* (c. 1500 B.C., 18 pp.); *Berlin* (c. 1300 B.C., 24 pp.); *Chester Beatty VI* (c.1300 B.C., 10 pp.); *London* (1350 B.C., 19 pp.; mainly magical). English translations available: *Kahun*, Griffith 1898; *Smith*, Breasted 1930 (an all-time classic); *Ebers*, Ebbell 1937 (readable but not sufficiently critical); Bryan 1930 (unusable, GMÄ II 92); *Chester B. VI* is available in French (Jonckheere 1947). The contents of all papyri are available in the German translation by Grapow (GMÄ IV/1 and IV/2, 1958) but regrouped by subject. Quotations from other sources should always be compared with GMÄ, which is also the most recent.

Hieroglyphs: Gardiner's grammar is excellent even in the hands of an intruder. Egyptian chemistry, technology, and drugs: Lucas and Harris (supplemented by Harris 1961) is an essential and so far unique source, striving to "replace wild conjecture by sober facts." General background on Egyptian medicine: very useful are Ghalioungui 1973, 1963 and Leca 1971. See also Sigerist 1955 and Wilson 1946 on Egypt in general.

Alexander, J. W., Kaplan, J. Z., and Altmeier, W. A., 1967: Role of Suture Materials in the Development of Wound Infection. Ann. Surg. *165*, 192–199.

Amonkar, S. V., and Banerji, A., 1971: Isolation and Characterization of the Larvicidal Principle of Garlic. Science *174*, 1343–1344.

Bibliography

Bell, H. I., 1948: *Egypt from Alexander the Great to the Arab Conquest*. London, Oxford University Press.

Bengtson, H., and Milojčić, V., 1963: *Grosser Historischer Weltatlas*. Munich, Bayerischer Schulbuch-Verlag (vol. I).

Berard, C. W., Herrmann, J. B., Woodward, S. C., and Pulaski, E. J., 1964: Healing of Incisions Closed with Surgical Adhesive Tape. Am. J. Surg. *107*, 591–594.

Berlin Papyrus. Abbr. Bln. Quoted as in GMÄ.

Biggs, R., 1969: Medicine in Ancient Mesopotamia. In *History of Science*, A. C. Crombie and M. A. Hoskin, eds. Cambridge, Heffer (vol. VIII, pp. 94–105).

Blomfield, R., 1973: Honey for Decubitus Ulcers. J. Am. Med. Ass. *224*, 905.

Breasted, J. H., 1906: Reign of Neferkirere: Tomb Inscriptions of the Vizier, Chief Judge, and Chief Architect Weshptah. In *Ancient Records of Egypt*. Chicago, University of Chicago Press (vol. I, pp. 111–113).

————, 1930: *The Edwin Smith Surgical Papyrus*. Published in facsimile and hieroglyphic transliteration with translation and commentary. Chicago, Ill., University of Chicago Press (2 vols.). [The original is now at the New York Academy of Medicine.] Abbr. Sm.

Browning, E., 1969: *Toxicity of Industrial Metals*. London, Butterworths (2nd ed.).

Brothwell, D., and Higgs, E., 1969: *Science in Archaeology*. London, Thames and Hudson (2nd ed.). [An important reference volume.]

Brunius, U., 1968: *Wound Healing Impairment from Sutures: A Tensiometric and Histologic Study in the Rat*. Doctoral thesis; University of Göteborg, Sweden.

Brunius, U., Zederfeldt, B., and Åhrén, C., 1967: Healing of Skin Incisions Closed by Non-Suture Technique. Acta Chir. Scand. *133*, 509–516.

Bryan, C. P., 1930: *The Papyrus Ebers*. Bles, London (trans. from the German version). [Unusable! Based on the 1890 Joachim translation.]

Buchheim, L., 1958: Der "Fleischverband" im alten Ägypten. Sudhoffs Arch. f. Gesch. der Med. *42*, 97–116.

————, 1960: Die Verordnug von "lebendem" Fleisch in altägyptischen Papyri. Sudhoffs Arch. f. Gesch. der Med. *44*, 97–116.

Budge, E. A. W., 1960: *The Book of the Dead: The Hieroglyphic Transcript of the Papyrus of Ani, the Translation into English and An Introduction*. New Hyde Park, N.Y., University Books.

Bulman, M. W., 1955: Honey as a Surgical Dressing. Brit. Bee Journal, pp. 664–665.

Caley, E. R., and Richards, J. F. C., 1956: *Theophrastus on Stones*. Columbus, Ohio, Columbus University Press.

Carpendale, M. T. F., 1964: Reduction of Surgical Wound Infection by Tape Closure. Surgical Forum *XV*, 58–60.

Carpendale, M. T. F., and Sereda, W., 1965: The Role of the Percutaneous Suture in Surgical Wound Infection. Surgery *58*, 672–677.

Cavallito, C. J., and Bailey, J. H., 1944: Allicin, the Antibacterial Principle of *Allium sativum*. I: Isolation, Physical Properties and Antibacterial Action. J. Am. Chem. Soc. *66*, 1950–1951.

Celsus: *De medicina*. Trans. W. G. Spencer. Loeb Classical Library, Cambridge, Mass., Harvard University Press; London, Heinemann (3 vols.; 1935–1938). Abbr. CDM.

Černý, J., 1927: *Quelques Ostraka hiératiques inédits de Thèbes au musée du Caire*. Ann. du Service des Antiquités de l'Egypte, XXVII, Cairo, Impr. de l'Inst. Français d'Archéol. Orientale, 183.

Chauvin, R., 1968: *Traité de la biologie de l'abeille*. Paris, Masson (5 vols.).

Chester Beatty Papyri. Abbr. CB. See Gardiner 1935.

Columella, L. J. M.: *De re rustica*. Trans. H. B. Ash and others. Loeb Classical Library, Cambridge, Mass., Harvard University Press, and London, Heinemann. (1960–1968; 3 vols.).

Comrie, J. D., 1909–1910: Die ältesten chirurgischen Instrumente. Arch. f. Gesch. d. Med. *3*, 269–272.

Connolly, W. B., Hunt, Th. K., Zederfeldt, B., Cafferata, H. T., and Dunphy, J. E., 1969: Clinical Comparison of Surgical Wounds Closed by Suture and Adhesive Tapes. Am. J. Surg. *117*, 318–322.

Coulthard, C. E., Michaelis, R., Short, W. F., Sykes, G., Skrimshire, G. E. H., Standfast, A. F. B., Birkinshaw, J. H., and Raistrick, H., 1945: Notatin: An Antibacterial Glucose-aerodehydrogenase from *Penicillium notatum* Westling and *Penicillium reticulosum* sp. nov. Biochem. J. 39, 24–36.

Crum, W. E., 1939: *A Coptic Dictionary.* Oxford, Clarendon (repr. 1962).

Cumont, F., 1937: *L'Egypte des astrologues.* Brussels, Edit. de la Fond. Egyptol. Reine Elisabeth.

Daumas, F., 1965: *La civilisation de l'Egypte pharaonique.* Paris, Arthaud. [A well-illustrated reference work.]

Dawson, W. F., 1930: *The Beginnings: Egypt and Assyria.* No. 1 in the Clio Medica Series. New York, Hoeber. [Good but outdated in parts.]

Dawson, W. R., 1924: The Mouse in Egyptian and Later Medicine. J. Egypt. Archaeol. 10, 83–86.

———, 1927: Making a Mummy. J. Egypt. Archaeol. 13, 40–49.

———, 1929: Studies in Medical History: (a) The Origin of the Herbal. (b) Castor-oil in Antiquity. Aegyptus 10, 47–72.

Dioscorides. See Gunther 1934.

Diringer, D., 1968: *The Alphabet. A Key to the History of Mankind.* London, Hutchinson (3rd ed; 2 vols.).

Dixon, M., 1969: The Transplantation of Punt Incense Trees in Egypt. J. Egypt. Archaeol. 55, 55–65.

Dold, H., Du, D. H., and Dziao, S. T., 1937: Nachweis antibakterieller, Hitze- und Lichtempfindlicher Hemmungsstoffe (Inhibine) im Naturhonig (Blütenhonig). Z. Hyg. 20, 155–167.

Dollfus, M. A., 1937: L'Ophtalmologie dans l'ancienne Egypte. Arch. Ophtalm. 11, 985–1001.

Dorveaux, P., 1915: Historique de l'eau d'Alibour [*sic*]. Bull. des Sci. Pharmacol. 22, 234–248.

Ebbell, B., 1937: *The Papyrus Ebers: The Greatest Egyptian Medical Document.* Copenhagen, Levin and Munksgaard. [Should not be used without comparing with GMÄ.]

———, 1938: *Alt-Ägyptische Bezeichnungen für Krankheiten und Symptome.* Skrifter utgitt av Det Norske Videnskaps-Akademi i Oslo, II Hist.-Filos. Klasse, No. 3.

———, 1939: *Die alt-ägyptische Chirurgie. Die chirurgischen Abschnitte der Papyrus E. Smith und Papyrus Ebers übersetzt und mit Erläuterungen versehen.* Skrifter utgitt av Det Norske Videnskaps-Akademi i Oslo. II. Hist.-Filos. Klasse, No. 2.

Ebers Papyrus. Abbr. Eb. Quoted as in GMÄ. See also Ebbell 1937.

Engelbach, R., and Derry, D. E., 1942: Mummification. Ann. du Serv. des Antiquités de l'Egypte 41, 235–265 (in English).

Erman, A., and Grapow, H., 1929: *Wörterbuch der Ägyptischen Sprache.* Leipzig. Hinrichs (vol. III).

Ernout, A., and Meillet, A., 1959: *Dictionnaire étymologique de la langue latine.* Paris, Klincksieck (4th ed.).

Flückiger, F. A., and Hanbury, D., 1879: *Pharmacographia: A History of the Principal Drugs of Vegetable Origin.* London, Macmillan. Abbr. FH.

Forbes, R. J., 1950: Professions and Crafts in Ancient Egypt. Arch. Internat. d'Hist. des Sci. 12, 599–618.

———, 1965(a): Chemical, Culinary and Cosmetic Arts. Ch. 11 in Singer and others, *A History of Technology* (vol. I, pp. 238–250).

———, 1965(b): *Studies in Ancient Technology.* Leiden, Brill (vol. III; 2nd ed.).

Forrester, J. C., Zederfeldt, B. H., Hayes, T. L., and Hunt, T. K., 1970: Tape-Closed and Sutured Wounds: A Comparison by Tensiometry and Scanning Electron Microscopy. Brit. J. Surg. 57, 729–737.

Franco, M., and Sartori, L., 1940: Sull' azione antibatterica del miele. Annali d'Igiene 50, 216–227.

Frankfort, H. A., Wilson, J. A., and Jacobsen, T., 1946: *Before Philosophy.* Baltimore, Penguin Books (repr. 1968).

Gabra, S., 1956: Papaver Species and Opium through the Ages. Bull. Inst. d'Egypte 37, 39–56.

Gardiner, A. H., 1935: *Hieratic Papyri in the British Museum*. Third Series: Chester Beatty Gift, ed. A. H. Gardiner, London, British Museum.

———, 1957: *Egyptian Grammar: Being an Introduction to the Study of Hieroglyphs*. London, Oxford University Press. (3rd ed.; repr. 1966). Abbr. EG.

Ghalioungui, P., 1963: *Magic and Medical Science in Ancient Egypt*. London, Hodder and Stoughton.

———, 1973: *The House of Life (Per Ankh)*. Amsterdam, Israël. [Very useful book—essentially a new edition of Ghalioungui 1963.]

Gipsen, J. G. W., 1968: Is the Origin of our Concept of "Inflammation" to be Found in the Ancient Egyptian Medical Texts? Verhandl. XX Internat. Kongr. f. Gesch. der Med., Hildesheim, 228–230.

Glenville, S. R. K., 1942: *The Legacy of Egypt*. Oxford, Clarendon (repr. 1963).

Glob, P. V., 1965: *Les hommes des tourbières*. Trans. from the Danish by E. Eydoux. Paris, Fayard.

Gonnet, M., 1966: Action inhibitrice de la propolis récoltée par l'Abeille (*Apis mellifica L.*) sur la germination et sur la croissance des jeunes plantules chez la Laitue (*Lactuca sativa*). C. R. Acad. Sci. Paris 262, 2281–2284.

Gonnet, M., and Lavie, P., 1960: Action antigerminative des produits de la ruche d'Abeilles (*Apis mellifica L.*) sur les graines et les tubercules. C. R. Acad. des Sci. Paris 250, 612–614.

Gonzenbach, W. von, and Hoffmann, S., 1936: Zucker, Honig und Wundbalsame in ihrer Wirkung auf infizierte Wunden. Eine experimentelle Studie. Schweiz. Med. Wchschr. I, 425–429.

Gourevitch, D., 1970: Some Features of the Ancient Doctor's Personality as Depicted in Epitaphs. Nordisk Medicinhistorisk Arsbok, 1–12.

Grapow, H., 1935(a): Über die anatomischen Kenntnisse der altägyptischen Ärzte. Morgenland, Heft 26. Leipzig, Hinrichs.

——— 1935(b): Die ägyptischen medizinischen Papyrus und was sie enthalten. Münch. med. Wchschr. 82, June 21, 958–962, 1002–1005.

———, 1935(c): Untersuchungen über die altägyptischen medizinischen Papyri. Teil I, Mitteilungen der Vorderasiatisch-Ägyptischen Ges. 40, 1–111.

———, 1936: *idem*, Teil II, 41, 1–138. [Excellent reviews but require knowledge of hieroglyphs.]

———, 1954–1962: *Grundriss der Medizin der alten Ägypter*. Berlin, Akademie-Verlag (in 10 parts). [The most recent, critical, comprehensive edition of all medical papyri. A colossal work. Fundamental.] Abbr. GMÄ.

Griffith, F. L., 1898: *Beni Hasan*. Part III: Archaeol. Survey of Egypt. London, Egypt Explor. Fund.

———, 1915: Note appended to an article by Weigall, A. E. P. B. J. Egypt. Archaeol. 2, 11–12.

Gross, M., and Greenberg, L. A., 1948: *The Salicylates: A Critical Bibliographic Review*. New Haven, Hillhouse.

Gunther, R. T., 1934: *The Greek Herbal of Dioscorides, Illustrated by a Byzantine A.D. 512, Englished by John Goodyear A.D. 1655* . . . London and New York, Hafner (repr. 1968).

Hagemann, E., 1904: Zur Hygiene der alten Ägypter. Janus 9, 214–229.

Hall, H. R., 1928: [Notices of recent publications] "Relazione sui lavori della Missione Archeologica Italiana in Egitto (Anni 1903-1920). II. La tomba intatta dell'architetto Cha. By E. Schiaparelli, Torino, R. Museo di Antichità, 1927." J. Egypt. Archaeol. 14, 203–205.

Harris, J. R., 1961: *Lexicographical Studies in Ancient Egyptian Materials*. Berlin, Akademie-Verlag.

Hassan, S., 1932: *Excavations at Giza*. Oxford, University Press (vol. I).

Hengen, O. P., 1971: Paléomédecine de l'Egypte ancienne. Image No. 45, 25–33.

Herodotus. Trans. A. D. Godley. Loeb Classical Library, Cambridge, Mass., Harvard University Press and London, Heinemann (1920–1925; repr. 1960–1966; 4 vols.).

Heyser, K., 1928: Die Alliumarten als Arzneimittel im Gebrauch der abendländischen Medizin. Kyklos. Jahrb. des Inst. f. Gesch. der Med. an der Univ. Leipzig, Band I, 64–102.

Hooton, E. A., 1917: Oral Surgery in Egypt during the Old Empire. Harvard African Studies *I*, 29–32 (+ 2 plates).

Hurry, J. B., 1926: *Imhotep: The Vizier and Physician of King Zoser and Afterwards the Egyptian God of Medicine.* Oxford University Press.

Jastrow, M., Jr., 1917: Babylonian-Assyrian Medicine. Ann. Med. Hist. *1*, 231–257.

Jayne, W. A., 1925: *The Healing Gods of Ancient Civilizations.* New Haven, Yale University Press.

Jensen, L. B., and Sherman, J. E., 1951: Antibiotic from Galingale Root as Food Preservative. U.S. 2.550.269, Apr. 24, 1951. Chem. Abstr. *45*, 7724 f.

Jonckheere, F., 1942: *Autour de l'autopsie d'une momie: le scribe royal Boutehamon.* Brussels, Edit. de la Fond. Egyptol. Reine Elisabeth.

———, 1945: Coup d'oeil sur la médecine Egyptienne. L'intérêt des documents non médicaux. Chronique d'Egypte 39–40, 24–32.

———, 1947: *Le Papyrus Médical Chester Beatty.* Brussels, Edit. de la Fond. Egyptol. Reine Elisabeth, No. 2.

———, 1950(a): La Place du prêtre de Sekhmet dans le corps médical de l'ancienne Egypte. Actes du IV Congrès d'Hist. des Sciences, Amsterdam, 324–333.

———, 1950(b): Médecins et malades dans l'ancienne Egypte. Arch. Internat. d'Hist. des Sci. *11*, 320–341. [See following ref.]

———, 1950(c): Le monde des malades dans les textes non médicaux. Chronique d'Egypte. *50*, 213–232. [Almost identical to the ref. above.]

———, 1951: A la recherche du chirurgien Egyptien. Chronique d'Egypte *51*, 28–45.

———, 1958: *Les médecins de l'Egypte pharaonique: Essai de prosopographie.* Brussels, Edit. de la Fond. Egyptol. Reine Elisabeth, No. 3.

Knudtzon, J. A., 1964: *Die El-Amarna Tafeln.* Aalen, Zeller.

Kovalenok, A., 1943: Action of Phytoncides upon Infusoria. Am. Rev. of Soviet Med. 239–241 (originally in Doklady Acad. Sci. USSR 1943, 38, No. 7, 218–220).

Lavie, P., 1960: Les substances antibactériennes dans la colonie d'abeilles (*Apis mellifica L.*). Ann. Abeille 3, 103–305.

———, 1963: Sur l'identification des substances antibactériennes présentes dans le miel. C. R. Acad. Sci. Paris 256, 1858–1860.

———, 1968: Propriétés antibactériennes et action physiologique des produits de la ruche et des abeilles. Ch. 1 in Chauvin, *Traité de la Biologie de l'Abeille* (vol. III, pp. 2–154; see ref.).

Lawick-Goodall, Jane van, 1971: *In the Shadow of Man.* London, Collins.

Leca, A.-P., 1971: *La médecine Egyptienne au temps des pharaons.* Paris, Dacosta.

Leek, F. F., 1969: Did a Dental Profession Exist in Ancient Egypt? The Dental Delineator, Spring fascicle, 1–4.

Lefebvre, G., 1952(a): Prêtres de Sekhmet. Archiv. Orientalni, Prague 20, 57–64. [In French.]

———, 1952(b): *Tableau des parties du corps humain mentionnées par les Egyptiens* (Ann. du Serv. des Antiquités, Suppl.; Cahier 17). Cairo, Impr. de l'Inst. Français d'Archéol. Orientale, No. 17.

———, 1955: *Grammaire de l'Egyptien classique.* Cairo, Impr. de l'Inst. Français d'Archéol. Orientale (2nd ed.).

———, 1956: *Essai sur la médecine Egyptienne de l'époque Pharaonique.* Paris, Presses Universitaires de France. [Useful booklet, more than an Essai; see review by R. O. Steuer in Isis 1960, 51, 583–587.]

Levin, S. S., 1970: *Adam's Rib: Essays on Biblical Medicine.* Los Altos, Calif., Geron-X.

Lewis, N., 1934: *L'industrie du papyrus dans l'Egypte Gréco-Romaine.* Doctoral Thesis, University of Paris. Paris, Rodstein.

Liddell, H. G., and Scott, R., 1968: *A Greek-English Lexicon.* Oxford, Clarendon. Abbr. LS.

Lindenfelser, L. A., 1967: Antimicrobial Activity of Propolis. Am. Bee Journal 107, 90–92 and 130–131.

Bibliography

London Papyrus. Abbr. L. Quoted as in GMÄ.

Lucas, A., 1962: *Ancient Egyptian Materials and Industries.* London, Arnold. (4th ed. revised and enlarged by J. R. Harris). Abbr. LH.

Mallowan, M. E. L., 1965: *Early Mesopotamia and Iran.* New York, McGraw-Hill.

McCord, C. P., 1965: The Early History of Ocular Prostheses, J. Occupational Med. 7, 61–68.

Mercer, S. A. B., 1939: *The Tell El-Amarna Tablets.* Toronto, Macmillan (2 vols.).

The Merck Index. An Encyclopedia of Chemicals and Drugs. Rahway, N.J., Merck, 1968 (8th ed.).

Merrillees, R. S., 1962: Opium Trade in the Bronze Age Levant. Antiquity 36, 287–292, Pl. XLII–XLIII.

———, 1968: *The Cypriote Bronze Age Pottery Found in Egypt.* Studies in Mediterranean Archaeology Vol. XVIII. Lund, Studies in Mediterr. Archaeology, Sölvegatan 2.

Myers, M. B., Cherry, G., and Heimburger, S., 1969: Augmentation of Wound Tensile Strength by Early Removal of Sutures. Am. J. Surg. 117, 338–341.

Naville, E., 1895–1898: *The Temple of Deir-el-Bahari.* London, The Egypt Exploration Fund (Part III).

Neolitzky, F., 1911: Nahrungs- und Heilmittel der Urägypter. Zeitschr. f. Untersuch. der Nahrungs- und Genussmittel *XXI*, 607–613.

Nickell, L. G., 1959: Antimicrobial Activity of Vascular Plants. Economic Botany *13*, 281–318.

Oppenheim, A. L., 1964: *Ancient Mesopotamia: Portrait of a Dead Civilization.* Chicago and London, University of Chicago Press (repr. 1965).

Ordman, L. J., and Gillman, T., 1966: Studies in the Healing of Cutaneous Wounds. Arch. Surg. *93*, 911–928.

Otto, E., 1960: *Das Ägyptische Mundöffnung Ritual.* Wiesbaden, Harassowitz.

Petrie, Hilda, 1927: *Egyptian Hieroglyphs of the First and Second Dynasties.* London, Quaritch.

Petrie, W. M. Flinders, 1892: *Medum.* London, Nutt.

Piankoff, A., 1930: *Le "coeur" dans les textes Egyptiens, depuis l'Ancien jusqu'à la fin du Nouvel Empire.* Doctoral thesis, Paris. Paris, Geuthner.

Pliny [The Elder]: *Natural History.* Trans. H. Rackham, W. H. S. Jones, and D. E. Eichholz. Loeb Classical Library, Cambridge, Mass., Harvard University Press and London, Heinemann (1956–1966: 10 vols.). Abbr. PNH.

Quibell, J. E., 1913: *Excavations at Saqqara (1911–12): The Tomb of Hesy.* Service des Antiquités de l'Egypte. Cairo, Impr. de l'Inst. Français.

Rosengarten, F., Jr., 1969: *The Book of Spices.* Wynnewood, Pa., Livingston; Macrae and Smith distr., Philadelphia.

Ruffer, M. A., 1921: *The Palaeopathology of Ancient Egypt.* R. L. Moodie ed. Chicago University Press.

Sackett, W. G., 1919: Honey as a Carrier of Intestinal Diseases. Bulletin 252, The Agricultural Experiment Station of the Colorado Agricultural College, Fort Collins, Colo., 3–18.

Sandison, A. T., 1969: The Study of Mummified and Dried Human Tissues. Ch. 42 in Brothwell and Higgs, *Science in Archaeology* (pp. 490–502, see ref.).

Saunders, J. B. de C. M., 1963: *The Transition from Ancient Egyptian to Greek Medicine.* Logan Clendening Lectures on the History and Philosophy of Medicine, 10th series. Lawrence, University of Kansas Press.

Schepartz, A. I., and Subers, Mary H., 1964: The Glucose Oxidase of Honey. I: Purification and Some General Properties of the Enzyme. Biochim. Biophys. Acta *85*, 228–237.

Schiaparelli, E., 1927; *Relazione sui lavori della Missione Archeologica Italiana in Egitto.* Anni 1903–1920. II: La tomba intatta dell' architetto Cha. Torino, R. Museo di Antichità (see review by Hall 1928).

Schmidt, A., 1924: *Drogen und Drogenhandel im Altertum.* Leipzig, Barth.

Schneider, O., 1967: *In C. Plinii Secundi Naturalis Historiae Libros Index.* Hildesheim, Olms.

Bibliography

Sestieri, P. C., 1956: An Underground Shrine at Paestum. Archaeology 9, 22–23.

Sethe, K., 1916: *Von Zahlen und Zahlworten bei den alten Ägyptern und was für andere Völker und Sprachen daraus zu lernen ist.* Strasbourg, Trübner.

Sigerist, H. E., 1944: Ambroise Paré's Onion Treatment of Burns. Bull. Hist. Med. *15,* 143–149.

———, 1955: Ancient Egypt. Ch. III in *A History of Medicine.* New York, Oxford University Press (vol I, pp. 215–373).

Simpson, G. G., 1967: *The Meaning of Evolution.* New Haven and London, Yale University Press.

Singer, C., Holmyard, E. J., and Hall, R. A., 1965: *A History of Technology.* Oxford, Clarendon (5 vols.).

Skinner, H. A., 1961: *The Origin of Medical Terms.* Baltimore, Williams and Wilkins (2nd ed.).

Smith, G. E., 1908: The Most Ancient Splints. Brit. Med. J. *1,* 732–734 (+ 2 pp. of illustr.).

———, 1912: *The Royal Mummies.* In *Catalogue général des antiquités Egyptiennes du musée du Caire,* Nos. 61051–61100. Cairo, Impr. de l'Inst. Français d'Archéol. Orientale.

———, 1914: Egyptian Mummies. J. Egypt. Archaeol. *I,* 189–196.

Smith, G. E., and Dawson, W. R., 1924: *Egyptian Mummies.* London, Allen and Unwin.

Smith, M. R., McCaughey, W. F., and Kemmerer, A. R., 1969: Biological Effects of Honey, J. of Apicultural Res. 8, 99–110.

Smith, W. S., 1958: *The Art and Architecture of Ancient Egypt.* Baltimore, Maryland, Penguin.

Smith Papyrus. See Breasted 1930. Abbr. Sm.

Spencer. See Celsus.

Spöttel, W., 1950: *Honig und Trockenmilch. Biochemie und therapeutische Bedeutung.* Leipzig, Barth.

Steuer, R. O., 1948: *Wḥdw: Aetiological Principle of Pyaemia in Ancient Egyptian Medicine.* Bull. Hist. Med., Suppl. 10.

Steuer, R. O., and Saunders, J. B. de C. M., 1959: *Ancient Egyptian and Cnidian Medicine.* Berkeley, Calif., University of California Press.

Sudhoff, K., 1932: Zum Papyrus Edwin Smith und anderen medizinischen Papyri. Janus 36, 218–233.

Tokin, B., 1943: Phytoncides or plant bactericides. Effect of Phytoncides upon Protozoa. Am. Rev. of Soviet Med. 237–239 (originally in Doklady Acad. Sci. USSR 1943, 38, No. 7, pp. 215–217).

Toroptsev, I., 1943: Effect of Phytoncides on Rabbits. Am. Rev. of Soviet Med. 242–244 (originally in Doklady Acad. Sci. USSR 1943, 38, No. 8, pp. 254–257).

Toroptsev, I. V., and Filatova, A. G., 1943: The Use of Phytoncides in the Treatment of Infected Wounds. Am. Rev. of Soviet Med. 244–250 (originally in *Khirurgia,* 1943, No. 5–6, pp. 15–22).

Trease, G. E., and Evans, W. C., 1972: *Pharmacognosy.* London, Baillière Tindall (10th ed.).

Villanueva, V. R., Bogdanovsky, D., Barbier, M., Gonnet, M., and Lavie, P., 1964: Sur l'isolement et l'identification de la 3,5,7-trihydroxy flavone (galangine) à partir de la propolis. Ann. Inst. Pasteur 106, 292–302.

Wainwright, G. A., 1932: Iron in Egypt. J. Egypt. Archaeol. *18,* 3–15.

Wall, O. A., 1917: Origin of the Sign ℞ . In Wall, O. A., *The Prescription Therapeutically, Pharmaceutically, Grammatically, and Historically Considered.* St. Louis, Mosby (4th ed.; pp. 263–268).

Walsh, J. J., 1907: First Pictures of Surgical Operations Extant. J. Am. Med. Ass. *49,* 1593–1595.

Weber, H., 1937: Honig zur Behandlung vereiterter Wunden. Therapie der Gegenwart 78, 547–550.

Weigall, A.E.P.B., 1915: An ancient Egyptian Funeral Ceremony. J. Egypt. Archaeol. 2, 10–12.

Wells, C., 1964: *Bones, Bodies, and Disease. Evidence of Disease and Abnormality in Early Man.* New York and Washington, Praeger.

White, J. W., Jr., Riethof, M. L., Subers, M. H., and Kushnir, I., 1962: *Composition of American honeys.* Superintendent of Documents, U.S. Govt. Printing Office, Technical Bulletin No. 1261.

White, J. W., Jr., Subers, M. H., and Schepartz, A. I., 1962: The Identification of Inhibine. Am. Bee Journal *102*, 430–431.

————, 1963: The Identification of Inhibine, the Antibacterial Factor in Honey, as Hydrogen Peroxide and Its Origin in a Honey Glucose-Oxidase System. Biochim. Biophys. Acta *73*, 57–70.

White, J. W., Jr., and Subers, M. H., 1964: Studies on Honey Inhibine. 4: Destruction of the Peroxide Accumulation System by Light. J. Food Sci. *29*, 819–828.

Wiedemann, A., 1920: *Das alte Ägypten.* Heidelberg, Winters.

Wilson, J. A., 1946: Egypt. In Frankfort, Wilson, and Jacobsen, *Before Philosophy* (pp. 39–133; repr. 1968; see ref.).

————, 1962: Medicine in Ancient Egypt. Bull. Hist. Med. *36*, 114–123.

Woldering, I., 1967: *Gods, Men and Pharaohs: The Glory of Egyptian Art.* Fribourg, Switzerland, Office du Livre.

Yang, K. L., 1944: The Use of Honey in the Treatment of Chilblains, Non-specific Ulcers, and Small Wounds. Chinese Med. J. *62*, 55–60.

Zaiss, 1934: Der Honig in äusserlicher Anwendung. Münch. med. Wchschr. *81*, 1891–1893.

4. The Iatrós

In the text, quotations from Hippocratic works always refer to the French translation of Littré (LTT), preceded by an English version when available (A = Adams, LB = Loeb edition). I translated the title Perì Helkón *On Wounds* (Adams has *On Ulcers*).

Ackerknecht, E. H., 1970: *Therapie - von den Primitiven bis zum 20. Jahrhundert. Mit einem Anhang: Geschichte der Diät.* Stuttgart, Enke.

————, 1971: The End of Greek Diet. Bull. Hist. Med. *45*, 242–249.

Adams, F., 1844–1847: *The Seven Books of Paulus Aegineta: Translated with a Commentary Embracing a Complete View of the Knowledge Possessed by the Greeks, Romans and Arabians on All Subjects Connected with Medicine and Surgery.* London, Sydenham Soc. (3 vols.).

Aeschines: *The Speeches.* Trans. C. D. Adams. Loeb Classical Library, Cambridge, Mass., Harvard Univ. Press, and London, Heinemann (1948).

Albarracín Teulón, A., 1971: La cirugía homérica. Episteme 5, 83–97.

Allbutt, T. C., 1905: *The Historical Relations of Medicine and Surgery to the End of the Sixteenth Century.* London, Macmillan.

Anagnostakis, A., 1872: *Contributions à l'histoire de la chirurgie oculaire chez les anciens.* Athens, Perris.

Aristotle: *Problems.* Trans. W. S. Hett. Loeb Classical Library. Cambridge, Mass., Harvard University Press and London, Heinemann (1953–1957; repr. 1961–1965; 2 vols.).

————, *Aristotele: Problemi di Medicina.* Trans. G. Marenghi. Milano, Ist. Editoriale Italiano (1965).

Baffoni, A., 1943: La cura delle ferite toraco-polmonari nella "Collectio Hippocratica" ed un preteso trattamento pneumotoracico. "Lotta contro la Tuberculosi" (Rome) year XIV, 3–7.

Bailey, K. C., 1929: *The Elder Pliny's Chapters on Chemical Subjects.* London, Arnold (2 vols.).

Becker, P., 1950: Ueber die bactericide Wirkung des Rotweines. Doctoral thesis, Fac. of Medicine, University of Mainz (Hygien. Institut).

Belloni, L., 1956: Dall'elleboro alla reserpina. Arch. psicol. neurol. e psichiat. Suppl. to 17, 115–148.

Benedicenti, A., 1947: *Malati, medici e farmacisti*. Milan, Hoepli.

Benedum, J., 1970: Fibula—Naht oder Klammer? Gesnerus 27, 20–56.

Billingham, R. E., and Russell, P. S., 1956: Studies on Wound Healing, with Special Reference to the Phenomenon of Contracture in Experimental Wounds in Rabbits' Skin. Ann. Surg. 144, 961–981.

Blegen, C. W., 1958: *Troy*. Princeton University Press.

Bourgey, L., 1953: *Observation et expérience chez les médecins de la Collection Hippocratique*. Paris, Vrin.

Brock, A. J., 1929: *Greek Medicine, Being Extracts Illustrative of Medical Writers from Hippocrates to Galen*. London and Toronto, Dent.

Broneer, O., 1962: The Apostle Paul and the Isthmian Games. The Biblical Archaeologist 25, 2–32.

Burnet, J., 1923: L'expérience et l'observation dans la science Grecque. Scientia (Rivista di Scienza) 33, 93–102.

Caskey, J. L., 1962: The Goddess of Ceos. Archaeology 15, 223–226.

Castiglioni, A., 1935: *L'orto della sanità*. Bologna, Librerie Italiane Riunite.

Celsus, A. C.: *De medicina*. Trans. W. G. Spencer. Loeb Classical Library, Cambridge, Mass., Harvard University Press, and London, Heinemann (1960–1961; 3 vols.). Abbr. CDM.

Cerney, C. V.: *Athletic injuries*. Springfield, Ill., C. C. Thomas, 1963.

Chantraine, P., 1933: *La formation des noms en Grec ancien*. Paris, Champion.

Charaka Samhita. Trans. A. C. Kaviratna. Calcutta (pub. by the trans.; 1912; 2 vols.).

Cignozzi, G., 1690: *Libro d'Ipocrate dell' Ulcere. Con le Note pratiche Chirurgiche*. Firenze, Pier Matini.

Cohn-Haft, L., 1956: *The Public Physicians of Ancient Greece*. Northampton, Mass., Smith College Studies in History (vol. XLII).

Cook, A. B., 1914: *Zeus. A Study in Ancient Religion. I: Zeus God of the Bright Sky*. Cambridge, Cambridge University Press.

Cope, Z., 1958: The Treatment of Wounds Through the Ages. Med. Hist. 2, 163–174.

Daland, J., 1935: Depressed Fracture and Trephining of the Skull by the Incas of Peru. Ann. Med. Hist., N. S. 7, 550–558.

D'Arcy Power, Sir, 1925: The Scamnum Hippocratis. Proc. Roy. Soc. Med. (Sect. Med. Hist.) 18, 15–17.

Daremberg, C., 1869: *Etat de la médecine entre Homère et Hippocrate*. Paris, Didier.
———, 1869: Etudes d'archéologie médicale sur Homère. Rev. Archéol., N. S. 12, 95–111; 249–267; 338–355. (Plate XXIII). (Also as a monograph, *La Médecine dans Homère*. Paris, Didier, 1865).

Devoto, G., 1966: *Avviamento alla etimologia Italiana: Dizionario etimologico*. Florence, Le Monnier.

Dierbach, J. H., 1824: *Die Arzneimittel des Hippokrates, oder ein Versuch einer systematischen Aufzählung der in allen Hippokratischen Schriften vorkommenden Medikamenten*. Heidelberg, Groos (facsimile reprod. 1969, Olms, Hildesheim).

Dioscorides. See Gunther 1934.

Dodds 1959. See Plato, *Gorgias*.

Dorvault, F. L. M., 1936: *L'Officine, ou répertoire général de pharmacie pratique*. Paris, Vigot (17th ed.).

Draczynski, M., 1951: Ueber die bakterizide Wirkung von Wein und Traubenmost, mit Bacterium Coli als Test. Wein und Rebe [Mainz] 1950–1951, 25–42.

Dumortier, J., 1935: *Le vocabulaire médical d'Eschyle et les écrits Hippocratiques*. Paris, Soc. d'Edit. "Les Belles Lettres."

Eckmann, L., ed., 1966: Principles on Tetanus (Proc. of the Internat. Conf. on Tetanus, Bern, July 15–19, 1966). Bern, Stuttgart, Huber.

Edelstein, E., 1952: The Relation of Ancient Philosophy to Medicine. Bull. Hist. Med. 26, 299–316.

Edelstein, E. J., and Edelstein, L., 1945: *Asclepius. A Collection and Interpretation of the Testimonies*. Baltimore, Johns Hopkins Press (2 vols.). Abbr. EE.

Edelstein, L., 1935: The Development of Greek Anatomy. Bull. Hist. Med. *III*, 235–248.

Ehrismann, G., 1918: *Geschichte der deutschen Literatur bis zum Ausgang des Mittelalters. I: Die Althochdeutsche Literatur.* Munich, Beck.

Flückiger, F. A., and Hanbury, D., 1879: *Pharmacographia. A History of the Principal Drugs of Vegetable Origin Met with in Great Britain and British India.* London, Macmillan (2 vols.). Abbr. FH.

Franke, P. F., and Hirmer, M., 1964: *Die Griechische Münze.* Munich, Hirmer.

Fredrich, C., 1899: Hippokratische Untersuchungen. Die Lehre von den vier Temperamenten. Heft 15 of *Philologische Untersuchungen*, A. Kiessling and U. von Wilamowitz-Möllendorff, eds. Berlin, Weidmann.

Frölich, H., 1877: Baracken im trojanischen Kriege. [Virch.] Arch. f. path. Anat. u. Physiol. *71*, 509–514.

————, 1879: *Die Militärmedicin Homer's.* Stuttgart, Enke.

Gabra, S., 1956: Papaver Species and Opium Through the Ages. Bull. Inst. d'Egypte 37, 39–56.

Gärtner, H., 1966: "TERESIS TOU HELKOUS": Ein Nachtrag zu Rufus von Ephesos. CMG Suppl. IV 41, 10 f; Hermes 94, 251–252.

Galen: *Claudii Galeni Opera Omnia*, G. C. Kühn, ed. Lipsiae, Off. Libr. C. Cnoblochii (1821–1833; 22 vols.). Abbr. K.

————, See also May 1968.

Gardiner, E. N., 1930: *Athletics of the Ancient World.* Oxford, Clarendon.

Garrison, F. H., 1969: *History of Neurology.* Springfield, Ill., Thomas.

Ghyka, M. C., 1931: *Le nombre d'or. Rites et rythmes pythagoriciens dans le développement de la civilisation occidentale. I: Les rites; II: Les rythmes.* Paris, Gallimard.

————, 1971: *Philosophie et mystique du nombre.* Paris, Payot.

Ginsburg, J., 1965: Clubbing of the fingers. *Handbook of Physiology*, Sect. 2, *III.* Baltimore, Williams and Wilkins (for the Am. Physiol. Soc.), 2377–2389.

Goodman, L. S., and Gilman, A., 1965: *The Pharmacological Basis of Therapeutics.* New York, Macmillan (3rd ed.).

Grapow, H., and others, 1954–1962: *Grundriss der Medizin der alten Ägypter.* Berlin, Akademie-Verlag (10 vols.). Abbr. GMÄ.

Grot, R. von, 1887: *Über die in der Hippokratischen Schriftensammlung enthaltenen pharmakologischen Kenntnisse.* Doctoral thesis, Dorpat.

Guidi, Guido, 1544: *Chirurgia e Graeco in Latinum conversa, Vido Vidio Florentino interprete . . .* Excudebat P. Galterius Lutetiae Parisiorum.

Gunther, R. T., 1934: *The Greek Herbal of Dioscorides, Illustrated by a Byzantine* A.D. *512, Englished by John Goodyear* A.D. *1655 . . .* London and New York, Hafner (repr. 1968).

Hagers, 1958: *Hagers Handbuch der pharmazeutischen Praxis.* Zweiter Ergänzungsband—Spezieller Teil. Berlin, Springer.

Harris, C. R. S., 1973: *The Heart and the Vascular System in Ancient Greek Medicine from Alcmaeon to Galen.* Oxford, Clarendon.

Harvey, S. C., 1929: The History of Hemostasis. Ann. Med. Hist. (New Ser.) *I*, 127–154.

Heistero, L., 1782: *Instituzioni Chirurgiche. II.* Venezia, F. Pitteri. [Italian translation.]

Herrmann, J. B., and Woodward, S. C., 1972: An Experimental Study of Wound Healing Accelerators. The Am. Surgeon 38, 26–34.

Herzog, R., 1931: Die Wunderheilungen von Epidauros. Philologus, Suppl. 22, Heft 3. Leipzig, Dietrich.

Hippocrates: *The Genuine Works of Hippocrates.* Trans. F. Adams. London, Sydenham Soc. (1849; 2 vols.). Abbr. A.

————, *Hippocrates.* Trans. W. H. S. Jones and B. T. Withington. Loeb Classical Library, Cambridge, Mass., Harvard University Press and London, Heinemann (1923–1931; repr. 1959–1967; 4 vols.). Abbr. LB.

————, *Oeuvres complètes d'Hippocrate: traduction nouvelle avec le texte grec en regard.* Trans. E. Littré. Paris, Baillière (1839–1861; 10 vols.). Abbr. LTT.

————, *Die Werke des Hippokrates.* Die hippokratische Schriftensammlung in neuer deutschen Übersetzung . . . Trans. R. Kapferer and G. Sticker. Stuttgart and Leipzig, Hippokrates-Verlag (1934–1939; 7 vols.). [The seven volumes are all printed in Gothic . . . The passages I checked were not as accurate as in Littré's translation.]

——, See also Cignozzi 1690.

Hodges, H., 1970: *Technology in the Ancient World.* London, Penguin.

Homer: *The Iliad.* Trans. A. T. Murray. Loeb Classical Library, Cambridge, Mass., Harvard University Press (1967; 2 vols.). Abbr. Il.

——, *The Odyssey.* Trans. A. T. Murray. Loeb Classical Library, Cambridge, Mass., Harvard University Press (1966; 2 vols.). Abbr. Od.

Hurlbutt, F. R., 1939: Perí Kardíes: A Treatise on the Heart from the Hippocratic Corpus. Introduction and Translation. Bull. Hist. Med. 7, 1104–1113.

Ilberg, J., 1911: Verbände in der griechischen und römischen Heilkunde. Ztschr. f. Samariter- und Rettungswesen (Leipzig), *XVII*, 185–190.

Inscriptiones Graecae, 1929. Berlin, de Gruyter (vol. IV). Abbr. IG.

Iversen, E., 1953: Wounds in the Head in Egyptian and Hippocratic Medicine. Studia Orientalia Ioanni Pedersen (*Festschrift*). Copenhagen, Munskgaard (pp. 163–171).

Jaeger, W., 1944: *Paideia: The Ideals of Greek Culture.* New York, Oxford University Press (vol. III).

Joly, R., 1966: *Le niveau de la science hippocratique: Contribution à la psychologie de l'histoire des sciences.* Paris, Les Belles Lettres. [Interesting and factual booklet—attitude is "let us keep level-minded about Hippocrates."]

Jones, W. H. S., 1946: Philosophy and Medicine in Ancient Greece. Bull. Hist. Med., Suppl. No 8, Baltimore, Johns Hopkins Press.

——, 1947: *The Medical Writings of Anonymus Londinensis.* Cambridge, Cambridge University Press.

Kapferer and Sticker. See Hippocrates.

Kass, E. H., and Sossen, H. S., 1959: Prevention of Infection of the Urinary Tract in Presence of Indwelling Catheters. J. Am. Med. Ass. 169, 1181–1183.

Kattlove, H., and Alexander, B., 1970: Effect of Cold on Bleeding. Lancet, Dec. 26, p. 1359 (letter to editor).

Kitto, H. D. F., 1951: *The Greeks.* Middlesex, Penguin.

Klibansky, R., Panofsky, E., and Saxl, F., 1964: *Saturn and Melancholy: Studies in the History of Natural Philosophy, Religion and Art.* London, Nelson.

Kraft, E., 1970: *Die Geschichte der Gefässunterbindung bis zu den Anfängen der modernen Chirurgie.* Doctoral thesis, Giessen (Veröff. aus dem Inst. für Gesch. der Medizin der Justus-Liebig-Univ. Giessen, M. Michler u. J. Benedum, Nr 1).

Krause, J. H., 1841: *Gymnastik und Agonistik der Hellenen.* Leipzig, Barth.

Kritikos, P. G., and Papadaki, S. N., 1967: The History of the Poppy and of Opium and their Expansions in Antiquity in the Eastern Mediterranean Area. Bull. Narcotics 19/3, 17–38 and 19/4, 5–10.

Krug, A., 1968: *Binden in der griechischen Kunst. Untersuchungen zur Typologie.* (6.—1. Jahrh. v. Chr.). Doctoral thesis, University of Mainz.

Kühn. Abbr. K. See Galen.

Laënnec, R. T. H., 1804: *Propositions sur la doctrine d'Hippocrate relativement à la médecine-pratique.* Doctoral thesis, Paris, Didot.

——, 1819: *De l'auscultation médiate* (repr. 1965, Monumenta Medica, Paris).

Lammert, F., 1938: *Pfeil.* In *Real-Encyclopädie der Classischen Altertumwissenschaft.* Stuttgart, Metzler (vol. 19/2, col. 1425–1430).

Leboucq, G., 1944: Une anatomie antique du coeur humain. Rev. des Etudes Grecques 57, 7–40.

Lewin, L., 1894: Die Pfeilgifte. Historische und experimentelle Untersuchungen. [Virch.] Arch. f. path. Anat. u. Physiol. 136, 83–126 and 402–443.

Lichtenthäler, C., 1963: Sur l'authenticité, la place véritable, et le style de l' "Epilogue" du IIIe Epidémique . . . La première clinique Hippocratique: Essai de synthèse. Quatrième série d'études Hippocratiques. Geneva, Droz.

Liddell, H. G., and Scott, R., 1968: *A Greek-English Lexicon.* Oxford, Clarendon. Abbr. LS.

Littré. Abbr. LTT. See Hippocrates.

Livingstone, R. W., 1921: *The Legacy of Greece*. Oxford, Clarendon (repr. 1962).

Lucas, A., and Harris, J. R., 1962: *Ancient Egyptian Materials and Industries*. London, Arnold (4th ed.). Abbr. LH.

Lund, F. B., 1935: Hippocratic Surgery. Ann. Surg. *102*, 531–547.

Majno, G., Shea, S. M., and Leventhal, Monika, 1969: Endothelial Contraction Induced by Histamine-Type Mediators. J. Cell. Biol. *42*, 647–672.

Marenghi. See Aristotle.

Martindale, 1958: *The Extra Pharmacopoeia*. London, The Pharmaceutical Press (vol. I; 24th ed.).

Masquelier, J., and Jensen, H., 1953: Recherches sur le pouvoir bactéricide du vin. Bull. Soc. Pharm. Bordeaux *91*, 24–29 and 105–109.

Mattioli, P. A., 1558: Matthioli Senensis . . . Commentarii . . . in Libros Sex Pedacii Dioscoridis, Venetiis, Ex. Off. Erasmiana V. Valgrisij.

May, M. T., 1968: *Galen: On the Usefulness of the Parts of the Body. Translated from the Greek with an Introduction and Commentary*. Ithaca, N. Y., Cornell University Press (2 vols.).

Michler, M., 1968: *Die Alexandrinischen Chirurgen. Eine Sammlung und Auswertung ihrer Fragmente*. Wiesbaden, Steiner.

Milne, J. S., 1907: *Surgical Instruments of Greek and Roman Times*. Oxford, Clarendon (also doctoral thesis, Aberdeen).

Moodie, R. L., 1927: Studies in Paleopathology. XXI: Injuries to the Head Among the Pre-Columbian Peruvians. Ann. Med. Hist. *IX*, 227.

Müri, W., 1953: Melancholie und Schwarze Galle. Museum Helveticum *10*, 21–38.

Neuburger, A., 1919: *Die Technik des Altertums*. Leipzig, Voigtländer.

Oberti, A., 1966: *Il Trattato sulle fasciature di Galeno, tradotto in Latino da Vido Vidi, fiorentino, e illustrato con adatte figure*. Pisa, Giardini. [Latin text with Italian translation.]

Paré, A., 1678: *The Works of that Famous Chirurgeon Ambroise Parey, Translated out of* LATIN, *and Compared with the* FRENCH, *by Th. Johnson* . . . London, Clark.

Paulus Aegineta. See Adams 1844–1847.

Phillips, E. D., 1973: *Greek Medicine*. London, Thames and Hudson.

Phillips, I., Fernandes, R. and Gundara, N. S., 1968: Acetic Acid in the Treatment of Superficial Wounds Infected by *Pseudomonas aeruginosa*. The Lancet, Jan. 6, 11–13.

Pick, A., 1892: Über den Einfluss des Weines auf die Entwickelung der Typhus- und Cholera-Bacillen. Vorläufige Mittheilung. Centralbl. f. Bakt. u. Parasitenkunde *12*, 293–294.

Plato: *Gorgias*. A Revised Text with Introduction and Commentary by E. R. Dodds. Oxford, Clarendon (1959).

————, *The Republic*. Trans. P. Shorey. Loeb Classical Library, Cambridge, Mass., Harvard University Press, and London, Heinemann (1963; 2 vols.).

Pliny [The Elder]: *Natural History*. Trans. H. Rackham and others; Loeb Classical Library, Cambridge, Mass., Harvard University Press, and London, Heinemann (1967; 10 vols.). Abbr. PNH.

Preuss, J., 1894: Der Arzt in Bibel und Talmud. Eine historische Studie. [Virch.] Arch. f. path. Anat. u. Physiol. *138*, 261–283.

Price, P. B., 1939: Ethyl Alcohol as a Germicide. Arch. Surg. *38*, 528–542.

Ribéreau-Gayon, J., and Peynaud, E., 1961: *Traité d'Oenologie*. Paris, Libr. Polytechn. C. Béranger (2 vols.).

Rochard, J., 1875: *Histoire de la chirurgie française au XIX siècle*. Paris, Baillière.

Rollinat, R., 1934: *La vie des reptiles de la France centrale*. Paris, Delagrave.

Rosenfeld, A., 1965: *The Inorganic Raw Materials of Antiquity*. London, Weidenfeld and Nicolson.

Roulet, F. C., 1952: L'Asklepieion de Pergame. Gesnerus *IX*, 1–8.

Sabatier, A., 1883: *Des méthodes antiseptiques chez les anciens et chez les modernes*. Doctoral thesis, Fac. de Médecine de Lyon. Paris, A. Delahaye and E. Lecrosnier.

Sabrazès, J., and Marcandier, A., 1907: Action du vin sur le bacille d'Eberth. Ann.

Inst. Past. *21*, 312–320.

Saggs, H. W. F., 1962: *The Greatness That Was Babylon*. New York, Hawthorn.

Saunders, J. B. de C. M., 1963: *The Transitions from Ancient Egyptian to Greek Medicine*. Logan Clendening Lectures on the History and Philosophy of Medicine, Tenth Series. Lawrence, Kansas, University of Kansas Press.

Schmiedeberg, O., 1918: *Über die Pharmaka in der Ilias und Odyssee*. Strasbourg, Trübner.

Schöne. H., 1896: *Apollonius von Kitium*. Illustrierter Kommentar zu der hippokratischen Schrift *Perí Arthrón*. Leipzig, Teubner.

Schöner, E., 1964: Das Vierschema in der antiken Humoralpathologie. Sudhoffs Arch. f. Gesch. d. Med., suppl. 4. Wiesbaden, Steiner.

Senn, G., 1929: Über Herkunft und Stil der Beschreibungen von Experimenten im Corpus Hippocraticum. Sudhoff's Arch. f. Gesch. der Med. *22*, 217–289.

Sharpe, W. D., 1962: Lung Disease and the Greco-Roman Physician. Am. Rev. Resp. Dis. *86*, 178–192.

Siegel, R. E., 1964: Clinical Observation in Hippocrates: An Essay on the Evolution of the Diagnostic Art. J. Mt Sinai Hosp. *31*, 285–303.

Sigerist, H. E., 1961: *A History of Medicine. II: Early Greek, Hindu and Persian Medicine*. New York, Oxford University Press.

Singer, C., 1921: *Medicine*. A chapter in *The Legacy of Greece*, R. W. Livingstone, ed. Oxford, Clarendon (pp. 201–248).

Singer, C., Holmyarder, E. J., and Hall, A. R., 1965: *A History of Technology*. Oxford, Clarendon (5 vols.).

Souques, A., 1937–1939: La douleur dans les livres hippocratiques. Diagnostics rétrospectifs. I: Affections du système nerveux, 1937, *31*, 209–244 and 279–309. II: Aff. de l'appareil respiratoire, 1938, *32*, 178–186 and 222–242. III: Aff. du tube digestif et péritoine, 1939, *33*, 37–48 and 131-144.

Sourlangas, M., 1894: *Etude sur Hippocrate, son oeuvre, ses idées sur l'infection et ses moyens antiseptiques*. Doctoral thesis, Fac. de Médecine de Paris. Paris, Steinheil.

Spencer. See Celsus.

Steuer, R. O., 1948: *Wḥdw: Aetiological Principle of Pyaemia in Ancient Egyptian Medicine*. Baltimore, Johns Hopkins Press. (Bull. Hist. Med., Suppl. No 10).

Steuer, R. O., and Saunders, J. B. de C. M., 1959: *Ancient Egyptian and Cnidian Medicine: The Relationship of Their Aetiological Concepts of Disease*. Berkeley and Los Angeles, University of California Press.

Stucky, G., 1949: Über die bactericide Wirkung des Rheinweines. Doctoral thesis, Fac. of Medicine, University of Mainz (Hygien. Institut).

Sutor, A. H., Bowie, E. J. W., and Owen, C. A., Jr., 1970: Effect of Cold on Bleeding: Hippocrates Vindicated. Lancet, Nov. 21, p. 1084.

———, 1971: Effect of Temperature on Hemostasis: A Cold-Tolerance Test. Blut *22*, 27–34.

Temkin, O., 1953: Greek Medicine as Science and Craft. Isis *44*, 213-225.

Theophrastus: *Enquiry into Plants* (*And Minor Works on Odours and Weather Signs*). Trans. A. Hort. Loeb Classical Library. Cambridge, Mass., Harvard University Press, and London, Heinemann (1961; 2 vols.).

Thompson, C. J. S., 1924: The Scamnum, as Described by Guido Guidi, Illustrated by an Actual Specimen of the Sixteenth Century. Proc. Roy. Soc. Med. (Section of Med. Hist.) *18*, 13–17.

Thorwald, J., 1962: *Histoire de la médecine dans l'antiquité*. Paris, Hachette.

Torr, E., 1964: *Ancient Ships*. Chicago, Argonaut.

Verdelis, N. M. (Trans. O. Broneer), 1962: A Sanctuary at Solygeia. Archaeology *15*, 184–192.

Walton, A., 1894: *The Cult of Asklepios*. Cornell Studies in Classical Philol. No. 3. Ithaca, N. Y., Ginn.

Watts, G. T., 1960: Wound Shape and Tissue Tension in Healing. Brit. J. Surg. *47*, 555–561.

Wellmann, M., 1895: Die Pneumatische Schule bis auf Archigenes in ihrer Entwicklung dargestellt. Heft 14 of *Philologische Untersuchungen*, A. Kiessling and U. v. Wilamowitz-Möllendorf, eds. Berlin, Weidmann.

Whibley, L., 1963: *A Companion to Greek Studies*. New York and London, Hafner (4th ed.).

Winckelmann, 1808: *Winckelmann's Werke*. Band II. C. L. Fernow, ed. Dresden, Walther.

———, 1811: *Winckelmann's Werke*. Band IV. H. Meyer and J. Schultze, eds. Dresden, Walther.

Wulfsberg, N., 1887: Geschichtliche Notizen über Oesypum und therapeutische Versuche mit dem reinen wasserfreien Lanolin. Therap. Monatshefte (Berlin), year I. 92–97.

Xenophon: *Memorabilia and Oeconomicus*. Trans. E. C. Marchant. Loeb Classical Library, London, Heinemann and New York, Putnam (1923).

Zervos, C., 1956: *L'Art de la Crète néolithique et minoenne*. Paris, Ed. Cahiers d'Art.

5. The Perfumes of Arabia

André, J., 1951: Murrina "Vin Myrrhé"? Ann. Fac. de Lettres d'Aix 25, 45–62.

Apicius: *De re coquinaria: L'art culinaire, texte établi, traduit et commenté par Jacques André*. Paris, Klincksieck (1965).

Beek, G. W. van, 1952: Recovering the Ancient Civilization of Arabia. The Biblical Archaeologist 15, 2–18.

———, 1958(a): Ancient Frankincense-Producing Areas. In *Archaeological Discoveries in South Arabia*. Bowen R. LeB. and Albright, F. P., eds. Baltimore, Johns Hopkins Press (pp. 139–142).

———, 1958(b): Frankincense and Myrrh in Ancient South Arabia. J. Am. Oriental Soc. 78, 141–152.

———, 1960: Frankincense and Myrrh. The Biblical Archaeologist 23, 70–95.

———, 1961: South Arabian History and Archaeology. In *The Bible and the Ancient Near East, Essays in the Honor of William Foxwell Albright*. London, Routledge and Kegan Paul (pp. 229–248).

Bowen, R. LeB., Jr., 1958(a): Ancient Trade Routes in South Arabia. In *Archaeological Discoveries in South Arabia*. Bowen R. LeB. and Albright, F. P., eds. Baltimore, Johns Hopkins Press (pp. 35-42).

———, 1958(b): Irrigation in Ancient Qatabân (Beihân). In *Archaeological Discoveries in South Arabia*. Bowen R. LeB. and Albright, F. P., eds. Baltimore, Johns Hopkins Press (pp. 43–131).

Bowen, R. LeB., Jr., and Albright, F., P., 1958: *Archaeological Discoveries in South Arabia*. Baltimore, Johns Hopkins Press.

Burkill, I. H., 1935: *A Dictionary of the Economic Products of the Malay Peninsula*. London, Crown Agents for the Colonies (2 vols.).

Carter, H. J., 1848: Frankincense in Arabia. J. of the Bombay Branch of the Roy. Asiatic Soc. 2, 380–390.

Celsus: *De medicina*. Trans. W. G. Spencer. Loeb Classical Library, Cambridge, Mass., Harvard University Press and London, Heinemann (1935–1938; 3 vols.).

Columella: *De re rustica*. Trans. H. B. Ash, E. S. Forster, and E. Heffner. Loeb Classical Library, Cambridge, Mass., Harvard University Press and London, Heinemann (1941–1955; 3 vols.).

Déonna, W., 1939: *Euodía*: Croyances antiques et modernes. L'odeur suave des dieux et des élus. Genava 17, 167–262.

Détienne, M., 1972: *Les jardins d'Adonis*. Paris, Gallimard.

Devoto, G., 1967: *Avviamento alla etimologia Italiana. Dizionario etimologico*. Florence, Le Monnier.

Dictionary of the Bible (The Interpreter's), 1962: An Illustrated Encyclopedia. G. A. Buttrick and others, eds. New York, Abingdon (4 vols.). Abbr. DB.

Drake-Brockman, R. E., 1912: *British Somaliland*. London, Hurst and Blackett.

Ernout, A., and Meillet, A., 1959: *Dictionnaire étymologique de la langue latine. Histoire des mots*. Paris, Klincksieck.

Filliozat, J., 1949: *La doctrine classique de la médecine Indienne. Ses origines et ses parallèles Grecs*. Paris, Impr. Nat.

Flückiger, F. A., and Hanbury, D., 1879: *Pharmacographia. A History of the Principal Drugs of Vegetable Origin Met with in Great Britain and British India*. London, Macmillan. Abbr. FH.

Garoglio, P. G., 1959: *La nuova enologia*. Florence, Istituto di Industrie Agrarie.

Griffith, F. Ll., 1900: *Beni Hasan*. Part IV. Archaeological Survey of Egypt, VII. London, Kegan Paul, Trench, Trübner.

Günther, E., 1950: *The Essential Oils*. New York, Van Nostrand (vol. IV).

Gunther, R. T., 1934: *The Greek Herbal of Dioscorides, Illustrated by a Byzantine* A.D. *412, Englished by John Goodyear* A.D. *1655* . . . London and New York, Hafner (repr. 1968).

Harding, G., 1964: *Archaeology in the Aden Protectorates*. London, Dept. of Technical Cooperation, Her Majesty's Stationery Office.

Harley, G. W., 1941: *Native African Medicine (With Special Reference to its Practice in the Mano Tribe of Liberia)*. Cambridge, Mass., Harvard University Press.

Hennig, R., 1939: *Kinnámomon* und *kinnamophóros chóra* in der antiken Literatur. Klio, N. F. *14*, 325–330.

Hepper, F. N., 1969: Arabian and African Frankincense Trees. J. Egyptian Archaeol. *55*, 66–72.

Herodotus. Trans. A. D. Godley. Loeb Classical Library, Cambridge, Mass., Harvard University Press and London, Heinemann (1961–1966; 4 vols.).

Hippocrates. See Littré.

Hornell, J., 1946: *Water Transport. Origins & Early Evolution*. Cambridge, Cambridge University Press.

Imbesi, A., 1964: *Index Plantarum* . . . [Indice delle piante finora ammesse nelle farmacopee ufficiali dei diversi Stati del mondo]. Messina (pub. by the author).

Lanteaume, M.-T., Ramel, P., Jaulmes, P., and Manin, D., 1969: Détermination et comparaison des DL 50 du métabisulfite de potassium, de l'éthanal, et de leur combinaison . . . par voie orale sur le rat de la souche Wistar. Ann. des falsific. et de l'expertise chim. *686*, 231–241.

Lederer, E., 1941: Sur les constituants du castoréum. I: Les acides. Trav. des membres de la Soc. Chim. Biol. *23*, 1457–1462.

Lewis, C. T., and Short, C., 1879: *A Latin Dictionary*. Oxford, Clarendon (repr. 1962).

Liddell, H. G., and Scott, R., 1968: *A Greek-English Lexicon*. Oxford, Clarendon. Abbr. LS.

Littré, É., 1839–1861: *Oeuvres complètes d' Hippocrate, traduction nouvelle avec le texte grec en regard* . . . Paris, Baillière (10 vols.). Abbr. LTT.

Lucas, A., and Harris, J. R., 1962: *Ancient Egyptian Materials and Industries*. London, Arnold. Abbr. LH.

Marchand, L., 1867: *De l' organisation des Burséracées*. Doctoral thesis, Fac. des Sciences de Caen . . . Paris, Martinet.

Marescalchi, C., and Dalmasso, G., 1937: *Storia della Vite e del Vino in Italia*. Milan, Gualdoni.

Masson, E., 1967: *Recherches sur les plus anciens emprunts sémitiques en Grec*. Paris, Klincksieck.

Miller, J. I., 1969: *The Spice Trade of the Roman Empire (29* B.C. *to* A.D. *641)*. Oxford, Clarendon.

Moldenke, H. N., and Moldenke, A. L., 1952: *Plants of the Bible*. New York, Ronald.

Naville, E., 1898: *The Temple of Deir el Bahari*. London, Egypt. Explor. Fund (vol. XVI, part 3).

Needham, J., 1965 - : *Science and Civilisation in China*. Cambridge, Cambridge University Press. Abbr. NEED.

Pasteur, L., 1866: *Études sur le vin, ses maladies, causes qui les provoquent, procédés nouveaux pour le conserver et pour le vieillir*. Paris, Imprim. Impériale.

Pauly-Wissowa, 1894–1972: *Paulys Real-Encylopädie der classischen Altertumwissenschaft*. Herausgeg. von G. Wissowa. Stuttgart, Metzler. Abbr. PW.

Phillips, W., 1955: *Qataban and Sheba. Exploring Ancient Kingdoms on the Biblical Spice Routes of Arabia*. London, Victor Gollancz.

Pirenne, J., 1956: *Paléographie des inscriptions sud-Arabes*. (Contribution à la chronologie et à l'histoire de l'Arabie du Sud antique). I: Des origines jusqu'à l'époque hymarite. Brussels, Paleis der Academien, Hertogelijke Straat 1.

———, 1960: *La Grèce et Saba*. Mém. présentés par divers savants à l'Acad. des Inscr. et Belles-Lettres de l'Inst. de France. Paris, Impr. Nat. (vol. XV/1).

Pliny [The Elder]: *Natural History*. Trans. H. Rackham, W. H. S. Jones and D. E. Eichholz. Loeb Classical Library, Cambridge, Mass., Harvard University Press and London, Heinemann (1956–1966; 10 vols.). Abbr. PNH.

Plutarch: *Lives. Demosthenes and Cicero. Alexander and Caesar*. Trans. B. Perrin. Vol. VII of *Plutarch's Lives*. Loeb Classical Library, Cambridge, Mass., Harvard University Press, and London, Heinemann (1919; repr. 1967; 11 vols.).

Pories, W. J., Henzel, J. H., Rob, C. G., and Strain, W. H., 1967: Acceleration of Healing with Zinc Sulfate. Ann. Surg. 165, 432–436.

Rawlinson, H. G., 1928: *Intercourse between India and the Western World (From the Earliest Times to the Fall of Rome)*. Cambridge, Cambridge University Press.

Ribéreau-Gayon, J., 1947: *Traité d'oenologie. Transformations et traitements des vins*. Paris et Liège, Librairie Polytechnique Ch. Béranger.

Rosengarten, F., Jr., 1969: *The Book of Spices*. Wynnewood, Pa., Livingston; Macrae and Smith, distr. Philadelphia. [Beautifully illustrated and very useful for the history of spices.]

Rudhardt, J., 1958: *Notions fondamentales de la pensée religieuse et actes constitutifs du culte dans la Grèce classique*. Geneva, Droz.

Ryckmans, G., 1951: *Les religions arabes préislamiques*. Louvain, Publications Universitaires (2nd ed.).

———, 1957: Petits Royaumes Sud-Arabes d'Après les Auteurs Classiques. Le Muséon, revue d'études orientales 70, 75–96.

Samarawira, I. St. E., 1964: Cinnamon. World Crops 16, 45–59.

Schäfer, H., 1902: *Ein Bruchstück altägyptischer Annalen*. Berlin, Verlag der Königl. Akad. der Wiss.

Schanderl, H., 1956: Die Schweflige Säure des Weines in hygienischer Sicht. Zeitschr. f. Lebensmittel-Unters. u. Forsch. 103, 379–386.

Schoff, W. H., 1912: *The Periplus of the Erythraean Sea. Travel and Trade in the Indian Ocean by a Merchant of the First Century. Translated from the Greek and Annotated*. New York, London, Bombay and Calcutta, Longmans, Green and Co.

Singer, C., and others, 1965: *A History of Technology*. Oxford, Clarendon (5 vols.).

Smith, G. E., 1912: *The Royal Mummies*. (Catal. gén. des antiquités égypt. du Musée du Caire, Num. 61051–61100). Le Caire, Impr. de l'Inst. Français d'Archéol. Orientale.

Sophocles, Trans. F. Storr. Cambridge, Mass., Harvard University Press and London, Heinemann (1951; 2 vols.).

Strabo: *Geography*. Trans. H. L. Jones. Loeb Classical Library, Cambridge, Mass., Harvard University Press and London, Heinemann (1966–1970; 8 vols.).

Theophrastus: *Enquiry into Plants and Minor Works on Odours and Weather Signs*. Trans. A. Hort. Loeb Classical Library, Cambridge, Mass., Harvard University Press and London, Heinemann (1961; 2 vols.).

Thorwald, J., 1963: *Science and Secrets in Early Medicine*. New York, Harcourt Brace and World.

Trease, G. E., and Evans, W. C., 1972: *Pharmacognosy*. London, Baillière Tindall (10th ed.).

Vallery-Radot, R., 1900: *La vie de Pasteur*. Paris, Flammarion.

Vogel, V. J., 1970: *American Indian Medicine*. University of Oklahoma Press (paperback: New York, Ballantine Books, 1973).

Wiedemer, H. R., 1966: Ein Augensalbenstempel aus Vindonissa. In Jahresbericht 1965, Vindonissa-Museum, Brugg, Switzerland, 56–58.

Bibliography

Wissmann, H. von, 1964: *Zur Geschichte und Landeskunde von Alt-Südarabien.* Wien, H. Böhlaus.

——, 1968: *Zur Archäologie und Antiken Geographie von Südarabien. Hadramaut, Qataban und das Aden-Gebiet in der Antike.* Istanbul, Nederlands Historisch-Archaeologisch Instituut in het Nabije Oosten.

World Health Organization, 1967: *Toxicological Evaluations of Some Antimicrobials, Antioxidants, Emulsifiers, Stabilizers, Flour-Treatment Agents, Acids and Bases* (9th Report of the FAO/WHO Expert Committee on Food Additives). Geneva, Switzerland.

——, 1971: *A Review of the Technological Efficacy of Some Antimicrobial Agents* (14th Report of the Joint FAO/WHO Expert Committee on Food Additives). Geneva, Switzerland.

6. The Yang I

Bengtson, H., and Milojčić, V., 1963: *Grosser Historischer Weltatlas.* Vorgeschichte und Altertum. Munich, Bayerischer Schulbuch-Verlag. [An excellent historical atlas.]

Biot, E., 1851: *Le Tcheou-li ou Rites des Tcheou.* Paris, Impr. Nat. (3 vols.; also phot. reprint by Ch'eng Wen Publ. Co., Taipei, 1969).

Bourgey, L., 1953: *Observation et expérience chez les médecins de la Collection Hippocratique.* Paris, Vrin.

Breasted, J. H., 1930: *The Edwin Smith Surgical Papyrus. Published in facisimile and Hieroglyphic Transliteration with Translation and Commentary.* Chicago, Ill., University of Chicago Press (2 vols.). Abbr. Sm.

Burkill, I. H., 1935: *A Dictionary of the Economic Products of the Malay Peninsula.* London, publ. on behalf of the Governments of the Straits Settlements and Federated Malay States by the Crown Agents for the Colonies (2 vols.).

Celsus: *De medicina.* Trans. W. G. Spencer. Loeb Classical Library, Cambridge, Mass., Harvard University Press and London, Heinemann (1935–1938; 3 vols.). Abbr. CDM.

Chamfrault, A., 1957–1964: *Traité de médecine chinoise.* Angoulême, éd. Coquemard (5 vols.). I: Acupuncture, Moxa, Massage, Bleeding; II: Transl. of the Nei Ching in Collab. with Ung Kang-Sam (see ref. below); III: Chinese Drugs; IV: Chinese Prescriptions (by disease); V: Man and Cosmos in Chinese Philosophy.

Chamfrault, A., and Ung Kang-Sam, 1957: *Les livres sacrés de médecine chinoise.* Angoulême, éd. Coquemard. [Actually a translation of the Nei Ching. and vol. II of the series cited in the ref. above.]

Chang, K.-C., 1968: Archeology of Ancient China. Science *162,* 519–526.

Chou-Li. See Biot 1851.

Cohn-Haft, L., 1956: *The Public Physicians of Ancient Greece.* Northampton, Mass., Smith College Studies in History *42.*

Confucius. See Waley 1938.

Cowdry, E. V., 1921(a): A Comparison of Ancient Chinese Anatomical Charts with the "Fünfbilderserie" of Sudhoff. Anat. Rec. *22,* 1–25.

——, 1921(b): Taoist Ideas of Human Anatomy. Ann. Med. Hist. *3,* 301–309.

Creel, H. G., 1970: *The Origins of Statecraft in China.* I: *The Western Chou Empire.* Chicago and London, The University of Chicago Press. [Pages 1–27 include discussions of the origin of examinations in China and their influence in the West.]

Diringer, D., 1968: *The Alphabet: A Key to the History of Mankind.* London, Hutchinson (2 vols.).

Drabkin, I. E., 1944: On Medical Education in Greece and Rome. Bull. Hist. Med. *15,* 333–351.

Bibliography

Filliozat, J., 1949: *La doctrine classique de la médecine Indienne*. Paris, Impr. Nat.

Flückiger, F. A., and Hanbury, D., 1879: *Pharmacographia. A History of the Principal Drugs of Vegetable Origin Met with in Great Britain and British India*. London, Macmillan. Abbr. FH.

Forke, A., 1925: *World Conception of the Chinese: Their Astronomical, Cosmological and Physico-Philosophical Speculations*. London, Probsthain.

Forrest, R. A. D., 1948: *The Chinese language*. London, Faber and Faber.

Grapow, H., 1954–1962: *Grundriss der Medizin der alten Ägypter*. Berlin, Akademie-Verlag (10 vols.). Abbr. GMÄ.

Gwei-Djen. See Lu Gwei-Djen.

Hall, A. J., 1974: A Lady from China's Past. (With color photographs from *China Pictorial*, a magazine of the People's Republic). Nat. Geographic Magazine *145* No. 5, 660–681.

Hartner, W., 1941–1942: Heilkunde im alten China. Sinica *16*, 217–265 (1941); *17*, 266–328 (1942). [Two very useful papers.]

Hennig, R., 1939: Kinnámomon und kinnamophóros chóra in der antiken Literatur. Klio, N. F. (New Series) *14*, 325–330.

Hightower, J. R., 1951: [Review of] Ilza Veith, *Huang Ti Nei Ching Su Wên, the Yellow Emperor's Classic of Internal Medicine . . .* Harvard J. of Asiat. Studies *14*, 306–312.

Hsieh, E. T., 1921: A Review of Ancient Chinese Anatomy. Anat. Rec. *20*, 97–127.

Huang Man. See Wong Man.

Huang Ti Nei Ching. Trans. Chamfrault and Ung Kang-Sam 1957; Veith 1966. See also Huang Wên 1950.

Huang Wên, 1950: The *Nei Ching*, The Chinese Canon of Medicine. Chin. Med. J. *68*, 1–33. [Contains a useful summary by chapters.]

Huard, P., 1957: Quelques aspects de la doctrine classique de la médecine Chinoise. In *La biologie médicale*. Paris.

Huard, P., and Wong, M., 1956: Bio-bibliographie de la médecine chinoise. Bull. Soc. Etudes Indochinoises, Nlle série *31*, 181–246.

————, 1957: Structure de la médecine chinoise. Bull. Soc. Etudes Indochinoises, Nlle série *32*, 299–376.

————, 1958(a): Cautérisation ignée et moxas. Histoire de la Méd., July 1958.

————, 1958(b): La chirurgie chinoise et les spécialités chirurgicales. Concours médical (Paris) *80*, 1857–1864.

————, 1959(a): *La médecine chinoise au cours des siècles*. Paris, Ed. Roger Dacosta.

————, 1959(b): Histoire de l'Acupuncture chinoise. Bull. de la Société des Etudes Indochinoises, Nlle Série *34*, 403–423.

————, 1964: *La médecine chinoise*. Coll. "Que Sais-Je?" No. 1112. Paris, Presses Universitaires de France.

Hudson, G. F., 1931: *Europe and China. A Survey of their Relations from the Earliest Times to 1800*. London, Arnold.

Hume, E. H., 1940: *The Chinese Way in Medicine*. Baltimore, The Johns Hopkins Press.

Huong Man. See Huang Wên.

Jeanselme, E., 1917: *De la protection de l'enfant chez les Romains*. Paris, Masson.

Jung, C. G., 1944: *Psychologie und Alchemie*. Zürich, Rascher.

Kleine Pauly. See Pauly.

Lassen, C., 1867: *Indische Alterthumskunde*. Leipzig, Kittler and London, Williams and Norgate (4 vols.).

Lu Gwei-Djen, and Needham, J., 1963: China and the Origin of Examinations in Medicine. Proc. Roy. Soc. Med. *56*, 63–70.

————, 1967: Records of Diseases in Ancient China. Ch. 17 in *Diseases in Antiquity*, D. Brothwell and A. T. Sandison, eds. Springfield, Ill., Thomas (pp. 222–237).

Mahdihassan, S., 1952: The Chinese Origin of Three Cognate Words: Chemistry, Elixir and Genii. J. Univ. Bombay *20*, 107–131.

————, 1959: Alchemy, a Child of Chinese Dualism as Illustrated by its Symbolism. Iqbal *8*, 15–37.

————, 1960: Alchemy in the Light of its Names in Arabic, Sanskrit and Greek. Janus *49*, 79–100.

Maspéro, H., 1965: *La Chine Antique*. Paris, Presses Universitaires de France (New ed.; Ann. du Musée Guimet, Tome 71).

McCrindle, J. W., 1885: *Ancient India as Described by Ptolemy*. Calcutta, Thacker, Spink and Co.; Bombay, Educ. Soc. Press; London, Trübner.

Miller, J. I., 1969: *The Spice Trade of the Roman Empire (29 B.C. to A.D. 641)*. Oxford, Clarendon.

Morse, W. R., 1934: *Chinese Medicine*. Coll. "Clio Medica." New York, Hoeber.

Needham, J., 1964: Science and Society in East and West. Centaurus *10*, 174–197.

————, 1965–(a): *Science and Civilisation in China*. Cambridge, Cambridge University Press. [Reviews: Pong 1972, de Solla Price 1968. A key work.] Abbr. NEED.

————, 1965(b): The Dialogue Between Asia and Europe. In *The Glass Curtain*, Raghavan Iyer, ed. Oxford University Press (p. 279).

————, 1968: Skin-Colour in Chinese Thought: An Extract from a Letter to the Editor. Race, p. 249.

Needham, J., and Lu Gwei-Djen, 1962: Hygiene and Preventive Medicine in Ancient China. J. Hist. Med. *17*, 429–478.

————, 1969: Chinese Medicine. In *Medicine and Culture*, F. N. L. Poynter, ed. London, Wellcome Institute of the Hist. of Medicine (pp. 255–284).

Nei Ching. See *Huang Ti Nei Ching*

Pálos, S., 1971: *The Chinese Art of Healing*. New York, Herder and Herder.

Pauly, Der Kleine, 1964 - : *Lexikon der Antike . . .* K. Ziegler, ed. Stuttgart, Druckenmüller. [A condensed version of Pauly's Realencyclopädie; 4 vols. up to 1972.]

Pauly, 1894–1972: *Real-Encyclopädie der classischen Altertumswissenschaft*. G. Wissowa, ed. Stuttgart, Metzler and Munich, Druckenmüller. Abbr. PW.

Peking Review, 1973: Preliminary Results from Study of 2,100-Year-Old Corpse. (Anon.). No. 32, 16–17.

Pliny [The Elder]: *Natural History*. Trans. H. Rackham, W. H. S. Jones, and D. E. Eichholz. Loeb Classical Library. Cambridge, Mass., Harvard University Press, and London, Heinemann (1956–1966; 10 vols.). Abbr. PNH.

Pong, D., 1972: [Review of Needham's *Science and Civilisation in China*, Vol. IV] Science *175*, 50–51.

Porkert, M., 1973: *The Theoretical Foundations of Chinese Medicine. Systems of Correspondence*. Cambridge, Mass., and London, M.I.T. Press.

Read, B. E., 1926: Gleanings from Old Chinese Medicine. Ann. Med. Hist. 8, 16–19.

Schliemann, H., 1885: *Ilios: Ville et pays des Troyens*. Trans. from the English. Paris, Firmin-Didot.

Schuchhardt, C., 1891: *Schliemann's Ausgrabungen in Troja . . .* Leipzig, Brockhaus.

Sharma, P. V., 1972: *Indian Medicine in the Classical Age*. The Chowkhamba Sanskrit Series Office, Varanasi, India.

Siegel, R. E., 1968: *Galen's System of Physiology and Medicine*. Basel, Karger.

Singer, C., Holmyard, E. J., and Hall, R. A., 1965: *A History of Technology*. Oxford, Clarendon (5 vols.).

Siu, G. H., 1968: *The Man of Many Qualities. A Legacy of the I Ching*. Cambridge, Mass., and London, England, M.I.T. Press.

Solla Price, D. J. de, 1968: Joseph Needham and the Science of China. Horizon *10*, No. 1, 52–63.

Trease, G. E., and Evans, W. C., 1972: *Pharmacognosy*. London, Baillière Tindall (10th ed.).

Ung Kang-Sam. See Chamfrault and Ung Kang-Sam 1957.

Veith, I., 1966: *Huang Ti Nei Ching Su Wên. The Yellow Emperor's Classic of Internal Medicine*. Berkeley, University of Calif. Press (new ed.) Abbr. Ve.

Waley, A., 1938: *The Analects of Confucius*. London, Allen and Unwin (repr. 1971).

Wang Chi Min, 1926: China's Contribution to Medicine in the Past. Ann. Med. Hist. 8, 192–201.

Bibliog-
raphy

Wang, Chi-Min, and Wu, Lien-Tê, 1932: *History of Chinese Medicine. Being a Chronicle of Medical Happenings in China from Ancient Times to the Present Period.* Tientsin, China, Tientsin Press.

Wieger, L., 1924: *Caractères chinois. Etymologie. Graphies. Lexiques.* Hien-hien, China. Imprimerie de Hien-hien (4th ed.).

Wilhelm, H., 1960: *Change. Eight Lectures on the I Ching.* Trans. from the German by C. F. Baynes. New York, Pantheon Books (repr. 1964 by Harper and Row, New York).

Wilhelm, R., 1950: *The I Ching or Book of Changes.* Trans. C. F. Baynes. New York, Bollingen Series XIX, Pantheon Books (2 vols.).

Wong, K. C., and Wu, L-T., 1932: See Wang and Wu.

Wong Man. See Huang Wên.

Wu, Lien-Tê, 1938: Past and Present Trends in the Medical History of China. The *Chinese Med. Journal* 53 (4), 313–322.

Yang, W. S.-Y., 1973: The Chinese Language. *Scientific American* 228, 51–60.

7. The Vaidya

Ackerknecht, E. H., 1946: Contradictions in Primitive Surgery. *Bull. Hist. Med.* 20, 184–187.

———, 1967: Primitive Surgery. Ch. 51 in *Diseases in Antiquity*, D. Brothwell and A. T. Sandison, eds. Springfield, Ill., C. C. Thomas (pp. 635–650).

Aristotle: *Parts of Animals. Movement of Animals. Progression of Animals.* Trans. A. L. Peck. Loeb Classical Library, Cambridge, Mass., Harvard University Press and London, Heinemann (1961; 1 vol.).

Arrian. Trans. E. I. Robson. Loeb Classical Library, Cambridge, Mass., Harvard University Press and London, Heinemann (1949; 2 vols.).

Atharva Veda. Abbr. AV. See Whitney 1962.

Auboyer, J., 1955: *La vie publique et privée dans l'Inde ancienne (IIe siècle avant J.-C.—VIIIe siècle environ).* Fasc. VI: *Les jeux et les jouets.* Paris, Presses Universitaires, Publ. du Musée Guimet (vol. VI).

———, 1961: *La vie quotidienne dans l'Inde ancienne (environ IIe siècle avant J.-C.—VIIe siècle).* Paris, Hachette. [Very informative—though it reads much like a novel.] Abbr. AUB.

Aymard, A., and Auboyer, J., 1953: *L'Orient et la Grèce Antique.* In *Histoire générale des civilisations.* M. Croizet, ed. Paris, Presses Universitaires (vol. 1).

Bagchi, A. K., 1968: The Influence of Sanskrit on Modern Medical Vocabulary. *Surg. Gynecol. Obst.* 126, 1327–1328.

Basham, A. L., 1954: *The Wonder That Was India: A Survey of the Culture of the Indian Sub-Continent Before the Coming of the Muslims.* London, Sidgwick and Jackson.

Beal, S., 1869: *Travels of Fah-hian and Sung-yun: Buddhist Pilgrims from China to India.* Trans. from the Chinese. London, Trübner.

Beebe, W., 1921: *The Edge of the Jungle.* New York, Holt.

Bhishagratna. See *Sushruta Samhita.* Abbr. SS.

Bingham, C. T., 1903: *The Fauna of British India, Including Ceylon and Burma.* II: *Hymenoptera.* London, Taylor and Francis.

Bloch, J., 1950: *Les inscriptions d' Asoka.* Paris, Les Belles Lettres.

Bühler, G., 1886: See Manu.

Burr, M., 1939: *The Insect Legion.* London, Nisbet.

Caland, W., 1900: *Altindisches Zauberritual. Probe einer Übersetzung der wichtigsten Theile des Kauśika Sutra.* Amsterdam, Müller.

Capeller, C., 1887: *Sanskrit-Wörterbuch.* Strassburg, Trübner.

Celsus: *De medicina.* Trans. W. G. Spencer, Loeb Classical Library, Cambridge, Mass., Harvard University Press and London, Heinemann (1935–1938; 3 vols.).

Chakravorty, R. C., 1969: The Treatment of Wounds and Abscesses in the Sutra-sthanam of the Sushrutasamhita. Indian J. of Surgery *31*, 261–266.

———, 1970: Surgical Principles in the Sūtrasthānam of the Suśruta Saṃhitā. Management of Retained Foreign Bodies. Indian J. of History of Science *5*, 113–118.

Chalmers, A. J., and Marshall, A., 1918: Notes on Minor Cutaneous Affections Seen in the Anglo-Egyptian Sudan. J. Tropical Med. and Hyg. *21*, 198–199.

———, 1919: Oedema of the Eyelids Caused by Ants. J. Tropical Med. and Hyg. *22*, 117 (with page plate).

Charaka Saṃhita. Trans. A. Ch. Kaviratna. Calcutta [pub. by the trans.; in 51 fascicles—about 2 vols.—between 1897 and 1912. Includes a fair amount of notes, but no index or table of contents, *see note 8.*] Abbr. ChS.

Childe, V. G., 1939: India and the West before Darius. Antiquity *13*, 5–15.

Converse, J. M., 1959: Reconstruction of the Nose by the Scalping Flap Technique. Surg. Clin. of North Am. *39*, 335–365.

———, 1964: *Reconstructive Plastic Surgery.* Philadelphia and London, Saunders (repr. 1967).

Coomaraswamy, A. K., 1913: *The Arts and Crafts of India and Ceylon.* London and Edinburgh, Foulis.

———, 1931: *Yakṣas.* Washington, D. C., Smithsonian Institution Publication No. 3059 (Part II).

Darmesteter, J., 1892: *Le Zend-Avesta. Traduction nouvelle . . . . II: La loi (Vendidad)* etc. Paris, Leroux.

Dart, R. A., 1955: Cultural Status of the South African Man-Apes. Ann. Report, Smithsonian Inst., pp. 317–338.

Deoras, P. J., 1971: The Story of Some Indian Poisonous Snakes. Ch. 22 in W. Bücherl and E. E. Buckley, eds., 1971: *Venomous Animals and Their Venoms.* New York and London, Acad. Press (vol. II, pp. 19–34).

Dibbell, D. G., 1970: Split Earlobe Deformities. J. Plast. and Reconstr. Surg. *45*, 77. [A short note].

Doflein, F., 1905: Beobachtungen an den Weberameisen (*Oecophylla smaragdina*). Biol. Centralbl. *25*, 497–507.

Duke-Elder, S., 1969: *Diseases of the Lens and Vitreous; Glaucoma and Hypotony.* In *System of Ophtalmology,* S. Duke-Elder, ed. London, Kimpton (vol. XI).

Elliot, R. H., 1918: *The Indian Operation of Couching for Cataract.* New York, Hoeber.

Fa-Hsian. See Beal 1869.

Fergusson, J., 1868: *Tree and Serpent Worship: or Illustrations of Mythology and Art in India in the 1st and 4th Centuries after Christ from the Sculptures of the Buddhist Topes at Sanchi and Amravati.* London, India Museum.

Filliozat, J., 1949: *La doctrine classique de la médecine Indienne. Ses origines et ses parallèles Grecs.* Paris, Impr. Nat. [Very important study of rare depth as regards East-West cultural links.]

———, 1956: *Les relations extérieures de l'Inde.* Pondichéry, Publ. de l'Inst. Français d'Indologie, No. 2.

Forbes, R. J., 1965: Extracting, Smelting and Alloying. Ch. 21 in C. Singer and others, *A History of Technology.* Oxford, Clarendon (vol. I, pp. 572–599).

Furnari, S., 1845: Notes sur un mode particulier de réunion des plaies, usité chez les Arabes. Journal de Chirurgie *3*, 118–119.

Giboin, L. M., 1949: *Epitomé botanique et de la matière médicale de l'Inde (et spé-cialement des établissements français dans l'Inde).* Doctoral thesis, Marseille (Fac. mixte de Méd. Gén. et Pharmacie).

Gnudi, M. T., and Webster, J. P., 1950: *The Life and Times of Gaspare Tagliacozzi, Surgeon of Bologna.* New York, Reichner.

Goodman, L. S., and Gilman, A., 1970: *The Pharmacological Basis of Therapeutics.* London and Toronto, Macmillan (4th ed.).

Grassmann, H., 1873: *Wörterbuch zum Rig-Veda.* Leipzig, Brockhaus.

Gudger, E. W., 1925: Stitching Wounds with the Mandibles of Ants and Beetles: A

Bibliog-
raphy

Minor Contribution to the History of Surgery. J. Am. Med. Ass. *84*, 1861–1864.

Hackin, J., 1954: *Nouvelles recherches archéologiques à Begram.* Paris, Presses Universitaires (2 vols.).

Hallade, M., and Hinz, M., 1968: *Un millénaire d'art bouddhique.* Fribourg, Switzerland, Office du Livre.

Harley, G. W., 1941: *Native African Medicine. With Special Reference to its Practice in the Mano Tribe of Liberia.* Cambridge, Mass., Harvard University Press.

Heath, J. M., 1839: On Indian Iron and Steel. J. Roy. Asiat. Soc. *5*, 390–397.

Henry, V., 1909: *La magie dans l'Inde antique.* Paris, Emile Nourry (2nd ed.).

Hippocrates: *Oeuvres complètes d'Hippocrate: traduction nouvelle avec le texte grec en regard.* Trans. E. Littré. Paris, Baillière (1839–1861; 10 vols.). Abbr. LTT.

Hultzsch, E., 1925: *Corpus Inscriptionum Indicarum.* I: *Inscriptions of Asoka.* Oxford, Clarendon (new ed.).

India Committee on Indigenous Systems of Medicine, 1948: *Report.* I: *Report and Recommendations.* Ministry of Health, Gvt. of India.

Jain, S. K., 1967: Plants in Indian Medicine and Folklore Associated with Healing of Bones. Indian Journal of Orthopaedics *1*, No. 1, 95–104.

Jee, B. S., 1896: *A Short History of Aryan Medical Science.* London, Macmillan.

Jolly, J., 1901: *Grundriss der Indo-Arischen Philologie und Altertumskunde.* Strassburg, Trübner (vol. III, article *Medicin*, pp. 1–140).

Kausika Sutra. See Caland 1900. Abbr. KS.

Kaviratna. See *Charaka Samhita.* Abbr. ChS.

Kennedy, J., 1898: The Early Commerce of Babylon with India - 700–300 B.C. J. Royal Asiatic Society of Great Britain and Ireland 1898, pp. 241 f.

Kirfel, 1949: Die Leistungen der altindischen Chirurgie. Grenzgeb. der Medizin *2*, 176–178.

Kosambi, D. D., 1965: *The Culture and Civilisation of Ancient India in Historical Outline.* London, Routledge and Kegan Paul (repr. 1970).

Lindblom, G., 1920: *The Akamba in British East Africa.* Uppsala, Appelbergs (Arch. d'Etudes Orientales, J. A. Lundell, ed.; vol. 17).

Lint, J. G. de, 1927: The Treatment of the Wounds of the Abdomen in Ancient Times. Ann. Med. Hist. *9*, 403–407.

Littré. See Hippocrates. Abbr. LTT.

Lu Gwei-Djen and Needham, J., 1967: Records of Diseases in Ancient China. Ch. 17 in *Diseases in Antiquity*, D. Brothwell and A. T. Sandison, eds. Springfield, Ill., C C Thomas (pp. 222–237).

Manu: *The Laws of Manu.* Trans. G. Bühler. Vol. 25 in *The Sacred Books of the East*, F. Max Müller, ed. Oxford, Clarendon.

McCrindle, J. W., 1885: *Ancient India as Described by Ptolemy.* Calcutta, Thacker, Spink & Co.; London, Trübner & Co.; Bombay, Education Society's Press.

————, 1887: *Ancient India as Described by Megasthenes and Arrian . . .* Calcutta, Thacker, Spink & Co.

————, 1901: *Ancient India as Described in Classical Literature; Being a Collection of Greek and Latin Texts Relating to India . . .* Westminster, Constable. [The last of 6 works collecting Greek and Latin texts related to India.]

McDowell, F., 1969: Ancient Ear-Lobe and Rhinoplastic Operations in India. (From the Sushruta Samhita, c. 800 B.C. Translated from the Sanskrit and published by K. K. L. Bhishagratna, Calcutta, 1907). Plastic and Reconstructive Surgery *43*, No. 5, 515–522.

Megasthenes. See McCrindle 1887.

Menninger, K., 1969: *Number Words and Symbols. A Cultural History of Numbers.* Cambridge, Mass., M.I.T. Press.

Merker, M., 1904: *Die Masai.* Ethnographische Monographie eines ostafrikanisches Semitenvolkes. Berlin, Reimer.

Minton, S. A., and Minton, M. R., 1969: *Venomous Reptiles.* New York, Scribner.

Monier-Williams, M., 1899: *A Sanskrit-English dictionary.* Oxford, Clarendon.

Müller, R. F. G., 1951: *Grundsätze altindischer Medizin.* Copenhagen, Munskgaard.

Mukhopadhyaya, G., 1913: *The Surgical Instruments of the Hindus. A Comparative*

Study of the Surgical Instruments of the Greek, Roman, Arab and the Modern European Surgeons. Calcutta, Calcutta University Press (2 vols.).

Navmed. See U.S. Government.

Needham, J., 1965– : *Science and Civilisation in China*. Cambridge, Cambridge University Press. Abbr. NEED.

Neuburger, M., 1910: *History of Medicine*. Trans. E. Playfair. London, Frowde (2 vols.). [Vol. 1 pp. 43–60 is a good summary of ancient Hindu medicine.]

Paré, A., 1564: *Dix Livres De Chirurgie Avec Le Magasin des Instrumens necessaires à icelle*. Paris, le Royer. (repr. 1964, Cercle du Livre Précieux, Paris, C. Tchou).

Pelt, J. -M., 1971: *Drogues et Plantes Magiques*. Strasbourg, Horizons de France. [Beautifully illustrated.]

Plutarch: *Lives: Alexander*. Trans. B. Perrin. Loeb Classical Library, Cambridge, Mass., Harvard University Press and London, Heinemann (Vol. VII of 11).

Raignier, A., 1960: Les Doryles africains. In Parcs nationaux (Belgium). Bull. trimestr. de l'A.S.B.L. Ardenne et Gaume 15, 3–19.

Rawlinson, H. G., 1916: *Intercourse between India and the Western World, From the Earliest Times to the Fall of Rome*. Cambridge, Cambridge University Press.

Rây, P., and Gupta, H. N., 1965: *Caraka Samhitā. A Scientific Synopsis*. New Delhi, Nat. Inst. of Sciences of India.

Read, B., 1926: Gleanings from Old Chinese Medicine. Ann. Med. Hist. 8, 16–19.

Reddy, D. V. S.,.1938: The Art of Surgery in Ancient Indian Sculptures. Bull. Hist. Med. 6, 81–87.

Reid, H. A., 1968: Symptomatology, Pathology, and Treatment of Land Snake Bite in India and Southeast Asia. Ch. 20 in *Venomous Animals and their Venoms*, W. Bücherl, E. Buckley and V. Deulofeu, eds. New York and London, Acad. Press (Vol. I, pp. 611–642).

Renou, L., 1946: Sushruta. In *Littérature sanskrite* (Glossaires de l'Hindouisme, fascicule V). Paris, A. Maisonneuve and Neuchâtel, Delachaux et Niestle.

————, 1957: *Vedic India*. Trans. P. Spratt. Calcutta, Susil Gupta.

Renou, L., and Filliozat, J., 1953: *L'Inde Classique. Manuel des Etudes Indiennes*. Paris, Imprimerie Nationale, Hanoi, Ecole Française d'Extrême-Orient (2 vols.).

Rig-Veda. See Wilson 1850–1866.

Schlitter, E., and others, 1954: Chemistry of *Rauwolfia* Alkaloids Including Reserpine. Ann. N.Y. Acad. Sci. 59, 1–7.

Schlumberger, D., Robert, L., Dupont-Sommer, A., and Benveniste, E., 1958: Une bilingue gréco-araméenne d' Asoka. J. Asiat. 246, 1–48.

Schoff, W. H., 1912: *The Periplus of the Erythraean Sea. Travel and Trade in the Indian Ocean by a Merchant of the First Century*. Trans. from the Greek . . . London, Bombay and Calcutta, Longmans, Green and Co.

Schröder, L. von, 1884: *Pythagoras und die Inder*. Eine Untersuchung über Herkunft und Abstammung der Pythagoreischen Lehren. Leipzig, Otto Schulze.

Schulberg, L. (and eds. of Time-Life), 1968: *L'Inde Classique*. (Coll. "Les Grandes Epoques de l'Homme"). Time Inc.

Senart, E., 1896: *Les castes dans l'Inde. Les faits et le système*. Paris, Leroux.

Sharma, P. V., 1972: *Indian Medicine in the Classical Age*. Chowkhamba Sanskrit Studies 85. Varanasi, India.

Singhal, G. D., and Gaur, D. S., 1963: *Surgical Ethics in Ayurveda*. The Chowkhamba Sanskrit Studies Vol. 60. Varanasi, India.

Smith, V. A., 1901: *Asoka, the Buddhist emperor of India*. Oxford, Clarendon.

————, 1920: *The Oxford History of India. From the Earliest Times to the End of 1911*. Oxford, Clarendon.

Sushruta Samhita. Trans. by K. L. Bhishagratna. Chowkhamba Sanskrit Series Office, Varanasi, India (1907–1911; repr. 1963; 3 vols.). [Handy edition, with notes, glossaries, and indexes; see notes 98, 280.] Abbr. SS.

Tarn, W. W., 1938: *The Greeks in Bactria and India*. Cambridge, Cambridge University Press.

Tennent, J. E., 1860: *Ceylon. An Account of the Island, Physical, Historical and Topographical* . . . London, Longman, Green, Longman and Roberts (vol. I; 4th ed.; 2 vols.).

Topoff, H. R., 1972: The Social Behavior of Army Ants. Scient. American 227, 71–79.

U. S. Govt. Printing Office, 1966: *Poisonous Snakes of the World. A Manual for Use by U. S. Amphibious Forces.* Washington, D.C. Navmed P-5099.

Vakil, R. J., 1961: *The Romance of Healing and Other Essays.* Bombay, Calcutta, New Delhi, Madras, London, and New York, Asia Publishing House.

Veda. See *Rig Veda; Atharva Veda.*

Veith, I., 1961: The Surgical Achievements of Ancient India. Surgery 49, 564–568.

Vogel, C., 1965: *Vāgbhata's Aṣṭāṅgahrdayasaṃhitā. The First Five Chapters of its Tibetan Version. Edited and Rendered into English Along with the Original Sanskrit.* Wiesbaden, Steiner (Abhandlungen f. die Kunde des Morgenlandes 37, 2). [For complete German translation see W. Kirfel and L. Hilgenberg, Leiden, 1937–1941.]

Vogel, J. P., 1926: *Indian Serpent-Lore or the Nāgas in Hindu Legend and Art.* London, Probsthain.

Wheeler, W. M., 1910: *Ants, Their Structure and Behavior.* New York, Columbia University Press (repr. 1960).

Whitney, W. D., 1962: *Atharva-Veda Saṁhitā, Translated with a Critical and Exegetical Commentary.* Delhi, Patna, Varanasi, Motilal Banarsidass (reprint of the American edition; 2 vols.). Abbr. AV.

Wilson, H. H., 1850–1866: *Rig-Veda Sanhitá . . . Trans. from the Sanskrit.* London, W. H. Allen (4 vols.).

Yazdānī, G., 1930–1955: *Ajanta. The Colour and Monochrome Reproductions of the Ajanta Frescoes . . .* London, Oxford University Press (4 vols.).

Zimmer, H. R., 1948: *Hindu Medicine. Edited with a Foreword and Preface by L. Edelstein.* Baltimore, Johns Hopkins Press.

8. Alexandria the Great

Aleotti D'Argenta, G. B., 1589: *Gli Artifitiosi et Curiosi Moti Spiritali Di Herrone.* Ferrara, Baldini.

Amman, J. C., 1709: *Caelii Aureliani Siccensis de Morbis Acutis & Chronicis Libri VIII.* Amstelaedami, Ex Officina Wetsteniana.

Anonymus Londinensis [Papyrus]. See W. H. S. Jones 1947.

Bell, H. I., 1948: *Egypt from Alexander the Great to the Arab Conquest.* Oxford, Clarendon.

Bernand, A., 1966: *Alexandrie la Grande.* Paris, Arthaud.

Blancard, S., 1697: *The Physical Dictionary. Wherein the Terms of Anatomy, the Names and Causes of Diseases, Chyrurgical Instruments and their Use; are accurately Describ'd,* etc. London, Crouch.

Buess, H., 1946: Die Injektion. Ciba Zeitschrift 100, 3594–3648.

Bushnell, G. H., 1928: The Alexandrian Library. Antiquity 2, 196–204.

Caelius Aurelianus. See Amman 1709.

Commandino, F., 1575: *Heronis Alexandrini Spiritalium liber. A Federico Commandino . . . ex Graeco, nuper in Latinum conversus.* Urbini.

David, M., and Groningen, B. A. van, 1952: *Papyrological Primer.* Leyden, Brill.

Dobson, J. F., 1927: Erasistratus. Proc. Roy. Soc. Med. 20, 825–832.

Drachmann, A. G., 1948: *Ktesibios, Philon and Heron. A Study in Ancient Pneumatics.* Copenhagen, Munskgaard, 1948 (repr. 1968, Amsterdam, Swets and Zeitlinger).

———, 1963: The Mechanical Technology of Greek and Roman Antiquity. Acta Historica Scientiarum Naturalium et Medicinalium Vol. 17. Bibliotheca Universitatis Hauniensis, Munksgaard.

———, 1967: *Grosse Griechische Erfinder.* Zürich, Switzerland, Artemis.

Eco, U., and Zorzoli, G. B., 1963: *The Picture History of Inventions - From Plough to Polaris.* New York, Macmillan.

Fåhraeus, 1957: Empty Arteries. 15th Internat. Congress on the History of Medicine (cited by Harris 1973 p. 93).

Fayûm Papyri. See Grenfell, Hunt and Hogarth 1900.

Finlayson, J., 1893: Herophilus and Erasistratus. The Glasgow Medical Journal *39*, 321–352.

Fuchs, R., 1892: *Erasistratea quae in librorum memoria latent congesta enarrantur. Dissertatio inauguralis philologica . . .* Lipsiae, Fock.

Galen. See Kühn.

Grenfell, B. P., and Hunt, A. S., 1898: The *Oxyrhyncus Papyri.* London, Egypt Exploration Fund; Kegan Paul, Trench, Trübner (Part I).

———, 1906: *The Hibeh Papyri.* London, Egypt Exploration Fund; Kegan Paul, Trench, Trübner (Part I).

Grenfell, B. P., Hunt, A. S., and Hogarth, D. G., 1900: *Fayûm Towns and their Papyri.* London, Egypt Exploration Fund; Kegan Paul, Trench, Trübner.

Hall, M. B., 1971: *The Pneumatics of Hero of Alexandria. A facsimile of the 1851 Woodcroft edition.* London, McDonald, and New York, Am. Elsevier.

Harris, C. R. S., 1973: *The Heart and the Vascular System in Ancient Greek Medicine from Alcmaeon to Galen.* Oxford, Clarendon.

Harrison, T. R., 1966: *Principles of Internal Medicine.* New York, McGraw-Hill (5th ed.).

Heron of Alexandria. See Aleotti 1589; Commandino 1575; Schmidt 1899; Woodcroft 1851.

Hibeh Papyri. See Grenfell and Hunt 1906.

Howard-Jones, N., 1949: The Origins and Early Development of Hypodermic Medication. J. Hist. Med. ii, 201–249.

Hurlbutt, F. R., Jr., 1939: *Perì Kardíes. A Treatise on the Heart from the Hippocratic Corpus: Introduction and Translation.* Bull. Hist. Med. 8, 1104–1113.

Jones, W. H. S., 1947: *The Medical Writings of Anonymus Londinensis.* Cambridge, Cambridge University Press.

Jones, D. E. H., 1971: The Great Museum at Alexandria: Its Ascent to Glory. The Smithsonian Magazine, Dec. 1971, pp. 53–60.

———, 1972: A Final Creative Gasp and then the Museum Fell. The Smithsonian Magazine, Jan. 1972, pp. 59–63.

Kenyon, F. G., 1893: *Greek Papyri in the British Museum.* London, British Museum and Longmans.

Kühn, C. G., 1821–1833: *Claudii Galeni Opera Omnia.* Lipsiae, Cnoblochii (22 vols.). Abbr. K.

Liddell, H. G., and Scott, R., 1968: *A Greek-English Lexicon.* Oxford, Clarendon. Abbr. LS.

Littré, E., 1839–1861: *Oeuvres complètes d'Hippocrate, traduction nouvelle avec le texte grec en regard . . .* Paris, Baillière (10 vols.). Abbr. LTT.

Lonie, I. M., 1973: The Paradoxical Text "On the Heart." Med. Hist. *17.* Part I, 1–15; Part II, 136–153.

Macht, D. I., 1916: The History of Intravenous and Subcutaneous Administration of Drugs. J. Amer. Med. Ass. 66, 856–860.

Mahaffy, J. P., 1893: *On the Flinders Petrie Papyri.* "Cunningham Memoirs" No. XI. With Eighteen Autotypes. Dublin, Academy House (Part II).

Mahaffy, J. P., and Smyly, J. G., 1905: *The Flinders Petrie Papyri, with Transcriptions, Commentaries and Index.* Dublin, Academy House.

Malgaigne, J. F., 1840: *Oeuvres complètes d' Ambroise Paré.* Paris, Baillière.

Michler, M., 1968: *Die Alexandrinischen Chirurgen. Eine Sammlung und Auswertung ihrer Fragmente.* Wiesbaden, Steiner Verlag GmbH.

———, 1969: *Das Spezialisierungsproblem und die antike Chirurgie.* Bern, Stuttgart, and Vienna, Huber.

Milne, J. S., 1907: *Surgical Instruments of Greek and Roman Times.* Doctoral thesis, University of Aberdeen. [A classic work.]

Morgan. See Vitruvius.

Needham, J., 1965– : *Science and Civilisation in China.* Cambridge, Cambridge University Press. Abbr. NEED.

Ogg, O., 1940: *An Alphabet Sourcebook.* New York and London, Harper.

Oxyrhyncus Papyri. See Grenfell and Hunt 1898.

Bibliography

Papyri. See *Fayûm, Oxyrhyncus, Petrie, Hibeh;* Kenyon 1893.

Paré, A., 1678: *The Works of that Famous Chirurgeon Ambrose Parey, Translated out of latin, and compared with the French . . . by T. Johnson . . .* London, Clark.

Parsons, E. A., 1952: *The Alexandrian Library.* New York, Am. Elsevier (repr. 1967).

Petrie Papyri. See Mahaffy 1893; Mahaffy and Smyly 1905.

Phillips, E. D., 1973: *Greek Medicine.* London, Thames and Hudson.

Picard, C., 1952: Quelques représentations nouvelles du Phare d'Alexandrie. Bull. Corr. Hell. 78, 61–95.

Pliny [The Elder]: *Natural History.* Trans. H. Rackham, W. H. S. Jones, and D. E. Eichholz. Loeb Classical Library, Cambridge Mass., Harvard University Press and London, Heinemann (1956–1966; 10 vols.). Abbr. PNH.

Plutarch: *Lives. Demosthenes and Cicero. Alexander and Caesar.* Trans. B. Perrin. Vol. VII of *Plutarch's Lives.* Loeb Classical Library, Cambridge, Mass., Harvard University Press and London, Heinemann (1919; repr. 1967; 11 vols.).

Préaux, C., 1939: *L'économie royale des Lagides.* Brussels, Edition de la Fond. Egyptologique Reine Elisabeth.

Rostovtzeff, M., 1941: *The Social and Economic History of the Hellenistic World.* Oxford, Clarendon (vol. III).

Sarton, G., 1927: *Introduction to the History of Science.* Baltimore, Williams and Wilkins (vol. I).

Schmidt, W., 1899(a): *Herons von Alexandria Druckwerke und Automatentheater.* Griechisch und Deutsch herausgegeben. Leipzig, Teubner.

———, 1899(b): *Heron von Alexandria.* Repr. from Neue Jahrbücher f. das klassische Altertum, Geschichte, u. Deutsche Literatur. Leipzig, Teubner.

Siegel, R. E., 1968: *Galen's System of Physiology and Medicine.* Basel and New York, Karger.

Singer, C., 1957: *A Short History of Anatomy and Physiology from the Greeks to Harvey (The Evolution of Anatomy).* New York, Dover.

Sprengel, K., 1815: *Histoire de la médecine, depuis son origine jusqu'au dix-neuvième siècle, . . . traduite de l'allemand.* Paris, Deterville (vol. I).

Sudhoff, K., 1909: *Ärztliches aus griechischen Papyrus-Urkunden: Bausteine zu einer medizinischen Kulturgeschichte des Hellenismus.* Leipzig, Barth. [A precious collection of texts, grouped by subject—law, sex, crime, etc.—with useful comments.]

Tarn, W. W., 1948: *Alexander the Great. II: Source and Studies.* Cambridge, Cambridge University Press.

Thiersch, H., 1909: *Pharos, antike Islam und Occident.* Leipzig and Berlin, Teubner.

Vitruvius: *The Ten Books on Architecture. With Illustrations and Original Designs.* Trans. M. H. Morgan. Cambridge, Mass., Harvard University Press (1914).

———, *De architectura.* Trans. F. Granger. Loeb Classical Library, Cambridge, Mass., Harvard University Press and London, Heinemann (1931–1934; repr. 1970; 2 vols.).

Wellmann, M., 1907: *Erasistratos.* In *Pauly's Realencyclopädie,* Stuttgart, Metzler, Band 11, col. 333–350.

Wilcken, U., 1899: *Griechische Ostraka aus Ägypten und Nubien.* Leipzig and Berlin, Giesecke and Devrient (2 vols.).

———, 1932: *Alexander the Great.* Trans. G. C. Richards. London, Chatto and Windus.

Wilson, L. G., 1959: Erasistratus, Galen and the pneuma. Bull. Hist. Med. 33, 293–314.

Woodcroft, B., 1851: *The Pneumatics of Hero of Alexandria.* See Hall 1971.

9. The Medicus

Allbutt, T. C., 1921: *Greek Medicine in Rome: The Fitzpatrick Lectures on the History of Medicine Delivered at the Royal College of Physicians of London in 1909–1910.* London, Macmillan. (Also printed in The Lancet, 1909, 1565–1578; 1910, 1325–1332, 1395–1409). [Outdated as regards archaeology, but still fundamental.]

Anon., 1900?: *Bäder von Baden bei Zürich. Ein römischer Militärspital*. Zürich, Polygraphisches Institut A.-G. [A well-compiled pamphlet, unsigned, undated; it is now uncertain that this was a military hospital.]

Anon., 1971: Lead in the Wines of Antiquity. Bull. Hist. Med. 45, 493.

Asclepiades. See Green 1955.

Auboyer, J., 1961: *La vie quotidienne dans l'Inde ancienne (environ IIᵉ s. avant J.-C.—VIIᵉ s.)*. Paris, Hachette.

Baatz, D., 1970(a): Krankenhäuser bei den Römern. Kurz und Gut 4, 8–10.

———, 1970(b): *Die Saalburg, Ein Führer durch das römische Kastell und seine Geschichte*. Saalburg-Kastell über Bad Homburg v. d. H., Saalburgmuseum (2nd ed.).

Bailey, K. C., 1929: *The Elder Pliny's Chapters on Chemical Subjects*. London, Arnold (2 vols.).

Ball, G. V., 1971: Two Epidemics of Gout. Bull. Hist. Med. 45, 401–408.

Becker, R. O., Spadaro, J. A., and Berg, E. W., 1968: The Trace Elements of Human Bone. J. Bone & Joint Surg. 50-A, 326–334.

Beek, G. W. van, 1960: Frankincense and Myrrh. The Biblical Archaeologist 33, 70–95.

Benveniste, E., 1945: La doctrine médicale des Indo-Européens. Rev. de l'Hist. des Religions 130, 5–12.

Bessone, L., 1969: Sulla morte di Plinio il Vecchio. Rivista di Studi Classici 17, 166–179.

Biot, E., 1851: *Le Tcheou-Li ou Rites des Tcheou, traduit pour la première fois du Chinois . . .* Paris, Impr. Nat. (3 vols.; also phot. reprint by Ch'eng Wen Publ. Co., Taipei, 1969).

Blinkenberg, C., 1926: *Fibules grecques et orientales*. Det Kgl. Danske Videnskabernes Selskab. Historisk-filologiske Meddelelser 13, 1. Copenhagen, Høst.

Bosanquet, R. C., 1904: Excavations on the Line of the Roman Wall in Northumberland. The Roman Camp at Housesteads. Archaeol. Aeliana (Second Ser.) 25, 193–300.

Briau, R., 1866: *Du service de santé militaire chez les Romains*. Paris, Masson.

———, 1869: *L'assistance médicale chez les Romains*. Paris, Masson.

———, 1877: *L'archiatrie romaine, ou la médecine officielle dans l'empire romain*. Paris, Masson.

Cagnat, R., 1909: *Les deux camps de la légion IIIᵉ Auguste à Lambèse d'après les fouilles récentes*. Mém. de l'Inst. Nat. de France, Acad. des Inscript. et Belles-Lettres 38, 1. Paris, Impr. Nat.

———, 1913: *L'armée Romaine d'Afrique et l'occupation militaire de l'Afrique sous les Empereurs*. Paris, Impr. Nat.

Casal, J. M., 1950: Fouilles de Virampatnam-Arikamedu. C. R. Acad. des Inscript. et Belles-Lettres, 142–147.

Castelli, B., 1682: *Castellus renovatus, hoc est, Lexicon Medicum . . .* Norimbergae, J. D. Tauberi . . . [One of many editions of this classic medical dictionary.]

Castiglioni, A., 1936: *Storia della Medicina*. Milan, Mondadori.

Catling, H. W., 1964: *Cypriot Bronzework in the Mycenaean World*. Oxford, Clarendon.

Cato: *On Agriculture*. In Cato and Varro, *De re rustica*. Trans. W. D. Hooper and H. B. Ash. Loeb Classical Library, Cambridge, Mass., Harvard University Press and London, Heinemann (1934; repr. 1967; 1 vol.).

Celsus: *De medicina*. Trans. W. G. Spencer. Loeb Classical Library, Cambridge, Mass., Harvard University Press and London, Heinemann (1935–1938; 3 vols.). Abbr. CDM.

Charaka Samhita. Trans. A. C. Kaviratna. Calcutta (pub. by the trans., 1912; 2 vols.). Abbr. ChS.

Chen, K. K., and Schmidt, C. F., 1930: Ephedrine and Related Substances. Medicine (Baltimore) 9, 1–117.

Chiappelli, A., 1881: *Le condizioni dell'esercizio medico nell'antica Roma*. Pistoia, Frat. Bracali.

Codex Iustinianus. See Mommsen and Krueger 1954.

Cohn-Haft, L., 1956: *The Public Physicians of Ancient Greece.* Smith College Studies in History 42.

Collingwood, R. G., and Richmond, I., 1969: *The Archaeology of Roman Britain.* London, Methuen.

Columella: *De re rustica.* Trans. H. B. Ash, E. S. Forster, and E. Heffner. Loeb Classical Library, Cambridge, Mass., Harvard University Press and London, Heinemann (1941–1955, 3 vols.).

Como, J., 1925: Das Grab eines römischen Arztes in Bingen. Germania 9, 152–162.

Corpus Iuris Civilis. See Mommsen and Krueger 1954.

Coturri, E., 1959: *Claudio Galeno: De theriaca ad Pisonem.* Florence, Olschki [Latin text with Italian translation.]

Crişan, I. H., 1957: O Trusă Medicală Descoperită la Grădiştea Muncelului. *In* Istoria Medicinei. Studii şi Cercetări. Bucuresti, Editura Medicală (in Rumanian; pp. 45–56).

Daniels, C., 1968: A Hoard of Iron and Other Materials from Corbridge. Archaeol. Aeliana (Fourth Ser.) 46, 115–126.

Daremberg, C., 1847: Etudes sur quelques points de la chirurgie de Celse, à l'occasion de la nouvelle édition de M. le Docteur des Etangs. Gaz. méd. Paris 2, 104–106.

Davies, R. W., 1969: The Medici of the Roman Armed Forces. Epigraphische Studien, Düsseldorf, Rheinland-Verlag 8, 83–99.

———, 1970(a): Some Roman Medicine, Medical History 14, 101–106.

———, 1970(b): A Note on the Hoard of Roman Equipment Buried at Corbridge. Durham Univ. Journal (New Series) 31, 177–180.

———, 1970(c): Review of J. Scarborough, "Roman Medicine." J. Roman Studies 60, 224–225.

———, 1970(d): The Roman Military Medical Service. Saalburg Jahrbuch (Bericht des Saalburg Museums) 27, 84–104. Berlin, de Gruyter.

———, 1971: Medicine in Ancient Rome. History Today 21, 770–778.

———, 1972: Some More Military Medici. Epigraphische Studien, Düsseldorf, Rheinland-Verlag 9, 1–11.

———, 1974: Medicus Duplicarius. Orvostörténeti Közlemények–Communicationes de Historia Artis Medicinae, Budapest, vols. 73–74.

Dechelette, J., 1910: *Manuel d'archéologie préhistorique celtique et gallo-romaine.* II: *Archéologie celtique ou protohistorique.* Paris, Picard.

Deneffe, V., 1896: *Les oculistes gallo-romains au IIIe siècle.* Anvers, Caals; Paris, Baillière; Leipzig, Hedeler.

De Pasquale, A., 1965: Le Efedre di Sicilia. I: Ricerche farmacognostiche sulla "Ephedra altissima" Desf. Lavori dell' Istituto di Farmacognosia dell'Università di Messina, vol. III.

D'Erce, 1969: La mort de Germanicus et les poisons de Caligula. Janus 56, 123–148.

Deringer, H., 1954: Die medizinischen Instrumente des Ennser Museums. Forschungen in Lauriacum. Bd. 2, 144–155. Linz, Jenny, Vetters, Kloiber.

Dioscorides. See Gunther 1934.

Dollfus, M.-A., 1958: Les instruments d'ophtalmologie chez les galloromains. Arch. Ophtalmologie 18, 633–651.

———, 1964: Nos confrères, les ophtalmologistes gallo-romains. Bull. Soc. Ophtalmol. de France 11, 1–12.

———, 1966: L'étonnante instrumentation des ophtalmologistes gallo-romains. Archeologia 10, 16–19.

Drabkin, I. E., 1944: On Medical Education in Greece and Rome. Bull. Hist. Med. 15, 333–351.

Du Chaliot, C., 1943: Studi per la valorizzazione della flora medica sarda. Nota III. Sulla possibilità di usare con vantaggio, nella terapia dell' asma bronchiale, le efedre sarde (*Ephedra vulgaris Rich.–Ephedra nebrodensis Tin.*). Riforma Medica 6, 1–8.

Duke-Elder, S., 1969: *System of Ophthalmology.* London, Kimpton (vol. XI).

Edelstein, E. J., and Edelstein, L. E., 1945: *Asclepius. A Collection and Interpretation of the Testimonies.* Baltimore, Johns Hopkins Press (2 vols.).

Elias, S., and Chvapil, M., 1973: Zinc and Wound Healing in Normal and Chronically Ill Rats. J. Surg. Res. *15*, 59–66.

Elliot, R. H., 1918: *The Indian Operation of Couching for Cataract (Incorporating the Hunterian Lectures Delivered . . . 1917).* New York, Hoeber.

Ernout, A., and Meillet, A., 1959: *Dictionnaire étymologique de la langue latine. (Histoire des mots).* Paris, Klincksieck (4th ed.).

Fellmann, R., 1958: *Die Principia des Legionslagers Vindonissa und das Zentralgebäude der römischen Lager und Kastelle.* Brugg (Schweiz), Vindonissamuseum.

Filliozat, J., 1956: Les relations extérieures de l'Inde. I. Pondichéry, Publ. de l'Inst. Franç. d'Indologie No. 2.

Flückiger, F. A., and Hanbury, D., 1879: *Pharmacographia. A History of the Principal Drugs of Vegetable Origin Met with in Great Britain and British India.* London, Macmillan. Abbr. FH.

Frölich, H., 1880: Über die Kriegschirurgie der alten Römer. Arch. f. Klin. Chir. *25*, 285–321.

Galen: *Claudii Galeni Opera Omnia.* C. G. Kühn, ed. Lipsiae, Off. Libr. C. Cnoblochii (1821–1833; 22 vols.). Abbr. K.

———, See also Coturri.

Garoglio, P. G., 1959: *La nuova enologia. Trattato di scienza enologica applicata alla tecnologia e all' analisi del vino.* Florence, Istituto di Industrie Agrarie.

Giboin, L., 1949: *Epitomé de botanique et de matière médicale de l'Inde (et spécialement des Etablissements Français de l'Inde).* Doctoral thesis, Marseille (Fac. mixte de Méd. Gén. et Pharmacie).

Gilfillan, S. C., 1965: Lead Poisoning and the Fall of Rome. J. Occupational Med. 7, 53–60.

Glasbergen, W., 1965–66: Het eerste jaartal in de geschiedenis van West-Nederland. Jaarboek der koninklijke Nederlandse Akademie van Wetenschappen, 102–121.

Goffres, 1858: *Précis iconographique de bandages, pansements et appareils.* Paris, Méquignon-Marvis.

Goodman, L. S., and Gilman, A., 1970: *The Pharmacological Basis of Therapeutics.* London and Toronto, Macmillan (4th ed.).

Green, R. M., 1955: *Asclepiades. His Life and Writings.* (A translation of Cocchi's *Life of Asclepiades* and Gumpert's *Fragments of Asclepiades*). New Haven, Licht, and Baltimore, Waverly Press.

Gunther, R. T., 1934: *The Greek Herbal of Dioscorides, Illustrated by a Byzantine* A.D. *512, Englished by John Goodyear* A.D. *1655 . . .* London and New York, Hafner (repr. 1968).

Haberling, W., 1909: Die Militärlazarette im alten Rom. Deutsche Militärärztl. Zeitschr. *11*, 441–467.

———, 1912: Die Entdeckung eines kriegschirurgischen Instrumentes des Altertums. Deutsche Militärärztl. Zeitschr. *17*, 657–660.

Hall, M. B., 1971: *The Pneumatics of Hero of Alexandria* (Facsimile of the 1851 Woodcroft Edition). London, MacDonald, and New York, Am. Elsevier.

Harig, G., 1971: Zum Problem "Krankenhaus" in der Antike. Klio *53*, 179–195.

Harley, G. W., 1941: *Native African Medicine.* Cambridge, Mass., Harvard University Press.

Helmreich. See Scribonius Largus.

Hippocrates. See Littré. Abbr. LTT.

Höfer, F., 1842: *Histoire de la Chimie depuis les temps les plus reculés jusqu'à notre époque.* I. Paris, Hachette (2 vols.).

Hofmann, K. B., 1885: *Das Blei bei den Völkern des Alterthums.* Berlin, Habel.

Hogg, A. H. A., 1968: Pen Llystyn: A Roman Fort and Other Remains. The Archaeol. Journal *125*, 101–192.

Imbesi, A., 1964: *Index plantarum quae in omnium populorum pharmacopoeis sunt adhuc receptae* [index of plants that have been accepted, to this date, in the pharmacopoeae of all countries]. Messina, Italy.

Inscriptiones Graecae. Consilio et auctoritate Acad. Litt. Reg. Borussicae ed. A. Kirchhoff. Berolini, apud Georgium Reimerum, 1873–.

Iustinianus, Codex. See Mommsen and Krueger 1954.

Jaworowski, Z., 1967: *Stable and Radioactive Lead in Environment and Human Body*. Warsaw, Nuclear Energy Information Center.

Jeanselme, 1921: L'emploi des sels de cuivre dans le traitement des plaies remonte à la plus haute antiquité. Bull. Soc. Fr. Hist. Méd. *15*, 105–106.

Jerome, St.: *Select Letters of St. Jerome*. Trans. F. A. Wright. Loeb Classical Library, London, Heinemann, and New York, Putnam's Sons (1933).

Jetter, D., 1966: Geschichte des Hospitals. Sudhoffs Arch., Suppl. 5.

Kleine Pauly. See Pauly.

Knörzer, K.-H., 1963: Römerzeitliche Heilkräuter aus Novaesium (Neuss/Rh.). Sudhoffs Arch. *47*, 311–316.

———, 1965: Römerzeitliche Heilkräuter aus Novaesium (Neuss/Rh.). Nachtrag. Sudhoffs Arch. *49*, 416–422.

———, 1970: Römerzeitliche Pflanzenfunde aus Neuss. *Novaesium IV* (Rheinisches Landesmuseum Bonn). Berlin, Mann.

Kobert, R., 1909: Chronische Bleivergiftung im klassischen Altertume. In *Beiträge aus der Geschichte der Chemie, dem Gedächtnis von Georg W. A. Kahlbaum*, Leipzig and Vienna, Deuticke (pp. 103–109).

Kühn. See Galen. Abbr. K.

La Floresta, A., 1940: Studi per la valorizzazione della flora medica sarda. Nota II: Sull'Ephedra vulgaris Rich. e sull'Ephedra nebrodensis Tin. Archivio di Farmacol. Sperim. e Scienze aff. *69*, 41–56.

Lanteaume, M.-T., Ramel, P., Jaulmes, P., and Manin, D., 1969: Détermination et comparaison des DL50 du métabisulfite de potassium de l'éthanal et de leur combinaison (hydroxy-éthane-sulfonate de potassium) par voie orale sur le rat de souche Wistar. Ann. Fals. Exp. Chim. *686*, 231–241.

Liddell, H. G., and Scott, R., 1968: *A Greek-English Lexicon*. Oxford, Clarendon (9th ed.). Abbr. LS.

Liebl, H., 1902: Zum Sanitätswesen im römischen Heere. Wiener Studien *24*, 381–385.

Littman, R. J., and Littman, M. L., 1969: The Athenian Plague: Smallpox. Amer. Philological Assoc. *100*, 261–275.

Littré, E., 1839–1861: *Oeuvres complètes d'Hippocrate*, traduction nouvelle avec le texte grec en regard . . . Paris, Baillière (10 vols.). Abbr. LTT.

Liversidge, J., 1968: *Britain in the Roman Empire*. London, Routledge and Kegan Paul.

Livy. Trans. B. O. Foster and others. Loeb Classical Library, Cambridge, Mass., Harvard University Press and London, Heinemann (1962–1969; 14 vols.).

Lorger, F., 1919: Vorläufiger Bericht über Ausgrabungen nächst Lotschitz bei Cilli. Jahreshefte des österreichischen archäologischen Institutes in Wien *19–20*, Beiblatt, 107–134.

Maiuri, A., 1938: Statuetta eburnea di arte indiana a Pompei. Le Arti I, 111–115.

———, 1964: *Pompei ed Ercolano, fra case e abitanti*. Milan, Martello.

Marcellus Empiricus: *Marcelli de medicamentis liber*. Recensuit M. Niedermann. Corpus Medicorum Latinorum, V. Lipsiae et Berolini, in aed. B. G. Teubneri, 1916.

Margotta, R., 1968: *Histoire illustrée de la médecine*. Paris, Ed. Deux Coqs d'Or.

Martial: *Epigrams*. Trans. W. C. A. Ker. Loeb Classical Library, Cambridge, Mass., Harvard University Press and London, Heinemann (1968, 2 vols.).

Marx, F., 1915: A. Corneli Celsi quae supersunt. In *Corpus Medicorum Latinorum, I*. Leipzig., Teubner.

McDaniel, W. B., 1972: A Sempiternal Superstition: For a Dislocated Joint, a Split Green Reed, and a Latin Charm. Perspectives in Biol. and Med. *15*, 295–306 (partial reprint of a paper in The Classical J. *45*, 1950).

Meyer-Steineg, T., 1912: Chirurgische Instrumente des Altertums. Ein Beitrag zur antiken Akiurgie. Jenaer medizin-hist. Beiträge, Heft I. Jena, Fischer.

Miller, J. I., 1969: *The Spice Trade of the Roman Empire* (29 B.C. to A.D. 641). Oxford, Clarendon.

Milne, J. S., 1907: *Surgical Instruments in Greek and Roman Times*. Oxford, Clarendon. (Also: Doctoral thesis, Aberdeen, 1907.)

Mommsen, T., 1934: *Theodosiani Libri XVI cum Constitutionibus Sirmondianis.* Berolini, apud Weidmannos.

Mommsen, T., and Krueger, P., 1954: *Corpus Iuris Civilis. Editio sexta decima . . .* Berolini, apud Weidmannos (2 vols.).

Mortillet, A. de, 1912: Evolution et classification des fibules. Comptes Rend. Ass. Franç. pour l' Avancem. des Sci. (Mém. hors volume, Congrès de Nîmes), 1–27.

Needham, J., 1965– : *Science and Civilisation in China.* Cambridge, Cambridge University Press. Abbr. NEED.

Neumann, A., 1950: *Die Römischen Ruinen unter dem Hohen Markt.* Vienna, Verlag für Jugend und Volk.

——, 1965: Spital und Bad des Legionslagers Vindobona. Jahrbuch des Römisch-Germanischen Zentralmuseums Mainz *12*, 99–126. (publ. in 1967).

Nissen, H., Könen, C., Lehner, H., and Strack, M. L., 1904: *Novaesium.* Bonner Jahrb. *111/112.*

Nutton, V., 1969: Medicine and the Roman Army: A Further Reconsideration. Medical History 13 (3), 260–270.

Olivier, E., 1944: Cachets d'oculistes, ou cachets à collyres? A propos du cachet de Q. Postumius Hermes. In *Mélanges d'histoire et de littérature offerts à Monsieur Charles Gilliard á l'occasion de son 65ᵉ anniversaire.* Lausanne, Librairie de l'Université (pp. 73–81).

Ovid: *Tristia. Ex Ponto.* Trans. A. L. Wheeler. Loeb Classical Library, Cambridge, Mass., Harvard University Press and London, Heinemann (1924; repr. 1965).

Oxé, A., 1941: Von römischen Augenärzten. Germania 25, 23–30.

Paré, A., 1678: *The Works of that Famous Chirurgeon Ambrose Parey, Trans. out of Latin, and compared with the French,* By T. Johnson . . . London, Clark.

Paribeni, R., 1926–27: *Optimus Princeps. Saggio sulla Storia le sui Tempi dell'Imperatore Traiano.* Messina, Principato (vol. I).

Paulus Aegineta: *The Seven Books of Paulus Aegineta, Translated from the Greek with a Commentary. Embracing a Complete View of the Knowledge Possessed by the Greeks, Romans and Arabians on All Subjects Connected with Medicine and Surgery.* Trans. F. Adams. London, The Sydenham Society (1844–1847; 3 vols.) [Contains precious notes just as the title promises].

Pauly, 1964– : *Der Kleine. Lexikon der Antike . . .* K. Ziegler, ed. Stuttgart, Druckenmüller [a condensed version of Pauly's *Realencyclopädie*; 4 vols. up to 1972].

Pauly's Real-Encyclopädie der Classischen Altertumswissenschaft. G. Wissowa, ed. Stuttgart, Metzler; Munich, Druckenmüller, 1894–.

Pazzini, A., 1967: A. C. Celso visto da Caio Plinio Secondo e dal mondo culturale romano. Riv. di Storia della Medicina, anno XI, 2, 155–166.

——, 1971: Ancora sulla possibilità o meno di autopsie umane in Roma antica. Riv. di Storia della Med. *15*, 131–150.

Petrikovits, H. von, 1960: Das römische Rheinland. Archäologische Forschungen seit 1945. In *Arbeitsgemeinschaft f. Forsch. des Landes Nordrhein-Westfalen*, Heft 86, Cologne and Opladen, Westdeutscher (pp. 5–175; 17 tables).

——, 1970: Die Spezialgebäude Römischer Legionslager. In *Legio VII Gemina* (Colóquio Internaciónal de Romanistas, Ciudád de León, Sept. 16–21, 1968), pp. 229–252.

Phillips, E. D., 1973: *Greek Medicine.* London, Thames and Hudson.

Plautus: *Menaechmi.* In *Plautus.* Trans. P. Nixon. Loeb Classical Library, Cambridge, Mass., Harvard Univ. Press, and London, Heinemann (1917; repr. 1965; 5 vols.).

Pliny [The Elder]: *Natural History.* Trans. H. Rackham, W. H. S. Jones and D. E. Eichholz. Loeb Classical Library, Cambridge, Mass., Harvard University Press and London, Heinemann (1956–1966; 10 vols.). Abbr. PNH.

Pliny [The Younger]: *Letters and Panegyricus.* Trans. B. Radice. Loeb Classical Library, Cambridge Mass., Harvard University Press and London, Heinemann (1969; 2 vols.).

——, *Plinii Secundi de medicina libri tres. Nunc primum editi a V. Rose.* Lipsiae, in aed. B. G. Teubneri (1875). [Latin text only.]

Pories, W. J., Henzel, J. H., Rob, C. G., and Strain, W. H., 1967: Acceleration of Healing with Zinc Sulfate. Ann. Surg. 165, 432-436.

Realencyclopädie. See *Pauly's.*

Ramel, P., Lanteaume, M. -T., Jaulmes, P., and Bodin, G., 1971: Comparaison des effets physiologiques à long terme sur le rat Wistar de l'acide sulfureux libre ou combiné à l'acétaldehyde. Action sur la thiamine apportée par le régime. Ann. Fals. Exp. Chim. 693, 38–47.

Rawlinson, H. G., 1916: *Intercourse Between India and the Western World from the Earliest Times to the Fall of Rome.* Cambridge, Cambridge University Press.

Râ

y, P., and Gupta, H. N., 1965: *Caraka Saṃhitā (A Scientific Synopsis).* New Delhi, Nat. Institute of Sciences of India.

Reallexikon der Vorgeschichte. Berlin, 1925.

Renou, L., and Filliozat, J., 1953: *L'Inde Classique,* Paris, Impr. Nat.

Richmond, I. A., 1968: *Hod Hill. Excavations Carried Out between 1951 and 1958 for the Trustees of the British Museum.* London, The Trustees of the British Museum (vol. II).

Richmond, I. A., and Gillam, J. P., 1952: Further Exploration of the Antonine Fort at Corbridge. Archaeol. Aeliana (Fourth Ser.) 30, 239–266.

Richmond, I. A., and McIntyre, J., 1939: The Agricolan Fort at Fendoch. Proc. Soc. of Antiquaries of Scotland 73, 110–154.

Richmond, I. A., and St. Joseph, J. K., 1957 and 1961: [On the legionary fortress at Inchtuthil]. J. Roman Studies 47, 198–199; 51, 160.

Roberts, C. H., 1950: An Army Doctor in Alexandria. In *Aus Antike und Orient.* Festschrift Wilhelm Schubart zum 75. Geburtstag. S. Morenz, ed. Leipzig, Harrassowitz.

Rossi, L., 1969: Il corpo sanitario dell'armata romana nel medio Impero. Physis XI, 534-551.

———, 1971: *Trajan's Column and the Dacian Wars.* London, Thames and Hudson.

Sabbadini, R., 1900: Sui codici della medicina di Corn. Celso. Studi ital. filol. class. 8, 1–32.

Sandys, J. E., 1963: *A companion to Latin Studies.* New York and London, Hafner (repr. of 3rd ed., 1935).

Sarton, G. G., 1959: *A History of Science: Hellenistic Science and Culture in the Last Three Centuries* B.C. Cambridge, Mass., Harvard University Press.

Scarborough, J., 1968: Roman Medicine and the Legions: A Reconsideration. Medical History 12, 254–261.

———, 1969: Roman Medicine. London, Thames and Hudson.

———, 1970: Romans and Physicians. The Classical Journal 65, 296–306.

Schefold, K., 1967: *La Grèce classique.* Paris, Albin Michel.

Scherz, G., 1969: *Steno: Geological Papers.* Trans. A. J. Pollock. Odense University Press.

Schoff, W. H., 1912: *The Periplus of the Erythraean Sea. (Travel and Trade In the Indian Ocean by a Merchant of the First Century).* New York, London, Bombay, and Calcutta, Longmans, Green & Co.

Schönberger, H., 1969: The Roman Frontier in Germany: An Archaeological Survey. J. Roman Studies 59, 144–197.

Schönberger, H., and Herrman, F. R., 1971: Das Römerkastell Künzing-Quintana. Jahresber. der Bayerischen Bodendenkmalpflege 8, 37–86.

Schulten, A., 1933: Masada, die Burg des Herodes und die römischen Lager. Zeitschr. des D. Palästina-Vereins 56, 1–185.

Schultze, R., 1934: Die römischen Legionslazarette in Vetera und anderen Legionslagern. Bonner Jahrb. 139, 54–63 (+ separate tables).

Scribonius Largus: *Conpositiones.* Compositions de remèdes, écrites et rassemblées au 1er s., . . . Introduction de G. Helmreich. Leipzig, Teubner (1887).[Latin text only.]

Sédille, A. -M., 1956: *Les ophtalmologistes gallo-romains.* Doctoral thesis. Faculté de médecine, Paris. Rabat, Ecole du Livre.

Bibliography

Senn, N., 1895: Pompeian Surgery and Surgical Instruments. The Medical News, December 28, 1–8.

Simonett, C., 1937: Vindonissa—Valetudinarium und Kasernen. Grabungen der Gesellschaft Pro Vindonissa und des archaeologischen Arbeitsdienstes der Schweiz, 1935-36. Anzeiger für Schweiz. Altertumskunde 39, Heft 2/3.

Simpson, F. G., and Richmond, I. A., 1941: The Roman Fort on Hadrian's Wall at Benwell. Archaeol. Aeliana (Fourth Ser.) 19, 1–43.

Simpson, J. Y., 1854: Notes on Some Ancient Greek Medical Vases for Containing Lykion. Pharm. Journ. xiii, 413–418.

Singer, C., 1924: [Roman] Science. In *The Legacy of Rome.* Bailey, C., ed. Oxford, Clarendon (pp. 265–324).

Sophocles. Trans. F. Storr. Loeb Classical Library, Cambridge, Mass, Harvard University Press and London, Heinemann (1913; repr. 1951; 2 vols.).

Spencer, W. G., 1926: Celsus's *De medicina*—A Learned and Experienced Practitioner upon What the Art of Medicine Could then Accomplish. Proc. Roy. Soc. Med. *XIX*, 129–139.

Stieren, A., 1928: Die neuen Grabungen in Haltern. Germania 11, 70–76.

———, 1930: Die römischen Lager bei Haltern in Westfalen. Neue Deutsche Ausgrabungen, Heft. 23/24, 190–198.

St. Joseph, J. K., 1961: Air Reconnaissance in Britain, 1958–1960. J. Roman Studies 51, 119–135.

Strabo: *Geography.* Trans. H. L. Jones. Loeb Classical Library, Cambridge, Mass., Harvard University Press and London, Heinemann (1966–1970; 8 vols.).

Suetonius. Trans. J. C. Rolfe. Loeb Classical Library, Cambridge, Mass., Harvard University Press and London, Heinemann (2 vols.; 1951 and 1914 repr. 1970).

Sushruta Samhita. An English Translation. Based on Original Sanskrit Text . . . by K. K. Bhishagratna. Chowkhamba Sanskrit Series Office. Varanasi, India (1912; repr. 1963; 3 vols.). Abbr. SS.

Szilágyi, J., 1956: *Aquincum.* Budapest. Verlag der Ungarischen Akademie der Wissenschaften. Berlin, Henschelverlag.

Tabanelli, M., 1958: Lo strumento chirurgico e la sua storia (dalle epoche Greca e Romana al secolo decimosesto). Forlí, Italy, Romagna Medica Ed.

———, 1963: *La medicina nel mondo degli Etruschi.* Florence, Olschki.

Tacitus: *The Histories.* Trans. C. H. Moore. *The Annals.* Trans. J. Jackson. Loeb Classical Library, Cambridge, Harvard University Press, and London, Heinemann (1931–1937, 4 vols.).

Trease, G. E., and Evans, W. C., 1972: *Pharmacognosy.* London, Baillière (10th ed.).

Trisolieri, V. N., 1969: Elenco di interessanti reperti di medicina Etrusca in alcuni musei Italiani inerenti all' epoca. Pagine di Storia della Med. 13, 72–87.

Varro. See Cato.

Vitruvius: *De architectura.* Trans. F. Granger. Loeb Classical Library, Cambridge, Mass., Harvard University Press and London, Heinemann (1931; repr. 1970; 2 vols.).

Vogel, Z., 1963: *Wunderwelt Terrarium.* Leipzig, Jena, and Berlin, Urania Verlag (Melsungen, J. Neumann-Neudamm).

Vulpes, B., 1847: *Illustrazione di tutti gli strumenti chirurgici scavati in Ercolano e in Pompei.* Naples, Stamperia Reale.

Watermann, R., 1970: *Ärztliche Instrumente aus Novaesium.* Cologne, Hang.

Wellmann, M., 1913: A. Cornelius Celsus: Eine Quellenuntersuchung. Philolog. Untersuchungen, Kiessling-Wilamowitz/Möllendorff. Berlin, Weidmann (Heft 23).

Wheeler, R. E. M., 1955: *Rome beyond the Imperial Frontiers.* London, Bell.

Wheeler, R. E. M., Ghosh, A., and Deva, K., 1946: Arikamedu: An Indo-Roman Trading Station on the East Coast of India. Ancient India 2, 17–124.

Winckelmann, G., 1767: *Monumenti Antichi Inediti.* Rome (pub. by author; 2 vols.).

Zereteli, G., and Jernstedt, P., 1930: *Papyri russischer und georgischer Sammlungen* (P. Ross-Georg) Bd. III. Tiflis, Universitätslithographie.

Bibliography

10. Galen—and into the Night

Ackerknecht, E. H., 1970: *Therapie von den Primitiven bis zum 2O. Jahrhundert. Mit einem Anhang: Geschichte der Diät.* Stuttgart, Enke.

——, 1971: The End of Greek Diet. Bull. Hist. Med. 45, 242–249.

Amman. See Caelius Aurelianus

Atiya, A. S., 1968: *A History of Eastern Christianity.* London, Methuen.

Bernhard, J., 1893: *La Thériaque. Etude historique et pharmacologique.* Paris, Baillière.

Briau, R., 1877: *L' Archiatrie romaine, ou la médecine officielle dans l' Empire romain.* Paris, Masson.

Brock. See Galen, *On the Natural Faculties.*

Caelius Aurelianus: *Caelii Aureliani Siccensis de morbis acutis & chronicis libri VIII.* Trans. J. C. Amman. Amstelaedami, Ex Officina Wetsteniana (1709).

Calza, G., 1953: *Scavi di Ostia.* Rome, Libreria dello Stato (vol. I).

Celsus: *De medicina.* Trans. W. G. Spencer. Loeb Classical Library, Cambridge, Mass., Harvard University Press and London, Heinemann (1935–1938; 3 vols.). Abbr. CDM.

Charaka Samhita. Trans. by A. C. Kaviratna. Calcutta (pub. by trans.; 1912; 2 vols.). Abbr. ChS.

Charas, M., 1753: *Pharmacopée Royale et Galénique.* Lyon, Bruyset.

Charles-Picard, G., 1965: *La Carthage de Saint-Augustin.* Paris, Fayard.

Dalton, J. C., 1873: *Galen and Paracelsus.* New York, Appleton.

Daremberg, C., 1854–1856: *Oeuvres anatomiques, physiologiques et médicales de Galien.* Paris, Baillière (2 vols.).

Daremberg, C., and Saglio, E., 1877–1919: *Dictionnaire des antiquités grecques et romaines, d'après les textes et les monuments* . . . Paris, Hachette (11 vols.).

Dioscorides: *The Greek Herbal of Dioscorides. Illustrated by a Byzantine* A.D. 512, *Englished by J. Goodyear* A.D. 1655, *Edited and First Printed by R. T. Gunther* . . . London and New York, Hafner (1934, repr. 1968).

Duckworth. See Galen, *On Anatomical Procedures.*

Duthoy, R., 1969: *The Taurobolium. Its Evolution and Terminology.* Leiden, Brill.

Elgood, C., 1938: Jundi Shapur—A Sassanian University. Proc. Roy. Soc. Med. 32, 57–60.

Figuier, L., 1866: *Vies des Savants Illustres.* Paris, Librairie Internationale.

Galen: *Claudii Galeni Opera Omnia.* C. G. Kühn, ed. Lipsiae, Off. Libr. C. Cnoblochii (1821–1833; Greek text with Latin trans.; 22 vols.). Abbr. K.

——, *On Anatomical Procedures. The Later Books.* Trans. W. L. H. Duckworth. Cambridge, Cambridge University Press (1962).

——, *On Medical Experience.* First edition of the Arabic version, with English trans. and notes by R. Walzer. London, New York, etc., Oxford University Press (1944).

——, *On the Natural Faculties.* Trans. A. J. Brock. Loeb Classical Library, Cambridge, Mass., Harvard University Press and London, Heinemann (1963; 1 vol.).

——, *On the Usefulness of the Parts of the Body (De Usu Partium).* Trans. M. T. May. Ithaca, N.Y., Cornell University Press (1968; 2 vols.).

Galeni Librorum septima classis, . . . Venetiis, apud Iuntas, 1609.

Gourevitch, D., 1970: Some Features of the Ancient Doctor's Personality as Depicted in Epitaphs. Nordisk Medicinhistorisk Arsbok 1970, 1–12.

Hacard, J., 1947: *La Thériaque et la Société de la Thériaque des Apothicaires de Paris.* Doctoral thesis, Strasbourg (Fac. of Pharmacy). Paris, Le François.

Hazard, H. W., 1952: *Atlas of Islamic History.* Princeton University Press.

Jargy, S., 1969: Les fondements théologiques du dialogue Islamo-Chrétien. Rev. de Théol. et de Philos. 6, 362–375.

Kraft, E., 1970: *Die Geschichte der Gefässunterbindung bis zu den Anfängen der modernen Chirurgie.* Doctoral thesis, University of Giessen (Fac. of Med., Inst. for the Hist. of Med., publ. No. 1).

Kühn. See Galen (*Opera Omnia*).

Major, R. H., 1954: *A History of Medicine*. Oxford, Blackwell Scient. Publ. (2 vols.).

May. See Galen, *On the Usefulness of the Parts of the Body*.

Mencken, H. L., 1958: *The Bathtub Hoax*. New York, Knopf.

Needham, J., 1965– : *Science and Civilisation in China*. Cambridge, Cambridge University Press. Abbr. NEED.

Oribase: *Oeuvres. Texte grec . . . traduit par les docteurs Bussemaker et Daremberg.* Paris, Impr. Impériale (1862).

Pazzini, A., 1971: Ancora sulla possibilità o meno di autopsie umane in Roma antica (con speciale riguardo ad un eventuale "jus cadaveris"). Riv. di Storia della Med. *15*, 131–150.

Petrikovits, H. von, 1961: Die Ausgrabungen in Neuss (Stand der Ausgrabungen Ende 1961). Bonner Jahrb. *161*, 449–485.

Phillips, E. D., 1973: *Greek Medicine*. London, Thames and Hudson. [A valuable account, from the point of view of a Greek scholar.]

Pliny [The Elder]: *Natural History*. Trans. H. Rackham, W. H. S. Jones and D. E. Eichholz. Loeb Classical Library, Cambridge, Mass., Harvard University Press and London, Heinemann (1956–1966; 10 vols.). Abbr. PNH.

Prüsmann, F., 1900: *Die Behandlung des Geschwürs nach Galen*. Doctoral thesis, Berlin (Fac. of Med.).

Rather, L. J., 1971: Disturbance of Function (*functio laesa*): The Legendary Fifth Cardinal Sign of Inflammation, Added by Galen to the Four Cardinal Signs of Celsus. Bull. N.Y. Acad. Med. *47*, 303–322.

Rây, P. and Gupta, H. N., 1965: *Caraka Samhitā. A Scientific Synopsis*. New Delhi, Nat. Inst. of Sciences of India.

Sarton, G., 1954: *Galen of Pergamon*. Lawrence, Kansas, University of Kansas Press.

Scarborough, J., 1971: Galen and the Gladiators. Episteme *2*, 98–111.

Schöner, E., 1964: *Das Vierschema in der Humoralpathologie*. Suppl. 4 to Sudhoff's Arch. f. Gesch. der Med. u. Naturwiss.

Schröder, E., 1901: *Die Allgemeine Wundbehandlung des Galen*. Doctoral thesis, University of Berlin (Fac. of Med.).

Schwartz, S. I., 1969: *Principles of Surgery*. New York, Toronto, Sydney and London, The Blakiston Division, McGraw-Hill (vol. I).

Scribonius Largus: *Scribonii Largi Conpositiones*. G. Helmreich, ed. Lipsaiae, in aed. B. G. Teubneri (1893).

Seidmann, P., 1936: Galien. In Laignel-Lavastine. *Histoire générale de la médecine*. Paris, Michel (vol. I, pp. 395–432).

Siegel, R. E., 1968: *Galen's System of Physiology and Medicine. An Analysis of his Doctrines and Observations on Bloodflow, Respiration, Humors and Internal Diseases*. Basel and New York, Karger.

————, 1970: *Galen on Sense Perception. His Doctrines, Observations and Experiments on Vision, Hearing, Smell, Taste, Touch and Pain, and their Historical Sources*. Basel and New York, Karger.

Sushruta Samhita, An English Translation. Based on Original Sanskrit Text . . . by K. K. Bhishagratna. Varanasi, India. Chowkhamba Sanskrit Series Office (1912; repr. 1963; 3 vols.). Abbr. SS.

Tacitus: *The Histories*. Trans. C. H. Moore. *The Annals*. Trans. J. Jackson. Loeb Classical Library, Cambridge, Harvard University Press, and London, Heinemann (1931–1937; 4 vols.).

Temkin, O., 1951: On Galen's Pneumatology. Gesnerus, *8*, 180–189.

————, 1973: *Galenism: Rise and Decline of a Medical Philosophy*. Ithaca, Cornell University Press.

Temkin, O., and Straus, W. L., Jr., 1946: Galen's Dissection of the Liver and of the Muscles Moving the Forearm. Translated from the "Anatomical Procedures." Bull. Hist. Med. *19*, 167–176.

Virchow, R., 1863: *Cellular Pathology, as Based upon Physiological and Pathological Histology*. Translated from the 2nd German ed. by F. Chance. (Repr., with an Introd. Essay by L. J. Rather, New York, Dover, 1971).

Bibliog-
raphy

Walsh, J., 1926: Galen's Discovery and Promulgation of the Function of the Recurrent Laryngeal Nerve. Ann. Med. Hist. 8, 176–184.

———, 1934–1937: Galen's Writings and Influences Inspiring them. Ann. Med. Hist. Part I: 1934, 6, 1–30; Part II: 1934, 6, 143–149; Part III: 1936, 8, 65–90; Part IV: 1937, 9, 34–61.

Watson, G., 1966: *Theriac and Mithridatium. A Study in Therapeutics.* London, The Wellcome Historical Medical Library.

Whipple, A. O., 1936: Role of the Nestorians as the Connecting Link Between Greek and Arabic Medicine. Ann. Med. Hist. 8, 313–323.

Wilson, L. G., 1959: Erasistratus, Galen and the Pneuma. Bull. Hist. Med. 33, 293–314.

Wortmann, D., 1971: *Von römischen Neuss.* Cologne, Rheinischer Verein f. Denkmalpflege u. Landschaftsschutz.

Bibliography

Abbreviations and Phonetic Notations

ḫ   should be read *ch* as in *Bach*
š   should be read *sh* as in *shell*
ṣ, ṭ   harder sounds than *s* and *t*
ṁ, ṃ   nasalize the preceding vowel (much like *n* in the French *sans*)
ṇ   a "retroflex" n, pronounced with the tongue bent back

A   Adams translation of Hippocrates
AMT   *Assyrian Medical Texts*, Thompson 1923
AUB   Auboyer, *La vie quotidienne dans l'Inde ancienne*, 1961
CAD   *Chicago Assyrian Dictionary*
CB   *Chester Beatty VI Medical Papyrus* (Jonckheere 1947)
CDM   Celsus, *De Medicina*
ChS   *Charaka Samhita*
CU   Chamfrault and Ung Kang-Sam translation of the *Nei Ching*
DB   *Dictionary of the Bible* [*The Interpreter's*]
Eb   *Ebers Papyrus* (+ paragr. + No., as standard in GMÄ)
EE   Edelstein and Edelstein, *Asclepius*, 1945
EG   *Egyptian Grammar*, Gardiner 1966 (+ page)
FH   Flückiger and Hanbury, *Pharmacographia*, 1879
GMÄ   *Grundriss der Medizin der alten Ägypter*, Grapow 1954–1962
IG   *Inscriptiones Graecae*
Il   *Iliad*
K   Kühn edition of Galen (+ vol. + page)
L   *London Papyrus* as quoted in GMÄ
LB   Loeb Classical Library edition (of any author previously mentioned)
LH   Lucas and Harris, *Ancient Egyptian Materials and Industries*, 1962
LS   Liddell and Scott, *Greek-English Lexicon*
LTT   Littré edition of Hippocrates
MEA   *Manuel d'Épigraphie Akkadienne*, Labat 1952
NC-LS   *Nei Ching, Ling Shu*
NC-SW   *Nei Ching, Su Wên*
NEED   Needham, *Science and Civilisation in China*, 1965–
Od   *Odyssey*
PNH   Pliny the Elder, *Natural History*
PW   Pauly-Wissowa, *Realencyclopädie*
Sm   *Smith Papyrus*
SS   *Sushruta Samhita*
Ve   Veith translation of the *Nei Ching*
W   *Wörterbuch der Ägyptischen Sprache*, Erman and Grapow

Notes to the Text

1. Prelude

1. An eminent pathologist, Burt S. Wolbach, wrote, "I get satisfaction in believing that the adaptation of marine creatures to terrestrial conditions was the result of eons of responses in myriads of survivors of non-lethal injuries" (Wolbach 1954). The thought that disease helped life is definitely flattering to a pathologist.

2. Jaeger 1944

3. For more details on wound healing see e.g. Florey 1970 Ch. 2, 3, 17; Ross 1969.

4. Majno and others 1971; Gabbiani and others 1972

5. Guex 1967

6. In Dart's original works the australopithecines of South African caves are estimated to be about 750,000 years old. Means of absolute dating are not available in South African sites. I have adopted the more recent estimations, which assign to the earliest australopithecines an age of about five million years (Howells 1973 p. 51), to those of South African caves about three million (Howells 1973 p. 61).

7. See all refs. to Dart; also Ardrey 1967, a highly readable but now seriously outdated account.

8. Dart 1949 p. 11; Ardrey 1967 p. 192 ff.

9. Dart 1949, 1957; Ardrey 1967 p. 194

10. Ardrey 1967 p. 31: "weapon fathered man." Ibid. p. 186: "a philosophical bomb, a positive demonstration that the first recognizably human assertion had been the capacity for murder."

11. Howells 1973 p. 45

12. A recent poll of opinions among anthropologists, regarding Dart's interpretation of australopithecine "culture," gave this odd result: of fifty scholars, only seven replied, and only one was clearly against (Wolberg 1970).

13. Kortlandt and van Zon 1969; Howells 1973 p. 46

14. Teleki 1973 plate 5

15. As of 1973, I find in Howells' *Evolution of the Genus Homo* (p. 129) this accepted fact: "australopithecines . . . began the expansion of cerebral control of manipulation (with the making of stone tools)."

16. Leakey 1932

17. PNH 11. 159/LB III 531

18. At first a British pathologist diagnosed the lump as a sarcoma (Lawrence 1935). Microscopic sections, however, show a "large number of fragments of lamellar bone, well-organised and scattered throughout the mass." This is not consistent with a malignant tumor, nor is it typical of a simple callus: the likeliest alternative is a fracture followed by osteomyelitis. I am indebted to Dr. P. V. Tobias for allowing me to quote this unpublished story.

19. Some sort of language communication may have started as far back as the australopithecines (Howells 1973 pp. 135, 144).

20. Howells 1973 p. 3

21. Howells 1967 p. 202; Solecki 1960

22. Only the skull of the Shanidar cripple has been published in detail (Stewart 1959); a description of the withered arm should follow (Stewart, personal communication).

23. Solecki 1960 p. 619

24. Solecki 1957 p. 63

25. Solecki 1971 p. 196

26. Solecki 1960 p. 619; 1963 p. 187; 1971 p. 196

27. Stewart 1969 p. 52

28. Solecki 1960 p. 619

29. Wells 1965 p. 48. Arrowheads and spearheads stuck in human bones have been found all over the world. See e.g. Cartailhac 1889; Miller 1913; Rouillon and Baudouin 1924; Morel and Baudouin 1928; Pales 1930; Morel 1951; Underwood 1951; Klindt-Jensen 1957 p. 55; Tasnádi-Kubacska 1962; Wells 1965.

30. Wells 1965 p. 33

31. Lorenz 1952

32. Ackerknecht 1946

33. For the references on apes I am indebted to Dr. Konrad Lorenz and to his collaborator Dr. Margret Schleidt. Bourne (II 273) on chimpanzees adds no new facts. The episode of dental care described later in the text seems to be the only new observation since Miles.

34. Goodall 1965; van Lawick-Goodall 1971

35. Excerpts of personal letters (13 April 1969, 30 November 1973) with kind permission of Baroness van Lawick-Goodall.

36. Miles 1963 pp. 841–842

37. Koehler 1927 p. 308

38. Barbers (or surgeons) wishing to refute the comparison with apes should address their complaints to Prof. Jean Posternak, Dept. of Physiology, University of Geneva. It was he who suggested the link, at first as an after-dinner joke.

39. McGrew and Tutin 1972, 1973

40. McGrew and Tutin 1973

41. Schultz 1939

42. Schultz 1969 p. 195

43. Bartels 1893 p. 283; Morice 1901 p. 22; Lindblom 1920 p. 312; Ackerknecht 1946; 1967; 1971 p. 95 ff.

44. Howells 1967 p. 206

45. The oldest bandage from the New World comes from Peru and may be 1500 years old. It is a cotton roll about 1 inch high, which was wound around the skull and held in place by strands of a woollen cord (Moodie 1926).

46. On the historic role of resins see Ch. 5. Neolithic man definitely used resin to fix in place the flint teeth of sickles (LH 1–9; see also Levey 1959 p. 77).

47. Discussed in Ch. 7.

48. Ackerknecht 1967 p. 636

49. The earliest evidence of cauterization is rather shaky: a strange type of lesion found on certain Neolithic skulls and shaped like a *T*, hence called "Syncypital T" (Manouvrier 1904).

50. Hare 1967 p. 115

51. Simpson 1967 pp. 79, 12

52. Barghoorn 1971

53. Correspondence with Dr. J. W. Schopf, author of the electron micrograph shown in Fig. 1.11, convinced me that these tiny bodies are indeed bacteria; color, resistance to mineral acids, electron transmissibility, combustibility, etc., all suggest a biogenic origin (see also Schopf and others 1965; Barghoorn 1971). Previous experience had made me skeptical, for the "fossilized bacteria" (Bradley 1968) of which I requested a photograph turned out to be grains of dust by the time my letter reached the author.

54. Gilmore 1912; Moodie 1923 p. 245

55. Moodie 1923

56. While the evidence for *free* fossilized bacteria is convincing, there is no good evidence of bacteria in fossilized, infected bones (i.e. bones deformed by osteomyelitis). The "fossilized bacteria" described by Moodie in his classic *Paleopathology* (1923) could be a variety of artifacts.

57. Clement 1956; Hengen 1967a, b. The age of the carious teeth as earlier published was 500–600,000 years; I increased it to fit the new data on australopithecines (Howells 1973).

58. Weidenreich 1939

59. Straus and Cave 1957; Gorjanović-Kramberger 1906; Hengen 1969

60. McKenzie and Brothwell 1967

61. Leroi-Gourhan 1971

62. Leroi-Gourhan 1964 p. 95

63. Leroi-Gourhan 1958 p. 390

64. Verbrugge 1956; 1965; 1969

65. Leroi-Gourhan 1967

66. Janssens 1957 p. 320

67. Verbrugge 1969 pp. 237, 240

68. Leroi-Gourhan 1967 p. 110

69. Hands—prehistoric, mutilated, or just artistic—have become an almost full-time calling for Father Verbrugge of Compiègne (Paris), who assembled a vast literature (Verbrugge 1965; 1969; 1970), including a monograph on 4000 hand imprints from Australian caves. In Europe, prehistoric imprints of hands have been found, strangely enough, only in France and Spain; "mutilated" imprints are clearly demonstrable in only 2 of the 22 caves. Some of the facts are certainly intriguing: at Gargas, for instance, of 138 hands, 124 are left hands, and the *left* hands are 67 to 1 on the *left* side of the cave (Verbrugge 1969 p. 62)—but then it might be impossible to tell right imprints from left if some were made backward, as Leroi-Gourhan suggested. One also has to be aware of fanciful interpretations, such as vertical imprints of stumps showing the scar (!) where the finger had been disarticulated (Sahly in Verbrugge 1969 p. 302). Skeletal remains might help, but nothing relevant has been found.

70. Janssens 1957; Verbrugge 1965

71. Sollas 1911 p. 240

72. Gardner 1963; Gardner and Heider 1968

73. For these details I am much indebted to my friend Robert Gardner. When the Dani were visited by the Harvard-Peabody New Guinea Expedition in 1961, they were Neolithic warrior-farmers almost virgin of contact with the outer world. The main body of the expedition departed in August 1961; within two weeks the Dutch police had "pacified" the area (Gardner and Heider 1968 p. xiv).

74. Gardner and Heider 1968 p. 101

75. Mennerich 1968

76. Bössneck 1971

77. Clark 1965 p. 63 ff., 76 ff.; Zeuner 1963 p. 55; Protsch and Berger 1973

78. The problem: not enough bones. Drew and others (1971) found the idea intriguing but could provide no supporting evidence.

79. For trepanation see the chapters by Lisowski and Margetts in Brothwell and Sandison 1967, which includes photographs of contemporary trepanations in Africa. For pre-Neolithic trepanation, see Dastugue 1959.

80. Wells 1965 p. 146

81. MacCurdy 1923 p. 260

82. Muniz and McGee 1897 p. 11; Daland 1936

83. MacCurdy 1923 p. 259

84. MacCurdy 1923

85. Hilton-Simpson 1922

86. Margetts 1967 p. 691

87. Stewart 1966

88. Fischer 1864 p. 598

2. The Asu

1. Gelb 1963. The invention of writing is usually credited to the Sumerians, but according to Oppenheim it is fairly certain that the Sumerians inherited the principle of writing from local, unknown predecessors (Oppenheim 1964 pp. 49, 237, see also Diringer 1968: I 17). Doubts were cast on the Sumerian priority by three mysterious "Tartaria Tablets" found recently in the ruins of a Neolithic village in the Balkans. They bear a few signs similar to those of the earliest Sumerian tablets but could be as many as 1000 years older (Hood 1968; Laki 1969).

2. Jacobsen 1968 p. 137

3. Contenau 1938 p. 1. This is the traditional view, supported by the fact that Sumerian settlements have not been found much downstream of Eridu; but see Parrot 1968 p. 39.

4. *Qanū*, the Akkadian word for reed, has the same root as the Greek *kánna*, the Latin *canna*, and the English *cane*. Many words of this Semitic language have roots that are familiar to us. Fat was *lipû*, which corresponds to the Greek *lípos*, hence the biochemical term *lipid*; *ellu* was oil, in Greek *élaion*.

5. Oppenheim 1964 p. 325

6. Piggott 1968. Wheeled transport seems to have appeared first in Mesopotamia. The event is neatly preserved in the evolution of a Sumerian pictogram, showing at

first the royal sledge,   then the same but with two wheels

added below   (Salonen 1951; Piggott 1968). Actual carts were found recently a few hundred miles east in Soviet territory (Piggott 1968); they do raise problems of priority, but they are not quite as old as the above pictogram. The Egyptians were unaware of wheeled transport until the Hyksos chariots stormed in about 1700 B.C.

7. Oppenheim 1964 p. 282

8. Saggs 1962 p. 152

9. Neugebauer 1957 p. 229

10. Parrot 1949

11. Ceram 1967 p. 223

12. Parrot 1953 p. 78

13. Kramer 1956

14. Not much was thought of this "mythical" deluge until Sir Leonard Woolley made an awesome finding in the remains of Ur, the city of Abraham. His team had dug a deep pit through millennia of stratified debris. Suddenly, at a depth of forty

feet, all trace of human life disappeared: the spades hit a layer of pure clay. At first
Sir Leonard thought that he had reached the virgin soil preceding human settlement.
Its level, however, did not fit with his estimations, so he ordered the digging to
resume, and eight feet deeper more pottery and stone implements reappeared.
Presumably these represented people who had been wiped out by a tremendous
flood, enough to bury much of Sumer under eight feet of alluvial deposit (Woolley
1965 p. 26; Ceram 1967 p. 309 ff.). Sir Leonard believed this to be the Flood echoed in
the seventh chapter of Genesis. But later excavations in the same general area
uncovered other deposits of the same kind, so that now we have too many Floods. Sir
Max Mallowan recently concluded that Sir Leonard's flood (about 3500 B.C.) is too
old; the right one should be another, dated about 2900 B.C. (Mallowan 1964). Others
are not so sure (Raikes 1966), but what remains undeniable is that the Book of
Genesis has its roots in the Sumero-Babylonian myth. For details see also Lambert
and Millard 1969. For the actual Sumerian story of the Flood, see Civil 1969. For flood
myths in other parts of the world and a skeptical view on Ut-Napishtim, see De
Santillana and Dechend 1969.

15. See Lambert and Millard 1969; Ceram 1967 p. 275.

16. Biggs 1969 p. 102. An oft-quoted set of surgical instruments was first shown
by Meyer-Steineg and Sudhoff in an illustration where nothing was said about them
except that they were "found at Nineveh"—too little to work with, let alone to
conclude that Akkadian surgeons "performed *cystectomies*" [*sic*, Thorwald 1962 p.
158].

17. Most of Assurbanipal's library is now at the British Museum. It is a
worrisome fact that the soil of Mesopotamia preserves the tablets better than many
museum shelves. Unbaked tablets must be de-salted and baked; otherwise, if they are
allowed to dry, crystals form on the surface, break it up, and obliterate the writing.
Only the great museums are equipped as required; scores of tablets turn to dust
without ever having been read (Neugebauer 1957 p. 61). In any event, only a small
fraction of the tablets found so far has been read and published; blame no one, they
amount to nearly half a million, with more coming every year (Oppenheim 1967 p.
9).

18. Oppenheim 1964 p. 15

19. Oppenheim 1962

20. Thompson 1923—all in cuneiform!

21. Labat 1966 p. 93

22. Thompson 1907; Labat 1959

23. Labat 1951

24. Ritter 1965 p. 300

25. The exception is Biggs 1969.

26. Köcher 1963; 1964

27. Oppenheim 1964 p. 288

28. Labat 1957 p. 115

29. Thompson 1937 p. 235

30. Thompson 1907 p. 345

31. AMT 74, 11, 23; AMT 23, 10, 8; AMT 16, 5, 7. Trans. courtesy of Prof. Labat
and Pablo Herrero.

32. von Soden 1965 p. 169

33. Labat 1964(b)

34. Ritter 1965

35. Thompson 1930 p. 1 No. 4

36. Thompson 1930 p. 2 No. 9

37. *Asû* or *azû* (long *û* but tonic accent on the *a*) is written as shown above the
title of this chapter (the two parts stand for *a* and *su*). It does not mean "he who
knows water," as usually stated (Contenau 1938 p. 30; Saggs 1962 p. 460). *A* does
mean water, but this *zu* is not written like the *zu* that means "to know" (CAD 1968,
asû A, p. 344, see also p. 347; Biggs 1969 p. 97).

38. Labat 1953 p. 17

39. Contenau 1947 p. 103

40. Ritter 1965

41. Oppenheim 1964 p. 295

42. Thureau-Dangin 1921; Contenau 1947 pp. 95, 180

43. Biggs 1969 p. 295

44. *Asa-* and *Rapha-* recall the names for physician in the Bible and the Talmud: *âsjâ, assîa* (Preuss 1923; 1894) and *rōphē*. The name of Rapha, a Biblical figure, was probably also short for Rapha-El (Buttrick 1962). In the episode of the Bible (2 Chron. 16:12), Asa did not live up to his name of "God-heals": being "gravely affected with gangrene in his feet, he did not seek guidance of the Lord but resorted to physicians."

45. Oppenheim 1964 p. 293

46. Labat 1954 p. 207

47. All the techniques of the Akkadian physician, including cutting, have been gathered and analyzed by Pablo Herrero, whose thesis on this subject is forthcoming.

48. Labat 1954

49. Oppenheim 1964 p. 324

50. Scheil 1902

51. Trans. by T. J. Meek in Pritchard 1950, quoted by permission of Princeton University Press.

52. Harper 1904; Johns 1905

53. CAD A II 346, 5

54. Labat 1951 p. xxii

55. Labat 1954, Akkadisches Handwörterbuch

56. One silver shekel weighed about 8.5 grams (Hastings 1909 p. 627; Labat 1954 p. 209). To measure what it took to earn 10 shekels, according to law 228 of Hammurabi's Code: "If a builder construct a house for a seignior . . . he shall give him two shekels per sar of house." One sar was 42.2 square yards. According to law 274, if a seignor hired a carpenter, the fee was 4 se per day (one shekel = 180 se; Thompson 1925(b) p. 128).

57. Mendenhall 1954 pp. 32, 35

58. Biggs 1969 p. 100

59. Cardascia 1969

60. CAD Z 126: *sha zigni*, "bearded"

61. Oppenheim 1964 pp. 24, 276

62. Civil 1960; 1961

63. Kramer and Levey 1955; Kramer 1959; Civil 1960

64. The prescriptions from the Sumerian tablet, as quoted, are English versions of Civil's original French, corrected by Civil himself (two plant names had changed).

65. Civil 1960 prescr. 1.7

66. Forbes 1965 p. 277; Röllig 1970

67. Civil 1960 prescr. 3.1

68. Levey 1959

69. Civil 1960 prescr. 1.5

70. Contenau 1938 p. 68

71. Ritter 1965 p. 313

72. Labat 1961

73. Thompson 1924(b) p. 26 No. 28

74. Köcher 1955; Glotz 1968

75. Kramer and Levey 1955 p. 370; Levey 1959 p. 128; Forbes 1965 p. 261

76. Labat 1959 p. 5 No. 20–21

77. Levey 1955; 1959 p. 31 ff.

78. The evidence for soap making in the Sumerian tablet, though mentioned in Kramer and Levey 1955 p. 370, is thin. In Civil's latest translation, prescriptions 3.1 and 3.2 do contain products of the naga plant, which was used—fresh—as a source of saponine or—burned—as a source of alkali (personal communication from Dr. Civil; Civil 1960 pp. 64, 70). Neither plaster includes much fat, but both are followed by rubbing with oil, and the second one may include a resin. Essence is mentioned in prescr. 2.1 (ibid. p. 63).

79. Herrero, see note 47

80. Labat 1954 p. 216

81. Labat 1954 p. 217

82. Littré 1851 p. 227

83. Thompson 1937 p. 234; Labat 1954 p. 212

84. These two Akkadian operations, scraping the skull and cutting into the chest, are amply discussed in the Hippocratic works. Whether the Greeks learned them from the Akkadians is unknown. For actual trepanation of the skull there is no acceptable evidence from Mesopotamia, though instances are known for the first millennium B.C. in Palestine (Biggs 1969 p. 100). It is strange that this operation, which was fairly current in prehistoric times, encountered no favor in Mesopotamia and Egypt (the Greeks made up for it).

85. Labat 1954 p. 215

86. Labat 1954 p. 212

87. Labat 1954 p. 213

88. Isaiah 6

89. Preliminary experiments by Dr. D. Kekessy, Geneva.

90. DB III 592

91. This version of Arad-Nana's letter is a composite of three original translations: Labat's to French (Labat 1953 p. 10) and two others to English (Waterman 1930 p. 73; Johnston 1898 p. 163). The translation of Ritter (1965 p. 319) reads somewhat differently, but the essence remains the same. Unaccountably, "⅚ of a double hour" is explained as "80 minutes"; I took the liberty of changing this to 100 minutes.

92. Johns 1904 p. 375

93. Labat 1953 p. 11

94. Labat 1951

95. As translated by Saggs 1962 p. 462

96. Saggs 1962 p. 350

97. Limet 1960 p. 121; von Soden 1965 p. 739

98. Because of a passage in the History of Technology of Singer and others (1965 I 251), I thought for a while that the Akkadian word for inflammation might still be alive in our word *naphtha*, as "the burning thing" (naphtha surfaces spontaneously in Mesopotamia). According to those authors, the greek word *naphtha* goes back to an old Babylonian *naptu*, used as early as 2000 B.C., "from a verb meaning to *flare up, to blaze.*" Alas, they were wrong; there is no such verb. *Naptu* certainly became *naphtha*, but it has no known relationship to *napāḫu*.

99. AMT 35, 2, 2, trans. courtesy of Prof. Labat and Pablo Herrero

100. That *ummu* means the "hot thing" is certain: its first meaning is "heat," and it has the same root as the verb *emému*, "to be hot." There are other words for "fever," such as *la'bu, li'bu, ḫumṭu,* and *ḫimṭu* (Labat 1964a). Another word that can be rendered as "inflammation" is *ishātu*, originally meaning "fire"; sometimes it may be translated as "abscess" (Labat and Herrero, personal communication). *Kuraru* originally meant "(hot) embers"; when it is a skin disease it is usually translated as "eczema." Note that *carbuncle* is also a former "hot coal" that became a "furuncle."

101. Flower pot: Contenau 1927 p. 444; brasero: Contenau 1940 p. 59.

102. Thompson 1907 p. 345; Labat 1954 p. 212

103. Thompson 1931 p. 54 No. 4, ibid. No. 8

104. Labat 1951 pp. 79, 123

105. Labat 1951 p. xxv

106. Labat 1953 p. 21; 1951 p. xxii; White 1969

107. Labat 1951 p. 229 No. 96

108. Oppenheim 1964 p. 295

109. Labat 1962

110. Waterman 1930 p. 415 letter 586. See also Townend 1938.

111. Denton 1943

112. Labat 1951 p. xxii

113. Oppenheim 1964 p. 176

114. Thompson 1924(a)

115. Labat 1953 p. 18; 1966 p. 102

116. Jastrow 1917 p. 237. The Akkadian way of saying "anything" was "everything that has a name." For the importance of names in antiquity, see Contenau 1947 p. 127.

117. Jastrow 1917 p. 237

118. Labat 1959 p. 5

119. Oppenheim 1964 p. 314

120. Thompson 1924(b) p. 10; Levey 1959 p. 36

121. Levey 1959 pp. 65, 69; Oppenheim 1964 p. 81

122. Levey 1959 p. 69

123. This is the basic problem of antisepsis: to find a poison for bacteria (= bacterial cells) that is less of a poison for human cells. To some extent, all antiseptics are also harmful to the tissues. The best antibiotics have a special key to the bacterial cell. For example, penicillin prevents bacteria from building a new cell wall (a coating that man's cells do not have); thus, existing bacteria are unaffected, but new ones cannot form. A definition of antibiotic is difficult to give, but essentially it is a product of living cells that in low concentrations is able to inhibit the growth of other cells.

124. Thompson 1930 p. 11 No. 3

125. Osborn 1943

126. Nickell 1959

127. Nickell 1959 p. 282

128. Maksymiuk 1970

129. Ivánovics and Horváth 1947

130. Flückiger and Hanbury 1879 p. 165

131. Labat 1953 p. 8

132. Ramparts were the distinguishing mark of cities in the Near East (with the possible exception of Egypt) from the third millennium B.C.; "it was the duty of the King to keep the walls in good repair and—correspondingly—to tear down those of conquered cities" (Oppenheim 1964 p. 127). The walls were made of brick, mostly unbaked.

133. Jean 1950 p. 211. For the reading "sling-stone" rather than "stone" as in the original translation, see CAD 1968, I, A, Part II, under asû A [a,2'] p. 345.

134. Oppenheim 1962

135. Thompson 1937 p. 235

136. Thompson 1937 p. 235

137. Herodotos I. 195/LB I 251; translation retouched. Whether Herodotos had been to Babylon on one of his travels or wrote about it by hearsay is not known. His remark may mean that physicians in his day were few, so that the man in the street was left to his own means (Saggs 1962 p. 460).

138. Mesopotamian science certainly provided the background for Greek mathematics and astronomy (Neugebauer 1957 p. 145). For medicine a legacy is much more difficult to prove. The Greek concern with prognosis may bear distant echoes of the Akkadian Prognoses (Labat 1951 p. xxviii, xxxv); the notion of "critical days" in the course of diseases has an Akkadian precedent (Labat 1966 p. 1000); and it is possible, but not proven, that some of the 250-odd Mesopotamian drugs were taken over by the Greeks.

The little that is said about wounds in the Talmud (which is far more recent, from the third to the fifth centuries A.D.) is in part reminiscent of Mesopotamian practices, as are the names of skin sores, mursa, simta (Preuss 1923 pp. 222–223). Local treatments for wounds included lint, binding on a sponge, onion leaves, garlic, and chewed grains of wheat. The people also used pieces of dung. Mar Samuel, the most famous Babylonian physician (165–257 A.D.), treated wounds with oil and water. Buried in the Talmud is also the statement that "the hand can cause inflammation" (Preuss 1923 p. 277 ff.; Lods 1925; Humbert 1964). For a survey of Biblical medicine, see Levin 1970 (although he has practically nothing on wounds and surgery).

139. Oppenheim 1962 p. 105; 1964 pp. 274, 301
140. Jeremiah 51:8

3. The Swnw

1. Bell 1948 p. 2
2. Wilson 1946 p. 40
3. Wilson 1946 pp. 41–47
4. Contacts between Egypt and Mesopotamia did of course exist: Sumerian cylinder seals were found in Egypt (Mallowan 1965 pp. 56, 57), and some 400 cuneiform tablets turned up in El Amarna on the Nile. They come from the archives of Pharaoh Amenophis IV (1375–1358), who corresponded with various rulers of the Near East (Mercer 1939). Almost all these tablets are letters; some are long inventories of unbelievably rich and varied presents.
5. Herodotos II 84/LB I 369
6. Whether Egyptian or Sumerian writing came first is not yet settled (Diringer 1968 pp. 29–31). Another mystery is that the Egyptians had plenty of clay, which they used for building but never for writing. And what were the early stages of the hieroglyphs, before the unification of Egypt under the first dynasty? This date too is uncertain: it has slowly shifted closer, from the fourth millennium to 2900 B.C. (Diringer 1968 pp. 29–31).
7. Quibell 1913
8. Hooton 1917
9. Leek 1969
10. Hooton 1917; Ruffer 1921 p. 314
11. Smith 1908
12. GMÄ II 3, 62
13. Ebbell's translation certainly has merit but it is replete with precise medical terms like Lepra maculo-anaesthetica, Anevrysma arterioso-venosum—which is about as precise as using sterile instruments to work in mud.
14. Late in Egypt's history the number of hieroglyphs grew to a few thousand (Diringer 1968 p. 146). The 753 most common signs have been classified by shape and species in this standard list (EG 438–548), which makes it relatively easy to look them up individually. Translation is another matter.
15. The hieroglyphs did undergo some evolution, as shown in Fig. 3.6. The sign for axe, for instance, was brought up to date as the axe changed shape. Also the scribe had some latitude at all times. For example, he felt free to change the sex, headgear, and dress of the sign for statue as he fancied. The object represented by a given hieroglyph is often obvious, especially when painted in great detail. In other cases it is obscure, and it was equally obscure to all but the earliest Egyptian scribes, because either the objects themselves or the way they were represented had become obsolete (EG 438, 439).
16. EG 28, 428
17. EG 5, 6
18. EG 512
19. Jonckheere 1958
20. Grapow 1936 p. 65
21. The word ankh, usually spelled ⚭ (ankh + n + kh) meant "sandal strap" as well as "to live" (EG 508). Hence, the ankh became a symbol of life; this is why Egyptian gods are often clutching it.
22. EG 47, 54
23. "Atemnot," GMÄ VII/1 109. The translation is not absolutely certain. A word that seems to mean "asthma" has some sort of lizard as a determinant, which Ebbell saw as a reference to the wheezing noise that a chameleon makes when he deflates his lungs in anger! (Lefebvre 1956 p. 121, GMÄ VII/2 922).

24. Lefebvre 1955 p. 19

25. GMÄ VII/2 584; haty can also mean "heart," but then other determinatives are used (GMÄ VII/2 577).

26. In practice, not all conceivable variants were used for each word; some never appeared.

27. EG 465

28. Diringer 1968 pp. 32ff., 146

29. Lefebvre 1955 p. 42

30. There was an even more cursive form of writing, *demotic*, which at the latest count only eight people in the world are able to decipher. Demotic was used as late as 452 A.D.; hieroglyphs had gone out of use some sixty years earlier (EG 11).

31. Jonckheere 1958 p. 149

32. W III 365

33. EG 444

34. Leca 1971 p. 373

35. Jonckheere 1958 p. 97

36. Jonckheere 1958 p. 152

37. EG 34

38. For whatever it is worth, the feminine version of *swnw* is my single original contribution to Egyptology. I cautiously submitted it to an eminent Egyptologist, Dr. Robert O. Steuer, who confirmed it. Beyond this, my ignorance is far too great to understand how a man of the competence of Jonckheere would have missed or disregarded this reading, *swnw-t*. He probably knew too much, and therefore came up with a more far-fetched interpretation as follows (Jonckheere 1958 p. 152). Note first that the same wording occurs three times on the same stele. In two cases the relevant words, *overseer + physician*, are side by side, *mr + swnw* [+ *t*]; in the third case (Fig. 3.9) they are aligned vertically. Jonckheere suggested that the feminine ending

◁ *t* belonged to *overseer* (which would give ◁ *mr-t*, "overseer-ess") but that each time the ◁ *t* somehow slipped sideways, or down, to contaminate the *swnw*. This would be a lot of slipping for even such casual fellows as the Egyptian scribes.

39. Cumont 1937 p. 30

40. Smith 1958

41. For female physicians in Mesopotamia, see Oppenheim 1964 p. 304; Biggs 1969 p. 98. For Greece and Rome, see Gourevitch 1970, who drew from the *Corpus Inscriptionum Latinorum* and from *Inscriptiones Graecae*. The Greeks had several ways of feminizing *iatrós* (ἡ ἰατρός, ἰατρίνη—*he iatrós, iatríne*—etc.), but the use is rare and applied sometimes to a healing goddess (Liddell and Scott 1968, *iatrós*).

42. Sm XIV

43. Gardiner 1935 p. 42

44. Gardiner 1935 p. 41

45. Sm 11

46. GMÄ II 124

47. Cumont 1937 p. 64; Lefebvre 1956 p. 168

48. Jonckheere 1950c p. 219

49. Jonckheere 1950c pp. 220, 221

50. Černý 1927 pp. 186, 191

51. GMÄ VII/2 887

52. Herodotos II 84/LB I 369. Jonckheere and others took the trouble to list all the names of physicians mentioned anywhere (monuments, tombs) in ancient Egypt. They came up with 103 (Jonckheere 1958 p. 17, 169). The list is dedicated to Imhotep, the great architect-physician of the Third Dynasty, later deified and identified by the Greeks with Asklepios (Aesculapius—Hurry 1926), but does not include him because, besides tradition, "no evidence remains to prove that Imhotep had any medical knowledge"!

53. Jonckheere 1958 p. 99

54. Historians searching for the Egyptian surgeon once identified him with the priests of Sekhmet; this is almost certainly wrong (Jonckheere 1950a; 1951).

55. Bronze is copper and tin (about 9:1). The ancient Egyptians had plenty of copper but probably no tin; therefore, their Bronze Age had to be based on imports (LH 217 ff.). For iron in Egypt, see the excellent article by Wainwright 1932; LH 235; Harris 1961 p. 166; Singer and others 1965 p. 592. Bronze surgical knives from Egypt have been described, but their origin is either uncertain (Comrie 1909–1910) or late (Leca 1971 Pl. XI).

56. LH 235

57. In Greek, *síderos* is "iron"; in Latin, *sidus, sideris*, is "star."

58. Budge 1960 p. 246; Otto 1960; Daumas 1965 p. 347

59. I base my discussion of *bya* as "iron" on Wainwright's well-documented article (1932), so captivating as to convince me that it is not delirious to read signs like ⬚⬚ ⬚⬚ as "meteorites on sledges." Gardiner speaks of a "sledge bearing a load of metal (?)" (EG 517). In Erman and Grapow's *Wörterbuch*, Vol. 2 (1928), *bya-n-pt* is "iron" but *bya* is "copper (?)"; however, this translation was done before Wainwright's study; and Gardiner, who wrote later, apparently missed it: EG 517, 492, also has *bya* as "copper."

60. Crum 1939 p. 41

61. LH 240

62. Wainwright 1932 p. 15

63. GMÄ III 104

64. EG 515; GMÄ III 105, VII/2 989

65. GMÄ VII/2 105, 836, 682, 1000

66. Eb 876/Ebbell 1937 p. 127; GMÄ III 105; Jonckheere 1951 p. 41

67. EB 876/Ebbell 1937 p. 127; GMÄ III 105; Jonckheere 1951 p. 41

68. Columella 12.49, 50/LB III 297, 305

69. Wilson 1962; Ghalioungui 1973 p. 89

70. For a discussion of the "tumors" in the Ebers papyrus, see Ghalioungui 1973 p. 81. The "serpentine windings" are in EB 876 = GMÄ IV/1 229; for the reading "varicose veins," see Ghalioungui 1973 p. 83.

71. Ghalioungui 1973 p. 89

72. Sm 22

73. Mustapha Aga's performance was flawless, considering what he might have done. The first recorded find of Egyptian papyri dates from 1778; there were fifty in all. One was bought; the others remained unsold and were eventually burned by the disgruntled natives (Bell 1948 p. 14).

74. The oldest written medical document is the Sumerian tablet mentioned in Ch. 2, which is some five-hundred years older than the Smith papyrus. However, the extant copy of this papyrus reproduces a text that may already have been centuries old when the Sumerian tablet was written.

75. Sm 73

76. Breasted says 3000 and 2500 B.C., but since he wrote, the dates of Egyptian history have been moving closer to us. That medical books did exist during the Old Kingdom is attested by an inscription, in which King Neferkirere (Fifth Dynasty) called for books and physicians in an effort to rescue his dying architect (Breasted 1906; Jonckheere 1945 p. 29).

77. Sm 225

78. The spelling of *ydr* is bizarre. Unfortunately the determinatives, which could be so useful in this case, are of no help (Sm 230). The "ear" may be there for purely phonetic reasons (its name is *ydn*). The other determinative is not understood; EG has "bandage (?)" (EG 527).

79. Sm 227

80. Sm 421

81. Ebbell 1939 p. 11

82. Sm 233

83. Nobody argues about the "two strips"; it is the "adhesiveness" that remains unproven philologically (GMÄ VII/I 2), though it seems almost inevitable medically.

84. LH 5, 7, 316 ff.

85. LH 6

86. GMÄ VI 516

87. Carpendale and Sereda 1965; Alexander and others 1967; Myers and others 1969

88. For the clinical advantages of tapes over sutures, see Connolly and others 1969. For experimental studies (generally in favor of tapes), see Berard and others 1964; Carpendale and Sereda 1965; Ordman and Gillman 1966; Brunius and others 1967; Brunius 1968; Myers and others 1968; Connolly and others 1969; Forrester and others 1970.

89. Sm 139, Case 4

90. Sm 134, 139

91. Wilson 1962 p. 118

92. LH 299

93. Eb 871 (107, 6; 108, 3); GMÄ VI/1 227

94. Eb 872 (108, 3–9); GMÄ VI 227

95. Eb 876 (109, 11–18); GMÄ VI 229

96. Sm 365

97. Sm 415

98. Sm 385

99. Sm 388; GMÄ VII/1 482, 779, 854. See also Gispen 1968.

100. Grapow 1936 p. 64; GMÄ VII/2 1003

101. Budge 1960 p. 318

102. Sm 374

103. Sm 56, 92; GMÄ III 113

104. Ebbell 1939 p. 63

105. Sm 384

106. GMÄ VII/2, 248, 589

107. GMÄ VII/2, 521

108. Sm 84

109. Sm 367; GMÄ VII/1 249; Jonckheere 1947 p. 16 note

110. Sm 368

111. Eb 522 = GMÄ IV/1 205, IV/2 157

112. GMÄ VII/1, 172; Sm 81

113. EG 453

114. Steuer 1948 p. 8

115. Eg 539; Steuer 1948 p. 6 and *passim*

116. GMÄ VII/1 208, 215; VII/2 631

117. EG 539, 540

118. Steuer 1948

119. A "bad-type" wound, determined by ◌, occurs only once in the Smith papyrus (Sm 298, case VIII 18). It is a simple wound of the ear, to be stitched immediately. When the scribe repeats the word *wound* in the diagnosis, he uses the "clean-type" determinative (◌) (Sm 300 line 19). Had he slipped up the first time?

120. Steuer 1948 p. 18

121. Sm 141 case 4

122. Sm 404 case 45

123. Sm 104 case 1

124. Sm 165 case 6

125. Hagemann 1904

126. Eb 456e; GMÄ IV/1, 8

127. GMÄ III 7, 8

128. Forbes 1965(b) p. 187

129. Singer and others 1965 p. 260. Some remedies were prepared by boiling fat with alkali, but the resulting soap is never mentioned; in fact, there seems to have been no word for it. Real soap was first mentioned in the third century B.C. in Greece, then by Pliny and by Galen, who was the first to state its use to keep man clean (Forbes 1965, p. 187).

130. Sm 422 case 47

131. Van Lawick-Goodall 1971 p. 240

132. Sm 96 ff.

133. GMÄ III 49 note

134. e.g. Eb 86 (23, 2–4); GMÄ IV/1 104; Buchheim 1960 p. 103

135. Buchheim 1960 p. 103

136. Buchheim 1960

137. Weigall 1915

138. Griffith 1915

139. Dawson 1929

140. GMÄ VI 526

141. GMÄ VI 883

142. Sm 379

143. Sm 9, 59

144. Salicylic *acid* does have antiseptic properties; in fact, it was once proposed as a substitute for phenol (Gross and Greenberg 1948 p. 5). But *salicin*, which is salicyl alcohol glycoside, is less effective; and it is not known whether it is contained in significant amounts in willow leaves, as recommended here (it is traditionally obtained from the bark).

145. Sm 9, 59

146. GMÄ VI 358 ff.

147. Gabra 1956

148. Trease and Evans 1972 p. 426

149. Daumas 1965 p. 556

150. Merrillees 1962, 1968

151. Gabra (1956) accepts *shepenn* as opium. The word occurs in Eb 782; in Ebbell's translation of this passage (p. 108) *shepenn* is left untranslated. Its meaning is discussed in GMÄ VI 490.

152. This startling discovery (?) of Egyptian morphine is described rather succinctly by Schiaparelli 1927 (note 4 pp. 154–158). I was highly skeptical, but a chemist who specializes in Egyptian materials, Dr. John Winter of University Museum, Philadelphia, assured me that the actual persistence of morphine as described is not impossible.

153. Sm 383

154. Harris 1961; LH 344

155. LH 344

156. Forbes 1965(a) p. 239

157. Harris 1961 p. 143

158. Personal communication from Dr. J. R. Harris, Institute of Egyptology, University of Copenhagen.

159. Harris 1961 p. 102

160. Forbes 1965(a) p. 293

161. Forbes 1965(a) p. 293

162. I owe this information to my friend Dr. R. S. Cotran.

163. Forbes 1965(a) pp. 292–293

164. Harris 1961 p. 224

165. Harris 1961 p. 224

166. Browning 1969 p. 147

167. For pilot experiments I am indebted to Dr. D. Kekessy of the Institute of Hygiene, and for the definitive experiments to Dr. E. Schorer and her assistant Mme S. Dersi, Département de Biologie Végétale, University of Geneva. Forbes wrote that the use of verdigris was unknown in Egypt, though attested for Mesopotamia (in Singer 1965 I, 239). This is inaccurate (personal comm. from Dr. J. R. Harris). It is true, however, that we do not know how the Egyptians made their "copper green." Several ways to obtain it were described much later by Pliny (PNH 34. 110/LB IX 209).

168. Gunther 1934 p. 629

169. Gunther 1934 p. 636

170. The Eau Dalibour (often misspelled D'Alibour) included in the 1972 *Pharmacopoea Helvetica* as "Solutio zinco-cuprica composita": copper sulphate 0.1%, zinc sulphate 0.4%, dissolved in a 0.1% watery solution of camphor. I understand that

some dermatologists leave out the camphor. The original formula included saffron. The Eau Dalibour was saved from oblivion by the French dermatologist Sabouraud, who says that as such it is painful, and that on wounds it should be diluted to $\frac{1}{3}$. For these data I am indebted to Prof. R. Laugier, Head, Dept. of Dermatology, University of Geneva (see Dorveaux 1915).

171. Sm 101; GMÄ VI 210

172. *Ftt* could not be cotton, for the plant did not reach Egypt from India until much later, being first mentioned in papyri of the second century A.D. (LH 147). When used as a contraceptive, the pad of *ftt* was duly enriched: in one case with a salve based on honey and three pounded plants; in another with crocodile dung (GMÄ IV/1 277).

173. Sm 316

174. It is impossible to tell which *mrht* (animal fat or vegetable oil) was meant in each case (GMÄ VI 250–279; Sm 100). Grapow prefers to translate each time "Fett/Oel." Of the twenty-two known animal varieties, goose grease is one of the commonest; cats, fish, crocodiles, and snakes provide their share.

175. Lefebvre 1956 p. 13

176. The proportion of grease to honey may have been too well-known to mention. Once only in the Ebers papyrus, in a remedy for the ear, "when the vessel (*met*) shivers," it is said: "lint, grease $\frac{2}{3}$, honey [?], apply to it many times" (Eb 766 = GMÄ IV/1 61, IV/2 65). The missing fraction for honey was filled in by Breasted, reasonably enough, as $\frac{1}{3}$ (Sm 101).

177. Lefebvre 1956 p. 62

178. Sethe 1916 p. 74; EG 197

179. In six cases grease alone is recommended; in six others, honey alone (Sm 101).

180. Sm 100

181. Lavie 1960 p. 105. This experiment of Lavie does not mean that bees are sterile; they have a rich intestinal flora (Lavie 1960 p. 105 ff.).

182. Sackett 1919

183. Average composition of 490 honeys: water 17.2%, sugars 79.59%, ash 0.169%. Honey is quite acid: pH 3.91 (White, Riethof and others 1962 p. 11).

184. Dold, Du, and Dziao 1937; Franco and Sartori 1940

185. Sestieri 1956

186. White and others 1962; 1963; 1964; Schepartz and Subers 1964

187. Coulthard and others 1945

188. Lavie 1960; 1963

189. Lavie 1960 p. 165; Villanueva and others 1964; Lindenfelser 1967

190. Gonnet and Lavie 1960; Gonnet 1966

191. Villanueva and others 1964

192. Jensen and Sherman 1951

193. Villanueva and others 1964

194. Yang 1944

195. Weber 1937

196. von Gonzenbach and Hoffmann 1936

197. Zaiss 1934; Spöttel 1950; Bulman 1955; Blomfield 1973. Published data on the use of pure honey on wounds are not very critical, and a well-controlled experiment is still missing. However, the procedure seems to be harmless, and reports of successful treatment of ulcers continue to appear. We tried to apply pure honey on wounds in guinea pigs: on the whole, the healing was somewhat delayed, but the experiment was unsatisfactory for technical reasons (the difficulty of keeping honey on the wound without using a stiff corset that interferes with the experiment).

198. For these bacteriological tests I am indebted to H. L. Wildasin, Ph. D., Director of Laboratories and Quality Control, H. P. Hood & Sons, Boston, Mass., and to Messrs. F. Bridges, F. Hubbard, and A. Frazer, also at H. P. Hood & Sons. Details of the experiments quoted are given in the notes to Figs. 3.27 and 3.28.

199. Lefebvre 1956 p. 113

200. Lavie 1963, 1968 p. 109

201. Simpson 1967 pp. 12, 31

202. In this account I made an arbitrary choice. The letter from Milkili is addressed to "The King," which could have been either Amenophis III or IV. I chose the son, because it was he who built the new capital at El Amarna. But anyway, as far as the episode is concerned, they were both married to the same woman, perhaps Nefertiti (Daumas 1965 p. 90), and the El Amarna letters show that they *both* received myrrh from Tushratta as a wedding gift!

203. Knudtzon 1964 I 833; Mercer 1939 II 681

204. Knudtzon 1964 II 1325

205. LH 316

206. Knudtzon 1964 I 189, 221

207. Dixon 1969 p. 60

208. GMÄ VI 99–104

209. GMÄ VI 452

210. Eb 529; GMÄ IV/1 204

211. Eb 508; GMÄ IV/1 219

212. GMÄ II 13 ff.

213. GMÄ III 94

214. Sm 203

215. This incantation and the following (Eb 1 and 2) are retranslated from the German version of GMÄ IV/1 308 and IV/2 231. The translation is literal almost to the word. Figure of Isis: from an illustration in the Papyrus of Ani (c. 1250 B.C.; about half actual size). By permission of the Trustees of the British Museum, London.

216. EB 499 = GMÄ IV/1 215, IV/2 165. Figures of Thoth and Horus: from an illustration in the Papyrus of Anhai (c. 1150 B.C.; about half actual size). By permission of the Trustees of the British Museum, London.

217. Ghalioungui 1973 p. 14

218. GMÄ III 94, II 12, 20; Lefebvre 1956 pp. 168–170

219. GMÄ IV/2 232

220. L 37 = GMÄ IV/1 158, IV/2 134

221. The Chester-Beatty VI papyrus is an all-anus treatise; it contains forty-one remedies.

222. CB 61

223. Jonckheere 1947 p. 44

224. Herodotos II 77

225. In Grapow's *Wörterbuch der Ägyptischen Drogennamen* (= GMÄ VI) we counted about 660 drug names. Whether 3, 10, or 30 of these drugs may have had a real pharmacological effect is a moot question. Hidden among them should be the cathartics of which Egyptian soil was, and still is, a generous source. The only one that is reasonably well identified is the *dgm* plant, which should be *Ricinus* (the castor oil plant), but there is also a *kaka* plant that might be it (GMÄ VI 583, 526). *Colocynth* is a small gourd "found in immense quantities in Upper Egypt and Nubia" (Flückiger and Hanbury 1879 p. 295); if it corresponds to *djart*, then it was used in many ways that have nothing to do with its typical action. *Aloes* is not well identified and neither is *senna*, until recently a monopoly of the Egyptian government and source of cathartic acid.

226. *Ukhedu* is written as a plural, but syntactically it is not a plural (personal communication of Dr. R. O. Steuer, the world expert on ukhedu, who very much regrets the disregard of GMÄ, where *ukhedu* is translated as a plural).

227. GMÄ VII/1 215

228. GMÄ IV/1 208; Eb 130

229. GMÄ I 82

230. GMÄ I 21

231. Sm 112

232. GMÄ VII/1 400 ff.; Sm 99

233. GMÄ I 73

234. Eb 856a; GMÄ IV/1 7

235. Bln 163a; GMÄ IV/1 7

236. For an excellent, critical review of embalming and especially of its chemistry, see Lucas and Harris 1962, Ch. 12 pp. 270–326; see also Engelbach and Derry 1942; Jonckheere 1942; Dawson 1927 (old!). For a summary, see Singer and others 1965 I 256–270. For histological studies, see Sandison 1969.

237. Alum is said to be *astringent*. Chemically, this property depends upon protein denaturation; hence the use of alum in leather tanning (known in ancient Egypt, LH 34). Egypt's alum was much praised by the Greeks (Hippocrates refers to it), and very old mines are known (LH 257).

238. LH 303

239. Columella XII 4/LB III 199

240. LH 283

241. Singer and others 1965 I 264

242. LH 272. See also Engelbach and Derry 1942 p. 263

243. LH 493–494, 263 ff.

244. For this formula I am indebted to Prof. P. Favarger.

245. LH 267

246. LH 291

247. LH 282

248. Engelbach and Derry 1942 p. 239

249. Engelbach and Derry 1942 pp. 255, 260

250. LH 293

251. See also LH 275.

252. LH 293

253. LH 309–312

254. LH 308

255. Rosengarten 1969 p. 15

256. LH 316

257. GMÄ VI 388

258. Wilson 1962

259. Toroptsev 1943; Toroptsev and Filatova 1943

260. Nickell 1959 p. 284

261. Cavallito and Bailey 1944; *Merck Index* 1968 p. 33. There is a large literature on onions in medicine, uncritically reviewed by Heyser 1928. Ambroise Paré, advised by "a certaine old countrey woman," treated burns with onions and found them very effective, which is probably worth investigating (Sigerist 1944).

262. Amonkar and Banerji 1971

263. Smith 1914

264. Smith 1912 p. 84

265. LH 324

266. Smith 1912 p. 110

267. Smith 1912 p. 66

268. Daumas 1965 p. 557

269. Smith 1912 p. 60

270. Engelbach and Derry 1942 p. 260

271. Smith 1914 p. 191; Sandison 1969 p. 490. In fairness to the embalmers, though they did not improve on nature's process chemically, they did so "aesthetically" with their artificial eyes, stuffing, etc.; and they certainly reached the goal of preventing the total, unsightly decay of the body laid in a coffin rather than in sand.

272. Neolitzky 1911

273. The mouse as a drug, especially for children, has a long, uninterrupted history down to the present day (Dawson 1924). In Pliny's *Natural History* it is quoted dozens of times (see Schneider's index 1967, *Mures*). Pliny also explains that the flooding of the Nile occasions "a marvel that surpasses them all: that is that, when the river withdraws its covering, water-mice are found with the work of generative water and earth uncompleted—they are already alive in a part of their body, but the most recently formed part of their structure is still of earth" (PNH 9.179/LB III 283).

274. Glob 1965; Wells 1964 p. 59

275. LH 34

276. Smith and Dawson 1924

277. Steuer and Saunders 1959 p. 4

278. For this information I am indebted to Prof. C. Maystre.

279. Sm 224

280. LH 26

281. Josephus, *Antiquities*, XIV 7:4; quoted by Levin 1970 p. 147

282. Another view holds that *ammoniacum* is the gum of an African shrub, which comes in drops gritty with sand, in Greek *ammi* (PNH 12, 107; Dioscorides 3, 98/Gunther 1934 p. 331). Yet another view: Mesopotamian tablets mention a "salt of Amanus," which is the name of a mountain range in northern Syria; this salt (which gave its name to today's *ammoniac* salt) was imported into Egypt, and the resemblance with Amon the god is a coincidence (Jastrow 1917 p. 242 note 55).

283. For some of the theories on the origin of the word *chemistry*, see Skinner 1961 p. 101. The name *Chemía*, "Black Land," for Egypt, is mentioned first by Plutarch (*Moralia*, Isis and Osiris 364c): "they call it so for much of it is black as the black of the eye [*the pupil*]." For a possible Chinese origin of the word, see Mahdihassan references in Ch. 6.

284. The Greek word for papyrus was *byblos*, probably a softened version of *papyrus*, which means that the word *Bible* now contains the word *Pharaoh*. For the spelling of *pa-pr-aa*, I am again indebted to Prof. Maystre.

285. Lewis 1934

286. A persistent legend holds that the modern physicians' symbol ℞ has evolved from the Egyptian symbol for the Horus eye, ℞ (cf. Wall 1917, McCord 1965). I have been unable to find the evidence.

287. Formulas found on tombs and statues (Sm 111 note).

4. The Iatrós

1. These are but a few of the modern medical terms that occur in the Greek text of the Hippocratic Collection. Whether any one was new at the time we do not know, but some at least were recent, because Socrates and Glaucon, in a dialog, agree that "breaths and catarrhs are strange and newfangled names," conjured up by the clever sons of Asklepios for the maladies of decadent citizens (Plato, *Republic*, III p. 405). Several medical terms occur in poetry and literature before Hippocrates (Daremberg 1865; 1869; Dumortier 1935), having possibly originated in common speech (Dumortier 1935; Temkin 1952). In most cases the meaning has remained about the same, but there are notable exceptions: *typhos* was sometimes a form of malaria (LB I p. lviii), *stómachos* rather meant esophagus, and a *thrómbos* in the *artería* could have meant a lump in the windpipe!

2. Phillips 1973 p. 182 ff.; Jones 1946; Cohn-Haft 1956; Sigerist 1961 II 84. The existence of an advanced medical art at the time of the Collection is also proven by the criticism in the Collection itself, where the Hippocratic method is presented as a better variant but not as a radical novelty. For example, the cautery for recurrent luxation of the shoulder was used, but "in the wrong place" (*On Joints*, #11/LB III 223 = LTT IV 107); and even the complicated method shown in Fig. 4.20 for reducing the dislocated femur was already being applied, but sometimes for the "wrong variety" of dislocation (*On Joints*, #77/LB III 381 = LTT IV 309).

3. Xenophon, *Memorabilia*, IV II 10

4. Temkin 1952 p. 213

5. Frölich 1879 p. 58; Albarracín Teulón 1971

6. Il. XI, 828. For the *klisíai* see Frölich 1877. The word *klisía* suggests "a place to lie," hence "barracks" (*klíno*, "I lie"); it has the same root as *clinic*. LS, however, translates it "hut."

7. Il. XI 638

8. Plato, *Republic*, III 406/LB I 273

9. Il. XIV 6

10. Il. XI 829

11. Od. XIX 456. The use of charms for hemostasis continued into the Middle Ages. See the *Strassburger Blutsegen* of the eleventh century "ad stringendum sanguinem" (Ehrismann 1918 p. 102) and the Italian thirteenth-century hemostatic formula: "Sangue sta in te come stette Cristo in sè" (Benedicenti 1947 p. 14).

12. Il. IV 123

13. Il. V 393

14. Il. IV 214

15. Il. XI 844

16. The method of pushing the arrow through (*diosmós*) is not clearly mentioned in the *Iliad* (Frölich 1879 p. 61) but is described by Celsus (CDM VII 5; see also Daremberg 1865 p. 79).

17. This is the informed guess of a famous German pharmacologist (Schmiedeberg 1918 p. 6), but without any real evidence. It is true, though, that the onion has antiseptic properties (Ch. 3).

18. Il. V 795

19. E.g. *On Wounds*, #1/A II 794 = LTT VI 401; see also notes 210 and 223 and pertinent text.

20. Galen, *De antidotis*, I v/K XIV 29–30

21. ChS I 313

22. Sigerist 1961 II 27

23. For references on wounds left undressed see note to Plate 4.3. I could find no reference to the scab as a natural dressing; this, too, is too obvious to put in writing!

24. Il. XIII 599

25. *On Diseases of Women*, II 144/LTT VIII 319

26. The second Homeric passage in which a bandage is mentioned refers simply to "binding up skillfully" (Od. XIX 455–457). Slings *as weapons* are not mentioned in Homer (Frölich 1879 p. 54).

27. Il. IV 190, XI 828, XV 393

28. Il. XI 639, XIV 5

29. Kritikos and Papadaki 1967 p. 30

30. Verdelis 1962

31. Beware of excessive enthusiasm: a poppy capsule slit vertically may be difficult to tell from another popular symbol, the pomegranate (Gabra 1956 p. 40 ff.; Kritikos and Papadaki 1967 p. 30). In some cases there is enough detail to leave no doubt, as in the clay model of Fig. 4.4.

32. Od. IV 221; see also Schmiedeberg 1918 p. 9; Kritikos and Papadaki 1967 p. 18

33. Il. IV 217

34. Daremberg 1865 p. 78

35. See Ackerknecht 1970 p. 5. The sucking out of snakebite wounds is mentioned also in the Talmud (Joma 83[b], Toseft. Sabb. XIV, 14 quoted by Preuss 1894 p. 265).

36. Od. I 261

37. Schmiedeberg 1918 pp. 14–25

38. This passage, actually the first to derive *toxic* from *tóxon*, should be found in Dioscorides Mat. Med. Lib. VI 20 (Lewin 1894 p. 87 and Lammert 1938). However, this book VI is probably not by the real Dioscorides (Lammert 1938). I have been unable to lay my hands on it. Pliny proposes an entirely different derivation of *toxic* from the earlier *taxic*, "the yew," which is a very poisonous tree (PNH 16 51/LB IV 421). The yew, *Taxus baccata*, is still associated with danger and mourning, and its leaves do contain poison, but the idea seems far-fetched.

39. Plato: Protagoras 311 B–C; Phaedrus 270 C-E (LB I xxxiii). Aristotle: *Politics* VII, 4 (1326a).

40. The most accepted view is that a century or so after the death of Hippocra-

tes a collection of scrolls, left over from the books of the medical school at Cos, found its way to the great library of Alexandria. Another and rather unsettling view is that a collection of works was arbitrarily ascribed to Hippocrates by the Alexandrian librarians, and that the only reliable testimonies of the historical Hippocrates are the quotation in Plato's *Phaedrus* and a passage in the *Papyrus Anonymus Londinensis*, written in the second century A.D. (Jones 1947 p. 20). See the excellent chapter in Sigerist (1961 II 260); Phillips 1973 p. 34 ff.; Harris 1973 p. 29 ff.

41. Ever since the earliest commentators the Hippocratic books have been subdivided into categories, from the "likeliest" to the "unlikeliest" writings of the Master himself. Littré recognizes eleven classes! (LTT I 293).

42. Phillips 1973 p. 185; Cohn-Haft 1956 p. 26

43. *In the Surgery*, #3/LB III 59 = LTT III 279

44. *On the Physician*, #1/LB 311 = LTT IX 205

45. *Precepts*, #10/LB I 327 = LTT IX 267

46. *In the Surgery*, #4/LB III 63 = LTT III 285

47. May 1968 I p. 74

48. *In the Surgery*, #10/A II 479 = LTT III 305

49. *In the Surgery*, #3/LB III 61 = LTT III 279

50. A II 469 = LB III 53

51. Allbutt 1905 p. 11

52. *Cheirurgía: On the Physician*, #6/LTT IX 212, etc. *Cheirurgéin: Breaths*, #1/LB II 227 = LTT VI 91, etc. *Cheirurgós*, "he who is working with the hand" (but not a surgeon) appears first in Plutarch, first century A.D. (LS 1986).

53. In piecing together each case and its treatment from several Hippocratic works, I chose to disregard the grading of the various books: after all, the entire set reflects the medical practices of the time. For the kinds of patients that Hippocrates may have received see LTT X xxix # xi.

54. *Epidemics II*, #14/LTT V 115

55. *Aphorisms V*, #23/LB IV 165 = LTT IV 541

56. The Hippocratic principle of not applying cold directly to a wound seems to be right: but the data are still fragmentary. The latest work of Sutor and others (1971) showed only that cold water, when applied over a tiny wound 1 mm wide and 1 mm deep, makes bleeding worse. The effect of cold on the surroundings is not discussed. Cold applied around such small wounds does help a little in hemophiliacs (Sutor and others 1970): it halves the blood loss, and bleeding time drops by about 10%. The effect of cold on *larger* bleeding wounds is still unclear, though chilling is often recommended (lit. in papers above). A satisfactory study should distinguish between hemorrhage from large vessels, capable of contracting, and capillary bleeding, an entirely different matter. Gaping capillaries are rapidly plugged by platelets, and cold prevents platelets from aggregating (Kattlove and Alexander 1970).

57. *Epidemics II*, #17/LTT V 131

58. Theophrastus, *Enquiry into Plants*, IX VIII 2/LB II 255

59. *Epidemics VI*, sect. 7 #2/LTT V 337

60. As always with the Collection, it is not to be taken for granted that this practice (wetting the bandage) was universal. However: "[*The bandages*] will not be applied dry, but wetted with the fluid appropriate to each case" (*In the Surgery*, #11/A II 480 [*translation not accurate*] = LTT III 309). Dipping in black "astringent" wine: *On Fractures*, #29/A II 537 = LTT III 515; *On the Use of Liquids*, #5/LTT VI 129. Affusion of wine on dressings or bandages: *On Joints*, #63/A II 634 ff = LTT IV 269 ff. Bandaging in general: passages too many to quote. See esp. *In the Surgery*, 7–12 and LTT X Index 479 ff. Bande, Bandage.

61. *Regimen in Acute Diseases*, [*App.*] #27/LTT II 515; Dierbach 1824 p. 31

62. Il. V 902–904

63. *On Diseases IV*, #52/LTT VII 591

64. LS 1241

65. *Epidemics II*, #14/LTT V 117

66. *On Joints*, #69/LB III 361 = LTT IV 283; repeated in *Mochlicon*, #35/LB III 433 = LTT IV 379

67. Scribonius Largus (discussed in Ch. 10)

68. Paré 1678 p. 303 (a late English edition)

69. E.g. Harvey 1929; Cope 1958; Michler 1968; Kraft 1970

70. LTT I 293

71. *Epidemics II*, sect. 3#14/LTT V 117

72. *Mochlicon* (or *Instruments of Reduction*) #35/LB III 433 = LTT IV 377. The second statement is almost identical, with small changes in wording. In Littré's edition the meaning emerges clearly: "Quant aux sphacèles des chairs, la compression d'une plaie compliquée d'hémorragie qu'on étreint fortement, dans une fracture trop serrée, et dans d'autres constrictions violentes, fait tomber les parties interceptées chez beaucoup de patients." Littré, however, retouched three words to make the text identical with the similar passage in Mochlicon (LTT IV 282 note 21). The Loeb edition preserves the standard text, and the translation becomes somewhat clouded: "As for gangrene in tissues occurring in wounds with supervening hemorrhage, *or much strangulation* . . . the intercepted parts come away in many cases [*italics mine*]" (*On Joints*, #69/LB III 361 = LTT IV 283). In any event, it is clear that the text in both cases means to convey that gangrene can develop in three situations that have in common excessive compression caused by the physician.

73. *On the Surgery*, #13/LB III 73 = LTT III 317

74. *On the Use of Liquids*, #1/LTT VI 121

75. Water on a wound or sore may seem to contradict the oft-quoted beginning of the treatise *On Wounds*: "Avoid wetting all wounds except with wine, unless they are on a joint. For the dry state is nearer to the sound, and the wet to the unsound" (*On Wounds* #1/A II 794 = LTT VI 401). There are two exceptions already in the injunction, and scores of other passages simply ignore this veto against moist applications. The affusion of warm water was definitely used upon the removal of bandages, as fully explained by Galen (*Meth. Med.* xiv quoted in A II 483 note 1). This is but one of the many irksome contradictions that plague anyone trying to draw a single line of thought from the Hippocratic Collection.

76. *On the Use of Liquids*, #1/LTT VI 119; *Aphorisms V*, #19/LB IV 163 = LTT IV 539

77. *On Wounds*, #15/A II 808 = LTT VI 431

78. *On Wounds*/A II 804 #10 = LTT VI 423 #17

79. *On the Use of Liquids*, #4/LTT VI 129

80. *On the Use of Liquids*, #5/LTT VI 129

81. *Of Places in Man*, #38/LTT VI 329

82. *On the Physician*, #5/LTT IX 211

83. *On Wounds*/A II 802 #7 = LTT VI 417 #14. Enheme suggests "bloody" wounds: presumably fresh wounds, as Celsus writes (CDM V 19 1/LB II 33).

84. *Verdigris* (*iós*): I find it rather disturbing—pharmacologically—that dictionaries define *iós* as "rust on iron, verdigris on copper and bronze" (e.g. LS); but on the authority of Francis Adams (*Paulus Aegineta*, III p. 142), the identity of *iós* with *Aerugo Aeris*, or verdigris, "seems indisputable."

85. "Flower of copper" (*ánthos chalkoū*): first, there is a mistake in Littré's translation; it has *fleur d'argent* (litharge). Littré was obviously misled by the "flower of silver" that actually occurs in the Greek text two lines above. Littré at first defined flower of copper as "grains of copper produced when cold water is thrown on the hot metal ingot" (LTT VI 413 #12; same in Adams 1844–1847 III 404). Later he changed this to copper oxide, adding that the "copper scales" (*lepís* or *pholís chalkoū*) were another form of copper oxide (LTT IX 144; X page L). His authorities: K. Sprengel, Ad Dioscorid. Mat. Med. V, 88; Dioscorid. Mat. Med. V, 89.

86. *Molýbdaina*: Littré translates as *massicot*; Adams, "plumbago." This is a yellow, amorphous lead oxide, which when heated turns into a reddish crystalline lead oxide, litharge. Littré translates the Greek "flowers of silver" (*ánthos argýrou*) as "litharge."

87. Grease of wool (*óisypos*): Dioscorides gives a good account of it: "The greasinesse of unwasht wool is called Oesypum, which you shall prepare thus. Taking soft wool unwasht, (not) scowred with the herbe Sopeweed, wash in hott water,

withall squeesing out all the filth, and casting it into a broade-mouthed vessell, and powring water thereon, pour it from on high back againe with a great spoone, tumbling it downe forcibly till it foame, or with a stick stir it about lustily, till that much & a foul foame be gathered together. Afterwards sprinckle it with sea-water. And when the fat that did swim upon it, is settled, put it into another earthen vessell, & pouring water into the vessell, stirr it about againe . . . And do this, thill there be no more foam standing vpon it, the greasie matter being spent. Then tempering with ye hand ye Oesypum that is gathered, presently, if it haue any filth (remaining vpon) take it away . . . Put to the tongue, it do not bite, but somewhat bind, and it looks fatt, & cleane, & white, & soe put it vp into an earthen vessell . . . But that is best which is not made cleane . . . & is smooth, smelling of unwasht wool . . . Now it hath the power of warming, mollifying & of filling of ulcers, especially of those about the seate . . ." (Dioscorides II 84 / Gunther 1934 p. 112; see also Wulfsberg 1887).

88. Because applying the bandage tight enough to "dry up" the injury was very much in line with the thinking of the time, this had been the accepted interpretation (LTT III 344 ff.), but the scriptures are again sibylline. The statement, "Make most pressure over the lesion and least at the ends," is perfectly explicit; but four paragraphs above, the text reads "pressure . . . less at the ends and least in the middle" (*In the Surgery,* #12/LB III 73 = LTT III 313; #8/LB III 65 = LTT III 295 and note 18). Littré works his way out of the problem with the help of Galen, who also struggles with the riddle and translates very freely as if it were "especially important to avoid *pain* over the middle." Pressure on swellings is also recommended later, where Galen explains that "inflamed" cases are excluded (*In the Surgery,* #21, 22/LB III 77, 79 = LTT III 327 and note 11).

89. *Regimen in Acute Diseases*/LB II 103 #46 = LTT II 321 #12

90. *On Wounds,* #1/A II 794 = LTT VI 401

91. Paré 1678 p. 705

92. A II 797 note 5

93. I owe the turtle analogy to Dr. Hermes Grillo of the Massachusetts General Hospital, Boston (Dr. Grillo referred to two sets of people holding hands and seen from a helicopter). Although there must be some truth to it, the exact translation from turtles to tissues is not yet available.

94. Watts 1960 p. 560

95. Billingham and Russell 1956 p. 967

96. *In the Surgery,* #3/A II 475 = LTT III 279

97. CDM VII 4/LB III 309

98. *On Diseases,* #47/LTT VII 71

99. *Of Places in Man,* #14/LTT VI 307–309

100. *Coan Prenotions,* #424/LTT V 681

101. *On Diseases* II, #47/LTT VII 71; *On Diseases* III, #16/LTT VII 155. This maneuver, succussion, is still used for the diagnosis of hydropneumothorax. Obviously, to hear a splash, the pleural cavity must contain fluid as well as air, which is a rare combination. The entire passage is a marvel of clinical acumen: "If you hear no splash, but the patient breathes with difficulty, his feet are swollen and he has a little cough, do not let yourself be fooled: assuredly his chest is full of pus."

102. *On Diseases* III, #16/LTT VII 155. The clay method was used also to find collections of pus in the abdomen, which were recognized especially by the pain (how true), "but if potter's clay or something similar is applied on the spot, it dries up rapidly" (*On Diseases* I, #17/LTT VI 171). Celsus misunderstood the method (Ch. 9). A similar one is found in the Sushruta Samhita.

103. *On Diseases* II, #47/LTT VII 71. My translation, using Littré (VII 71) and Lund (1935) as guidelines.

104. "Tent" and "drain" in my translation correspond to one and the same Greek term, μοτός (*motós*), and to the corresponding verb μοτοῦν. Any item of dressing that went into a wound was called a *motós*; it was then specified whether the dressing was of linen, raw linen, etc. It would be tempting to translate the word as "drain," but not knowing what effect the physician had in mind when he introduced

the piece of linen, I twice use the old surgical term *tent*, which has exactly the same meaning as *motós*. Littré, who did the same, could not have used the term *drainage* anyway, because he published his Vol. VII in 1851, a couple of years too early to hear Chassaignac use that new surgical term (Rochard 1875 p. 780). However, the third time the text leaves no doubt as to the purpose of draining: "when the pus is fluid [enough] introduce a *kassiterínon kóilon motón* [*hollow motós of tin*]." This is clearly a tube, and the sense must be a drain.

105. Dr. Margaret Pittman of Harvard Medical School remembered injecting an oily preparation called *Gomenol* (Martindale 1958 p. 631).

106. *Regimen in Acute Diseases*, LB II 57 = LTT II 224.

107. *On Diseases I*, #21/LTT VI 181

108. *On Diseases II*, #47/LTT VII 71; ibid. #61 p. 97

109. Aeschines, *Speeches: Against Timarchus*, 41/LB 37.

110. *Pleurá* or *pleurón* (generally "flank," also of an army) was also used for "ribs." What is now called pleura is a microscopically thin membrane, which the Greeks could not possibly have recognized as a separate entity (Souques 1937 *31* p. 183).

111. The ending *-itis* to mean "inflamed" was a gradual, largely modern development. In classical Greek it had mostly a technical connotation: *ampelítis* = "concerning the upkeep of the vine (*ámpelon*);" *pharmakítis* = "concerning drugs (*phármaka*)" (Chantraine 1933 p. 340). For the veins *hepatítis* and *splenítis* see e.g. *On Diseases I*, #26/LTT VI 195. Ophthalmítis was the epithet for Athena as moon goddess (LS, *ophthalmitis*).

112. After Hippocrates, auscultation was forgotten. Hence, this now famous passage lost its meaning, was incorrectly transcribed, and finally became unintelligible. It was Littré who restored it (LTT VII 1–3, 1851) because he knew about auscultation, which had been rediscovered by Laënnec thirty-two years before (Laënnec 1819).

113. *On Diseases II*, #59/LTT VII 93

114. The assembling procedure of the *sýrinx* or "syringe" is described in detail only once (*On Sterile Women III*, #222/LTT VIII 431), where the bladder was definitely filled through a second opening, as in Heister's model of 1718 (Fig. 4.16); but I have seen medieval representations showing just a bag with a tube emerging from a single opening.

115. Lund 1935 p. 536; Souques 1937 p. 185; Baffoni 1943; Sharpe 1962 p. 185; Bourgey 1953 p. 158; Littré missed it too: LTT VII 1–3.

116. Anatomy in the Hippocratic Collection is, on the whole, the kind that could be learned from the kitchen, the sacrificial altar, the battlefield (Sigerist 1961 II 277), and a study of nudes. Systematic dissection did not begin until about a century later in Alexandria (see Edelstein 1935). One baffling exception is the treatise *On the Heart* (LTT IX 76 ff.; Hurlbutt 1939; Leboucq 1944) which seems to suggest the dissection of a human heart, possibly in Greek Sicily, 400–340 B.C.

117. *On the Nature of Women*, #14/LTT VII 333

118. *On Diseases III*, #14/LTT VII 137. This interpretation of the "fallen lung" is my own; it comes from reading Hippocrates with the eyes of a pathologist. The recoiling of the lung is an everyday observation in the autopsy room. One modern commentator (Baffoni 1943) prefers to read the passage as if the iatrós had fitted the air bag itself into the wound, like a plug, the best "evidence" for this being a modern inflatable rubber gadget, shaped like an hourglass, and used as a plug. I reject this interpretation on several grounds: it is technically unlikely; it makes difficult to understand the final step of introducing a solid plug of tin; it fails to explain the fallen lung and hence the reason to blow air into the chest; and it ignores the two other techniques based on blowing air into the body.

119. *Epidemics IV*, #11/LTT V 151

120. Wine for wounds could be red or white. Both wine and vinegar were often used on wounds (LTT X Index 842, *Vin, Vinaigre*).

121. *On Wounds*, A II 797 #2 = LTT VI 405 #4

122. *On Wounds*, #1/A II = LTT VI 403

123. *On Diseases II*, #36/LTT VII 53

124. *On Wounds*/A II 796 #1; 796 #3 = LTT 405 #2; 409 #10

125. Cignozzi 1690 pp. 108–110

126. *In the Surgery*, #7/LB III 65 = LTT III 293

127. *In the Surgery*, #8/LB III 65 = LTT III 295–297 and note 6; Benedum 1970 pp. 53, 55

128. *On Joints*, #35/LB III 265 = LTT IV 159

129. *On Diseases II*, #10/LTT VI 159

130. *On the Physician*, #4/LTT IX 211

131. *On Wounds*/A II 796 #2 = LTT VI 405 #3

132. von Grot 1887 pp. 31–38

133. Hydromel (honey boiled in water) and oxymel (honey and vinegar) were popular refreshing drinks (Sigerist 1961 II 216). Their merits are discussed at length in *Regimen in Acute Diseases*. In hydromel, the proportion of honey could vary from $\frac{1}{3}$ to $\frac{1}{9}$ (A I 299 note 1).

134. *On Affections*, #55/LTT VI 267. For anti-cheese remarks in Hippocrates, see LTT X 615, *Fromage*. Plato joined the chorus, as we saw earlier. Perhaps the opposition to cheese was also a matter of "delicate digestions of at least a great number of otherwise quite normal Greeks" (Jones 1946 p. 74).

135. *On Fractures*, #26/LB III 155 = LTT III 505

136. Actual sutures are mentioned only twice: once on the nose after the nostril has been slit to extract a polyp (*On Diseases II*, #36/LTT VII 53); once in the general statement that purging is good for wounds which require suture (*On Wounds* /A II 796 #2 = LTT VI 405 #3), obviously in the hope of fighting off suppuration. A third instance concerns stitches placed in the upper eyelid when it is abnormally folded inward (*trichiasis*; *Regimen in Acute Diseases* (*Appendix*), #29/LTT II 517). A transverse fold of the skin is stitched at its base. The method was said to work after a fashion (Anagnostakis 1872 p. 4).

137. I owe this information to Dr. John P. Remensnyder, Department of Surgery, Massachusetts General Hospital, Boston.

138. The bench is described twice in the Collection (see LTT X xii). There is no proof that Hippocrates invented it; but the idea caught on. Five centuries later there were at least seven models, and Celsus noted that they could "rupture the ligaments and muscles" (*De medicina*, VIII 20/LB III 577). In 1924 a real specimen of the *scamnum* was found, in a monastery tucked away in the mountains of central Italy, where it was used as a refectory table. It is now at the Wellcome Museum in London. Its date is uncertain, perhaps early 1500s, by which time it had become almost entirely obsolete (Thompson 1925; D' Arcy Power 1925).

139. *On Joints*, #3/LB III 205 = LTT IV 83

140. *On Joints*, #11/LB III 223 = LTT IV 107

141. *On Joints*, #11/LB III 223 = LTT IV 107

142. *On Joints*, #11/LB III 229 = LTT IV 113

143. Cignozzi 1690 pp. 254–257

144. *Epidemics V*, #16/LTT V 215

145. *On Wounds in the Head*, #10/LB III 21 = LTT III 213

146. *On Wounds in the Head*, #14/LB III 35 ff. = LTT III 235 ff.

147. *On Diseases II*, #13/LTT VII 25

148. The salve probably *was* cobbler's blacking, because for the same operation, Celsus prescribes just that: *atramentum sutorium*. It was made with green vitriol or ferrous sulphate mixed with oak bark or galls. In medicine it had several uses, including the treatment of wounds. It was supposed to be caustic and hemostatic (Spencer 1961 p. xvi, *Aes*; PNH/LB IX 210 note a).

149. A I 440. Greek physicians were very worried about humors seeping into the skull. This seems to be the reason that wounds in the head were left without a bandage, i.e. without compression (*On Wounds in the Head*, #13/A I 457 = LTT III 231): they felt that pressure on a bone could not help to wring out its bad humors and might even push them inward, so it was better to let them ooze out freely (Galen quoted by Cocchi 1754 quoted in LTT III xxx). Trepanation for skull contusions died away in the nineteenth century, although in 1849 Adams tried hard to defend it (see A I 431–442).

150. *On Wounds in the Head*, #21/LB 49 = LTT III 259

151. Theophrastus, *Enquiry into Plants*, V IX 6–7/LB I 473

152. *Epidemics V*, #16/LTT V 217

153. *On Wounds in the Head*, #21/LB 49 = LTT III 259

154. *Epidemics V*, #16/LTT V 217

155. *On Diseases II*, #61/LTT VII 95

156. This historic passage is the clearest of the two that mention auscultation (*On Diseases II*, #61/LTT VII 95; #59 p. 93). Laënnec, who rediscovered auscultation, was an expert on Hippocratic medicine and did acknowledge the priority of Hippocrates (though quite lefthandedly), but he adds that he had forgotten about it before making his discovery.

157. *Prognostic*, #1/LB II 7 = LTT II 111

158. *On Internal Affections*, #23/LTT VII 227

159. Urinoscopy, as this kind of inspection came to be called, played an important role in Greek medicine. The basic idea was right—that urine reflects happenings in the body—but the practice was mostly nonsense (see e.g. LTT X 826).

160. LB II 229 #2 = LTT VI 93

161. *Regimen in Acute Diseases (Appendix)*, #9 = LTT II 443

162. Ginsburg 1965

163. LTT VII 94 note 7; Laënnec 1819 II 118–119 note a

164. Siegel 1964 p. 293

165. Boiling vinegar occurs e.g. in our case 7 (*On Wounds in the Head*, #14/LB III p. 33 = LTT III 237).

166. Gardiner 1930 pp. 99–116

167. Gardiner 1930 pp. 197–211

168. Plato, *The Laws*, VIII p. 830

169. *On Joints*, #39/LB III 275 = LTT IV 171

170. *On Joints*, #35–39/LB III 265–275 = LTT IV 159–173

171. After the Egyptian fluff (or *ftt*, Ch. 3), this seems to be the world's first mention of *charpie* or lint, which was to become a standard dressing (and source of infection) for millennia. Adams translated the passage, "caddis scraped from a linen towel." The Greek text has "*áchne* [anything that comes off a surface, also chaff] from a *hemitýbion* [a stout linen cloth, actually an Egyptian word]." Cotton, an Indian good, was known but had not yet spread west as far as Greece (LH 147–8). Although wool was handier, it became customary to procure fluff for dressings by the peculiar procedure of scraping cloth.

172. Cerney 1963 p. 354

173. Krause 1841 p. 517

174. Aristophanes, *Fragm.* 98

175. Plato, *Protagoras*, 342–5; see also Dodds 1959 p. 357. Several specimens of broken ears are preserved in sculpture, including, it is said, one of the two colossi, Castor and Pollux, on the Capitol (Winckelmann 1808 p. 430 ff.; 1811 pp. 210–218; Krause 1841 p. 516–518; for ref. in classical literature see LTT IV 332–333). An equivalent of the modern expression "cauliflower ears" may have been the "ear mushrooms" of Tertullian (*De spectaculis* XXIII 7).

176. According to Galen, *syrmaisms* were mild means of evacuation "from above as well as from below" (LTT IV 174 note 3).

177. Gardiner 1930 p. 204

178. Whibley 1963 p. 513

179. *On Wounds*/A II 807 #13 = LTT VI 420 #23

180. *On Fractures*, #28/LB III 161 = LTT III 28

181. *On Affections*, #38/LTT VI 249

182. *Aphorisms I*, #22/LB IV 109 = LTT IV 469. See also LTT X 713, *Orgasme*.

183. This celery crown must have been exceedingly perishable, for the *sélinon* that I picked in Selinunte was already fading after ten minutes. There is some evidence that it was still used in the first century A.D., when the Apostle Paul was in Corinth; perhaps this was the "perishable wreath" of which he wrote (I Cor. 9:25; Broneer 1962 p. 16).

184. *On Affections*, #38/LTT VI 249

185. *On the Physician*, #11/LTT IX 217

186. *On Wounds*/A II 808 #13 = LTT VI 429 #23. The Greek has *spodón*, "ashes"; see also note 241.

187. *On Wounds*/A II 796 #1 = LTT VI 405 #2

188. *On Affections*, #38/LTT VI 249, 248.

189. Gardiner 1930; Whibley 1963

190. Jones 1946 p. 41

191. Jones 1946 pp. 28–31

192. *Airs Waters Places* #8/LB I 91 = LTT II 33. Among the fuzzy Hippocratic experiments, the shining exception are the observations on the embryos of "twenty or more hen's eggs given to hatch to two or more hens" (*On the Nature of the Child*, #29/LTT VII 531). Partial reviews of experiments in Hippocratic books: Senn 1929; Bourgey 1953. For rational versus scientific medicine see also Harris 1973 p. 30.

193. Edelstein 1952 p. 307; Joly 1966

194. Jaeger 1944 pp. 30 and 298 note 73; *Epidemics VI*, Sect. 5 #5, LTT V 317

195. Daremberg, see Kitto 1951 p. 190

196. No explicit statement of the doctrine of the four humors exists in the Collection, where definitions altogether are rare. It was Galen who gave it its full formulation and ascribed it to Hippocrates, which is not necessarily correct (Sigerist 1961 II 317 ff.; Bourgey 1953; LB I xlvi-liii; Schöner 1964).

197. *On Diseases IV*, #51/LTT VII 585

198. *On Diseases IV*, #52/LTT VII 591

199. The golden section refers to the division of a segment into two unequal parts in such a way that the ratio of the larger part to the whole is the same as of the smaller to the larger (1:1.618). The solution to the problem, which can be expressed $a:x = x:(a - x)$, is found in Euclid's *Elements* (third century B.C.). During the Renaissance the proportion was recognized as a key to Greek aesthetics (Ghyka 1931). The relations between the golden section and a pentagon are many. For example, in a regular pentagon *abcde*, if points *a* and *c* are connected, the segments *ab* and *ac* will be related as 1:1.618 (courtesy of Jacques Vicari).

200. The Greeks had three seasons until about 450 B.C., when summer and autumn were separated. Perhaps the separation of black bile and yellow bile was a similar process (Müri 1953; Sigerist 1961 II 334 note 13). For the "fourfold symmetry" in antiquity see Schöner 1964.

201. Schöner 1964 p. 100

202. Plato, *Gorgias*, 464-B

203. For the theory of residues see note 283.

204. I take full responsibility for this reconstruction. It seems to hold together, although it was difficult to assemble because the pieces are scattered over many books. As usual, the Collection takes much knowledge for granted and does not furnish explanations. The reader should keep in mind that these mechanisms of diseases were certainly not the only ones, for doctrines were loose, and different interpretations were possible and even compatible.

205. *The Art*, #11/LB II 209 = LTT VI 21

206. The nerves would be discovered by the Alexandrians. In the Collection, both *néuron* and *ténon* mean "tendon." There may be vague hints of nerves in such statements as "fire is inimical to *néura*" in cauterizing the armpit, where the problem is really the nerve plexus (*On Joints*, #11/LB III 229 = LTT IV 113). But there is an awfully large gap between the "two tendons coming from the brain" (*Epidemics IV*, #2/LTT V 125) and the statement that Hippocrates "gave a crude description of the sympathetic trunk" (Garrison 1969 p. 8).

207. On blood turning into pus: after injury, blood flows to the part and in time becomes pus (*On Diseases IV*, #50/LTT VII 583); clots of blood left in a bloodletting incision cause inflammation and suppuration (*On Wounds*/A II 809 #16 [*thrómbos* = clot] = LTT VI 431 #26); blood spilled into the belly becomes pus (*On Diseases I*, #17/LTT VI 171); if blood spills into a cavity, it must become pus (*Aphorisms VI*, #20/LB IV 185 = LTT IV 569); blood spilled into the lung decays;

the patient spits out pus (*On Diseases I*, #14/LTT VI 163); wound in the chest; blood decays and is expectorated as pus (phlegm does too) (*On Diseases I*, # 15/ LTT VI 167).

208. Galen, quoted in LTT V 569 note 7

209. Spasms played an important role among the symptoms to observe (*spasm* alone has over one-hundred entries in Littré's Index). There was also a vague term *tà spasmódea*, which can only be translated "spastic accidents" (e.g. *Epidemics VII*, #35/LTT V 402, 405). I suspect that cramps observed during gymnastics, which was a central feature of daily life, must have helped to focus attention on "spasms," but I found no text to support this idea.

210. Cold causing spasms: on certain wounds wine causes spasm if too cold (*On Joints*, #63/LB III 353 = LTT IV 271); cold makes blood become denser and causes veins to contract (*On Diseases I*, #24/LTT VI 189); cold makes veins taut (*On Places in Man*, #9/LTT VI 293; also *Aphorisms V*, #17, 20/LB IV 161, 163 = LTT IV 539). Some of these thoughts may reflect experience with severe frostbite (as mentioned in *On the Use of Liquids*, #1/LTT VI 121). For cold on wounds especially see note 223.

211. Spasms by bleeding (convulsions): e.g. the aphorism—*Spasmós* or hiccough supervening on a copious flux of blood is a bad sign (*Aphorisms V*, #3/LB IV 159 = LTT IV 533; see also *Aphorisms VII*, #9/LB IV 195 = LTT IV 581).

212. Spasms from purging were of course the convulsions of hellebore: see e.g. *Aphorisms V*, #1 and 4, where spasms from hellebore or excessive purging are dangerous (LB IV 159/LTT IV 533; see also *Aphorisms VII* #25/LB IV 197/LTT IV 583).

213. *On Diseases I*, #17/LTT VI 171

214. *Of Places in Man*, #9/LTT VI 239

215. *On Diseases I*, #26/LTT VI 195

216. Fatigue as a cause of disease: fatigue causes venules to break (*On Diseases I*, #14/LTT VI 163); fatigue causes blood to become fixed where the strain is greater, causing *pléthos*, "plethora" (*On Diseases IV*, #50/LTT VII 583); fatigue or gymnastics can cause a rupture, the blood is retained and decays (*On Diseases I*, #15/LTT VI 167; the rupture must be of a vessel, not to be confused with the "erup-tion" of lung abscesses as discussed in LTT V 576–579); fatigue is listed with heat, cold, etc., as a cause of disease (*On Diseases I*, #2/LTT VI 143).

217. *On Diseases I*, #17/LTT VI 171

218. *On Diseases I*, #14/LTT VI 163

219. *Epidemics V*, sect. 3 #11/LTT V 297, 298 note 2, 45

220. Majno and others 1969

221. *On the Use of Liquids*, #2/LTT VI 125

222. *On the Use of Liquids*. #2/LTT VI 123. In the text "tétanoi" is a plural, because tetanus was considered merely as a type of spasm (with three varieties), not a specific disease.

223. See also: cold on open fractures can cause chills, spasms, ulcers (*On Fractures*, #34/LB III 179 = LTT III 537); after cauterizing the armpit, hold the arm close to keep the wounds warm (*On Joints*, #11/LB III 229 = LTT IV 113).

224. *On Wounds in the Head*, #13/A I 457 = LTT III 233 also: the swelling around a wound is due to condensed blood (*On Diseases IV*, #50/LTT VII 583); after injury, blood flows to the part (*On Diseases IV*, #50/LTT VII 583); blood gathers at the site of pain (*On the Nature of Man*, #11/LTT VI 61).

225. When the surgeon Francis Adams translated this passage in 1849, he still approved of the treatment and regretted that in his time too many colleagues "stopped the flow of blood as quickly as possible" (*On Wounds* /A II 796 #1 [note 1] = LTT VI 403 #2).

226. *On Fractures*, #26/A II 535 = LTT III 507

227. *On Diseases IV*/LTT VII 583

228. The only English word that comes close to covering both wound and ulcer is *sore*. Classical Greek also had the word *tróma* or *tráuma* (which gave today's trauma), referring to wounds caused by external violence; it had nothing to do with the subsequent clinical course and merely suggested the cause. Thus, the treatise on

"*Trómata* in the head" was translated by Adams "Injuries in the Head" (A I 421). The word *tróma* is not used by Homer; before Hippocrates it occurs in Aeschylos; and Herodotos uses it in the sense of "disaster" (Hist. I 18). In modern Greek *trávma* and *hélkos* have come to mean "wound" and "ulcer." *Hélkos* and the Latin *ulcus*, "ulcer," come from the same Indoeuropean root ELK-, "wound, tear" (Devoto 1966 p. 444).

229. Cignozzi 1690 p. 15

230. *Ichór* was also—rather surprisingly—the blood of the gods.

231. *Aphorisms VII*, #44/LB IV 203 = LTT IV 591; *Prognostic*, #7/LB II 19 = LTT II 131, and *passim*

232. *On Wounds in the Head* #11/A I 454 = LTT III 221; #15/A I 461 =LTT III 245; *On Fractures*, #26/A II 535 = LTT III 505

233. *On Wounds*/A II 798 #3 = LTT VI 409 #10

234. *Aphorisms V*, #66/LB IV 179 = LTT IV 561; also in *Epidemics II*, LTT V 119 #18

235. It was standard surgical belief—from Hippocrates to the 1860s—that "suppuration prevents inflammation," which makes no sense in today's terms, because suppuration is in fact a form of inflammation. What was meant, on the clinical level, was that abundant suppuration (typically due to staphylococci) usually happened in wounds that did not develop more threatening complications, such as a "spreading inflammation" (typically due to streptococci). The underlying truth was that staphylococci are not as dangerous as streptococci. Adams wrote as late as 1849, "every person acquainted with practice is aware that a healthy suppuration is one of the best means of preventing inflammation" (A II 795 note k). Of course, there was little hope of replacing one type of infection with another, but it remained a Hippocratic principle to "oppose inflammation and favor suppuration" (*On Fractures* #31/LB III 175 = LTT III 531).

236. For *apóstasis* see Bourgey 1953 p. 240.

237. E.g. take the wound as fast as possible through suppuration (*On Wounds in the Head*, #15, 17/A I 461, 462 = LTT III 245, 251; see also *On Fractures*, #26/LB III 157 = LTT II 505).

238. Beware: in Adams' translation this drug does just the opposite: it *prevents* inflammation (*On Wounds*/A II 801 #5). Adams was a busy surgeon, whereas Littré, whose translation came ten years later, was a full-time scholar. It is wiser to follow Littré (ibid. /LTT VI 415 #12). But worse has yet to come, for in Adams this paragraph ends with the sentence: "These things in powder prevent recent wounds from suppurating." This is baffling, because they are not powders, but the general sense seems to confirm a pus-preventing action of the drugs described in the preceding paragraph. Now in Littré's version, the same sentence begins the next paragraph (LTT VI 417 #13), where the drugs discussed are actual powders. Thus, Adams had transformed into pus-preventing all the drugs in the preceding paragraph, which he had to do to achieve consistency, but the result is a mess. Littré's version makes much more sense.

239. *Téresis tou hélkous* (Gärtner 1966)

240. The text also mentions different combinations of these powders, plus a vegetable powder, *aristolochia*. It is striking that all inorganic salts (antiseptics?) should be mentioned together (*On Wounds*/A II 802 #7 = LTT VI 417 #13).

241. The translation of *spodium* (lit. "ashes") is difficult; I chose zinc oxide. Here the text reads *spódoi* from Cyprus, which Littré rendered "ashes of copper," Adams "copper recrement" (a vague word, by which he did not mean slag). Often the text has only *spodium*, which Littré maintained as "ashes of copper," Adams as his noncommittal "spodium" (e.g., *On Wounds*/A II 808 #13 = LTT VI 429 #23). Adams (*Paulus Aegineta*, III 352) believed that the spodium of later authors was impure zinc oxide, whereas in the Collection the word was used more generally "for various recrements of the metals."

242. *Chalcitis* is an impure form of copper sulphate, formed by evaporation of the water of copper mines (Adams, *Paulus Aegineta*, III 399–404; see also Grot 1887 p. 58).

Notes to pages 183–185

243. The enhemes were *chemically* antiseptic, but whether they did any good on wounds I do not know. I tried one on rats, with bad results: but the dose may have been excessive.

244. *On Wounds*/A II 802 #7 = LTT VI #14. Quantities of each drug are not given, as usual. Another moist enheme of this series was described in the case of the round ulcer.

245. *On Diseases II*, #33–37/LTT VII 51

246. Singer and others 1965 I p. 565

247. Spencer 1961 p. xxiii; Bailey 1929 I p. 209

248. Kass and Sossen 1959

249. Phillips and others 1968

250. Price 1939 p. 537

251. Ribéreau-Gayon and Peynaud 1961 p. 135

252. Draczynski 1951 p. 26

253. Stucky 1949

254. Ribéreau-Gayon and Peynaud 1961 p. 145

255. The experiments were carried out by Dr. D. Kekessy of the Institut d'Hygiène, University of Geneva. For the samples of Greek wine, I am much indebted to Isabelle Joris and Lise Piguet, who brought them from Crete, and to Dimitrios Nevrakis, who supplied them.

256. Ribéreau-Gayon and Peynaud 1961 p. 136

257. Draczynski 1951 pp. 26, 40

258. Ribéreau-Gayon and Peynaud 1961 p. 124 ff.

259. Masquelier and Jensen 1953 p. 107

260. Ribéreau-Gayon and Peynaud 1961 p. 142

261. Draczynski 1951 p. 37

262. Ribéreau-Gayon and Peynaud 1961 pp. 139, 143

263. Draczynski 1951 p. 32; Ribéreau-Gayon and Peynaud 1961 p. 137

264. Ribéreau-Gayon and Peynaud 1961 p. 145

265. Masquelier and Jensen 1953 pp. 106–107. In the experiment just quoted, the bacteria were still sensitive to phenol at 3.33 g/l, to oenidol at 0.1 g/l.

266. Both the history and the effects of the two hellebores overlap in a most confusing manner. The Collection mentions hellebore 69 times, but adds "black" only 13 times, "white" only 3 times (Schmiedeberg 1918 p. 19 note 77). The "black" kind, *Helleborus*, still mentioned in some pharmacopoeias (Dorvault 1936; Hagers 1958), is practically extinct as a drug. *Veratrum* alkaloids enjoyed a brief revival a few years ago, just in time for the second edition of Goodman and Gillman's textbook, but slumped again in the third (Goodman and Gillman 1965 p. 716): it proved too difficult to use them to lower the blood pressure without unpleasant side effects. In Germany *Veratrum* is called *Nieswurz*, "sneezing root." When Castiglioni wrote in 1935, sneezing powder of *Nieswurz* was still sold in Germany; elsewhere "hellebore" had retreated to the level of a pesticide (Dierbach 1824; Flückiger and Hanbury 1879; Schmiedeberg 1918 pp. 14–25; Castiglioni 1935; Belloni 1956).

267. See e.g. the aphorism: "Convulsion after hellebore, deadly" (*Aphorisms V*, #1/LB IV 159 = LTT IV 533; see also LTT X Index 628, *Hellébore*; 806, *Superpurgation*). The mechanism of spasms caused by *Veratrum* is now well known and physiologically very interesting (Goodman and Gilman 1965 p. 716 ff.).

268. Schmiedeberg 1918 p. 23

269. Quoted by Pliny: PNH 25.58/LB VII 179

270. *On Ancient Medicine*/LB I 17 #8/LTT I 575

271. *On Ancient Medicine*/LB I 25 #8/LTT I 587. This passage is rather garbled.

272. *Regimen in Acute Diseases*/LB II = LTT II

273. On Greek diet and its evolution, see Ackerknecht 1970, 1971

274. Herrmann and Woodward 1972.

275. *On Joints*, #69 = LTT IV 283/A II 639

276. *On Joints*, #69 = LTT IV 283/A II 639

277. *On the Nature of Women*, #108/LTT VII 423, and elsewhere.

278. See LTT X Index 692, *Miel*.

279. See LTT X Index 572, *Egypte*.

280. Saunders 1963

281. On the fixation of humors: phlegm and bile, see e.g. *On Affections*, #16/LTT VI 225; *On Hemorrhoids*, #1/LTT VI 437; phlegm, *On Fistulae* #7/LTT VI 455.

282. Concept of *fixation* in Egyptian pathology: the dreaded ukhedu could become "fixed" in the blood of the eye (Steuer 1948 p. 16). Various diseases could become "fixed" in one part of the body or another (GMÄ III 30). Sometimes they are "not yet fixed," e.g. Eb 193 (GMÄ IV/1 90), where feces are not yet fixed, or Eb 593 (GMÄ IV/1 157), where a prescription is given for removing a "blood-nest" that has not yet attached itself (repeated in *Papyrus Hearst* 143; GMÄ IV/1 157).

283. For the theory of residue (*períttoma*) see Sigerist 1961 II 262 ff.; for its possible connection with the ukhedu see Steuer and Saunders 1959. The Collection never mentions this theory. Besides Aristotle, the main source is the *Papyrus Anonymus Londinensis* of the second century A.D. Concerning possible connections between Egyptian and Greek surgery there is also a paper by Iversen comparing "Wounds in the Head in Egyptian and Hippocratic Medicine" (1953). Since the author seems to have misunderstood the meaning of *hédra* (assumed to be a hole in the skull, "like a puncture in a jar"), and since the paper is largely about the hedra, little can be gleaned from this study.

284. Translations are my own, based on Littré, and checked against the Greek with the precious aid of Mrs. Martine Vodoz. Some cases were recently summarized in Phillips 1973 pp. 70–71.

285. *Epidemics V*, #96/LTT V 257; repeated in *Epidemics VII*, #34/LTT V 403, where the names become Aydellos and Dyschytas

286. *Epidemics V*, #98/LTT V 257; repeated in *Epidemics VII*, #29/LTT V 401

287. *On Sevens*/LTT VIII 616

288. *Epidemics V*, #61/LTT V 241

289. *Epidemics V*, #21/LTT V 221

290. *Epidemics V*, #32, 33, 35/LTT V 231

291. *Epidemics VI*, sect. 8 #26/LTT V 353

292. LB I 141

293. *Epidemics IV*, #11/LTT V 151

294. *Epidemics V*, #26/LTT V 225

295. *Epidemics V*, #97/LTT V 257

296. *Epidemics VII*, #35/LTT V 403

297. *Epidemics VII*, #113/LTT V 461, repeated with slight change in *Epidemics V*, #100/LTT V 257. The word *siegón*, translated as "jaw," might also mean "cheek." A rapidly progressing gangrene of the mouth, cheek, and jaw, usually fatal, is well known under the ancient term *noma*; it occurs most frequently in children debilitated by infectious disease or by malnutrition. The banquets of the ancient rich are well known, but not the meals of the people at large, except that some Greeks ate only once a day (*On Ancient Medicine*, #10/LB I 29 = LTT I 591; Jones 1946 p. 74 note).

298. *Epidemics V*, #45, 46/LTT V 235. This is a remarkable passage: in the Collection arteries and veins are in a highly confused state (see e.g. LTT X 489, *Artères*; Fredrich 1899 p. 57 ff.). One case of *artería* is a definite trachea (*On the Nature of Bones*, #13/LTT IX 185), but in the treatise *On the Heart* there is reference to real arteries (LTT IX 91 #11). In another case the trachea is called *brónchos* and its branches are *artería* (*On Places in Man*, #14/LTT VI 303–305); in yet another the aorta becomes "the hollow vein" and all its branches are veins (*On the Flesh*; Fredrich 1899 p. 70). At this stage one wonders how to take the startling promise of "another book" in which "the communications between arteries and veins will be discussed in detail" (*On Joints*, #45/LB III 289 = LTT IV 191).

299. *Epidemics V*, #95/LTT V 255

300. PNH 77:198/LB III 557

301. *On the Sacred Disease*/LB II 181 #20 = LTT VI 393 #17; *On Virgins*, #1/LTT VIII 469

302. *Epidemics V*, #47/LTT V 235

303. Opisthótonos, which is a symptom of tetanus, was considered to be a disease of its own; or rather, one of three kinds of tetanus: tetanus from wounds; opisthotonos, which happens "when the tendons in the back of the neck are ill" (*On Internal Affections*, #53/LTT VII 301); and tetanus that occurs by falling on the back of the head (convulsions due to cerebellar injury?) (*On Internal Affections*, #52–54/LTT VII 299–303). The treatment for "tetanus and opisthotonos" is warmth, including warm fluids "by the nose" in case of lockjaw (*On Diseases III*, #12, 13/LTT VII 133; *On Internal Affections*, #53, 54/LTT VII 301); but "if you wish," you can also try cold water on opisthotonos (*On Diseases III*, #13/LTT VII 135).

304. The Greek text here is, "he caught a sprain at the big finger, below." Littré's version is, "he had a sprain at the lower part of the thumb." Since Greek has no special word for toe, I tried to change "below the thumb" to "the thumb below" and proposed to my Hellenist adviser the translation "stubbed his big toe," which better fits with tetanus. It was vetoed. The Greeks would have said "the thumb of the foot."

305. *Epidemics V*, #74, 75/LTT V 247, repeated with small changes in *Epidemics II*, #36, 37/LTT V 405

306. Eckmann 1966 p. 100

307. *Epidemics II*, #37/LTT V 405

308. *Epidemics V*, #76/LTT V 249; repeated with insignificant changes in *Epidemics VII*, #38/LTT V 407

309. *Epidemics VI*, sect. 5 #1/LTT V 315

310. EE I 423 #30

311. EE II 169

312. See EE I vii; II 139; Phillips 1973 p. 197.

313. EE II 154, 140

314. *Regimen IV* [*On Dreams*], #87/LB IV 423 = LTT VI 643

315. *Decorum*, #6/LB II 289 = LTT IX 235

316. EE II 158, 233, 193. The Asklepieia included, besides the temple, a whole precinct. It is often claimed that they became health resorts. They did include a source (Herzog 1931 p. 155), and the two most famous ones, those of Epidauros and Pergamon, did rise in magnificent surroundings; but the statement is not accurate, for the main requirement was that they be on a sacred site. In one case at least, this site was a swamp.

317. The connection between the snake and health goes back at least as far as **the Sumerian myth of Gilgamesh. The Mesopotamian god Ninazu ("Lord-physician") had a son, Ningizzida, whose symbol was a rod with two intertwined serpents** (Saggs 1962 p. 460; Thorwald 1962 p. 155). Explanations for the association of the snake with health are many: the snake may have represented rejuvenation (from the shedding of its skin), shrewdness, sharp-sightedness, vigilance, and healing power as such, since it was used as a remedy. *Elaphe longissima* also stood for mildness: it rarely strikes at man, and when it does, it is not dangerous (see EE II 227 ff.). As to the dog, one myth had it that the baby Asklepios was suckled by a bitch (ibid.).

318. Whibley 1963 p. 664; see also Sigerist 1961 II 60–61.

319. Herzog 1931 p. 6

320. Asklepios asked little but did not like to be cheated. When Echedorus kept for himself a gift that Pandarus had asked him to deliver to Asklepios, the god had him come to the temple and marked his face with the marks of Pandarus (EE I 231 #7). There is a parallel punishment in the Old Testament (Phillips 1973 p. 199).

321. EE I 423 #30

322. EE I 423 #40

323. EE I 235 #32

324. EE I 233 #177; *Inscriptiones Graecae* 1929 pp. 70–73 lines 113–119

325. "When Rome was troubled by a pestilence in 292 B.C. the envoys dispatched to bring over the image of Asclepius from Epidaurus to Rome fetched away a serpent which had crawled into their ship and in which it was generally believed that the god himself was present. On the serpent's going ashore on the

island of the Tiber, a temple was erected there" (Livy, *Periocha*, XI; EE I p. 431 No. 846, p. 432 No. 848).

326. Aristophanes, *Plutus*, pp. 676–681; EE I 179 #490

327. *Pepsis* and *sepsis* are explained by Aristotle as two stages of "breakdown": pepsis occurs in the upper belly, and the residue putrefies by sepsis in the lower. This was a perfect summary; the two processes are still called *peptic* and *septic*, one enzymatic, the other bacterial (Steuer and Saunders 1959 p. 9).

328. The ultimate catharsis of the four humors took place with "sense of humor."

329. Joly 1966 pp. 243, 130 ff. An excellent monograph on the "rational" versus "scientific" value of Hippocratic medicine.

330. Edelstein 1952

331. Plato, *Charmides*, 155–156/LB 15–21

5. The Perfumes of Arabia

1. The cosmetic use of cinnamon is well documented in the Bible and in Pliny. See also FH p. 519; Burkill 1935 p. 543; Moldenke 1952 p. 75; Rosengarten 1969 p. 188.

2. Dictionaries translate *arómata* as "herbs" or "spices," but the word has a broader meaning. E.g., Theophrastus, *Concerning Odours*, lists myrrh under aromata (#34/LB II 357).

3. The use of spices for endearment was no more bizarre than today's use of *honey* for the same purpose (see Lewis and Short under *cinnamomum*).

4. A readable, well documented book on the role of perfumes in antiquity is Détienne's *Les Jardins d'Adonis*.

5. Singer and others 1965 I p. 286

6. Proverbs XXVII 9

7. Plutarch, *Life of Alexander*, 4/LB VII 233; Détienne 1972 p. 28

8. Déonna 1939

9. Harley 1941 p. 177

10. See e.g. Pauly-Wissowa under *Rauchopfer*; Rudhardt 1958 pp. 293, 297. The idea recurs in Hindu religion and in China (Moldenke 1952 p. 57).

11. The word *perfumum*, however, came very late; it does not exist in classical Latin. The smoke in the word *perfume* is probably that of churches (incense), but it might also have something to do with the smoking of foodstuffs.

12. Détienne 1972 p. 95

13. On perfume and the gods see also Singer 1965 I p. 289

14. Aristophanes, *Birds*; Lucian, *Icaromenippos*, 26

15. According to the same passage, it was still common to offer as a sacrifice "fragrant woods cut in pieces" (Theophrastus, *On piety*, fragm. 2).

16. Lederer 1941

17. Trease and Evans 1972 p. 156

18. FH p. 164

19. CDM xxxviii. The peculiar method of harvesting ladanum is not unique. One modern technique of collecting *charas*, the resin of hemp, is to scrape it off the leather garments of men sent wandering in the plantation (FH p. 550).

20. LTT X Index 617

21. Ammonia is something of a language puzzle. There are two North African products of entirely different nature but with similar names: *ammoniacum*, a resin (FH 324) and salts of ammonia (see Ch. 2, 3; and p. 487 note 282).

22. PNH 12.77/LB IV 57

23. See FH; Trease and Evans 1972

24. Egyptians chewing papyrus: PNH 13.72/LB IV 143. In antiquity, the habit of chewing plant gums and resins is well documented (e.g. PNH 22.45/LB VI 323). Even nowadays, "the children in eastern lands often spend their coins for this material (mastic, from *Pistacia lentiscus*) which they use like chewing-gum" (Moldenke 1952 p. 177).

25. PNH 14.124/LB IV 267

26. See e.g. Smith's report on the Royal Mummies (1912): a "spicy odor" and "a strong pungent aromatic odor" (pp. 1, 110) alternate with horrible smells. Also LH p. 315.

27. The episode, told by Pliny (PNH 12 111/LB IV 79), refers to the shrubs that give Mecca balsam, *Commiphora opobalsamum*. These shrubs "paid tribute to Rome together with the race to which they belonged," the Jews; so the *Commiphorae*, in the end, meant more to either party than just balsam.

28. The name has nothing to do with bursae of resin; it was given "in memoriam Joachimi Burseri."

29. Until recently the history of pre-Muslim Arabia had been almost completely lost, also because after Mohammed this time was referred to as "period of ignorance" (Ryckmans 1951 p. 7; van Beek 1961 p. 230). For bibliography see note 105.

30. DB IV 405; Moldenke 1952 pp. 84, 85; van Beek 1958(b) p. 146

31. Van Beek 1958(b) p. 151

32. Van Beek 1958(b); Ryckmans 1957 pp. 86, 88. Reference to *the* Incense Route should not be taken literally; there were alternate pathways (Bowen 1958(a) p. 38).

33. PNH 12.32/LB IV 45

34. In 24 B.C., Augustus sent Aelius Gallus to Arabia on a campaign "to win wealthy friends or conquer wealthy enemies" (Strabo 16. 4. 22). Bad planning, disease, and the Nabataean guides led the expedition to disaster.

35. The destruction of Aden by "Caesar" is reported in the Periplus. This was doubted by Schoff (1912 p. 115), who read "Charibael" for "Caesar," but accepted by Miller 1969 p. 14 ff.

36. Carter 1848; also quoted in FH p. 138

37. In Greek, the word for incense is *ho líbanos*, or *libanotós* (Masson 1967 p. 54).

38. "Olibanum softens in the mouth; its taste is terebenthinous and slightly bitter, but by no means disagreeable. Its odour is pleasantly aromatic, but is only fully developed when the gum-resin is exposed to an elevated temperature. At 100° C, the latter softens without really fusing, and if the heat be further raised decomposition begins" (FH 138).

39. Günther 1950 p. 344

40. Masson 1967 p. 54. The similarity of the roots *mrr* and *mur*, "bitter," with the Latin *amarus*, is thought to be coincidence, amarus being probably related to the Sanskrit *amláh*, "sour" (Ernout and Meillet 1959, *amarus*). Words that travel usually represent material objects, not abstract ideas (Masson 1967).

41. The English text in the Loeb collection translates the last word freely as "ointments," but the Greek has "myrrh." See also LS *smyrna*.

42. This figure refers to all uses of myrrh, not only on wounds. In Littré's index of Hippocrates (LTT X), gums and resins are mentioned in prescriptions at least 131 times, probably an underestimate. I counted the number of times that each of 10 gums and resins was used: ammoniacum, 1; incense, 24; galbanum, 10; "gum," 4; ladanum, 1; myrrh, 54; opoponax, 1; "resin," 23; styrax, 5; turpentine, 8.

43. CDM V 27/LB II 125

44. Jeremiah 8:22, 46:11

45. This analogy has been suggested for the use of resin in Indian medicine (Filliozat 1949 p. 110).

46. Theophrastus, *Concerning Odours*, 8.35 (LB II 359).

47. Sophocles, *Philoctetes* 782, 890/LB II 429, 439

48. Trease and Evans 1972 p. 488

49. My warmest thanks to Dr. Elisabeth Schorer and Sylvie Dersi, who tested samples of myrrh from three different suppliers. These tests, to be reported elsewhere, showed that all three samples had bacteriostatic properties toward grampositive bacteria, not toward the gram-negative. An alcohol-soluble principle could also be demonstrated.

50. Trease and Evans 1972 p. 488

51. Vogel 1970 p. 219

52. Trease and Evans 1972 p. 438

53. Monardes 1574, quoted by Vogel 1970 p. 218

54. Trease and Evans 1972 p. 447

55. Pories and others 1967

56. Trease and Evans 1972 p. 448

57. I owe this information to Dr. P. S. Statkov.

58. LTT X Index 817

59. Rosengarten 1969 p. 439

60. Thorwald 1963 p. 65

61. Professor P. Favarger, Head of the Dept. of Biochemistry, University of Geneva, was kind enough to test the smoke of frankincense (gum olibanum) and myrrh, both obtained from Fritsche, Dodge & Olcott, Inc., New York. The smoke was bubbled through an alkaline solution, so as to trap the phenol, and then tested by several reactions (ferric chloride, diazotation, uranyl nitrate). Phenol was detectable but in very small amounts; a rough estimate from the ferric chloride reaction showed that 10.5g of frankincense yielded about 15mg of total phenols.

62. Rosengarten 1969 p. 188. Another source of confusion as regards cassia is a well-known but wholly unrelated *Cassia fistula*, a leguminosa, also growing in India; it produces long pods, commonly used to make a laxative. This double use of the name *cassia* goes back as far as Hippocrates, who mentions cassia (bark) as well as cassia pods (*kassíe karpós*, LTT VII 357, VIII 405).

63. Burkill 1935 p. 548; Samarawira 1964; Trease and Evans 1972 p. 386; Rosengarten 1969 p. 188

64. Miller 1969 pp. 153–172

65. Hennig 1939 p. 327. Cinnamon was used in aromatic wines (PNH 14.107/LB IV 257), but strangely enough, there is no reference to its use on solid foods in antiquity. In the famous cookbook of Apicius (*De re coquinaria*) I found neither cassia nor cinnamon, as bark. The leaves were used as a spice, known as *malabathrum*; but in the Mediterranean world of antiquity it was not realized that the two were parts of the same Indian plant, so malabathrum was not considered as a kind of cinnamon.

66. Exodus 30:22–32

67. Hippocrates, *On Diseases of Women II*, #51/LTT VII 111

68. Trease and Evans 1972 pp. 511–512

69. Burkill 1935 p. 543; FH p. 510

70. Trease and Evans 1972 p. 394, but with no reference. I have come across innumerable statements concerning the antiseptic properties of spices, but have not yet unearthed bacteriologic data, which surely exist.

71. The parallel with medicine is implied in the terminology of wine makers, who speak of *infected wines* and *wine diseases*. In a standard treatise on wine making (Ribéreau-Gayon 1947 p. xv), the first function of oenology is said to be *avoiding wine diseases*.

72. PNH 14.137/LB IV 277

73. The ABC of wine science was explained to me, with great patience and kindness, at the Swiss Federal Agronomic Station of Lausanne by Messrs. J. F. Schoepfer and A. Dufour. I am much indebted also to Silvio Cavallero, Geneva.

74. Columella XII 20.8/LB III 237

75. The oldest use of sulphur in wine making was to prepare the vats by burning a "mèche" or wick of sulphur inside them. This method of disinfecting the vats, still used, was the only one at the time of Pasteur (1866 p. 132). Perhaps this was the procedure that Pliny had in mind when he made his cryptic statement about "sulphur" in wine making. Exactly where and when the method originated is not known, but according to Mr. Schoepfer of Lausanne, it must be at least as old as the use of wooden casks in wine technology (the first centuries A.D.), because such casks cannot be used unless they are first disinfected inside. The method works well, but it is empirical and not sufficiently reliable. The "scientific" use of SO_2 came about only after 1899 (Garoglio 1959 p. 251). SO_2 is a colorless gas, responsible for the characteristic smell of burning sulphur. It can bleach a flower held above it; some wines are decolorized by it. In wine it is partly combined with sugars and aldehydes, but only the free SO_2 is antiseptic.

76. Wine is spoiled by exposure to air because: *Acetobacter* can only work in the presence of oxygen, which it needs in large amounts; exposure to air causes various oxidative reactions that spoil the bouquet; new bacteria drop into the wine; and the SO_2 is lost. Some evaporates, some becomes oxidized to sulphuric acid, which is much less antiseptic (Ribéreau-Gayon 1947 p. 323 ff.).

77. Maximum daily intake of free SO_2 admitted by the World Health Organization, in mg per kg of body weight: unconditional acceptance, 0-0.35; conditional acceptance, 0.35–1.5. Maximum amount of free SO_2 allowed in wine by USA standards: 70mg per liter (Schanderl 1956). For a 70kg adult, one bottle is therefore a large dose of SO_2. The lethal dose for rats, in 50% of the animals tested: 1040mg/kg (Lanteaume *et al.* 1969). But the problem transcends wine; for SO_2 in high doses is also used for the preservation of many other foods, especially dried fruits (WHO Report, 1971, pp. 33–40).

78. See e.g. *Etat actuel des techniques pour le remplacement de l'anhydride sulfureux,* 1971:481, p. 238; 1971:488, p. 926. There seems to be hope in purely physical methods, like pasteurization. It should not be forgotten that some wines can take care of themselves, i.e. fight off bacteria without outside help, especially the sweet wines, like Sauterne.

79. Columella 12.19 ff./LB III 229–235

80. PNH 14.131/LB IV 273

81. PNH 14.92/LB IV 249

82. Mark 15:23. "Drugged wine" is a free and inaccurate translation, as I have on the authority of Prof. R. Martin-Achard. For a study of *vin myrrhé* see André 1951.

83. The addition of resin to wines was perhaps born of the observation that wines from resinated casks kept better. Pasteur himself discussed the ancient use of resin and pitch as wine preservatives, whose effect was to cause "considerable disturbance to the development of wine parasites" (Pasteur 1866 p. 132).

84. PNH 14.107/LB IV 257

85. The "new wood" was boiled in the must, which presumably was then fermented (PNH 14.112/LB IV 261).

86. Columella 12.18/LB III 227; PNH 14.134/LB IV 275

87. PNH 14.129/LB IV 271

88. PNH 35.177/LB IX 391

89. Pliny also mentions a wine that had been kept for nearly two-hundred years, but it was "reduced to the consistency of honey with a rough flavor" (PNH 14.55/LB IV 223). The empirical Roman antiseptics have become obsolete, but several other Roman techniques are still used in wine making, such as chalking to correct the acidity, or saving a wine on the verge of turning into vinegar by making it ferment on lees of good wine (personal communication, Prof. C. Tarantola, Experimental Institute of Oenology, Asti, Italy; see also Marescalchi and Dalmasso 1937 pp. 307–320).

90. PNH 14.57/LB IV 225

91. Marescalchi and Dalmasso 1937 p. 317

92. Pasteurization of wine is still performed on a large scale. In France it is known as *thermolisation,* used mainly on ordinary wines. About half of the Italian wine produced is pasteurized, by showering the bottles with water of increasing temperature (personal communication Mr. J. F. Schoepfer, Lausanne).

93. As early as 1860, after his experiments on spontaneous generation, Pasteur had dropped the highly significant remark: "It would be most desirable to push these studies further, and to open the way to serious research on the origin of various diseases." But his work on human infections did not begin until about 1873, when he was fifty-one, after he had completed his studies on beer, wine. vinegar, and the silkworm (Vallery-Radot 1900 pp. 110, 298).

94. The ancient Egyptians have no reputation as sailors (Rawlinson 1916 p. 10), despite their naval jaunts down the Red Sea to the Land of Pwnt, like that of Queen Hatshepswt.

95. Herodotos III 107/LB II 135

96. Herodotos III 107/LB II 135; 109/LB II 137

97. Herodotos III 110/LB II 137

98. Herodotos III 111/LB II 139

99. Aristotle, *Historia Animalium*, IX 13 616–617

100. PNH 12.42/LB IV 63

101. PNH 12.42/LB IV 63

102. The tale of Ethiopia producing cinnamon caught on so well that in many old maps the name "Regio Cinnamomifera" can be found on the Horn of Africa (Drake-Brockman 1912 pp. 5–9; Schoff 1912 p. 87).

103. According to the Periplus, the secret of the monsoons was discovered by one Hippalus about 45 A.D. (Schoff 1912 pp. 227–230). Another blow to the economy of South Arabia came when the same Greco-Roman ships were stopping over at the South Arabian harbors and draining the Incense Route, so to speak, into the sea (Ryckmans 1957 p. 87). Commercial competition was fierce even in those old days. Witness the story told by Strabo of the Phoenician captain who was sailing to the "Tin Islands," the secret source of Phoenician tin (probably the Scilly Isles off the coast of Cornwall). Finding himself followed by a Roman vessel, he chose to shipwreck rather than to show the way; and when he eventually managed to return home, a grateful Phoenician government refunded his loss (Strabo 3.5.11/LB II 157).

104. The drainage of Roman gold is a matter of fact; just how critical it was is disputed (Needham 1965 I 183; Miller 1969 pp. 242 ff.).

105. The Marib dam was probably built around 750 B.C. (Bowen 1958(b) p. 75). South Arabia was greener and more populous in the distant past (Ryckmans 1957 p. 76; Bowen 1958(b); van Beek 1961; 1958(b)). Archeology of this area is just beginning; until 1951, only three Europeans had reported seeing the fabled Marib dam (Bowen 1958(b) p. 70). For literature see Bowen and Albright 1958; Phillips 1955; see also Ryckmans 1957; van Beek 1952; 1958(a, b); 1961; Pirenne 1956; 1960 (discussed by van Beek 1961); Harding 1964; Wissmann 1968.

106. Bowen 1958(a)

107. The expression "spice curtain" is my own, but the fact of Arabian secrecy in the spice trade is well established (see e.g. van Beek 1958(b) p. 147; 1960 p. 91). It must have implied the connivance of the Phoenicians, whose ships had a lot to do with the spice market. According to Herodotos, the name *kínnamon* or *kinnámomon* was "taught to the Greeks by the Phoenicians" (Herodotos III 111/LB II 139). The Phoenicians themselves might have made up the word from the Malaysian *kayu manis*, "sweet wood" (Burkill 1935 I p. 544).

108. Herodotos III 113/LB II 141

109. PNH 12.41/LB IV 61

6. *The Yang I*

1. Historians were a typical feature of Chinese courts (NEED I 74): hence the unmatched series of twenty-four official dynastic histories since 90 B.C. (Needham 1965(b) p. 282).

2. For the booklets of bamboo or wood, see NEED I 86, 111, 112. Silk was also used (ibid. p. 111).

3. Chinese writing seems to date from the beginning of the second millennium B.C. (Diringer 1968 p. 67; also Yang 1973). It was therefore developed much later than either cuneiform or Egyptian hieroglyphs.

4. NEED I 95

5. For book titles and dates I follow NEED I and II.

6. Lu Gwei-Djen and Needham 1967 p. 7; NEED I 86, II 307

7. NEED I 95; 500 to 250 B.C.

8. The *Lun Yü*, now known as the "Analects," were certainly compiled soon after the death of Confucius in 479 B.C. (NEED II 5). Translation: Waley 1938. The five-element theory was systematized by Tsou Yen about 350–270 B.C. from ideas that had been "floating about . . . for not more than a century at most before his time"

(NEED II 232). Instead of "five elements," Porkert (1973 p. 43 ff.) prefers "five Evolutive Phases."

9. NEED II 232 ff.

10. The yin-yang concept is probably not older than the sixth century B.C. (Needham and Lu Gwei-Djen 1962 p. 430). As philosophical concepts, the words appear in the early fourth century B.C. (NEED I 153–154, II 273 ff.). Oddly enough, the yin-yang equivalence male/hot–female/cold is typical also of Greek medicine (Bourgey 1953 p. 49; Siegel 1968 p. 230).

11. NEED II 277

12. NEED II 312–321; Wong and Wu 1932 p. 9

13. The I Ching probably originated from omen compilations in the seventh or eighth century B.C. but did not reach its present form before the end of the Chou dynasty, 221 B.C. (NEED II 307).

14. The I Ching was translated into German by R. Wilhelm; this version was then rendered into English by C. F. Baynes (1950). C. G. Jung was asked to write a foreword. Not being an expert on China, Jung had a brilliant idea: since the I Ching was an oracle book, he performed what he called an experiment and asked the book whether he, Dr. Jung, should accept the task of presenting it to a Western audience (R. Wilhelm 1950 p. vi). The I Ching replied: "There is food in the caldron . . . The handle of the caldron is altered. One is impeded in his way of life. The fat of the pheasant is not eaten." Jung took this to mean that the wisdom of the I Ching was going to waste in the West, being unusable in Chinese, and he wrote the preface. He also wrote, incidentally, a book entitled Psychology and Alchemy (Jung 1944).

15. NEED II 335. See also the recent attempt to edit the I Ching for the "Western man of affairs" (Siu 1968).

16. NEED II 310

17. Having read the I Ching, I find the words of Needham very descriptive: "the abstractness of the symbolism gives the book a deceptive profundity" (NEED II 304). However, it is interesting to see the impact that it had on H. Wilhelm (son of the translator), who published a series of lectures about it (H. Wilhelm 1960).

18. R. Wilhelm 1950 I 107

19. R. Wilhelm 1950 I ii

20. R. Wilhelm 1950 I 261

21. Needham and Lu Gwei-Djen 1962 pp. 438–439

22. NEED II 304

23. The compilation of the Chou Li must be considered a work of the early Han (2nd century B.C.), but much of the material may well date from the Chou period (Lu Gwei-Djen and Needham 1967 p. 6).

24. Biot 1851 p. 495 ff. I used the French translation of Biot 1851, which in modern Sinological circles is considered excellent.

25. Biot 1851 p. 8 ff.

26. Creel 1970

27. The four commentators are from the first, second, eighth, and twelfth centuries A.D. (Biot 1851 I lx [= 60]).

28. Thus in Needham and Lu Gwei-Djen 1969 p. 256; but in Wong and Wu (1932 p. 7) it is implied that Confucius still refers to a "priest-doctor." In Waley's translation the passage reads (Waley 1938 p. 177 No. 22): "Without stability a man cannot even make a good shaman or witch-doctor." The same passage occurs in another ancient text, the Li Chi; there the witch-doctor is replaced by a "diviner by the yarrow-stalks" (Waley 1938 p. 177 note 4).

29. Wong and Wu 1932 p. 7

30. Creel 1970 p. 17; also Lu Gwei-Djen and Needham 1963 p. 64

31. Creel 1970 p. 19 note 64; Needham and Lu Gwei-Djen 1969 p. 268

32. The evidence is gathered by Cohn-Haft 1956 p. 57. Vague hints about the procedure are found in Plato, Gorgias 455B, 456B, 514D-E and in Xenophon, Memorabilia, 4.2.5. See also Drabkin 1944 p. 344; Bourgey 1953 pp. 116, 120

33. The Chinese consider the color of their skin to be white (Needham 1968). In the tables of correlations by "fives," there is a different color for each of five rulers, and Huang Ti corresponds to yellow (NEED II 263).

34. NEED I 98

35. See Needham and Lu Gwei-Djen (1969 p. 263), who propose "The Yellow Emperor's Manual of Corporeal [Medicine]." This should be opposed to "magico-religious medicine," and in fact there had been such a book, now lost: *Huang Ti Wai Ching*, "The Yellow Emperor's Manual of Incorporeal (or Extra-Corporeal) [Medicine]" (ibid.).

36. Huang Wên 1950 (this paper, though not to be relied on for depth of scholarship, contains useful summaries of the *Nei Ching*); Lu Gwei-Djen and Needham 1967 p. 11

37. Breasted 1930 p. 61

38. The partial English translation is by Ilza Veith (1949; 1966), abbreviated henceforth as Ve; see the critique by J. R. Hightower (1951).

39. The French translation is by A. Chamfrault and Ung Kang-Sam 1957, abbreviated henceforth as CU. The passages quoted here are CU 75, 163.

40. Porkert 1973

41. CU 60; Ve 151

42. CU 64; Ve 155

43. The *Nei Ching* consists of two parts, each with 81 chapters: *Su Wên* (meaning uncertain, perhaps "Simple Questions and Answers") and a shorter *Ling Shu* ("Mysterious Pivot"), which is mainly a treatise on acupuncture. There is some confusion of names: the title *Su Wên*, for example, is sometimes applied to the whole. To compound the confusion, in the French version the two parts are correctly named in the preface, but in the text they are entitled *Su Wên* and *Nei Ching* (*Sou Ouenn, Nei King*). The English version covers only chs. 1–34 of *Su Wên*. In my text, quotations are from the English version; abbreviations are as follows: NC = *Nei Ching*; SW = *Su Wên*; number = chapter (disregarding the subdivision into books); LS = *Ling Shu*; CU = Chamfrault and Ung Kang-Sam version (+ page); Ve = Veith version (+ page). When the content of the two versions is generally comparable, the concordance is given as = ; otherwise as = ? It is possible that the original Chinese editions were not the same. Sometimes even the short summaries of Huang Wên (1950) have no precise equivalent in CU or Ve.

44. NC-SW 1/Ve 97 = CU 17

45. NC-SW 12/Ve 147 = CU 56

46. NC-SW 2/Ve 102 = CU 20

47. NC-SW 26/Ve 220 = CU 108

48. NC-SW 2/Ve 105 = CU 22

49. NC-SW 4/Ve 111 = ? CU 28

50. NC-SW 14/Ve 152 = ? CU 61

51. NC-SW 3/Ve 107 = ? CU 23–25 (?)

52. NC-SW 5/Ve 117 = CU 32: almost the same!

53. NC-SW 13/Ve 151 = ? CU 58 ?

54. NC-SW 14/Ve 152 = ? CU 60

55. The reconstruction is based almost entirely on the *Nei Ching* and the *Chou Li*, for other sources on wounds and ulcers are not available in translation. The next step should be to consult two anonymous, untranslated works of Han times: *Chin-ch'uang tsung-chih fang*, a treatise on wounds (ref. courtesy of Dr. Nathan Sivin), and *Chin-Ch'uang Hsi Ts'ang Fang*, a collection of recipes for wounds caused by weapons and dog bites (Huard and Wong 1959(a) p. 139).

56. NC-SW 77, 78/CU 293, 297 = Huang Wên 1950 p. 18

57. Quotations from Huang Wên pp. 6 (#7), 8 (#18, 19), 14 (#48)

58. NC-SW 10/Ve 144; CU 52 is different. . .

59. Huang Wên 1950 pp. 31, 33. *Tu quoque*, Huang Wên! It is a wild suggestion that the ancient Chinese had trained their fingers to detect "what the electro-cardiogram showed of changes in the heart." This kind of "mastery" was largely an exercise in self-deceit.

60. The *hot disease* is discussed at length in the *Nei Ching* (e.g. NC-SW 31–34/Ve 239 ff. = CU 120 ff.). Wong Man and Chamfrault translate it as "fever," but from the text I infer that it also covered "local heat" (inflammation). If it did not, there would be no mention of "local heat" in the whole book, a very unlikely

omission. In Chamfrault I, Index (*Traité de Médecine Chinoise*, largely based on the *Nei Ching*), the term *inflammation* is almost ignored, being used only once in relation to the kidneys. Inflammations of the skin are called "swellings"; on suppurations there is very little. It seeems that in ancient Chinese practice, as judged from the *Nei Ching*, today's syndrome of inflammation is rather broken down and de-emphasized.

61. For this fundamental piece of information—the lack of venesection in ancient China—I am once again deeply indebted to Prof. Needham. In his summary of the *Nei Ching* (p. 17) Huang Wên used the word *venesection*; but the surgical act must have been more like a puncture, Chinese style. See e.g. "puncture the point Ta-Tchong-4-kidneys . . . and make it bleed. After half an hour, if the patient is not relieved, puncture the opposite point" (NC-SW 63/CU 229). Other passages of the *Nei Ching* indicate that *some* blood was drawn; e.g. "Nowadays it is known that in order to cure completely the suffering of hand and foot, of yin and yang, one must first remove blood; and by such means one also removes the ailment which can then be examined" (NC-SW 24/Ve 210 = CU 104). However, there is no indication that veins were slit and that correspondingly large amounts of blood were drawn,—except in a passage of the English version, where blood is drawn by the *pint* (NC-SW 7/Ve 130). This is a mistranslation; the French version is altogether different (CU 42).

62. Porkert 1973 p. 167

63. Huang Wên 1950 p. 30

64. In NC-SW 27 the concept is translated as "draining" (Ve 224), "extraction" and "purging" (Huang Wên 1950 p. 10), or "dispersion" (CU 111). The basic idea remains the same.

65. E.g. Huard and Wong 1964 p. 8; Pálos 1971 p. 40. The fact that the needles were stone also suggests the Stone Age.

66. CU throughout

67. Ung Kang-Sam in Chamfrault II 14

68. For the nine needles see NC-LS/CU 305; for the choice of the flint needle in case of ulcers of the ankle see NC-LS 81/CU 560, 559 note 1; for the 365 points see NC-SW 58/CU 198.

69. CU p. 9

70. NC-LS 67/CU 519; NC-LS 1/CU 308

71. For an "abscess" on the inside of the ankle the *Nei Ching* recommends a flint needle on the "*Iu* point of the corresponding meridian" (NC-LS 81/CU 560).

72. Huard and Wong 1958(a) p. 8

73. For literature on the moxa see Veith 1966 p. 58 ff.; Huard and Wong 1958. Notice there on p. 12 the practice (how old?) of actively delaying the healing of the burn, as was common in Greek medicine.

74. Information from Dr. Chong Yu-ming, acupuncturist, Taipei, Taiwan; see also Pálos 1971 p. 121 ff.

75. Hume 1940 p. 94

76. Hints at purging in the *Nei Ching* are few but clear: "one should restore their bodies and open the anus, so that the bowels can be cleansed" (NC-SW 14/Ve 153; ibid. CU 61 has "purifier les entrailles"). "When a patient has been ill for more than three days, one can bring about [abdominal] dispersion" (NC-SW 31/Ve 241 = CU 122: "il faut purger au quatrième [jour]").

77. Perhaps the most famous Chinese drug is Ma Huang; for the world career of this drug see Ch. 9.

78. NEED II 264

79. Biot 1851 I 97

80. Needham and Lu Gwei-Djen 1962 p. 436. Incidentally: the *yang* of *yang i* is unrelated to the yin-yang couple.

81. The information (largely unpublished) contained in this paragraph was graciously provided by Prof. Needham. Western literature about ancient Chinese surgery contains many mistakes (such as the alleged use of opium and hemp for anesthesia), often due to erroneous readings of the Chinese. Regarding anesthesia: tradition maintains that Hua T'o improved methods that were already in use four

hundred years earlier by Pien Ch'io (Hume 1940 p. 88; Hartner 1941 p. 247), who is a semi-legendary figure (NEED II 54; Huard and Wong 1959(a) p. 139).

82. One passage is as follows: "weigh and consider carefully removal, as well as cutting and scooping out exposed and spoiled particles" (NC-SW 14/Ve 153; missing in CU). The disease is incomprehensible, but this is clearly minor surgery. The second surgical passage: "if a toe becomes red and black from suppuration [gangrene?] one should not hesitate to cut it off" (NC-LS 81/CU 560).

83. NC-SW 25/Ve 53 = CU 106; but CU reads rather differently, as if giving five precepts for the practice of acupuncture.

84. CDM VII *Prooemium*/LB III 295

85. Huard and Wong 1957 p. 15; 1960 p. 65

86. Hume 1940 p. 102 ff.

87. Wong and Wu 1932 p. 113

88. The use of wine for anesthesia should have come about naturally; consider the vast number of "Wine-Men" on the Chou staff and the opening paragraphs of the *Nei Ching* about wine intoxication.

89. Lucian, *De dea Syria*, § 51

90. Kleine Pauly I, *Castratio*

91. Jeanselme 1917 p. 85. The event occurred under Emperor Justinian (*Novella CXLII* in: *Corpus Iuris Civilis*, III, R. Schoell and G. Kroll, Berolini, apud Weidmannos, 1954, p. 7055).

92. Juvenal, *Saturae*, VI 366–378; also *Eunuchus* in PW Suppl. III.

93. NEED I 105

94. Translation courtesy of Prof. Needham.

95. Biot 1851 p. 97 note 7

96. Cinnabar (mercuric sulphide), though not mentioned in the Hippocratic books, was used in Roman medicine for cleansing sores; Celsus mentions it also as "erodent" (see CDM/LB II xliii, *Minium*). "Minium" is now lead oxide, but in antiquity it referred to several red pigments, including cinnabar (Singer and others, *History of Technology*, 1957 II 361).

97. Huard and Wong 1957 p. 23

98. "Important remedies have been made by the profit-seeking Greeks even with human offscouring from the gymnasia; for the scrapings from the bodies soften, warm, disperse" (PNH 28.50/LB VIII 37; also PNH 15.19/LB IV 301). Celsus agrees (CDM V 11/LB II 11). For Western examples of bizarre and revolting drugs, if necessary, see Pliny's home remedies, Ch. 9.

99. Chamfrault III 29

100. NEED I 203, II 350

101. See e.g. the use of resin to make lacquer. The lacquer tree of China and Japan is *Rhus verniciflua* (Burkill 1935 II 1904).

102. Burkill 1935 I 117 ff.

103. Trease and Evans 1972 p. 43

104. The Indians called storax by the Sanskrit name *rasamala*, "excrement." The Chinese were apparently skeptical (Burkill 1935 I 117; NEED I 203 note a). For Arabic tales about cassia and cinnamon see Ch. 5.

105. Data on the Han tomb courtesy of Peking Television. The tomb, found in Ma-wang-tui (Hunan), was thought at first to contain the wife of Li Tsang, who was made marquis of Tai in 193 B.C., but the identity of the lady is uncertain (see Hall 1974). The wealth of objects (over 1000) recalls the treasure of Tutankhamun.

106. Peking Review 1973 no. 32 p. 17

107. Biot 1851 I 111

108. According to Dr. Donald Tipper, Head, Dept. of Microbiology, University of Massachusetts Medical School.

109. Other factors that contributed in a major way to the preservation of the body were exclusion of air (and hence oxygen), prevention of evaporation, and cold (about 13°C). I learned from Prof. Needham that another possibility was discussed in recent Chinese publications. The coffin complex contained large amounts of methane, probably originating from the decay of food placed in the spaces between

coffins. It has been hypothesized that the low temperature may have favored the methane-forming bacteria while holding in check the bacteria of putrefaction. As for the mercury, the main compound was mercuric sulphide. See also the recent article by Hall (1974).

110. NC-SW 46/CU 173

111. Sharma 1972 p. 14

112. For comparison between the Greek and the Chinese element-theories see NEED II 245.

113. Veith 1966 p. 89

114. From the second to the fifteenth centuries A.D. China was technologically far in advance of Europe (Needham 1964 p. 174). For a long list of Chinese firsts, including paper (second century A.D.), printing, the magnet, gunpowder, and rockets, see NEED I 242.

115. NEED I 150 ff.; Filliozat 1949 p. 215

116. NEED I 83

117. Hudson 1931 p. 22

118. NEED I 183, 199

119. NEED I 195, 210

120. This historic voyage ended in 124 B.C. Chang Ch'ien returned home with much news and many novelties, including the grapevine (*Vitis vinifera*; Hudson 1931 p. 53 ff.; NEED I 172 ff.).

121. NEED I 176, 181

122. NEED I 191

123. NEED I 193–194

124. NEED I 195

125. Cassia trees grow wild throughout Indo-China and are cultivated in China (Burkill 1935 I 548). Cassia bark is an ancient and favorite Chinese drug, *kuei* (e.g. Hartner 1941 p. 244). The Chinese province of Kuei-lin means "Cassia forest" and has been so named since 216 B.C. (Miller 1969 p. 42).

126. I said a *faint chance*—but there is a chance. The name of *cassia* has been given three possible pedigrees: from the Chinese *kuei-shu*, "Cinnamon tree" (I have already discussed the near-synonymous use of cassia and cinnamon); from the Khasya Mountains in eastern Bengal, where the bark is also produced (FH 528; Miller 1969 p. 42); and from "a Semitic root meaning *cutting up, peeling*, and thus definitely Phoenician" (Lassen 1867 I 329). Burkill (1935 I 545) mentions "an untenable theory that Chinese bark reached ancient Egypt," but it is not untenable at all in view of the exploits of the Malaysian double outriggers in the second millennium B.C. (Fig. 5.4). I am also tantalized by a possible link between the Bengali *taj* for "cassia" or "cinnamon bark" (McCrindle 1885 p. 220) and the ancient Egyptian *tj-šps*, "perhaps cinnamon" (GMÄ VI 549); and between the Egyptian *khisit* ("equivalent to the Greek *kinnámomon*," Hennig 1939 p. 328) and *kwei-shu* + the feminine ending *t*. Spice names travel well: of the two or three words of Chinese that have penetrated into European languages, one is *tea* (Forrest 1948 p. 123; also Mahdihassan 1952; 1959; 1960).

7. *The Vaidya*

1. Arrian, *De expeditione Alexandri*, VI 1/LB II 103–104

2. The mouthwash, "called the Indian preparation," was made by pounding anis, dill, and myrrh in white wine (*On Diseases of Women II*, #185/LTT VIII 367). Mouth hygiene received much attention in ancient Indian writings (e.g. ChS I 60; SS II 480). Teeth were to be brushed twice a day (ChS I 60). Buddha planted one of his *dântakachta* (toothbrush twigs), and it became a tree (Beal 1869 p. 72).

3. Hippocrates, *On Diseases of Women II*, #205; I, #81/LTT VIII 395; 203

4. Data on Mohenjo-Daro: Renou and Filliozat 1953 p. 665. Origin of the word *Aryan*: other theories derive it from the Sanskrit *arya*, "noble," or from *ari*, "stranger," as a reference to the great hospitality of these "strangerly" people. (Courtesy of Gopal Sukhu).

5. AUB 227

6. ChS I 105. The word *vaidya*, however, is not the ancient Vedic word for "physician," although it is attested as early as the "epic" period of Sanskrit. The Vedic term is *bhishaj* (*bhishak-* and *bhisag-* in composite words). In classical Sanskrit, *bhisaj* and *vaidya* coexist, much as "physician" and "doctor" in modern Indo-European languages (information courtesy of Prof. H. Frei).

7. SS II ii ff.

8. *Sam-hita*, too, means "together-put." Both these classics are written in prose mixed with verse. Sushruta (whose name means "he who was well heard") comes to about 1700 pages; Charaka to twice as many. They are well preserved and agree in many points. The English translations are somewhat old and not wholly free of bias, but no others exist. For comments on the translator of Sushruta see notes 98, 280. An eminent French scholar called his work "unsure" (Renou 1946 p. 125). The translator of Charaka, a practitioner of Hindu medicine, stated in the preface that he needed help in the translation, because his knowledge of English was insufficient. For a critical study of the contents of Charaka see Rây and Gupta 1965.

9. ChS I 847

10. Smith 1920 p. xviii

11. SS I intro. i

12. SS I foreword 5

13. Smith 1920 p. xiv

14. AUB 20

15. Smith 1920 pp. 85–86

16. The main passage (Strabo 15.60) says that Indian physicians cure mainly by diet and plasters, use few drugs, practice fortitude and patience, and have charms that can bring about numerous offspring (male or female as preferred). Unfortunately, no mention is made of surgery. For fragments of Megasthenes' work, see McCrindle 1877.

17. Smith 1920 p. 95

18. Kosambi 1965 p. 157

19. Smith 1901 pp. 116, 114

20. Zimmer 1948 p. 173

21. Mukhopadhyaya 1913 I 8

22. Bloch (1950 p. 94) has "deux secours médicaux, secours pour les hommes, secours pour les bêtes." Hultzsch 1925 p. 52 has "two kinds of medical treatment . . . for men . . . for cattle."

23. Smith 1901 p. 115

24. Ironically, Ashoka's concern for animals caused such discontent that it may ultimately have contributed to the breakup of the empire after his death (Smith 1920 p. 107).

25. Smith 1920 p. 84

26. Sushruta's dates are a reasonable assumption because: modern criticism allows the *Sushruta Samhita* to have been composed perhaps "as far back as the last centuries B.C." (Renou and Filliozat 1953 p. 147); the Indian translator (admittedly not unbiased) argued for the sixth century B.C. (SS I iv); and Sushruta, much like Hippocrates, did not create his own surgery but largely codified the existing art, which was necessarily older (all the background works are lost). Note also that around 326 and 300 B.C. two Greeks, Alexander and Megasthenes, were impressed with Indian medicine.

27. Sushruta's opening paragraph explains that the work was "dictated to Sushruta" by the holy sage Dhanvantari (unlike the Hippocratic authors, Sushruta never appears in the first person).

28. ChS I 955

29. Bandits were a recognized pest in ancient India. There was even a special caste of outlaws (AUB 77 ff.).

30. SS I intro. xiii

31. Skill in archery was useful even in procuring a wife, through a contest (AUB 46).

32. SS I xiii 336

33. SS I 16

34. SS I 16

35. SS I 18

36. Teaching by recitation was and still is a typically Indian practice (AUB 225). Great stress is laid on learning first just the syllables (even backward!), then the meaning. I was told by Prof. J. Filliozat that still today the children of some Brahmans, between the ages of about five to eight, are given—to begin—a whole Sanskrit dictionary to learn by heart. Later, they are taught Sanskrit; and then they discover that a whole dictionary is available to them! For "oral reciters" see Whitney 1962 p. lxvi,

37. SS I 341

38. SS I 339

39. Steel was known in ancient India, but its beginnings cannot be dated (Forbes 1965 p. 597). It was probably made by the technique still used in Ceylon: melting pieces of iron in a crucible in the presence of bits of wood (Coomaraswamy 1913 p. 137). The British were much intrigued by this simple, unorthodox, and very effective method. The famous Damascus blades were made of Indian steel.

40. AUB 259

41. For bamboo shoots as probes see SS II 250; for facing north while gathering herbs see SS I 337; ChS II 1920

42. SS I 16

43. ChS I 422

44. Hippocrates, *The Physician*, LB II 311/LTT IX 205

45. SS I 71

46. SS I 242

47. SS I 74

48. SS I 270

49. SS I 270

50. SS II 723

51. SS I 76; ChS I 109

52. SS I 258. The two methods (pulling the arrow back or pushing it through) are not specifically Indian. See e.g. the Akamba people of East Africa (Lindblom 1920 p. 312) and the Romans (CDM VII 5/LB III 317).

53. SS I 258

54. SS I 259

55. Sushruta, who is meticulous in describing equipment, mentions no gadget of this kind. Yet it is hard to believe that the ancient Hindus, so familiar with arrow wounds, did not invent something like the spoon of Diokles. Mukhopadhyaya (1913 p. 110) does mention two such instruments, *pañcamukha* and *trimukha*, but they are more recent; they are described in Vagbhata's *Astangahrdayasamhita*, c. seventh century A.D.

56. SS I 261

57. SS I 261

58. SS I 260

59. E.g. pure honey-butter salve, made with clarified butter, was used on burns by the cautery (SS I 91), after extraction of a foreign body (I 260), and on wounds (II 240, 262).

60. Though clarified butter or *ghee* lasts longer than butter (almost indefinitely, like oil), Prof. Filliozat tells me that it has a rather rancid taste. Clarified butter "matured" from eleven to one hundred years was said by the Hindus to ward off monsters; beyond one hundred years it was called *Kumba Ghritam* (Great Clarified Butter) (SS I 443). Ghee made of woman's milk "should be regarded as the prototype of divine ambrosia on earth" (SS I 442). A traveler in the late 1600s speaks of tanks of ghee four hundred years old! (Schoff 1912 p. 177).

61. Jee 1896 p. 58

62. SS I 60, 66

63. SS I 57

64. SS II 250

65. SS I 252

66. SS I 252

67. Fragrant sandalwood is another typically Indian material. It is used for fine woodwork; distilled it gives an oil used in perfumes; as a powder or paste it is used in the pigments used by the Brahmans for their distinguishing caste-marks. It is now used extensively wherever Buddhism prevails.

68. SS I 251. A less attractive paste for this purpose was made of beans, wheat, barley, and cow dung (ibid.). The method was also used for a longevity test: "Men, on whose bodies sandal paste and similar preparations begin to dry up from the head downward . . . should be looked upon as persons endowed with an uncommonly longer duration of life" (SS I 309).

69. SS I 254

70. SS I 257

71. SS I 63

72. SS I 63

73. SS I 258

74. SS I 248. I have searched many a museum in vain for an Indian arrowhead of this kind.

75. SS I 169. The Hippocratic passage that has been interpreted as advising not to tie the knot over the wound is quite garbled (*On the Surgery*, #8/A II 478 and note 2 = LTT 296–297 and note 6).

76. SS I 176

77. SS I 179

78. SS I 180

79. SS I 180

80. SS I 180

81. SS I 182, 185; ChS II 1776

82. SS I 181

83. SS I 181

84. SS I 181

85. SS I 181

86. SS I 178

87. SS I 182

88. SS I 40. There were several ways to fumigate, e.g. by pouring over a hot brick sour gruel (SS II 558) or clarified butter and certain resins (SS II 255). See also the nadi-sveda below. The pain-killing was surely psychological.

89. SS I 44

90. SS I 44

91. See e.g. Read 1926 p. 18

92. SS I 305, II 263; ChS I 102

93. ChS I 130

94. SS I 3

95. ChS I 287; for list of Charaka's main principles see ChS I 276–289

96. SS II 172

97. It is a poor excuse that dogs do have a bone in the penis. Equally mystifying is Charaka's vaginal bone (ChS I 805). Neither of these skeletal anomalies appear in Sushruta. The neglect of the lungs (Zimmer 1948 p. 161) is remarkable, since consumption was described (ChS I 979). The share of fancy in Hindu anatomy is clearly apparent in Sushruta's account (SS II 159 ff.). However, remember that for all of their anatomic ignorance, the Hindus somehow knew enough about the eye to operate on cataracts.

98. SS II 191 ff. The literal meaning of *dosha* is not "principle" but "defect;" in fact *dosha* is related to the Greek *dys-*, "ill-" as in "ill-advised."—The comparison between the Hindu and the Greek four-humor theories is the subject of a classical study by J. Filliozat (1949). The Hindu theory is usually referred to as the *tridosha* (literally "three-defect" or three-principle) theory, but in reality

there were three principles plus blood—as in the Greek system. Filliozat's excellent book also deals with the relations between Greek and Indian cultures in general. Sushruta's translator, Dr. Bhishagratna, wrote at length to prove the absolute originality of the Hindu *doshas*, "principles": though they are often translated as air, bile, and phlegm, he warned, "nothing could be more misleading" (SS I xxxix). He treated Hippocrates as a confused plagiarist of Hindu medicine, but obviously knew nothing about his theories (SS I i note). On this score, he is not a reliable witness. (For Hindu medical theories see also Rây and Gupta 1965).

99. Bagchi 1968 p. 1328

100. The peccant humors—vayu, pitta, kapha—are in fact mentioned in Sushruta and Charaka at every step. I underplayed them in this chapter for fear of boredom.

101. Filliozat (1949 p. 215) concludes: if the Greek and Hindu ways of thinking had points of contact, "c' est qu' en sous-oeuvre ils communiquaient." Joseph Needham refers to the same phenomenon when he speaks of "capillary" exchange between ancient China and the West (NEED I 191).

102. SS II 181

103. SS II 173; ChS I 808

104. SS II 184

105. SS II 175

106. SS II 179

107. SS II 187

108. SS II 180, 176. Sushruta gives yet another explanation for death by injury in a marma (SS II 178): sometimes "The Vayu [wind] aggravated by an injury to the Marma, blocks up [the four classes of vessels] . . . throughout the organism and gives rise to great pain . . . all over the body." Note that death was sometimes expected to occur many days after the injury to the marma; this must have reflected past experience with infections, such as tetanus.

109. Kosambi 1965 pp. 73, 79

110. Wilson 1857 p. 48. For a list of marma in the *Rig Veda* see Grassmann 1873; also Filliozat 1949 p. 133.

111. I owe these details to Dr. G. Sambasivan, World Health Organization, Geneva.

112. SS II 172

113. The Greek "eye of the mind" occurs first in Hippocrates (*On Breaths* [also called *On Winds*] 3/LTT VI 95): "ἀλλὰ μήν ἐστί γε τῇ μὲν ὄψει ἀφανὴς, τῷ δὲ λογισμῷ φανερός." Galen uses the expression several times.

114. SS I 74

115. SS I 77

116. SS I 77

117. ChS II 1632 (*arishta*); SS II 715

118. SS II 700

119. ChS I 264

120. ChS II 1632

121. SS II 716

122. AV VI 12/Whitney 1962 I 289

123. SS II 704

124. SS II 715; ChS II 1632

125. SS II 706

126. ChS II 1653; SS II 707

127. ChS II 1653; SS II 707

128. SS II 715; ChS II 1667

129. SS II 715. One could also fill the mouth with barley meal, dust, or ashes (ChS II 1631).

130. The text says "one Muhurta," the thirtieth part of the day.

131. ChS II 1632

132. Sushruta says that incision, cauterization, and sucking should be highly recommended in *all* cases of snake bite (SS II 715). A note by the translator of Charaka

says that the cut (puncture) is made "in case the bitten part cannot be tied" (ChS II 1631). Cauterization, prescribed by both classics (ChS II 1632; SS II 715), was presumably applied with an iron rod; I assumed the vaidya had no cautery with him, and therefore used the red-hot coal method described in the *Kausika Sutra* (a catalog of rituals and gestures that had to accompany each magic formula found in the *Atharva Veda*: a sort of practical manual of the Atharvan priests). Note the reassuring gesture of "throwing away the poison" (KS 32. 20–25/Caland 1900 p. 106). In another ritual of the *Kausika Sutra* the bite is rubbed with grass, then the grass is lit and thrown toward the snake (KS 29.6/Caland 1900 p. 92).

133. SS II 719, 716

134. SS II 724

135. SS II 717

136. AUB 245

137. The ancient use of *Rauwolfia serpentina* for snake bite is mentioned by Vakil (1961 p. 97), who was responsible for bringing it to the West as a tranquilizer (Goodman and Gilman 1970 p. 171). Dr. Vakil mentioned Charaka as a source, but I was unable to find *Rauwolfia* (*Sarpagandha* in Sanskrit) in the chapters on snake bite in either of the Hindu classics; nor is *Rauwolfia* mentioned in the list of Charaka's plant-drugs (Rây and Gupta 1965 pp. 52–77). For the history of *Rauwolfia* see Schlitter and others 1964; Pelt 1971 p. 54.

138. Goodman and Gilman 1970 p. 170. *Sarpagandha* means "serpent fragrance."

139. SS I 77

140. SS II 707

141. SS II 711

142. ChS II 1627

143. ChS I 405

144. SS II 717

145. ChS II 1655

146. Sushruta has a whole chapter on antipoison drums (SS II 727). Dr. Bhisha-gratna, who translated it, should have known the topic. However, the translator of Charaka regarded this as an error of interpretation: in his opinion, it is true that drums are beaten to keep the patient awake, but the drugs are smeared on the patients, not the drums (ChS II 1640 note)!

147. SS II 702

148. SS II 716

149. Reid 1968 p. 614

150. Navmed 1966 p. 123

151. SS I 420

152. SS I 337; ChS II 1920

153. Although the Hippocratic Collection includes a passing reference to the principle of the hemostatic tourniquet, it never describes its application, for either bleeding or snake bite. As to a possible historical correlation between the two tourniquets, I have no data. However, it is tempting to speculate: someone *could* have noticed that a tight ligature for snake bite was also able to stop the bleeding.

154. Minton and Minton 1969 p. 69

155. SS II 673–762; ChS II 1624–1668; AV X 4/Whitney 1962 II 575 ff. and index.

156. Vogel 1926 p. 6

157. Aelian, see McCrindle 1901 p. 145

158. Arrian, *Indica*, VIII 15/LB II 353

159. Deoras 1971 p. 26

160. ChS II 1655; 1627

161. Harley 1941 p. 105 ff.

162. Harley 1941 p. 103

163. Harley 1941 pp. 98–104

164. AUB 216

165. SS III 141

166. SS I 141

167. SS I 141

168. Coomaraswamy 1931; AUB 200 ff.

169. SS I 141

170. SS I 143 (wording changed to the first person)

171. These famous caves, twenty-nine in all, are Buddhist temples and retreats carved into a cliff and decorated with paintings dated from the second century B.C. to the sixth century A.D. (Yazdani 1930–1955).

172. Stretched earlobes also existed in ancient Egypt, where they left traces in art and on mummies, not in medical history. See e.g. the large holes in the ears of the Egyptian head in Plate 3.5; Nefertiti and Akhenaton both had their earlobes pierced and somewhat stretched (Fig. 3.30). In a mummy of the Twenty-second Dynasty "the ears are pierced and the lobules drawn into long strings (16 cm.)" (Smith, *The Royal Mummies* [Cairo 1912], p. 109). In life, these ears must have looked much like those of the Indian girl in Fig. 7.19.

173. Having seen some Swiss male peasants wearing a ring in the right ear only, I learned from Prof. Jean Babel, Head, Dept. of Ophthalmology, University of Geneva, that worried mothers sometimes consulted him to find out whether they should have the ears of their children pierced, to protect their eyes against disease.

174. SS I 142

175. SS I 143

176. SS I 142–143

177. Basham 1954

178. Bühler 1886

179. Sharma 1972 p. 77

180. See also McDowell 1969

181. AUB 50

182. SS I 151

183. SS I 147

184. The vaidyas were positively unimpressed by the Brahman anathema against wine (ChS I 295, 363), though they realized that it was a cause of disease (ChS II 1668–1696!): "Wine is poison, but poison administered duly promotes nutrition" (ChS II 1676).

185. AUB 50

186. SS I 147

187. AUB 41

188. SS I 147

189. Converse 1964 p. 1118

190. SS I 147, 37

191. SS I 147–148

192. Hindu surgery was made known in Europe in the Middle Ages by the great Arab physicians (Rhazes, Avicenna, and others). It surely was related to the making of new noses in Sicily in the early 1400s and ultimately to the publication of Tagliacozzi's famous book *De curtorum chirurgia* in 1497 (Gnudi and Webster 1950).

193. SS I 153 ff.; Converse 1959 p. 339. I am much indebted to Dr. Denys Montandon, plastic surgeon, for advice on these topics.

194. Dibbell 1970

195. ChS I 168–171. Charaka also describes a lying-in room that should be built before the ninth month (ChS I 844 ff.). Otherwise, he never refers to the place where the patients are treated.

196. ChS I 901

197. ChS II 2145

198. ChS II 2060

199. This interpretation of Charaka's "hospital" as an infirmary built into a rich home is also that of Mukhopadhyaya (1913 I 8).

200. NEED I 120, 207

201. Beal 1869 pp. 3, 18

202. Beal 1869 p. 107

203. AUB 173

204. SS II 63
205. SS II 188
206. SS I 160
207. AUB 253. Charaka speaks often of the virtues of wine. His list of wines "that are beneficial to mind and body" comes to eighty-four (ChS I 291). Ashoka's edicts, which insist on meat prohibitions, never mention wine (Basham 1954 p. 214).
208. SS I 457–466
209. The preoperative meal was skipped before certain operations, e.g. on the mouth or anus (SS I 39). Anesthesia with wine is mentioned only once, in this passage.
210. SS I 160, italics mine.
211. The short Hippocratic treatise *On the Use of Liquids* (LTT VI 116) discusses wine only as a surgical dressing and as a vehicle for cathartics (ibid. pp. 129–131).
212. AUB 259
213. The place for the operation is my guess. Sushruta too never says where the patients are treated.
214. SS I 37–38
215. SS I 67–68
216. SS I 38
217. SS I 39
218. SS I 40
219. SS I 162
220. SS II 560
221. ChS I 160
222. ChS I 160
223. SS II 559–560
224. SS II 559 note; see also ChS I 160
225. Chs I 58
226. SS I 43–44
227. SS II 63
228. SS II 243–245
229. SS I 44
230. SS II 245
231. SS I 398
232. SS II 262, I 358
233. SS I 359
234. SS I 358
235. SS I 466
236. ChS I 27
237. SS I 467
238. SS II 260
239. SS II 627 ff.; see also ChS II 2036 ff.
240. SS II 207, italics mine; see also ChS I 259
241. AUB 195
242. The text merely says "two tubes open at both ends" (SS II 284). Tips for enema tubes were made of bamboo or bone (ChS II 2038).
243. SS II 284
244. SS II 284
245. Sharma 1972 p. 74
246. For *vrana* see SS II 241; for "instant ulcer" see SS I 240 (the transliteration *brana* in Chakravorty 1969 is less current). As *vrana* corresponds to the Greek *hélkos*, *sadyovrana* is equivalent to the Greek *tróma*, "recent wound due to violence." Sushruta observed very astutely that after one week there is no point in making the distinction between *sadyovrana* and *vrana*, because by that time the clean "instant sore" has become "associated with deranged Vayu, Pitta or Kapha" (= infected!), "hence at that stage the medical treatment of both forms of ulcer is (practically) the same" (SS II 240).

247. SS II 268

248. SS I 241

249. SS II 267

250. This is only one of several hemostatic charms (AV I 17.4/ Whitney I 18). Ancient commentators believe that the gesture accompanying the charm may have been to sprinkle sand or gravel on the wound as a "dam." Whitney and others rather believe that a sandbag was used (ibid.). Compare with the Homeric episode in the *Odyssey* (Ch. 4).

251. SS I 44

252. SS I 267 ff.

253. SS I 217

254. SS I 224

255. SS I 268. Lack of pain is indeed typical of many cancerous ulcers.

256. SS II 261

257. SS II 261

258. SS III 338 ff.

259. SS II 261

260. SS II 243

261. SS I 267

262. SS I 225

263. SS II 262

264. SS II 260

265. SS I 166

266. SS I 269

267. SS II 201

268. SS II 201

269. Sushruta leans over backward in compiling lists of accidents due to treatment: emetics have fifteen, enemas a whole chapter (SS II 577, 599). Sometimes he overdoes it; not all the troubles he describes seem iatrogenic.

270. AUB 133

271. SS II 180

272. SS II 189

273. SS I 69

274. SS I 241

275. SS I 19

276. SS I 339

277. SS II 189, 188

278. SS II 188

279. SS II 680

280. SS II 673. Dr. Bhishagratna actually believed this: "The poison operates through the perspiration, proving almost instantaneously fatal through the act of dalliance" (SS II 673 note). He also believed that the effect of planets on infectious diseases is "almost a proved fact" (SS I lxv), and that "Marriages with girls of prohibited description have been known . . . to have ushered in an epidemic which devastated a whole town or a country" (SS I 52 note). But these shortcomings must be seen in perspective, for Dr. Bhishagratna was a busy practitioner who undertook a huge work. His labor of love in translating Sushruta remains admirable.

281. SS II 253

282. SS II 676, 679

283. ChS II 2145. Elephant medicine was one of the ancient Hindu specialties (Sharma 1972 p. 101; Renou and Filliozat 1953 p. 138). On enemas for elephants, the position of the elephant, etc., see Mukhopadhyaya 1913 I 131–132.

284. SS II 254

285. SS III 169–211

286. SS III 170

287. SS III 210–211

288. SS III 170; ChS I 941

289. SS III 182

290. SS III 188

291. SS III 204. Charaka suggests the same erotic treatment but makes less fuss about it (ChS I 1140).

292. SS III 204

293. SS II 273

294. SS II 272

295. Ackerknecht 1946, 1967; for a review of insect sutures see Gudger 1925. For guidance in the world of ants I am indebted to Dr. Arthur T. Hertig, Harvard Medical School, and Dr. Marshall Hertig, University of Illinois.

296. Wheeler 1910 p. 10

297. Beebe 1921 p. 178

298. The entomologist was Dr. C. Baroni-Urbani, Museum of Natural History, Basel, Switzerland, to whom I also owe the following information: the ants used by the Hindus belonged most likely to the genus *Odontomachus*, found all over India. Recent news from Central Africa is that ant sutures are still a common and successful practice in the former Congo, possibly with termites. Dr. A. Raignier heard similar reports.

299. Wheeler 1910 p. 217

300. Doflein 1905

301. Ant sutures in Europe still bear a question mark. European surgeons of the Renaissance often mention them (Gudger 1925), but one cannot tell whether they really tried them or just repeated what they had read in Albucasis, who was quoting Sushruta. An ant suture was apparently witnessed in Smyrna on the Turkish coast in 1895 (Burr 1939 p. 222). If the report is true, this territory—and the ants—were within the range of Hippocrates. According to Dr. C. Baroni-Urbani, the best candidate in Europe would be *Camponotus vagus* (the carpenter ant is *Camponotus pennsylvanicus*), whose jaws cannot compete with *Eciton* or *Odontomachus*, but match *Oecophylla*; for small wounds they might do. Ant heads clinging by their jaws to the eye or in the throat can be a medical nuisance (Chalmers and Marshall 1919).

302. Dart 1955 p. 331

303. Judges 15:15–17

304. Furnari 1845

305. Lu Gwei-Djen and Needham 1967 p. 7

306. NC-SW 19/Ve 180 = CU 84

307. Filliozat 1949 pp. 64, 154 ff.

308. ChS I 222

309. Also translated *On Breaths* (LTT VI 88–115). A similar theory appears in Plato's *Timaeus* 85, where it is said that tetanus is due to air that enters from without and causes the sinews to swell and strain.

310. ChS II 1677

311. A comparative study of the two doctrines, so far as I know, has not been made; in fact, I have never seen a suggestion that the two may be related.

312. The *Zend-Avesta* is the sacred book of the ancient Persian religion called Mazdeism, Magism, or Zoroastrianism. Little is left of it since the impact of Mohammed. The *Zend-Avesta* cannot be accurately dated; it reflects the religious thought prevailing in Iran from roughly 500 B.C. to 800 A.D., with influence from the Koran, the Talmud, and the Gospels (Darmesteter 1892).

313. The text quoted is taken (with one retouch) from the first, 1880 translation of J. Darmesteter, generally considered obsolete, but this passage is almost identical in the improved 1892 French version (*The Vendîdâd* VIIa, 1880 p. 83; 1892 p. 105). The single change: in 1880 the penalty was "the same as for wilful murder"; in 1892 it was explained that the literal translation is "wilful injury"; a commentator adds that the corresponding penalty was the amputation of six fingers.

314. AUB 40

315. Singhal and Gaur 1963

316. ChS I 554

317. The operation for cataract, perhaps the most spectacular surgical feat of antiquity, is discussed in Ch. 9.

318. Veith (1961) says that there are 760 "healing plants" in Sushruta. For Charaka the figure varies from 500 (Neuburger 1910 p. 54) to "2,000 vegetable drugs plus a few mineral and animal remedies" (India Committee Report 1948 p. 538). A modern list of Indian *materia medica* has roughly 1000 plants (Giboin 1949). I prefer to adopt the figures of Rây and Gupta (1965), who compiled laborious tables of Charaka's drugs, and report a total of 582 (341 from plants, 177 from animals, and 64 mineral substances).

319. Notably lacking among the inorganic drugs are the various salts, more or less poisonous, that the Greeks powdered onto wounds as *énaima*. The Hindus also used powders, but made of plant products (SS I 242, II 252, 254). Copper, so important in Greek surgery, has little use in ancient Hindu medicine, like all the drugs of the inorganic group that are mentioned briefly by Sushruta (SS I 530). It is used in an eye salve as copper sulphate (SS III 53). There is also the passage: "Proper drugs or articles (such as sulphate of copper, etc.) powdered and pasted with honey should be applied for destroying soft marginal growths of an ulcer" (SS II 256). I suspect the parenthesis of being an addition of the translator. Copper had the reputation of being a poison (ChS I 12) and was used as an emetic (ChS II 1665). I found no mention of copper acetate (verdigris).

320. The caste system was of course another expression of this tendency to classify. Recently the number of castes was of the order of 4000 (Smith 1920 p. 37; Senart 1896). Incidentally, the Hindu skill with numbers produced something that is not widely recognized, the ancestors of "Arabic" numerals, which are really Hindu-Arabic. *Zero* comes from the Sanskrit *sunya*, "empty" (Menninger 1969 p. 400).

321. SS II 240 ff.

322. Ayurvedic medicine is officially practiced and taught by vaidyas in many institutions (India Committee Report 1948). It is now only one of three "Indigenous Systems" alive in India. One of the others stems from the Arabic influence. Ayurvedic medicine reached its peak in antiquity, then declined, especially in its best branch, surgery (Mukhopadhyaya 1913 I viii ff.).

8. Alexandria the Great

The title of this chapter, an obvious pun on Alexander the Great, is borrowed from André Bernand's *Alexandrie la Grande*.

1. Plutarch, *Lives*, 51 2–6/LB VII 373. Strictly speaking, Alexander was a Greek (definitely so by education). However, Macedonians spoke a dialect of their own and thought of themselves almost as barbarians in comparison with the Greeks. This inferiority complex is openly expressed in Plutarch's *Life of Alexander*.

2. Tarn 1948 pp. 232, 455

3. Plutarch, *Lives*, 26 1–5/LB 299–300

4. Plutarch, *Lives*, 8.2/LB VII 243

5. Bernand 1966 p. 27 ff.

6. Bernand 1966 p. 49

7. There was e.g. a museum in Athens (Sarton 1927 I 158). The Greek *mouseia* (museums) were sanctuaries for all activities of the mind, under the auspices of the nine Muses: such is the noble ancestry of today's museums. For the Alexandrian Museum see Jones 1971; 1972; Bernand 1966 pp. 112–122. As regards the ancestry of Greek museums, it is well to remember that the notion of "center of scholarship" had a very ancient and important precedent on Egyptian soil: the *Houses of Life* attached to the temples (see P. Ghalioungui 1973, *The House of Life*, Amsterdam, B.M. Israel, p. 28 and elsewhere).

8. Bernand 1966 p. 90

9. Measuring the earth's diameter was the feat of Erathosthenes (Jones 1971); but in all fairness the accuracy of the figure depends on the value selected today for the ancient measuring unit, the stadium (see Sarton 1927 p. 172).

10. No screws seem to have existed before Archimedes (287–212 B.C.), so he may well have been the first to cut a spiral groove in a round peg (Drachmann 1967 p. 25). He probably was at the the Museum about 260 B.C., then returned to his native Sicily (Jones 1971). Pliny's account of that great novelty, the Greek wine press (written about 75 A.D.), shows that a screw, in his time, was still unusual: "In the old days people used to drag down the press-beams with ropes and . . . by means of levers; but within the last 100 years the Greek pattern of press has been invented, with the grooves of the upright beam running spirally . . . an arrangement which is very highly approved" (PNH 18 317/LB V 387).

11. NEED I 95

12. NEED I 127

13. Bell 1948 p. 54

14. The system of *written accents* was another Alexandrian first; and the sciences of bibliography and literary criticism, in the West, started here (Bell 1948 p. 54).

15. Bernand 1966 p. 119

16. Bell 1948 p. 13

17. Thus, the fascinating science of papyrology should really be called Greek papyrology. Its materials, practically all Egyptian in origin, are mostly documents preserved on papyrus. Those written on potsherds, wood, and vellum are included; those on stone and bronze are not (Bell 1948 p. 19), and neither, as a rule, are those written in the Egyptian language. As to the *óstraka*, a most interesting collection of 1624 pieces has been published by Wilcken (1899). The word *óstrakon* referred originally to the shell or carapace of animals (cf. *oyster*, Ital. *ostrica*); later it was applied also to potsherds, since they too are "hard and convex" (ibid. p. 3). Because potsherds were so cheap, Athenians used them on a large scale as voting ballots, when they came to *ostracize* an unwanted citizen.

Geographically, most of the Greco-Egyptian papyri come from upper Egypt, where the soil is almost ideal as a preserver of documents. Unfortunately the whole region of the Delta is too damp and its west side is slowly sinking (Bernand 1966 p. 29), so that the level of ancient Alexandria is now underwater and hopeless (Bell 1948 p. 10). Not a scrap of papyrus has ever been recovered from it. The finds are usually made in ancient rubbish heaps, ruins and tombs. Many papyri are still unpublished. Discoveries of new sources are dwindling; but the science of Papyrology has grown to the extent of producing such specialized aids as a *Namenbuch* (list of personal names found) and the *Konträrindex* (Bell 1948 p. 19). The world at large does not realize that a poem, a tax law, a fact about Greek history may have turned up in a dump or in the mummy of a sacred crocodile (ibid. p. 19).

18. David and van Groningen 1952 p. 2

19. David and van Groningen 1952

20. This tax was levied on the priest, it seems, because private offerings represented a profit (Grenfell and Hunt 1906 p. 307).

21. *Fayûm Papyri 97, 25, 5–15.* For other scars see e.g. *Fayûm Papyri 24, 18; 29, 19; 36, 22; 39, 24, 26, 27;* for *ásemos* see ibid., *28, 13, 14; 96, 8; 97, 9;* etc. Many other examples of both labels are in the *Oxyrhincus Papyri.*

22. Scars are mentioned in a "high proportion" of legal documents—thus I am informed by an eminent papyrologist, Prof. Jean Rudhardt, University of Geneva. Precise figures are not available.

23. Kenyon 1893 p. 48; Sudhoff 1909 p. 260

24. To spoil the fun, an earlier papyrologist reads *iatrokáystes* instead of *iatroklýstes*, and therefore "the cauterizing physician" (Sudhoff 1909 p. 260).

25. Sudhoff 1909 pp. 238–239

26. Sudhoff 1909 pp. 248–249

27. Sudhoff 1909 pp. 249–250

28. *Hibeh Papyri* pp. 277–278

29. The *iatrikón* or physician tax, paid in support of public physicians, existed also in Greece (Wilcken 1899 p. 375; Greenfell and Hunt 1906 pp. 276–278; Préaux 1939 p. 132 ff.). There was also a *hetairikón* or prostitute tax (Wilcken 1899 p. 217), but that was paid *by* the prostitutes rather than to support them.

30. Wilcken 1899 p. 747

31. *Hibeh Papyri* pp. 276–277

32. Sudhoff 1909 p. 255

33. Drachmann 1968. The cult for robots certainly goes back to the third century B.C., when Philon of Byzantium, author of another *Pneumatics*, wrote a whole play for an "automatic theatre." Philon spent some time in Alexandria and must have been impressed by the lighthouse, because it was he who started the tradition of the seven wonders of the world (Schmidt 1899(b) pp. 8, 10).

34. Woodcroft 1851 p. 109

35. Did the huge statue on top of the lighthouse really rotate like a weather-vane? Thiersch did his best to work out a system of counterweights. For this statue see Picard 1952 pp. 71, 74.

36. Picard 1952 p. 75

37. For the dates of Ktesibios I follow Drachmann 1968 p. 3 (300–230 B.C.).

38. This passage is unclear: how could *one* lead ball run down several tubes? Prof. Drachmann preferred to ignore the ball and visualize a channel of square section, made of wooden planks (Drachmann 1967 p. 9, and personal communication). If we read the text to mean "one weight per tube," implying a battery of parallel tubes, the whole setup becomes so clumsy that Ktesibios would squirm in his tomb. Another translation renders *tubuli* as "small piping" (Morgan 1914 p. 273). This encouraged me to solve the riddle by taking the text literally: a *single* weight runs down *a series of tubes* aligned one above the other (Fig. 8.9). An advantage of this interpretation is that a slit between two segments could have worked as the outlet that produced the fateful sound.

39. Vitruvius, *De architectura*, IX viii 2–4/LB II 257. Vitruvius, who "writes an atrocius Latin, but knows his business," wrote *De architectura* around 25 B.C. Since he took his information from a book written by Ktesibios himself, we may accept his account as authentic (Drachmann 1963 p. 12; 1968 p. 3).

40. Drachmann 1963; 1967; 1968

41. Drachmann 1968 pp. 80, 81

42. *Pyulcus* comes from *pýon*, "pus," and *hélko*, "I pull." The invention of the syringe is often credited to the Arabs. I traced this mistake back as early as Gatenaria, a medieval Arabist, who apparently describes the syringe as an *instrument à clystères* but gives the credit to Avicenna. Malgaigne is sure that this is false modesty and concludes that the discovery of the syringe is Gatenaria's and deserves "imperishable fame" (Malgaigne 1840 p. xcix)!

43. Eco and Zorzoli 1963 p. 83

44. Paré 1678 p. 316

45. The Egyptians were giving themselves enemas well before the Alexandrian syringe: their clyster kit must have consisted of a tube, an animal bladder or skin, and a piece of string (Fig. 4.16), an assembly that did its job until the nineteenth century (Milne 1907 p. 105), competing with the real syringe. But in a dictionary published in 1675 (Blancard 1697) the syringe properly appears as "an Instrument which is used in injecting Liquors into the Fundament, Womb, Ears, etc."

46. The charge of human vivisection against the Alexandrian anatomists has caused much ink to flow. It rests mainly on the testimony of Celsus and Tertullian, but Galen's silence throws much doubt on the reliability of their sources, and there the matter lies (Finlayson 1893; Sarton 1927 p. 160).

47. The birth date of Erasistratos is placed between 310 and 300 B.C. (Wellmann 1907); Herophilos is usually taken to be slightly older (Finlayson 1893 p. 324; Wilson 1959 p. 297).

48. Wellmann 1907 cols. 333–350

49. Finlayson 1893 pp. 333–334

50. The comparison with a *calamus scriptorius* shows again that these Alex-

andrian scientists were Greeks, not Egyptians. Egyptian writing pens, as now seen in museums, were solid reeds. The Greeks introduced the *kálamos*, a hollow pen split down the middle, perhaps not long before Herophilos. The oldest known was found in an Aegean island, in a tomb of the third century B.C. (Ogg 1940 p. 39). Galen says that it was current in Alexandria (Finlayson 1893 p. 338). Another structure named by Herophilos is still known by (some) medical students as *Torcular Herophili*; for a delightful discussion of this cryptic name see Finlayson 1893 pp. 336–338.

51. Fuchs 1892. It is my impression that this count, taken from Fuchs's Latin thesis on Erasistratos, is an underestimate. Galen, who worshiped Hippocrates, had two major gripes against Erasistratos: he dared to ignore the four humors, and even opposed such a helpful treatment as venesection. It is true that Erasistratos belonged to the school of Cnidos, the rival of Cos, and therefore may have felt more free to depart from the teachings of Hippocrates (Finlayson 1893 p. 342). But when Galen goes as far as "doubting that Erasistratos ever read a single book of Hippocrates" (K II 132, X 159), he is merely being consistent with his own grouchy disposition.

52. Caelius Aurelianus, *De Morbis Chronicis*, III 65/Amman p. 454

53. *Papyrus Anonymus Londinensis*/Jones 1947 p. 127

54. Sprengel 1815 I 451; Phillips 1973 p. 155

55. Celsus was a brilliant compiler, not a surgical wizard, so the new operations cannot possibly be his own. Alexandria is the likeliest source; but one should not forget the East, especially India, either directly or through Alexandria.

56. See Harris 1973

57. *Perì kardíes*, #10/Hurlbutt 1939 p. 1112 = LTT IX 89; my translation. It is sometimes said that the same treatise recognizes the atrioventricular valves, which is probably not correct. There is a fuzzy reference to other membranes and structures like spiderwebs (certainly the A-V valves and their *chordae tendineae*), but they are vaguely interpreted as part of the "beginning of the aortae," not as another set of valves. See Lonie 1973 I 11–15.

58. A recent critical study places the treatise *On the Heart* no earlier than 350 B.C., more likely in 300–250 B.C., and somewhat before the work of Erasistratos (Lonie 1973 II 152).

59. Singer 1957 pp. 19–20; Lonie 1973 I 8, 11. Aristotle, too, came too early to hear of the pump: if he died in 322 B.C., that was perhaps 50 years too early.

60. Herophilos was for active contraction; Galen for active expansion, which caused a suction (Wilson 1959 pp. 296, 304).

61. See Harris 1973 p. 108

62. Wilson 1959 p. 295

63. Fårhaeus 1957; Harris 1973 p. 93

64. Tricuspid = *triglochín*. *Glochín* or *glochís* was any projecting point, hence also the end of a yoke strap, and the barb of an arrow (LS p. 353).

65. Lonie 1973 II 137. Galen's passage: *De placitis*, K V 548–550

66. If Wellmann and Drachmann (already quoted) are right, Ktesibios and Erasistratos were about the same age. I find the same guess in Lonie 1973 II 139 note 42.

67. Siegel 1968 p. 48 ff.

68. The branching "nerves" may possibly have been tendons ("sinews") (Wellmann 1907 col. 337 #30; Harris 1973 p. 220). In any event, they too were hollow, like vessels (Wellmann 1907 col. 337 #20). This famous passage is in Galen, K III 538 (Dobson 1927 p. 827; Harris 1973 p. 196 ff.).

69. Galen, K XIV 697; see discussion in Harris 1973 p. 217 ff.

70. For Erasistratos' theories see Wellmann 1907; Dobson 1927; Fuchs 1892; and esp. Harris 1973 ch. 4; Phillips 1973 ch. 6. For the *horror vacui* theory in Alexandria see Phillips 1973 p. 150.

71. Hippocrates, *On Joints*, #45/LTT IV 191

72. Hippocrates, LTT X index, *Pléthore*

73. Fuchs 1892; Harris 1973 p. 204

74. See discussion in Harris 1973 p. 204 ff. Erasistratos was almost unique in neglecting the four humors as a cause of disease (Wellmann 1907 col. 344).

75. Erasistratos has been mistakenly regarded as recommending the tourniquet

for hemostasis: e.g. he "employed ligatures upon the arteries . . . for haemorrhage" (Dobson 1927 p. 831). As for the invention of the ligatures, Caelius Aurelianus attributes the method to both Herophilos and Erasistratos (Caelius Aurelianus, *De Morbis Chronicis*, II 186/Amman p. 416; see also Michler 1968 p. 13).

76. I owe this information to Prof. Pierre Duchosal of Geneva.

77. Harrison 1966 p. 793.

78. For the hasty reader who might overestimate the intellectual gifts of King Ptolemy I and his progeny: Claudius Ptolemaeus of Alexandria, the mathematician, astronomer, and geographer, who worked in Alexandria during the second century A.D., had nothing to do with the ruling dynasty.

79. Jones 1972

80. The popular story of the Arabic sacrilege against the library has come under serious criticism (Bushnell 1928; Parsons 1952; Jones 1972). History has also cleared Julius Caesar of some of his guilt, for it seems that he did not really send the library up in flames, as usually stated. Perhaps only some dockyard warehouses of books awaiting shipment perished (Jones 1972).

81. Bernand 1966 p. 116

82. Bernand 1966 p. 108

9. The Medicus

1. PNH 29.16/LB VIII 193. Pliny specifies that the Roman forefathers lived "without physicians . . . but not without physic" (*sine medicis . . . nec tamen sine medicina*; PNH 29.11/LB VIII 191). As for the Etruscans, almost nothing is known of their medicine, except that they seem to have used gold on teeth as early as the seventh century B.C. (Tabanelli 1963 pp. 90–96; Trisolieri 1969 p. 83).

2. PNH 20.81/LB VI 49

3. Lighting fires to chase away an epidemic was an ancient method (whether the rationale was to purify the air, to frighten off evil influences, or both). According to Galen, this is how Hippocrates drove off an Ethiopian plague that was threatening Greece; flowers, unguents, and perfumes were burned in the fires (*De theriaca ad Pisonem*, 16/Coturri 1959 pp. 94–95). There is no record of this in the Hippocratic books.

4. The story is told by Livy and others (Edelstein and Edelstein 1945 I 431 ff.).

5. The thirty-five books of Livy are strewn with bloody battles, but physicians are never there to tend the wounds. The word *medicus* occurs only once, during the Punic Wars, and in a peculiar context (Livy 22. 18.9/LB V 261). Fabius, the general, is in Rome pleading for his famous delaying tactics. Livy makes him say that "*medici* also, at times, find it better to keep quiet rather than moving and acting." If Fabius really spoke those words, they would be evidence that *medici* were an established profession in the Roman world in 217 B.C., just two years after the arrival of Archagathus. However, Livy was writing two hundred years later, and he may well have put his own words in the mouth of Fabius. It is therefore impossible to quote this passage, as is often done, to prove that the Romans already had physicians during the Punic Wars.

6. PNH 29.13/LB VIII 191

7. PNH 29.14/LB VIII 191

8. Green 1955 pp. 121, 125, 111

9. Cato's treatment is not quite so absurd as my ancient and beloved master, Prof. Arturo Castiglioni, reports it. Cato recommends binding on a reed (*harundo*); Castiglioni makes it a swallow (*hirundo*; Castiglioni 1936 p. 182; Cato, *On Agriculture* 160/LB 153). The superstition of the green reed is still alive (McDaniel 1972).

10. PNH 29.11/LB VIII 189

11. PNH LB I intro. vii

12. PNH preface 17/LB I 13

13. PNH preface 18/LB I 13; Pliny the Younger, *Letters*, III 5/LB I 173

14. For instance, Pliny quotes treatments that exist also in Dioscorides, and by comparing the texts it is clear that Pliny must have confused *oúla* (gums) with *oulé* (scar), and *óta* (ears) with *ostá* (bones) (PNH LB VI intro. xix).

15. PNH preface 17/LB I 13

16. Pazzini 1967 p. 155

17. The mushroom cloud was "best expressed as being like a pine," in the words of Pliny the Younger, who lived to tell about it. He obviously meant the Mediterranean umbrella pine.

18. The tradition that Pliny the Elder was asphyxiated is based on the account of his nephew, who had not been an eyewitness. A careful study of the facts takes some of the punch out of the drama: it was probably a heart attack (Bessone 1969).

19. These personal letters are highly worth reading. Two contain first-hand accounts of the eruption (Pliny the Younger, *Letters*, VI 16 and VI 20/LB I 425 and 439). Another fascinating letter describes the working habits of the elder Pliny (ibid., III 5/LB I 173).

20. PNH 2.8/LB I 175

21. PNH 2.5–6/LB I 173

22. PNH 2.142/LB I 279

23. PNH 31.33/LB VIII 397

24. PNH 7.189/LB II 635

25. PNH 2.14/LB I 179

26. PNH 7.5/LB II 511

27. PNH 7.2/LB II 507

28. PNH 7.7/LB II 511

29. PNH 15.49/LB IV 321

30. PNH 10.171/LB III 401

31. PNH 7.1/LB II 507

32. PNH 13.68/LB IV 139

33. PNH 23.26/LB IX 23

34. PNH 14.4/LB IV 189; PNH 14.5/LB IV 189

35. PNH 34.5/LB IX 129

36. PNH 34.46/LB IX 161

37. PNH 23.33/LB VI 437

38. PNH 33.5/LB IX 5

39. PNH 19.24/LB V 435

40. PNH 37.49/LB X 201

41. PNH 22.14/LB VI 305

42. PNH 14.90/LB IV 247

43. PNH 7.63/LB II 547. This was a common belief in antiquity, mentioned by Plato (*Timaeus*, 91 C).

44. PNH 12.84/LB IV 63

45. PNH 28.76–77/LB VIII 55

46. PNH 13.3/LB IV 99

47. PNH 13.20/LB IV 111

48. PNH 23.85/LB VI 471

49. PNH 13.20/LB IV 111

50. PNH 23.41/LB VI 441. Modern rationale certified by Prof. M. Demole, Professor of Dietetics, University of Geneva.

51. PNH 31.88/LB VIII 433

52. PNH 12.29/LB IV 21

53. PNH 10.52/LB III 325

54. PNH 13.39/LB IV 121

55. PNH 12.32 /LB IV 23

56. PNH 28.133/LB VIII 93

57. PNH 9.168/LB III 277

58. PNH 32.64/LB VIII 503

59. PNH 31.40/LB VIII 401. At the court of the Chou emperors, whose rule ended almost three centuries before Nero, there was an Ice Service with about one

Notes to
pages
341–344

hundred employees in charge of cooling everything from wine to the body of the dead emperor (Biot I 10, 105).

60. PNH 14.130/LB IV 273
61. PNH 23.31–32/LB VI 435
62. PNH 3.43/LB II 35. For Roman mile see Sandys 1963 p. 437
63. PNH 3.122/LB II 91
64. PNH 36.77/LB X 61
65. PNH 36.83/LB X 67
66. PNH 7.210/LB II 647
67. PNH 6.84–85/LB II 401
68. PNH 16.203/LB IV 521
69. PNH 7.192/LB II 635
70. PNH 2.118/LB I 259
71. PNH 9.46/LB III 461
72. PNH 11.117/LB III 505
73. PNH 11.5/LB III 435
74. PNH 10.194/LB III 415. I owe this information to Prof. Eric G. Ball, Emeritus, Harvard Medical School. One of the leads for this development came by word of mouth: commercial fishermen in Florida, who caught sharks mainly for their livers, maintained that if they threw the carcasses overboard, eventually the sharks left the area and the boats had to seek new fishing grounds. "At any rate we found that decayed dogfish flesh was a good repellent to dogfish."
75. PNH 27.43/LB X 197
76. PNH 37.164/LB X 297. In the 1682 edition of Castelli's *Lexicon medicum* the *glossopetrae* are still said to have excellent medicinal properties, whether applied externally or internally. The man who recognized them as fossilized shark teeth was the Danish bishop-scientist Nicolaus Steno (Niels Stensen, 1638–1686), who also described "Stensen's duct" of the parotid (Scherz 1969 p. 20 etc.).
77. PNH 34.112/LB IX 211. The experiment shown in Plate 9.1 was performed by Dr. Isabelle Joris, with her usual love and care. Pliny used a sheet of papyrus "steeped in an infusion of [oak] gall," a rich source of tannin. Although his short account is garbled, it is easily reconstructed, because the reaction involved was the one to make shoemaker's blacking in his day: green ferrous sulphate plus tannic acid (from oak bark or galls) gives a black product. It remained one of the basic ways to make ink. Green copper acetate plus tannic acid gives a brown spot product (for the reagents see CDM II xvi, *Aes*; PNH/LB IX 210 note a).
78. PNH 33.63/LB VI 457
79. PNH 10.221/LB III 427
80. PNH 28.10/LB VIII 9. Pliny is quite ambivalent about magic. He reminds me of a prominent Italian lawyer who once told me, "The evil eye does not exist, but I believe in it."
81. PNH 28.23/LB VIII 17
82. PNH 28.29/LB VIII 23
83. PNH 30.17/LB VIII 289. For the Magi see PNH VI intro. xx
84. PNH 30.1–3/LB VIII 279
85. PNH 28.49/LB VIII 37

86. PNH 29.82/LB VIII 237
87. PNH 30.13/LB VIII 287
88. PNH 30.98/LB VIII 341
89. PNH 2.147/LB I 283
90. PNH 2.209/LB I 341
91. PNH 7.17/LB II 517
92. PNH 7.24/LB II 563
93. PNH 9.267/LB III 601; PNH 9.70/LB III 209
94. PNH 10.110/LB III 363
95. PNH 7.85/LB II 561
96. PNH 10.172/LB III 401
97. PNH 11.144/LB III 523

98. PNH 7.180/LB II 627
99. PNH 7.91/LB II 565
100. PNH 11.11/LB III 439
101. PNH 9.16/LB III 173
102. PNH 11.222/LB III 573
103. PNH 12.38/LB IV 29
104. PNH 13.31/LB IV 117
105. PNH 36.174/LB X 139
106. PNH 7.73/LB II 553
107. PNH 36.199/LB X 157
108. PNH 2.235/LB I 361
109. PNH 11.247/LB III 587
110. PNH 23.44/LB VI 445
111. PNH 23.45/LB VI 445
112. PNH 28.58/LB VIII 43
113. PNH 22.99/LB VI 365
114. PNH 16.194/LB IV 515
115. PNH 26.1/LB VII 265
116. PNH 7.172/LB II 621
117. PNH 7.171/LB II 621; PNH 29.4/LB VIII 185
118. PNH 24.1/LB VII 3
119. PNH 36.202/LB X 159
120. PNH 24.5/LB VII 7
121. PNH 29.18/LB VIII 195
122. PNH 29.4–8/LB VIII 185–187; for minimum living wage see van Beek 1960
p. 87
123. PNH 29.17–18/LB VIII 195. The Latin is beautiful: "adeo blanda est
sperandi pro se cuique dulcedo." The little we know about medical education in
Pliny's time is discussed in Ch. 10.
124. PNH 22.15/LB VI 305
125. PNH 1.24/LB I 15
126. PNH 16.4/LB IV 389
127. PNH 7.130/LB II 593
128. PNH 28.9/LB VIII 9
129. PNH 29.29, 31, 39, 41/LB VIII 201, 203, 209; PNH 30.115/LB VIII 353; PNH
24.15/LB VII 13; PNH 28.242/LB VIII 163; PNH 24.48/LB VII 41; PNH 23.4/LB VI 417;
PNH 28.241/LB VIII 163; PNH 29.58, 59/LB VIII 221; PNH 29.91/LB VIII 243; PNH
30.80/LB VIII 329; PNH 30.118/LB VIII 355; PNH 28.63/LB VIII 47
130. PNH 27.79/LB VII 437; Goodman and Gilman 1965 p. 1068
131. PNH 30.112/LB VIII 351
132. PNH 28.239/LB VIII 161
133. PNH 28.258/LB VIII 173
134. PNH 26.132–134/LB VII 365
135. Goodman and Gilman 1965 p. 507
136. Dr. Carl F. Schmidt was kind enough to write to me—with unabated enthusiasm, half a century later—the details of his trip to China, and the adventure of his
discovery of ephedrine through ma huang. Without his studies, Pliny's precious
infusion of "a plant that some call ephedron" might never have been revived.
137. Dioscorides IV 46/Gunther 1934 p. 438
138. NEED I 197
139. PNH 6.54/LB II 379
140. Charaka does not list Ephedra among the herbs recommended for asthma;
in fact, he declares that cough and asthma are incurable. He would not have said this
if he had known of Ephedra (ChS II 1476 ff.). Sushruta's chapter on asthma (SS III
319) contains a vast number of Sanskrit drug names, but the long list of English equivalents at the end of the volume (app. pp. 65–81) does not mention Ephedra, and the
same is true for the list of Charaka's plant drugs compiled by Rây and Gupta 1965 pp.
52–77.

141. De Pasquale 1965; La Floresta 1940; Du Chaliot 1943. For the literature on Italian *Ephedrae* I am indebted to Prof. Antonio Imbesi, Faculty of Pharmacology, University of Messina, Italy. As a folk remedy, *Ephedrae* have been used all over the world, and of course not only in the "proper" way but for practically any disease, from syphilis to rheumatism (Chen and Schmidt 1930 p. 4 ff.).

142. Among the minor sources: Scribonius Largus wrote a small book of *Conpositiones* (prescriptions), and Pliny the Younger wrote another booklet bearing the more pretentious title *De medicina libri tres*. It too is a collection of prescriptions, grouped by diseases, whose purpose is to save time and trouble for travelers who fall into the hands of incompetent doctors! Oddly enough, this work of Pliny the Younger—which I found in Geneva in a 1875 edition—is not mentioned in any bibliography or history of medicine that I know; I plan to investigate its authenticity.

143. For data on Celsus, see Spencer 1926; Allbutt 1921; Wellmann 1913; Marx 1915 (in Latin); Sabbadini 1900 (on the codices). The initial "A." of Cornelius Celsus is usually interpreted as Aulus, but according to Pazzini (1967) it should be Albinovanus. Whether Celsus was a physician is not certain; the question has been much debated (Pazzini 1967).

144. PNH 39.17/LB VIII 195

145. *Vir mediocri ingenio* in the words of Quintilian (Quintilian X 1, 123/Marx 1915 1 I). Elsewhere Quintilian makes up for this remark by saying that Celsus had written on philosophy "not without culture and elegance" (*non sine cultu ac nitore*; Quintilian X 1, 123/Marx 1915 2 XI). For other ancient references to Celsus see Pazzini 1967.

146. Pazzini 1967

147. PNH 29.1/LB VIII 183

148. Allbutt 1921 p. 202

149. Sabbadini 1900 pp. 310–311

150. Greek and Roman debts to Indian medicine are not usually acknowledged; it is customary to search instead for Greek influence in India. See e.g. Scarborough's recent book on Roman medicine, p. 37.

151. CDM *Prooemium* 25–36/LB I 15

152. CDM *Prooemium* 23–24/LB I 15

153. Sarton 1959 p. 133

154. This passage of Celsus has been a classical trap (Spencer 1926 p. 132). Another scholar fell into it recently (Phillips 1973 p. 141). Since Celsus begins by presenting the case for Alexandrian vivisection, the first paragraph may be mistaken for the author's own opinion.

155. CDM *Prooemium* 43/LB I 25. This method of learning anatomy as a by-product of accidental violence explains the casual remark of Celsus that the brain has no sensation (CDM IV 1.10/LB I 361). He says the same of the marrow and of the omentum. But some parts of the omentum are surely sensitive. As to the bone marrow, he may be referring to the diploe (deep part of the skull bone), which is in fact not sensitive.

156. CDM *Prooemium* 74–75/LB I 41, my translation

157. Pazzini 1971. Celsus must be quoting once again from Alexandrian sources rather than describing what was actually happening in Rome.

158. Galen, *De anatomicis administrationibus*, II 3/K II 289; Pazzini 1971 p. 148. The original Greek for *vulneraria speculatio* is τραυματικὴ θέα.

159. CDM VII 1/LB III 295; CDM VII 4/LB III 297

160. It is interesting to compare the three descriptions of the perfect surgeon—Greek, Indian, and Roman—as an expression of three cultures. Cf. pp. 148, 269

161. The actual proportion of Greeks among Roman physicians is impossible to assess. Pliny makes clear that medical fashion and practice in Rome were essentially Greek. I tried to draw more precise conclusions from the names of the eighty-five know physicians of the Roman army, but Prof. R. W. Davies kindly pointed out to me that this is both dangerous and inadequate.

162. PNH 39.17/LB VIII 195

163. For Roman surgical instruments see Milne 1907; Meyer-Steineg 1912;

Tabanelli 1958; Deringer 1954; Liebl 1902 (bas-relief); Liversidge 1968 p. 323 ff.; Davies 1970(d) pp. 89–91; Deneffe 1896; Dollfus 1958; 1964; Como 1925; Vulpes 1847; Senn 1895. More refs. are in Scarborough 1969 p. 203 note 4. Crişan (1957)—in Rumanian—describes a rare medical kit of the box type.

164. The fallen "surgeon" is described by Maiuri (1964 pp. 199–200). Maiuri, an archeologist of great renown who was in charge of the excavations at Pompeii, gives no further reference. A search for photographs at Pompeii and in Naples was fruitless.

165. The collyrium stamps found to date are usually called "oculist stamps." This would mean, however, that there were some 250 Roman oculists—surely far too many. A misunderstanding arose through the changed connotation of the word *collyrium*: because it now refers to eye medicine, the stamps were misnamed "oculist stamps"; they should be called "collyrium stamps" (Olivier 1944). The name *kollýrion* seems to mean "little roll," being the diminutive of *kóllyra*, probably the same as *kóllyx*, "roll of bread" (LS p. 972). Another suggested origin is from *kolobè ourá*, "truncated tail," on account of the conical shape. Hippocrates mentions kollyria as pessaries. As sticks for exploring wounds, Celsus mentions them twice (CDM VII 4/LB III 306; CDM V 28.12/LB II 158). Remains of many collyrium tablets (but not of the conical confection) have been found and analyzed (Deneffe 1896 p. 46 ff.). The best summary of collyria in antiquity is in the Adams translation of *Paulus Aegineta*, III 548–557. For chemical analyses see Sédille 1956; Dollfus 1966; Oxé 1941.

166. CDM VII 5.3A/LB III 319

167. Congratulations to my German colleague, for I myself would have been unable to understand the description of Celsus. As translated by W. G. Spencer (CDM VII 3B/LB III 318), it becomes even more confused, because the supposed spoon is described in a footnote as "similar to the present-day midwifery forceps."

168. CDM V 26.20/LB II 77

169. CDM IV 12/LB I 401

170. PNH 28.198/LB VIII 133

171. The Alexandrian physicians who performed autopsies might *possibly* have recognized gastric ulcers.

172. CDM V.21 ff./LB II 81 ff.

173. CDM V.21/LB II 81

174. PNH 31.125/LB VIII 457

175. CDM V.26 21C/LB II 81, my translation. In particular, I prefer to render *venae* as "veins," not "blood vessels," for Celsus probably believed that arteries contain air.

176. CDM VII 31.3–33/LB III 469

177. Paré 1678 p. 304

178. Deneffe 1896; Sédille 1956; Dollfus 1966. These "oculists" who used hemostatic forceps were more probably regular physicians and surgeons; the misunderstanding that led to calling them "oculists" was explained above.

179. This was still the current belief, reported by Pliny (PNH 11.219, 220/LB III 571), who adds that if an artery is severed, the part of the body concerned is paralyzed—a notion presumably derived from the fact that arteries and nerves often run together.

180. CDM V 26.22/LB II 83

181. CDM V 26.23/LB II 83

182. CDM VII 7.8C/LB III 339

183. I was told this by Prof. Jean Babel, who witnessed the sutures with hair.

184. CDM V 26.23/LB II 83

185. For fibulae see Déchelette 1910; Blinkenberg 1926; Catling 1964; *Reallexikon der Vorgeschichte*, Berlin 1925, *Fibel*.

186. CDM V 26.23/LB II 85, 87

187. Ovid, *Ex Ponto*, III epist. VII 25–26/LB 417. In the context, Ovid is complaining about moral wounds, and alludes to bodily wounds as a metaphor.

188. CDM V 26.23/LB II 87

189. CDM V 19/LB II 33

190. The thirty-four preparations are given in CDM V 19 1–28/LB II 33–45. The five plasters free of metals are nos. 9, 10, 13, 14, and 17 (numbering mine). They are essentially mixtures of resins (turpentine, myrrh, frankincense), pitch, wax, oils, fats, and soda. Plasters "for drawing out pus" are sometimes called by Celsus *epispastics*, from the Greek *epí–spáo*, "towards–draw." A precious dictionary of Celsian drugs, with comments, appears in the Loeb edition of Celsus (II xv–lxvii). It indicates that lead was used as an oxide (*spuma argenti*, "litharge"), as basic acetate (*cerussa*, "white lead," made with lead and vinegar), as sulphide (*plumbum combustum*, "galena," the Greek *molýbdaina*), and even as slag (*plumbi recrementum*). Copper was used as scales (*aeris squama*), as calcined ore (*aes combustum*), as acetate (*aerugo*, "verdigris"), as basic carbonate and sulphate (*chalcitis*, "copperas or green vitriol"), as red oxide (*flos aeris*), as black oxide (*squama aeris*, "chipped-off molten copper"), and in several other forms.

191. CDM V 19.28/LB II 45—no. 34 of the series

192. CDM V 27.12B/LB II 123; see also CDM/LB II xlviii (intro.)

193. PNH 33.124/LB IX 95

194. For lead poisoning in antiquity see Hofmann 1885; Kobert 1909. On lead in bones see also Jaworowski 1967; Becker and others 1968; Anon. 1971; Ball 1971. Gilfillan 1965 suggests that the fall of Rome may have been due largely to lead poisoning. However, the promised analyses of lead in Roman bones never followed. Correspondence with the author convinced me that lead poisoning surely existed but that the above theory is a flight of fancy. Water was delivered to many wealthy homes through lead pipes, a practice that was current until recently, as witnessed by the word *plumbing* (from *plumbum*, "lead").

195. Columella XII 20/LB II 233

196. PNH 14.136/LB IV 277

197. Pliny says of *sandarach*, red sulphide of arsenic: "it is useful for giving women a fair complexion; but like scum of silver [*lead oxide*] it is a deadly poison" (PNH 34.176/LB IX 255). *Cerussa*, basic lead acetate (white lead) was made by leaving pieces of lead in jars full of vinegar. The Greeks called it *psimýthion*. It was a popular white face-powder (Theophrastus, *On Stones*, pp. 55–56; Plato, *Lysis*, p. 217 d, etc.; see also LS p. 2024).

198. PNH XXXIV xiv, 152/LB IX 239

199. PNH 34.100/LB IX 201. For the technology, adulteration, and uses of verdigris and other copper compounds see PNH 34.110–127/LB IX 209–221; see also Davies 1970(b).

200. Pories and others 1967

201. Elias and Chvapil 1973

202. CDM V 26/LB II 97

203. Of course, the Roman dressing need not have been inspired by its Egyptian predecessor.

204. CDM V 8/LB II 9

205. CDM V 2/LB II 5

206. CDM V 25/LB II 59

207. CDM III 10/LB I 273

208. CDM III 10.2/LB I 273

209. CDM III 1/LB I 219.

210. Auboyer 1961 pp. 77, 146, 177, 204

211. The amphorae came from a known factory in Arezzo, Tuscany. They are described by Wheeler 1946 and discussed by Filliozat 1956 p. 15 ff.

212. Maiuri 1938; Filliozat 1956 p. 15

213. PNH 6.56 ff./LB II 379 ff.

214. PNH 7.23/LB II 521; PNH 7.11/LB II 513. Trust Pliny to record such marvelous tales; but many originated with the Indians themselves (Rawlinson 1916 p. 26).

215. PNH 13.90/LB IV 153; PNH 9.71/LB III 209

216. PNH 12.26 ff./LB IV 19 ff.; PNH 16.236/LB IV 477

217. PNH 16.162/LB IV 493

218. PNH 35.43, 46/LB IX 293, 295

219. PNH 9.106/LB III 235

220. Regarding *malabathrum*: the Greek ear, hearing *tamala pâtra*, probably separated *ta-mala*, interpreting *ta-* as the Greek article, neuter plural, *tá*. Another possible derivation of *malabathrum*: *mâlâ*, "garland," and *pâtra* (Schoff 1912 p. 220). The curious fact about malabathrum is that no secret was made of its Indian origin, whereas the source of the bark of the same tree, cinnamon, was kept secret (presumably because more lucrative). Romans never made the connection between the two (ibid.).

221. PNH 6.101/LB II 415

222. This fascinating book is usually known as *The Periplus of the Erythraean Sea*. It was written in Greek by an anonymous sea-captain, perhaps from Alexandria. Pliny may have drawn from it (Schoff 1912). For Roman trade relations with the East during this period see Miller 1969.

223. PNH 24.5/LB VII 5

224. PNH 12.71/LB IV 53. India is not now a producer of myrrh, and *Balsamodendron myrrha* is not described among the Indian flora (Giboin 1949). Arabian myrrh is now bought by Indian merchants, who process it and distribute it to the world markets. Prof. R. L. Cleveland of Regina University, Saskatchewan, one of the few historians expert on this topic, never heard of Indian myrrh (personal communication). However, a *Boswellia* ("Indian olibanum") is mentioned among the plant-drugs of Charaka (Rây and Gupta 1965 p. 72 #265).

225. The excellence of Indian lycium is testified by Pliny (PNH 24.125/LB VII 91), Scribonius Largus (#19), Galen (*De simplicibus medicamentis* K VII 64), and about 400 A.D. by Marcellus Empiricus (VIII) who draws from Scribonius.

226. J. Y. Simpson, Professor of Midwifery in Edinburgh, writes in 1854 that lycium "is still used extensively by the native medical practitioners of India, under the Hindu name of *Rusot* or *Ruswut* chiefly for inflammations of the eyes." It is prepared from the wood and roots of various species of *Berberis*. Whether it really works, I do not know; Prof. Simpson tried it on one eye, in patients with bilateral inflammation, and found it "interesting" that lycium worked better than the *usual treatments*: leeches and blisters applied to the other eye! (Simpson 1854 p. 417). See also Adams' comments in *Paulus Aegineta* III 234. The drug is still sold in Indian bazaars (Giboin 1949 p. 81).

227. Suetonius, *Caligula*, 1/LB I 405

228. SS III 701

229. PNH 9.187/LB III 549; D'Erce 1969

230. Elliot 1918 p. 15

231. Normally the light rays converge onto the retina thanks to the cornea and the crystalline lens. If the lens is removed, the image forms too far behind the retina—unless the eye is sufficiently elongated, as it is in the shortsighted.

232. CDM VII 7.14 ff./LB III 349 ff.

233. ChS II 1744

234. SS III 76

235. The Indian operation for couching was the subject of the Hunterian Lectures of 1917. The author, R. H. Elliot, a famous ophthalmologist, worked twenty-five years on the topic, spent much time in India, supervised one Indian ophthalmic hospital, and left his name to another—but evidently never heard of Sushruta or Charaka! He studied 550 patients who had been "couched." In 10.59% vision was ⅓ or better; some vision was restored in a total of 38.33%; the other patients became permanently blind. Since a cataract means blindness anyway, it is obvious that, *before modern eye surgery, about four patients in ten could thank their vaidya*. The main causes of failure are infection and sometimes loss of eyesight in later years through an increase of intraocular pressure—glaucoma—for unclear reasons. See also Duke-Elder 1969 XI 63, who recognizes the priority of Sushruta. The incidence of cataract, I am told, is very high in some parts of India.

236. CDM VII 9.1/LB III 363. This method of Celsus was discussed by Daremberg 1847.

237. CDM VII 8.3/LB III 361

238. One of the devices used in ancient India for stretching the earlobes were fish vertebrae of increasing size (Casal 1950). A set found in a tomb of the second century B.C. is exposed at the Musée Guimet in Paris. Small fish vertebrae, allegedly found in a tomb on the Palatine Hill in Rome, were also interpreted as earlobe dilators of Indian style (ibid. p. 146). Details on the find were not given. Until then, I prefer to adopt the suggestion of Prof. R. W. Davies that the Roman fish may have been food for the afterlife.

239. Exodus 20:22–21:6

240. Martial VI 64/LB I 399: "... if I brand you with the heat of my wrath, Cinnamus ... will not erase the marks."

241. CDM V 27 3A/LB II 115

242. It is highly unusual for Celsus to acknowledge the priority of foreigners in matters medical, especially an African tribe (CDM/LB II 114 note b).

243. Ligature for snake bite is also known nowadays by African people (Harley 1941 p. 98).

244. CDM/LB II 195, 201. Celsus also mentions lycium and malabathrum, but without reference to India (CDM/LB II xl, xli).

245. Livy II xlvii/LB I 381

246. Livy II xiv/LB I 267

247. Suetonius, *Tiberius*, 40/LB I 351

248. Tacitus, *Annals*, IV 63/LB III 113

249. Livy X xxxv/LB IV 491

250. Scarborough 1968 p. 259. References on military hospitals will be found in the note to Fig. 9.34. For help on military hospitals I am indebted to Prof. R. W. Davies of Sunderland College and Dr. J. K. S. St. Joseph, Director in Aerial Photography, Cambridge University.

251. Nutton 1969 p. 266 note 39

252. Davies 1970(d) pp. 93–98 and fig. 14.

253. The estimate is 3% in Richmond 1968 p. 66; it was later raised to 5%, possibly 10% in times of emergency (personal communication, Dr. J. K. S. St. Joseph). For calculations on number of beds per cubicle see also Davies 1970(d) note 150. The use of bunk beds could have doubled the number of occupants (personal communication, Prof. R. W. Davies).

254. Personal communication, Dr. J. K. S. St. Joseph.

255. Watermann 1970

256. Anon. 1900[?] p. 15

257. Knörzer 1963 p. 311

258. Knörzer 1965, 1970

259. CDM III 18.12/LB I 297

260. Goodman and Gilman 1965 p. 524 ff.

261. PNH 25.66/LB VII 185

262. See Ch. 4 (Homeric medicine). *Centaurium umbellatum* is not mentioned even in Flückiger and Hanbury, *Pharmacographia* (1879) and in Trease and Evans, *Pharmacognosy* (1971). *Centaurium umbellatum* = *Erythraea centaurium* = *Centaurium minus* (Imbesi 1964 p. 251) = the french *petite centaurée*.

263. PNH 34.153, 154/LB IX 239

264. Davies 1970(b)

265. The organization of medical care in the Roman army has been much debated recently. The rather negative view of Scarborough (1968) that there was no regular corps of doctors has been effectively refuted by Vivian Nutton 1969; see also Davies 1969; 1970(a, c, d).

266. Davies 1969 p. 95 ff.; 1972; 1973

267. The text of this letter is in Zereteli and Jernstedt 1966 pp. 1–8. It is discussed in Roberts 1950; Davies 1969 pp. 93–94. Translation revised with the aid of Mrs. M. Vodoz.

268. It is often reported that in 46 B.C. Julius Caesar, pressed by the need of physicians, granted Roman citizenship to the Greeks of that profession. In fact, he gave this right wholesale to all foreigners teaching any liberal art in Rome (Suetonius, *Divus Iulius*, 42.1/LB I 59).

269. This subtle (but still debated) observation was made by a fellow pathologist from Milan, Dr. Lino Rossi, an expert on the Roman army and author of a book on the Trajan Column (Rossi 1969; 1971 pp. 152–153). For the use of the scarf (*focale*) by the auxiliaries see Paribeni 1926–1927 p. 224.

270. PNH 39.17/LB VIII 193

271. The problem of public medical care in Rome has made little or no progress since Briau's studies almost a hundred years ago. These works are indispensable, but on one point they baffle me. On the one hand, the Romans were utterly unable to conceive of free medical care for the poor (Briau 1869 p. 5); on the other, there is no doubt that the archiatri cared for the poor (Briau 1877 p. 64). The overall conclusion is that "somehow, almost everybody was looked after" (Briau 1869 p. 108). For public physicians in Greece see Cohn-Haft 1956.

272. Pliny complains about the high fees of physicians (PNH 29.7, 29.22/LB VIII 187, 197).

273. The evidence for guild physicians is meager: two inscriptions on stone (Briau 1869 pp. 79, 85 ff.).

274. "Sell worn-out oxen, blemished cattle, blemished sheep . . . an old wagon, old tools, an old slave, a sickly slave, and *whatever else* is superfluous" (Cato II 7/LB 9). Legally, slaves were objects, not people. For sick slaves abandoned on the island and decree of Claudius see Suetonius, *Claudius*, 25/LB II 49.

275. Cohn-Haft 1956; Briau 1877 p. 64

276. The decree of Antoninus *regulates* the office of public physician in the provinces; Briau interprets this as suggesting that this office already existed but needed the firm hand of the law because it had entailed administrative abuse (Briau 1877 p. 55 ff.). Though Antoninus does not yet call these physicians *archiatri*, their function is the same. For the decree of Antoninus see Briau 1877 pp. 57–58; *Corpus Iuris Civilis*, L tit. IX; XXVII tit. I.

277. The name *archiatrus* is not well explained, however. Names with *arch-* usually meant "chief-," but then it is not clear of what they were chiefs. A less likely meaning is "physician-of-the-chief (= emperor)" (Briau 1877 pp. 14, 15).

278. Briau 1877 p. 64

279. Mommsen 1934

280. See Briau 1877 pp. 84–85; *Codex Iustinianus*, VI 43.3

281. Kleine Pauly 1964 I 506

282. CDM *Prooemium* 65/LB I 35. In this sweeping comment on dumb foreigners (*exterae gentes*) Celsus seems to forget the notoriously subtle Greeks; but maybe he did not mean to include them, since Greece, after all, was then a part of the Roman Empire.

283. These *servi medici* are attested on inscriptions (Briau 1869 p. 66 ff.), and in a late edict their price is set three times higher than for ordinary slaves (Chiappelli 1881 p. 17; *Codex Iustinianus*, VI 43.3).

284. Columella 12 III 8/LB III 193

285. Columella 12 III 7/LB III 191

286. For Seneca and valetudinaria, see Seneca, *Ep.* 27.1; *De ira* I, 16.4; *Quaest. nat. I. Praef. ante med.* 6. These passages, and the question of civilian infirmaries in general, are well discussed by Harig (1971).

287. Minuscule evidence for "private infirmaries" appears in a comedy of Plautus. Says the *medicus*, talking about a madman: "See that he is taken to me [*to my place*]." "Do you mean it?" "By all means: there I shall be able to cure him as I please" (*Menaechmi* V 946–949/LB II 461). Plautus was writing this about 200 B.C., so he could have had in mind the story of Archagathus and of the private office financed for him by the city. But he could also have lifted the idea from a Greek original, with no Roman relevance. It is sometimes said that Vitruvius mentions *hospitalia* in his books *On Architecture*, written about 25 B.C. Sure—but for him the word meant "places for guests" in homes and theaters (Vitruvius, *De architectura*, V 6, 7/LB I 284, 288).

288. Harig 1971

289. As evidence of Roman cruelty, Briau (1866 p. 28) quotes this gladiator's oath: "By the words of Eumolpius, we swear that we shall suffer to be burned, bound,

beaten, and killed by the iron, and anything else that Eumolpius might order. As regular gladiators, we most solemnly entrust our bodies and souls to the master" (Petronius, *Satyricon*, 117). The cruel status of the gladiators is not to be disputed; however, the *Satyricon* of Petronius can scarcely be quoted as a historical source.

290. How available it was, in any given time and place, is not in the books, as far as I know. Drabkin also notices that there are in antiquity "innumerable literary, epigraphic and papyrological evidences of the employment of doctors by the state to treat patients without charge" (Drabkin 1944 p. 347); but of course episodes do not make statistics.

291. St. Jerome, *Epistulae*, LXXVII, *Ad Oceanum De Morte Fabiolae*/LB 323

292. Edelstein and Edelstein 1945 II 176, I 739. Buildings attached to Asklepieia, to house the pilgrims, are known for Pergamon and other sites. In Pergamon the addition came under the Romans, as attested by Pausanias, who wrote in the second century A.D.: "The Epidaurians about the sanctuary were in great distress, because their women were not allowed to bring forth under shelter, and their sick were obliged to die under the open sky. To remedy the inconvenience he [*the Roman senator Antoninus*] provided a building where a man may die and a woman may give birth to her child without sin" (EE II 176, I 739).

293. The root of *medicina* was taken up by Russian and the other Slavic languages, as well as by Albanian, a separate language of Indo-European origin; but *not* by Finnish and Hungarian. See the excellent study by Benveniste (1945).

10. Galen—and into the Night

1. The famous Kühn edition of 1821–1833 (as illustrated above the title). Though not complete, this edition includes the Latin translation: so the photograph may somewhat overplay Galen's graphomania.

2. Walsh 1934 p. 1

3. English translations of Galen up to 1954 are listed in Sarton 1954 pp. 101–107; see also Duckworth 1962; Brock 1963; May 1968. I consulted the original text on many occasions, with the invaluable help of Mrs. Martine Vodoz; but I must confess that when it came to Galen I broke my own rule: I did *not* read the twenty-two volumes of the Kühn edition.

4. Siegel 1968 p. 29

5. PNH 13.70/LB IV 141

6. K XIV 17

7. K II 17

8. Gourevitch 1970 p. 7. Briau tries to make a case for the existence of a medical school in Rome during the first century (1877 p. 101 ff.), his evidence being two undated inscriptions in stone, one mentioning a *Tabularius scholae medicorum* and the other, a *Scriba Medicorum* (secretary to the medical school, secretary to the physicians). There the matter rests. Galen's tirade against Thessalus (K X 4) surely proves that medical education in Rome was not formalized. Galen likes to contrast the depth of his own preparation (e.g. K XIX 59) with the superficiality of his colleagues' (e.g. K X IX 804).

9. Sarton suggests that Galen knew Latin perhaps as well as a "European officer in Egypt" might have known Arabic (1954 p. 81). Although Seidmann says that Galen mentions learning Latin, he gives no reference (1936 p. 400), and I found none.

10. There is one possible exception (Sarton 1954 p. 79): the individuals to whom Galen dedicated his works must have been somehow close to him; but warmth was not his lot.

11. Phillips 1973 p. 172.

12. For Galen's experiments on the nervous system see Dalton 1873. For his ligature of the ureters see Brock 1963 p. 59.

13. May 1968 I 367

14. Walsh 1937 p. 35; see also Scarborough 1971

15. Daremberg and Saglio II 1565; Walsh 1936 p. 39

16. K XIII 599/Walsh 1937 p. 34

17. K XIII 600/Walsh 1937 p. 36

18. K XIII 633–644

19. K XII 226

20. Plain chimney soot was used as a wound disinfectant in 1870 by the French army besieged in Metz, upon the advice of one Dr. J. Jeannel, pharmacist of the Guard (information courtesy of Colonel Ferry, Service Historique de l'Armée, Vincennes, France). Dr. Jeannel may have based his suggestion upon the similarity between soot (obtained by burning coal in air) and coal tar (obtained by heating coal in the absence of air). Coal tar was then a common disinfectant.

21. Shoemaker's blacking (ferrous sulfate + tannic acid) is recommended by Celsus for cleansing sores and as a caustic (e.g. CDM V 2 and 8/LB II 5 and 9). Writing ink, made with the soot of torches, he recommends for bald spots (CDM VI 4/LB II 183): a harmless substitute for black hair.

22. K XVIII(2) 567/Walsh 1937 p. 40

23. Galen's treatment for wounds and ulcers is summarized in two German theses (Prüsmann 1900; Schröder 1901). Unfortunately both lack references in the text.

24. K X 378/Walsh 1937 p. 40

25. K XIII 601/Walsh 1937 p. 36

26. Walsh 1926 p. 183

27. K X 410 ff./Walsh 1937 p. 42

28. May 1968 I 215. After he lost his omentum, this gladiator remained very sensitive to cold, kept himself wrapped in wool, and "could not bear to have his abdomen uncovered." True or not, these symptoms misled Galen into concluding that the function of the omentum was to keep the intestines warm.

29. K VIII 304

30. K I 1–39/Walsh 1937 p. 50

31. Walsh 1937 p. 39

32. Charles-Picard 1965 p. 79

33. Human sacrifice in Rome, according to Pliny, had been abolished only in 97 B.C. (PNH 30.12/LB VIII 287).

34. Scribonius Largus, *Conpositiones*, 17/Helmreich p. 11

35. PNH 28.4/LB VIII 5

36. For the *taurobolium* see Duthoy 1969. One such pit (*fossa sanguinis*) was found at Ostia (Calza 1953). A well-preserved one is on display at Novaesium [Neuss] (Wortmann 1971). See also von Petrikovits 1961.

37. Dr. Walsh (1937 p. 44) was seriously mistaken here: Galen did not use the tourniquet. The word that he translates as "tourniquet" (K X 318) is *ánkistron*, "fishhook" or simply "hook." The text leaves no doubt: "hook the vessel, pull, and twist." Galen uses the same method for vivisection (Duckworth 1962 p. 16).

38. K X 318

39. Duckworth 1962 p. 16

40. Duckworth 1962 p. 16

41. K X 942

42. NEED I 197

43. K X 320

Notes to pages 398–405

44. If the Latin of Celsus is compared to a glass of sparkling wine, that of Scribonius is not far from dishwater.

45. That Scribonius is really talking about a tourniquet seems certain: the words are *artus constringere*, "to constrict the limb."

46. Scribonius Largus, *Conpositiones*, 84/Helmreich pp. 85–86

47. K II 537

48. Walsh 1937 p. 54

49. Duckworth 1962 p. 182. As for autopsies on "fresh" human cadavers in Rome, it is very unlikely that Galen ever performed any. Physicians may have felt

the need to dissect human bodies (Celsus says so quite clearly) and the law was not specifically against it; but custom was, and it seems to have prevailed (Pazzini 1971). Human autopsies were performed, if anywhere, in Alexandria. See also Temkin 1973 pp. 115, 136–140.

50. Duckworth 1962 p. 182
51. Duckworth 1962 p. 87
52. Duckworth 1962 p. 24
53. Duckworth 1962 p. 29
54. Duckworth 1962 p. 15
55. Walsh 1926; 1937 p. 52
56. Walsh 1926; Daremberg 1854 I 498
57. Duckworth 1962 p. 207
58. K VIII 55. Accidental injury to the recurrent laryngeal nerves is still a hazard during operations for goiter.
59. Walsh 1937 p. 55
60. The translator's comments here are misleading (SS II 185). To the "four Dhamani" he appends "arteries." But the sense of *Dhamani* is obviously more vague, for in his glossary he gives Dhamani as "vessel, artery, or duct" (SS III Appendix p. 46). There he also refers to SS II 209, where Dhamani is translated first "ducts," then "arteries," and finally "nerves." So it is false precision, and of no help, to label the four Dhamani in the neck as arteries; the sense actually points to nerves.
61. SS II 185
62. According to the original legend the Neela-Manya marma corresponds to the following structures: "*Superior* laryngeal–glossopharyngeal–hypoglossal–superior thyroid–lingual" [italics mine]. Galen's nerve is of course the *inferior* laryngeal.
63. From the translation of *Cellularpathologie* 1863, 2nd ed., reprinted in 1971, p. 430. The first edition (1858) has the same passage. The "more recent schools," said by Virchow to "agree" with the necessity of a fifth symptom, remain a question mark.
64. Quoted perfunctorily from textbook to textbook, the four cardinal signs of inflammation (plus one) have undergone a hilarious series of mistakes and permutations, well summarized by Dr. Rather (1971). Still missing in this delightful essay is the real father of the fifth symptom; the earliest and still "fatherless" mention that Dr. Rather could find was in Uhle and Wagner's *Handbuch* of pathology, 1864.
65. On Dec 28, 1917, H. L. Mencken published in the New York *Evening Mail* a completely fake account of the invention of the modern bathtub as it was supposed to have occurred in Cincinnati in 1842: "Alas . . . they swallowed it as gospel, gravely and horribly." The story ended up in reference books and encyclopedias, becoming undistinguishable from established fact. "*Despite all this extravagant frenzy for the truth, there is something in the human mind that turns instinctively to fiction*" (Mencken 1958 pp. 15–16).
66. Rather 1971
67. Sarton 1954 p. 65
68. For an excellent history of theriac see Watson 1966.
69. Today's figures are still high: in the U.S. alone, an estimated 2 million people are bitten by animals each year; of these, about .5 million are bitten by dogs, 3000–6000 by snakes; deaths by snake bite average 14 per year (Schwartz 1969 p. 165 ff.).

Notes to pages 405–414

70. For the thankless job of counting bites in the Gunther edition of Dioscorides I am indebted to Lise Piguet.
71. CDM V 27/LB II 111
72. K V 41
73. PNH 28.40/LB VIII 31
74. PNH 11.170/LB III 539
75. PNH 28.40/LB VIII 31
76. Schwartz 1969 p. 165 ff.
77. Watson 1966 p. 13
78. Scribonius Largus, *Conpositiones*, 163/Helmreich p. 67.

79. PNH XXV iii/LB VII 141

80. Watson 1966 p. 35

81. Tacitus, *Annals*, XII 66, XIII 15/LB III 413, IV 25; Watson 1966 p. 86

82. The similarity between *galene* and Galen is accidental. *Galenós* meant "calm"—a peace surely not unrelated to opium.

83. Some people, however, remained skeptical. Hear Pliny on *Mithridatium*: it is "composed of 54 ingredients, no two of them having the same weight . . . Which of the gods, in the name of Truth [*the goddess*], fixed these absurd proportions?" (PNH XXIX 24/LB VIII 1999).

84. K XIV 232/Watson 1966

85. Watson 1966 p. 87

86. K XIV 280/Watson 1966 p. 63

87. K XIV 219/Watson 1966 p. 63

88. NEED I 205

89. ChS II 1638

90. SS II 740

91. Watson 1966 p. 104

92. This statement is made with the usual reservations that apply to any data on China (meaning that it is third- or fourth-hand information), but it is generally believed that with Hua T'o, a contemporary of Galen's, Chinese surgery reached its peak.

93. PNH VI 23.100–147/LB VI 481–513

94. For Greek diet see Ackerknecht 1970 p. 170 ff.; 1971

95. K XI 147–378; K XIX 519–528

96. K V 119/Walsh 1934 p. 14

97. Caelius Aurelianus, *De morbis chronicis*, II. xiii. 183/Amman p. 415

98. Ackerknecht 1970 p. 109 ff.

99. Literature on this major episode is amazingly scant. See Whipple 1936; Elgood 1938; Major 1954 p. 227, on which I based my account. For the sad lot of today's Nestorians see Atiya 1968.

100. The tolerance of the early Muslims should be emphasized. They found little difference between their creed and that of the Nestorians; and to the Nestorians, the Islamic message did not sound very different from their own (Jargy 1969).

101. *On Medical Experience*, a ninth-century copy of the original Arabic translation by Hubaish of the Syriac version by the Nestorian scholar Hunain. The book had been written by Galen at the age of nineteen!

Notes to the Illustrations

FIGURES

1.1 Found in the Chubut Valley, Patagonia (Collection de la Vaulx, No. 12.282; see Pales 1930 p. 97). Black background added. Courtesy of the Musée de l'Homme, Paris.

1.4 Specimen found at Sterkfontein and published in Dart 1949 Plate 3 No. 26, as "endocranial cast" (i.e. a natural fossil cast of the inner cavity of the skull) of *Plesianthropus transvaalensis Broom*, which is the obsolete name given by Broom to *Australopithecus africanus* (see Ardrey 1967 p. 181). Courtesy of Prof. Phillip V. Tobias, Dept. of Anatomy, University of Witwatersrand Medical School, Johannesburg, South Africa, and of The Wistar Press.

1.5 Profiles of mandibles: *Gorilla*, Howells 1967 p. 91; *Kanam Fragment*, Tobias 1962 p. 345; *Sapiens and Pekin man*, Wells 1958 (in Howells 1962 pp. 460–465).

1.6 Though actual photographs of similar specimens are easily obtainable, this old drawing was chosen because the bony reaction is particularly well shown. Redrawn from Cartailhac 1889 p. 254. No date given.

1.7 These pictures are eight photographic steps removed from the original color slides (lost), hence their relatively poor quality. Dr. Miles is Emeritus Professor of Psychology, Yale University Medical School. Reproduced with permission from Dr. Miles and from the National Academy of Sciences.

1.8 Courtesy of Dr. W. C. McGrew and Miss Caroline E. G. Tutin, Gombe Stream Research Centre, Kigoma, Tanzania, and of the American Dental Association.

1.9 See 1.8

1.10 From Felkin 1884

1.11 The fossil-bearing rock was polished, etched with acid, and covered with an ultramicroscopic layer of carbon; this carbon film was then floated off and examined. Hence the picture shows a replica of the bacteria, not the bacteria themselves. From Schopf, J. W., and others, Science 1965: *149*, 1365. Courtesy of Dr. J. W. Schopf and of Science. Copyright 1965 by the American Association for the Advancement of Science.

1.12 Skeleton of *Dimetrodon*, courtesy of Mr. Gilbert Stucker, American

Museum of Natural History, New York. Latest dating: 230 million years. Background retouched. With permission from The American Museum of Natural History. Single bone: Plate XVa from Moodie, *Paleopathology*. Bone section: Plate XXI, ibid.

1.13 Upper left second molar of *Paranthropus crassidens*, Swartkrans. Estimated age 800,000 years according to the original publication, but these figures must be increased as explained in the text. From Clement, Brit. Dental J. 1956: *101*, 4; rephotographed with permission from the British Dental Journal and slightly retouched.

1.14 I owe this striking electron micrograph to Prof. R. M. Frank of the Centre de Recherches Odontologiques, Equipe de Recherche Associée au C.N.R.S., Faculté de Médecine, Strasbourg, France (for the electron microscopy of caries see Frank and Brendel 1966).

1.15 Original in reddish brown, height about 20 cm. The figure as reproduced in H. Breuil (1920 Plate III, detail) is a drawing of the original, not a photograph. Breuil interprets it as a man seen from the back, seemingly hit by eight arrows, and shown as if trying to "pull out the lines that pierce him" (p. 21). Courtesy of Masson and Co., Editors, Paris.

1.16 Rephotographed and enlarged from Fig. 11 in Malvesin-Fabre and others 1954. With permission from E. Privat, Editor, Toulouse.

1.17 Reproduced and slightly modified from Leroi-Gourhan 1967. With permission from Prof. A. Leroi-Gourhan and the Bull. de la Soc. Préhistorique Française.

1.18 Courtesy of Prof. A. Leroi-Gourhan (1964 Fig. 9D) and of the Presses Universitaires de France.

1.19 Redrawn from the color photographs in Howell 1970 pp. 184–185, with permission of the photographer, Prof. Irven DeVore. The original hand-signs, twenty-one in all, are extremely effective and should be seen in the original. Profiles of animals taken mostly from Smithers 1966 Plates 2, 6, 10. The choice of a female lion was my own liberty.

1.20 Rephotographed from a paper by R. Virchow, Zeitschr. f. Ethnol. 1886: XVIII, 221. The little girl is on Plate V Fig. 2; she missed the last phalanx of both little fingers (p. 224), but the drawings of hands correspond to two young males: N'Fim N'Fom, perhaps twenty-four (Fig. 2 p. 234) and N'Ko, nineteen (Fig. 1 p. 234). Virchow makes no comment on the missing phalanges.

1.21 Courtesy of Robert G. Gardner, Film Study Center, Harvard University; Random House, Inc.; and Alfred A. Knopf, Inc. (Figs. 253 and 23 in Gardner and Heider 1968).

1.22 See 1.21

1.23 Courtesy of Drs. G. Mennerich and J. Bössneck. (Unlike people, bovines have only one, large metacarpal per foot: the so-called *cannon bone*).

1.24 From Lisowski 1967 p. 661. Courtesy of Dr. F. P. Lisowski and of C. C. Thomas, Publisher, Springfield, Illinois.

1.25 Skull from Patallacta, Peruvian highlands (MacCurdy 1923 Plate XXVI and pp. 242–243). Courtesy of the American Journal of Physical Anthropology and of The Wistar Press.

1.26 Skull No. 283 from Moodie 1927 Fig. 19B and 1929 Fig. 8D. The vertical crack runs down the middle of the frontal bone; at top left, the coronal suture.

1.27 Courtesy of Prof. Enrico Atzeni, Cagliari, Sardinia. From the remains of a robbed grave.

1.28 Courtesy of Dr. T. D. Stewart, Dept. of Anthropology, U.S. National Museum, Washington, D.C.; of the Bull. of Med. History; and of the Johns Hopkins Press (Stewart 1966 p. 307).

Ch. 2 title page: the two cuneiform symbols stand for *a-su*, Akkadian for "physician" (see note 2.37).

2.1 Redrawn from Bishop 1939 p. 46, with permission from the American Oriental Society.

2.2 This aerial view comes from the eastern rim of Mesopotamia (Ghirshman and others 1966 Plate I). This area belonged first to Elam (now Iran) and was later conquered by the Assyrians (Ghirshman and others 1966 p. 8). The modern name of Dur-Untash is *Tchoga Zanbil*, "[upside-down] basket hill," from the aspect of the dilapidated Ziggurat (Ghirshman and others 1966 p. 10). The river is the Âb-è Diz, tributary of the Karun, which now joins its waters with those of the Tigris and the Euphrates in the Shatt-el-Arab, but once opened independently into the Persian gulf. With permission from Prof. R. Ghirshman.

2.4 Courtesy of Miss M.-L. Vollenweider, Musée d'Art et d'Histoire, Geneva. Hematite cylinder, No. 12688; actual dimensions 22 x 12 mm. Interpretation in Vollenweider 1967 p. 44 (No. 38).

2.5 Redrawn from examples chosen in MEA pp. 146, 230, 176, 240, 158, 90, 54, 150.

2.6 With permission from Prof. R. Ghirshman. From Ghirshman and others 1966 Plates II, IV.

2.7 See 2.6

2.10 Courtesy øf the Trustees, British Museum, London.

2.11 Courtesy of The Mansell Collection, London.

2.12 Known as the "Plaque des Enfers," height 14.5 cm. Courtesy of the Louvre Museum, Paris.

2.13 Photograph of the dagger courtesy of the Trustees, British Museum, London. The specimen came from the Royal Cemetery at Ur and is now in Baghdad. Montage and drawing by Mr. P. Duvernay.

2.14 The three Sumerian pictograms are redrawn from MEA pp. 46, 162, 98.

2.15 In my original plans, a cloaked Paris policeman should have posed next to the Code (actual height 225 cm) for scale. No live policeman would be allowed into the Louvre. Courtesy of Service de Documentation Photographique, Louvre Museum, Paris.

2.16 I identified this law on the monument by using Scheil's original photographs, transcription and translation, as well as Harper's edition. The law is in Col. XXXIV, 55 ff.; it is on the rear right, at about eye-level, and is written downward in the archaic style; the text should be turned 90 degrees counterclockwise to conform with the other cuneiform writings illustrated. Courtesy of Service de Documentation Photographique, Louvre Museum, Paris.

2.17 Transcription and translation courtesy of Pablo Herrero, Collège de France, Paris.

2.18 Courtesy of Dr. S. N. Kramer, University Museum, Philadelphia, Neg. 6783. Actual size: 150 x 97 mm.

2.19 Courtesy of Dr. F. Köcher and of Akademie-Verlag, Berlin (Köcher 1955 p. 77).

2.20 From Oeder, G. C., *Flora Danica . . .* , Havniae [Copenhagen], typis Claudii Philiberti, Vol. 2, pp. 1765–1767.

2.21 This presumed "distillation vessel" was found at Tepe Gawra, northern Mesopotamia. Such pots were found at levels IX to XI, i.e. at depths going back to about 3500 B.C. (Levey 1959 p. 33); the pottery wheel seems to appear just below, at level XII (Parrot 1953 p. 194). Actual dimensions of the pot: max. width 530 mm, height 480 mm, capacity 37.3 liters, capacity of the rim 2.1 liters. Others of this kind were found; some, which have the inner rim perforated, could also have been used as extraction apparatus (vapor trickling into the rim could have extracted material placed therein). There is a tablet describing perfumery operations about 1200 B.C., compatible with the use of such double-rimmed pots (Levey 1959 p. 36). Lids were not found; perhaps they were made of wood and glazed inside (Levey, personal communication). Much later Arabic apparatus for distillation and sublimation is based on similar double-rimmed containers with tall conical lids (Levey 1959 p. 40). Photograph courtesy of the University Museum, Philadelphia (neg. 44456). The scheme is my own but based on published data (Levey 1959 pp. 40–41).

2.22 The tablets are rephotographed from Thompson 1923; the numbers (3, 4, 5) are my own, adopted because they correspond to the explanations in Prof. Labat's letter (Fig. **2.23**): 3 = *18*, No. 3 (tablet K 10535); 4 = *22*, No. 2 (tablet K 3550, obverse); 5 = *21*, No. 2 (tablet K 6196). Slightly reduced. Minimal retouches on some defective lines and signs. Thompson's translations are found in *Assyrian Medical Texts*. Proc. Roy. Soc. Med. 1924: *19*; 3 = p. 52, 4 and 5 = p. 56. (With permission of the Clarendon Press, Oxford, and of the Trustees, British Museum, London.)

2.23   Reproduced with kind permission of the late Prof. R. Labat.

2.25   Redrawn from MEA pp. 110–111.

2.26   From Contenau 1927 p. 444 (with permission of Editions A. et J. Picard, Paris).

2.27   Redrawn from MEA pp. 112–113.

2.28   Redrawn from MEA pp. 67 and 175.

2.29   P. XIX of Thompson's *Assyrian Herbal*.

2.30   From Regnault, F., *La Botanique* . . . , Tome III, Paris, 1774.

2.31   The slingers are from a bas-relief found in Kouyounjik (ancient Nineveh) and dating from the period of Sennacherib, 705–681 B.C. Courtesy of the Trustees, British Museum, London (Relief No. 124775).

Ch. 3 title page: the three hieroglyphs spell the word *swnw*, "physician."

3.1   Based on Bengtson and Milojčić 1963 p. 26.

3.2   Courtesy of the National Aeronautics and Space Administration (NASA); kindly reproduced by EROS Data Center, Geological Survey, U.S. Dept. of the Interior (Scene Identification No: NASA ERTS E-1039-08001-7).

3.3   Ages of medical papyri acc. to GMÄ I. All dates prior to 2000 B.C. are uncertain (in recent years the First Dynasty has moved from 3500 to 2900 B.C.).

3.4   Courtesy of Henry Riad, Chief Curator, Egyptian Museum, Cairo. Letters added.

3.5   From Smith 1908 Fig. 7. The published reproductions were poor and had to be heavily retouched. With permission of the Editor, British Medical Journal.

3.6   From Petrie 1927 Plate VII, rearranged.

3.7   From p. 27 of A. Gardiner's *Egyptian Grammar*, with permission of Chicago University Press.

3.8   Parts of Plates XIII and XIII-A of Breasted 1930 Vol. II (reversed, left to right). With permission of Chicago University Press.

3.9   From Hassan 1932 Fig. 143.

3.10   Courtesy of the Museum of Fine Arts, Boston (Fourth Dynasty). The usual name *Mycerinus* is the ancient Greek rendering (Latinized) of Pharaoh Mn-ka-re.

3.11   My simplified summary of papyrus technology, from Lewis 1934, and especially Pliny the Elder as quoted in text. Width of one papyrus sheet about 40 cm.

3.12   Siderolite found in Texas. Courtesy of Prof. Marc Vuagnat, Institut des Sciences de la Terre, University of Geneva.

3.13   Courtesy of the Trustees, British Museum, London. Papyrus of Hunefer. For explanations see Budge 1960 p. 248, Daumas 1965 p. 313.

3.14   From Breasted 1930 I; part of Plate IV. Courtesy of Chicago University Press.

3.15   From Goffres, *Précis iconographique de Bandages* etc., Paris, 1858 (Plate 74).

3.16   Data on "flaming hieroglyphs": Wiedemann 1920 p. 190.

3.17   From Griffith 1898 Fig. 80 Plate V. In the text (p. 26) the instrument is "mistakenly explained as a bow drill" (Wiedemann 1920 p. 187). Courtesy of the Egypt Exploration Society, London, and of Routledge and Kegan Paul, Ltd., London.

3.18   Courtesy of Jane van Lawick-Goodall and of W. Collins Sons and Co., London. Phot. Hugo van Lawick (van Lawick-Goodall 1971 Fig. opp. p. 240).

3.19   From a relief in the Cairo Museum, Nineteenth Dynasty, as redrawn in Weigall 1915 Fig. 1.

3.20   Courtesy of Mrs. D. Darbois, Paris.

3.21   Courtesy of Dr. R. S. Merrillees, Australian Mission to the United

Nations, N.Y.; Prof. H. S. Smith, Dept. of Egyptology, University College of London; and the Editor of Antiquity.

3.22 Experiment by Dr. Elisabeth Schorer and Mme S. Dersi, Dépt. de Biologie Végétale, University of Geneva.

3.23 See 3.22

3.25 Experiments by Mrs. Jean M. Thurston, Harvard Medical School.

3.26 See 3.25

3.27 Experiments by Dr. H. L. Wildasin and coll. (see note 3.19). Honey: Florida Orange Blossom Honey, raw, kindly provided by R. B. Wilson, Inc., New York. Butter prepared from cream allowed to sour naturally overnight. Pathogenic bacteria kindly provided by Dr. E. H. Kass, Channing Laboratories, Boston City Hospital. Butter-honey mixture (with or without bacteria) blended by hand, then with a Waring blender, and kept at room temperature. Bacterial counts performed on solid media. In the case of *E. coli* the count included whatever members of the coliform group may have been present initially in the butter-honey mixture (i.e. in the soured cream).

3.28 See 3.27

3.29 From Chauvin 1968 III p. 109 Fig. 39. Beehive pattern added. Courtesy of P. Lavie and of Masson and Co., Editors, Paris.

3.30 New Kingdom, Seventeenth Dynasty; 15.7 x 21.6 cm. Courtesy of the Brooklyn Museum. Gift of the Estate of Charles Edwin Wilbour.

3.31 Original bas-relief: Temple of Deir el Bahari (Naville 1898 Vol. XVI Plate 74). Drawing rephotographed from Schmidt 1924 Taf. I, with permission from J. A. Barth, Publisher.

3.32 From Singer and others 1965 pp. 264–265 Figs. 164, 163, 165; p. 269 Fig. 170. Courtesy of Dr. T. I. Williams, Managing Editor for C. Singer and others, *A History of Technology*.

3.33 See 3.32

3.34 From Smith 1912 Plates 56, 29, 22, 68, and frontispiece plate. With kind permission of H. Riad, Chief Curator, Egyptian Museum, Cairo.

3.35 See 3.34

3.36 Published by permission of the Danish National Museum, Copenhagen; phot. Lennart Larsen.

Ch. 4 title page: the Greek letters spell the word *Iatrós*, physician.

4.2 One of very few weapons found in the Homeric (VII-a) layer of Troy, in 1935; "possibly one of the missiles discharged during the fighting that resulted in the burning of the town" (Blegen 1958 Vol. IV Part 1 p. 51 and Part 2 Fig. 219, invent. No. 35-486). Courtesy of Prof. J. L. Caskey, Dept. of Classics, University of Cincinnati, of Prof. Carl W. Blegen, American School of Classical Studies, Athens, and of Princeton University Press. Actual length 38 mm.

4.3 Coin: a *hékte*, courtesy of Franke and Hirmer (from Franke and Hirmer 1964 Plate 179, top right). Reconstruction of the headband: modified from Krug 1968 p. 134 ff. (Dr. A. Krug kindly agreed that the thin ends should be longer than in her own scheme of Plate I-9).

Illustrations

4.4 From Solygeia. Capsule is represented without slits. Fig. 18 in Kritikos and Papadaki 1967, slightly retouched. Courtesy of Dr. P. G. Kritikos and of the United Nations Bull. on Narcotics.

4.5 Poppy heads photographed in the dried state. Courtesy of Mr. D. Mack, Dépt. de Biologie Végétale, University of Geneva.

4.6 Courtesy of Editions "Cahiers d'Art," Paris (in Zervos 1956 Figs. 774, 775). Data in Kritikos and Papadaki 1967 p. 23 ff., Caskey 1962 pp. 224–225.

4.7 Apollo shooting arrows at the sons and daughters of Niobe. From a chalice dated 500–450 *B.C.* (G 341), courtesy of the Louvre Museum, Paris, and of M. Chuzeville, photographer.

4.9 Evidence that Achilles made a mistake in applying this bandage should be a loose end of the bandage under his left hand; this is shown in Singer's drawing (1921

Fig. 6), but is not well apparent on the original photograph of the vase as I obtained it from the Berlin Museum. Prof. K. Vierneisel, Director of the *Antikenabteilung*, kindly assured me that the white tip of the bandage is clearly visible on the vase: hence I took the liberty of retouching it slightly on this figure. Courtesy of Staatliche Museen, Preussischer Kulturbesitz, Berlin (#F 2278). Another "mistake" in this vase: the wound represented is not mentioned by Homer! (Daremberg 1865 p. 82).

4.10 Petri dishes with just enough commercial milk to cover the bottom (about 2 cc). With fresh cow milk the effect was identical.

4.14 The thread hanging from the drain is not mentioned in the text, but I added it because the linen "tents" inserted in the same position do have this safety device (*On Diseases II*, #47/LTT VII 71).

4.16 Drawing based on the following passages concerning ancient bladder-type syringes: manner of assembly, *On Barren Women III*, #222/LTT VIII 431 (confirmed by Heister 1782 II Plate XXXIIII Fig. 12 and pp. 265–266); silver model for gynecologic use, ibid.; feather shaft, *On Fistulae*/A II 819 #5 = LTT VI 453 #6.

4.17 My interpretation.

4.18 From Adams 1849 Vol. II Plate VII.

4.19 For details see Gardiner 1930 Fig. 156 and p. 187, where this throw is called a "flying mare." Courtesy of the Trustees, British Museum, London (*se-oi-nage* means "shoulder-lift-throw").

4.20 From LTT IV 311 and LTT X xiv. In discussing the first figure, Littré adds that for accuracy the ties on the ankle should extend all the way down the leg, and those on the thigh should be wider. He was not yet aware of the lateral levers (second figure); hence Adams calls this figure erroneous and adds the levers (A II Plate V 1). Note that with two cranks and two levers, it took four people to work the bench.

4.21 Plates IV and IX from H. Schöne 1896 (*Apollonius von Kitium*). With permission from B. G. Teubner Verlagsgesellschaft, Leipzig.

4.22 See 4.21

4.23 Drawing based on the description in *On Joints*, #11/LB III 223 = LTT IV 105.

4.24 Courtesy of Römisch-Germanisches Zentralmuseum, Mainz, Germany. Provenance uncertain, but acceptable as "Roman." Longest = 165 mm. Greek specimens are very much the same.

4.25 The twenty-odd dents in this skull were probably due to stones (sling-shot) or to the fearful Inca star-shaped war club (Daland 1935 p. 555). Three were full-blown depressed fractures, i.e. worse than simple *hédrae*. Moodie calls this man The Thickheaded Village Fool (Moodie 1927 p. 286).

4.27 From Adams 1849 Vol. I, Plate I Nos. 6, 7, 8. Adams, in turn, lifted these drawings from Guido Guidi (Vidus Vidius): *Chirurgia e Graeco in Latinum conversa, Vido Vidio interprete, Lutetiae Parisiorum* pp. 117–119 (1544).

4.28 Courtesy of Dr. Jean Ginsburg, Royal Free Hospital School of Medicine, University of London, and of the American Physiological Society (Fig. 1 in Handbook of Physiology Sect. 2 Vol. III).

4.29 Attic kylix (discussed in Gardiner 1930 p. 197 ff. and Fig. 173) and pana-thenaic amphora, Archonship of Pithodelos (discussed in Gardiner 1930 p. 187 ff. and Fig. 175; modern drill-holes retouched). Courtesy of the Trustees, British Museum, London.

4.30 From Guido Guidi (Vidus Vidius) *De Chirurgia* Lib. III p. 56 Fig. LIII. Courtesy of Biblioteca Nazionale Braidense, Milan.

4.31 Courtesy of the Soprintendenza alle Antichità, Rome.

4.32 Courtesy of Hirmer Verlag, Munich (Franke and Hirmer 1964 Plate 66).

4.33 Sources for ancient number-schemes: Schöner 1964; Ghyka 1931, 1971.

4.34 Actual Greek monument; redrawn from E. Mössel, *Die Proportion in der Antike und Mittelalter.* Munich, C. H. Beck, 1936 (p. 66). With kind permission from C. H. Beck Verlag.

4.37 Data redrawn from Fig. 3 and Fig. 9 of Draczynski 1951. Wines were ten to eleven years old; pH 3.12 (white) and 3.60 (red); alcohol tested at pH 7.48. If the alcohol was tested at pH 3.26, it killed the bacteria much faster (two hours), though not as fast as wine (ibid. Fig. 9). With kind permission of the author and of J. Diemer Verlag, Mainz.

4.39   From Mattioli, P. A., *Commentario alla Materia Medica di Dioscoride*, Venezia, 1568. Courtesy of Prof. Luigi Belloni.

4.40   See 4.39

4.41   Coin kindly selected by Mr. G. K. Jenkins of the British Museum and Mr. N. Dürr, Musée d'Art et d'Histoire, Geneva (publ. in L. Anson, *Numismata Graeca*, 1910 Part V/v Plate XIV 605). From Apollonia (Mysia). Courtesy of the Trustees, British Museum, London.

4.42   Courtesy of Mr. A. Küng, Observatoire de Sauverny, Geneva.

4.43   Courtesy of PhotoThomke, and of the Stadtverwaltung, Bingen am Rhein. Background retouched.

4.44   Courtesy of the Trustees, British Museum, London (Kylix E 86).

4.45   Bronze weapon inscribed PHILIP OF MACEDONIA (the father of Alexander). Found at Olynthus, besieged and sacked 348 B.C. Courtesy of the Trustees, British Museum, London (No. 1912 4–19 x).

4.46   From C. Bell, *The Anatomy and Philosophy of Expression As Connected with the Fine Arts*, London, G. Bell and Sons, 1890 (7th ed.), p. 146: a soldier wounded at the battle of Corunna in 1809, drawn by the author.

4.47   Courtesy of Mrs. H. Papadaki, Athens.

4.48   The beautiful photographs of this stele are the fruit of a complex task organized through the kindness of Mrs. R. Andreadi of Athens: Mr. N. Gialouris gave the permission of the Archeological Service and dispatched an archeologist (Dr. M. T. Mitsos) and a photographer (Mr. M. Vernardos) from Athens to Epidauros. To all—and to Martine Vodoz who alerted me to the existence of the stele—go my warmest thanks for this labor of love.

4.49   From Rollinat 1934 Fig. 5. With permission from Librairie Delagrave, Paris.

4.50   See 4.48 above.

4.51   From "the first German Calendar, Augsburg, about 1480" (Klibansky and others 1964 p. 299 Figs. 85, 87, 89a and b). Courtesy of Prof. R. Klibansky and of T. Nelson and Sons, Ltd., London.

Ch. 5 title page: drugs oozing from wounded trees. After a quaint woodcut of a wounded sandarach-tree, reproduced at the end of this chapter (from J. Meyden-bach's *Ortus sanitatis*, Moguntiae, 1491, a popular herbal in its time).

5.1   From *Beni Hasan*, Plate XVII (Griffith 1900). Some details removed.

5.2   From Schäfer 1902 p. 38. Explanations added (kindly checked by Prof. C. Maystre). With permission of Akademie-Verlag, Leipzig.

5.3   Bas-relief from the temple of Deir el Bahari. Scale: the heap in the original is about 32 inches high (Naville 1898 Plate LXXIX).

5.4   Map based on van Beek 1958 (b) p. 152 (also Pirenne 1960; von Wissmann 1964; Miller 1969 map 5; Hepper 1969 Plate XIV). Present distribution of trees kindly confirmed by Prof. Ray L. Cleveland (personal communication). Range of Malaysian outriggers: Miller 1969 pp. 171–172 and map 7; Hornell 1946 last map.

Illustrations   **5.5**   From color plate in Marchand 1867 (Plate 1).

5.6   Photographed in 1960 by Prof. Ray L. Cleveland, Dept. of History, University of Saskatchewan, Regina, Saskatchewan, to whom I owe these rare documents. Najd region of Dhofar, Sultanate of Oman. Height of tree shown in first photograph is 2–3 m; it was just north of the Qara mountains.

5.7   See 5.6

5.8   From Drake-Brockman 1912 p. 303; a Somali specimen ("Didin, the source of Guban myrrh"). With permission of Hutchinson Publishing Group Ltd., London.

5.9   Courtesy of Walther Paulsen GMBH, Hamburg, Germany, and of Fritsche, Dodge & Olcott Inc., New York.

5.10   Courtesy of Mr. M. Hartmann, Archéologue Cantonal, Brugg, Switzerland. Published by Wiedemer 1966. Actual dimensions c. 45 × 20 × 6 mm

5.11   Experiment performed by Dr. Elisabeth Schorer and Mme. Sylvie Dersi of the Dépt. de Biologie Végétale, University of Geneva. Myrrh was used in a concentration of 1 g/5 ml H_2O. Prediffusion was allowed to occur for six hours at room temperature.

5.13   From Rosengarten 1969 p. 197. Courtesy of F. Rosengarten Jr.

5.14   Cultures kindly provided by Dr. Elisabeth Schorer, Dépt. de Biologie Végétale, University of Geneva. *Saccharomyces cerevisiae* (1936 Fendant, Valais; phot. in dark field), and *Acetobacter aceti* (LBG-B 4106, Inst. Microbiol., Zürich; smear, negatively stained with nigrosine).

5.15   From Pasteur's book on diseases of wine (1866); Fig. 3, labeled "Maladie de l'acescence du vin (*Mycoderma vini* et *Mycoderma aceti* réunis.). La maladie est à son début . . ."

Ch. 6 title page: the Chinese characters read *Yang I*, "Ulcer Physician" or "Physician for External Diseases."

6.1   Redrawn from Bengston and Milojčić 1963 I c.

6.2   From the film of the discovery of the Han tomb (see Fig. 6.22).

6.3   From NEED I 86.

6.4   The map of China corresponds very roughly to the Warring States period; based on NEED I 92 Fig. 12 (beginning of third century B.C.). The walls were many more than sketched.

6.5   See e.g. Wong and Wu p. 11, NEED II 257.

6.6   Ancient forms: *Yin*, Wieger 1924 p. 246 No. 101 B; *Yang*, Wieger 1924 p. 232 No. 93 C. Modern forms: calligraphy by Mr. Lee Kwok-wing.

6.8   From *The I Ching* or *Book of Changes*, trans. by Richard Wilhelm, rendered into English by Cary F. Baynes, Bollingen Series XIX (copyright © 1950 and 1967 by Bollingen Foundation), Fig. I. Reprinted by permission of Princeton University Press and of Routledge and Kegan Paul, London.

6.9   From *Change: Eight Lectures on the I Ching*, by Hellmut Wilhelm, Bollingen Series LXII (copyright © 1960 by Bollingen Foundation), Fig. 2. Reprinted by permission of Princeton University Press.

6.10   Top: calligraphy by Mr. Lee Kwok-wing; (a) from NEED II p. 228; (b', b'') from Lu Gwei-Djen and Needham 1967 p. 3 #1; (c, d, e) ibid. #2/1, #5/1, #3/2.

6.13   From Kan 1920 Fig. 21 (Sketches of Confucius, With Illustrations; Shanghai, Commerical Press Ltd.).

6.14   From Cowdry 1921(b) Fig. 13.

6.15   Character as reported in Ve 239, 247, redrawn by Mr. Lee Kwok-wing.

6.17   From Morse 1934 p. 147 (source not given).

6.18   Photographs courtesy of Dr. Chong Yu-ming, Acupuncturist, Taipei.

6.19   From Wong and Wu Fig. 21; no details given, but a common Chinese vignette.

6.20   Most data from NEED II 262–263. Such tables are in practically all works on Chinese history.

6.22   From frames of a film produced by Peking Television on the discovery of the Han tomb, 1972. Courtesy of Peking Television.

6.23   Schuchhardt 1891 p. 53; see also Schliemann 1885 pp. 300–304.

Ch. 7 title page: the Sanskrit characters read *vaidya*, "physician."

7.1   From an old print, courtesy of Jacques Vicari, Geneva.

7.2   Adapted from Schulberg 1968 p. 75, plus another site mentioned by Schlumberger and others 1958.

7.3   From Smith 1901 Plate II. Courtesy of The Clarendon Press, Oxford.

7.4   Courtesy of the Office du Livre S. A., Fribourg, Switzerland (Fig. 143 in Hallade and Hinz 1968).

7.5   Courtesy of J. Auboyer and of Presses Universitaires de France. From Hackin 1954 Fig. 105, text p. 233, redrawn by J. Auboyer (1955 Plate VI).

7.6   From Tennent 1860 I p. 499. The method is mentioned by Arrian, *Indiká*, XVI (II cent. A.D.) in relation to Alexander's expedition. For Alexander's wound: Plutarch, *Lives: Alexander*, 63/LB VII 405.

7.7   These drawings represent methods described by Sushruta, but details are of course wholly imaginary (only source: SS I 71–72). An effort was made to draw the instruments according to Hindu models—but those too are reconstructions (Mukhopadhyaya 1913 II). Butcher-bird: ibid. II Plate XIV 6.

7.8   Based on Sushruta's description (SS I 261).

7.9   Composite from Mukhopadhyaya 1913 II Plates XI–XIV.

7.10   Mukhopadhyaya 1913 II Plate XIII, text Vol. I p. 103.

7.11   From Paré 1564 (repr. 1964, p. 4).

7.12   Redrawn after SS II, Plates I and II, pp. xix, xx. For the identification of anatomical structures I am indebted to Prof. J.-A. Baumann, Head, Dept. of Anatomy, University of Geneva.

7.14   I owe this striking photograph to Mr. Harry Miller, Madras, India, who was also the owner of this rare white cobra.

7.15   From R. Vira and L. Chandra 1965, end of fascicle 48 (text pp. 9–10). Courtesy of Prof. L. Chandra, International Academy of Indian Culture, New Delhi. I learned from Prof. Chandra that these mantras, written by the monk Zen-nin, bear no explanation in the original book. They are mantras simplified to the extreme, *bija-mantras* (*bija* = "seed"). Ordinary mantras may be a whole sentence or even a hymn; bija-mantras sum it up in a single, "nuclear" syllable. Typical is the mantra-syllable *om*; it is the traditional opening of most Sanskrit texts, somewhat like an invocation. Because its sound originates deep down in the throat, and terminates at the lips, it is thought to encompass all possible sounds: hence its symbolic value. (Information courtesy of Gopal Sukhu).

7.16   Granite figure, sixth century Pallava from Mahabalipuram. From a color slide kindly provided by Mr. Harry Miller.

7.18   From Coomaraswamy 1931 II Plate 25.1. Courtesy of the Indian Museum, Calcutta.

7.19   Courtesy of the Musée de l'Homme, Paris. Child of the *cheddoul* caste wearing heavy copper and silver earrings (Madras, Madurai). Cliché P. Monge, 1947.

7.20   From Merker 1910 p. 138 Fig. 47. Courtesy of D. Reimer Verlag (Andrews and Steiner), Berlin.

7.21   I had these fourteen ear-conditions drawn, to the best of my understanding, from Sushruta's descriptions, some of which are not clear. The fifteenth of Sushruta's list is the "ganda-karna" shown in Fig. 7.22.

7.22   Drawn after J. M. Converse, *Reconstructive Plastic Surgery*, 1968, Vol. III Fig. 28.52 ABC.

7.23   Drawn with the guide of the "bullock driver" illustration (Gnudi and Webster 1950 Fig. 47).

7.24   From Converse 1959 p. 339. Courtesy of Dr. J. M. Converse and of W. B. Saunders Co.

7.25   The drawing was made by combining Sushruta (SS II 159–160), who describes the superimposed pitchers and the use of "basket material" for making the pipe, and Charaka (ChS I 559–560), who says that the pipe should be made airtight with thick leaves. "Triple bend" and shape like an elephant trunk are specified in both sources. The diameter is anybody's guess: (1) Sushruta, no figure; (2) Charaka: circumference *or* caliber (sic) from 1/4 to 1/8 of a *Vyama* (width of outstretched arms!); (3) Mukhopadhyaya 1913 I p. 145 quotes Sushruta (??) as specifying the "circumference of a common pea". . .

7.26   Prepared with the help of Prof. D. Ingalls and of Gopal Sukhu.

7.28   Lotus flower courtesy of Jean Mohr, Geneva. Knife drawn by Mr. P. Duvernay.

7.29   From Fergusson 1868 Plate XXXIII.

7.30   Courtesy of Dr. Jean-Pierre Lamelin. From the Sun Temple of Konarak (Orissa).

7.31   From Neal A. Weber, "Fungus-Growing Ants," *Science*, 5 Aug. 1966: *153*,

587–604, Fig. 12 (top right). Copyright 1966 by the American Association for the Advancement of Science. With permission of Science and Prof. N. A. Weber. As to the "6 mm. wounds" caused by *Atta*, I owe this information to Prof. Weber (Swarthmore College, Penn.), who also feels sure that *Atta*, the leaf-cutting ant, could not suture wounds. I tend to agree. The mystery is Beebe's reference to clamping by *Atta*. Beebe wrote a book about ants and was a personal friend of Wheeler, top authority on ants: how could he go so wrong?

7.32 Originals in Doflein 1905 Figs. 3, 4 (redrawn in Wheeler 1910 Figs. 122, 123). With permission from G. Thieme Verlag, Leipzig, and of Columbia University Press.

7.33 See 7.32

7.34 Photographed in Mayidi, ancient Belgian Congo. *Anomma wilverthi* (Emery) is *Dorylus wilverthi* Em. Even very small workers, 33 mm long, brace themselves in this "cataleptic" sentinel attitude. Data and photograph courtesy of Prof. A. Raignier, S. J., Heverlee, Belgium. *Eciton* and *Dorylus* are the most important genera in the subfamily Dorylinae, one of eight in the family Formicidae. *Eciton* is typical of American tropics, *Dorylus* of the African; they are called army ants, soldier ants, driver ants, etc.

7.35 Photographed in my laboratory, with a specimen kindly provided by Dr. W. Wittmer, Naturhistorisches Museum, Basel, Switzerland (*Scarites buparius* Forst.; *pyracmon* is a synonym). With permission, Naturhistorisches Museum, Basel.

7.36 From "The Social Behavior of Army Ants" by Howard R. Topoff. Copyright © 1972 by Scientific American, Inc. All rights reserved.

The unnumbered drawing at the end of the chapter is another Mantra from the same group as those of Fig. 7.15. With kind permission from Prof. L. Chandra.

Ch. 8 title page: the Roman coin shows a ship approaching the lighthouse of Alexandria. Second century A.D. Courtesy Mr. R. A. Gardner, British Museum, London.

8.1 Based on the 1866 map reproduced by Bernand 1966 pp. 364–365.

8.2 Rephotographed from Sudhoff 1909 Plate III (number P. 3983 at bottom retouched off). The word *trauma* identified and redrawn with the help of Prof. Jean Rudhardt, University of Geneva. With permission from J. A. Barth Verlag, Leipzig.

8.3 From the Flinders Petrie Papyri, Plate XIII (Mahaffy 1893), with permission from The Royal Irish Academy. For other papyri with *iatrikón* see Mahaffy and Smyly 1905.

8.4 From Commandino edition of Heron, No. 44 and No. 33; and from Aleotti edition, No. 67.

8.5 From Eco and Zorzoli 1963 p. 59, with permission of Dr. U. Eco and of Casa Editrice V. Bompiani, Milan.

8.6 From Aleotti edition of Heron, No. 37.

8.7 From Commandino edition of Heron, No. 21.

8.8 From Thiersch 1909 p. 90 Fig. 71, with permission of B. G. Teubner Verlag, Stuttgart.

8.10 From Aleotti edition of Heron, No. 27.   Illustrations

8.11 From Drachmann 1967 Fig. 8 (letters added). Courtesy of Prof. A. G. Drachmann and of Artemis Verlag, Zürich.

8.13 From Aleotti edition of Heron, No. 57.

8.14 From Heron, *De machinis Bellicis*. Rephotographed from Eco and Zorzoli 1963 p. 83, with permission of Dr. U. Eco and of Casa Editrice V. Bompiani, Milan.

Unnumbered drawing at end of chapter: bronze coin struck at Alexandria, showing the lighthouse (144–145 A.D.). Courtesy of American Numismatic Society, N.Y.

Ch. 9 title page: the Latin words emphasize the importance of military medicine in Rome. They represent the beginning of a marble inscription found in Via Nomentana, Rome (Briau 1866 p. 25), and read: *Tiberius Claudius Iulianus, clinical physician to the fourth infantry battalion* ("cohors IIII"). The modern-sounding word *clinicus* had a somewhat different connotation: it probably meant "in charge of lying patients" (from the Greek *klíno*, "I lie") i.e. bedridden patients hospitalized in the wards, as opposed to ambulatory cases (see Davies 1969 p. 87).

9.1   Courtesy of Prof. Zdenek Vogel and of Urania-Verlag, Leipzig. From Vogel 1963 Fig. 164.

9.2   From Hall 1971 p. 68 No. 46.

9.3   Found by my daughter Corinne on the beach of Gay Head, Mass., where the fossils date from the Miocene (12–20 million years old).

9.4   Specimen kindly provided by Prof. A. Imbesi, Director, Istituto di Farmacognosia, Università di Messina, Italy.

9.5   From Hartner 1941 p. 217, with permission of the China-Institut, J. W. Goethe-Universität, Frankfurt am Main.

9.7   From Gunther 1934 p. 439, with kind permission of A. E. Gunther.

9.8   Stele at the Museum of Palestrina, with permission of the Soprintendenza alle Antichità del Lazio, Rome.

9.9   The bas-relief was found "South of the Acropolis, on the site of the Asklepieion, in the defense wall of Turkish times . . . It decorated a base that carried an ex-voto to Asklepios." Photograph and data courtesy of B. Kallipolitis, Director, National Museum, Athens.

9.10   From Vulpes 1847 Plate VII; text pp. 74–81.

9.11   From the Museo Nazionale, Naples, with permission of Prof. A. de Franciscis, Soprintendenza alle Antichità, Naples.

9.12   For the first draft of this drawing I had the stick of "swan collyrium" stamped with "the likeness of a swan," as suggested by an explanatory note in CDM/LB II 196. I then found that the swanness was only in the color; Galen explains that these collyria "are called by physicians *libiana* or *swans* because of their white color." Note the astonishing appearance of the Arabic *lubán*, "white" (*De compos. medicam.*/K XII 707–708; see also *Paulus Aegineta*/Adams III 549, 550). The swan-collyrium or *cygnarium* was meant especially for the eyes: surely its name and color had something to do with "whiteness" being good for "clear vision." There is a Greek inscription about a blind soldier to whom the God ordered a collyrium made with the blood of a white swan (I.G. XIV 966). Only tablet-shaped collyria have been found (duly stamped with the physician's seal).

9.13   From Vulpes 1847 Plate IV; text p. 39 ff.

9.14   From Frölich 1880, also reproduced by Haberling 1912.

9.15   Drawn after Meyer-Steineg 1912 Plate II No. 3 and pp. 26–27.

9.16   Courtesy of Dr. D. Baatz, Saalburgmuseum, to whom I owe the following data. The instrument was found in 1890 and not labeled until 1900; shortly thereafter someone (probably a physician) gave it the present interpretation. Also published by Davies 1970 p. 92 (Museum Inv. No. P 5603).

9.17   With permission of Max Parrish Publisher, London (Fig. 15.6 in *Roman Silchester* by G. Boon; also in Liversidge 1968 p. 342 Fig. 131 f). For similar Pompeian specimen see Vulpes 1847 Plate V Fig. 4.

9.18   From Vulpes 1847 Plate IV; text p. 39 ff.

Illustrations   **9.19**   Photograph (reversed) and text from the posthumous English edition of 1678 p. 304 (the original is from 1564).

9.20   Photograph courtesy of Dr. M.-A. Dollfus, retouched. The forceps is now at the Cabinet des Médailles, Paris. According to Dr. Dollfus, other such forceps have been found (Dollfus 1965 Figs. 4, 5).

9.21   From Blinkenberg 1926; (a) Crete (p. 40), (b) Arcadia, age uncertain (p. 41), (c) Mycenaean (p. 48), (d) Mycenaean (p. 44). Sizes not given for all; (c) is about $\frac{1}{2}$ of natural size. With permission from Det Kongelige Danske Videnskabernes Selskab, Copenhagen.

9.22   From Goffres 1858 Plate 77 Fig. 8; text p. 534.

9.23   From Paré 1564 p. 214.

9.24   From Vulpes 1847 Plate V; text pp. 49–54.

9.25   Bas-relief at the Museo Nazionale, Naples. Descriptions also in Winckelmann 1767 I p. 163 Fig. 122; Jeanselme 1921. With permission from Prof. A. de Franciscis, Soprintendenza alle Antichità, Naples.

9.26   Cod. Vatic. Lat. 5951, p. 41 verso. Courtesy of Biblioteca Apostolica Vaticana, Vatican City (codex described by Sabbadını 1900 p. 302).

9.27   See 9.26

9.28   Map based on Wheeler 1955. Amphorae: data in Wheeler 1946.

9.29   The ivory was found in a box with various bronze implements and glassware. A letter of the Indian *kharosthi* alphabet is carved beneath the base (see Maiuri 1938 Plate XLII). Courtesy of Le Arti, S.n.c., Milan.

9.30   From Simpson 1854. The writing on the first pot means "Lycium of Heracleus"; a physician of Tarentum by that name was actually named by Celsus and Galen (Simpson 1854 p. 415). This would date the pot (at the latest) from the first years A.D.; however, the name was a common one.

9.31   For advice concerning the cataract operation I am indebted to Dr. Jaqueline Starobinski, Geneva.

9.32   Drawing based on W. G. Spencer's illustration in CDM/LB III facing p. 362, and on comments by Daremberg 1847.

9.34   Sources on Roman military hospitals (the following list, with Davies 1970d, is a key to almost all the literature available). *In Germany and Austria* (general): Haberling 1909, Schultze 1934, Jetter 1966, von Petrikovits 1970, Baatz 1970. *Bonna* (Bonn): von Petrikovits 1960. *Haltern:* Stieren 1928, 1930. *Künzing:* Schönberger 1969, Schönberger and Herrman 1971. *Novaesium:* Nissen and others 1904; Waterman 1970. *Oberstimm:* publ. in local paper, Ingolstädter Heimatblätter, 34 Jahrg., No. 11, 1971, 37–40, and in Bayerische Vorgesichtsblätter 1972: 37, 31–37 (ref. courtesy of Prof. R. W. Davies). *Saalburg:* Baatz 1970(a, b). *Vindobona* (Vienna): Neumann 1950, 1965. *Carnuntum:* see Schultze 1934 (no new data since then, pers. comm. from Museum Carnuntinum). *Jugoslavia: Lotschitz,* Lorger 1919. *In Great Britain* (general): see Collingwood and Richmond 1969 pp. 15–59. *Benwell:* Simpson and Richmond 1941. *Corbridge:* Richmond and Gillam 1952, Arch. Aeliana 117 1968. *Fendoch:* Richmond and McIntyre 1939. *Hod Hill:* Richmond 1968 p. 85. *Housesteads:* Bosanquet 1940. *Inchtuthil:* Richmond and St. Joseph 1957, 1961. *Pen Llystyn:* Hogg 1968. *Switzerland: Baden,* Anon. 1900? (perhaps not a *military* hospital). *Vindonissa:* Simonett 1937, Fellmann 1958. *Holland, Valkenburg:* Glasbergen 1966. *Hungary, Aquincum* (Budapest): Szilágyi 1956 (evidence indirect). *Israel, Masada:* Schulten 1933. *Africa, Lambaesis:* Cagnat 1909, 1913; *Alexandria:* only from literary evidence.

9.35   From Baatz 1970(b) p. 24. Courtesy of Dr. D. Baatz, Saalburg Museum.

9.36   All from Schultze 1934 (slightly retouched). Vetera I: Plate IV Fig. 2; Vetera II: Plate I; Novaesium: Plate IV Fig. 3; Lotschitz: Plate V. Courtesy of the Rheinisches Landesmuseum, Bonn.

9.37   From J. of Roman Studies 1961: *51,* 158. With kind permission of Lady Richmond and of the J. of Roman Studies.

9.38   From J. of Roman Studies 1956: *46,* 199. With kind permission of Lady Richmond and of the J. of Roman Studies.

9.39   For this scheme I am much indebted to my friend Jacques Vicari of Geneva, architect, archeologist, and expert on hospital buildings.

9.40   Courtesy of Dr. K.-H. Knörzer (Knörzer 1963; *Hyoscyamus niger* p. 313; *Centaurium umbellatum Gilib.* pp. 32, 312). With permission from Gebr. Mann Verlag, Berlin.

9.41   See 9.40

9.42   From an amphora in Basel, Switzerland (Schefold 1967 p. 39). With kind permission from Holle Bildarchiv, Baden-Baden, Germany.

9.43   Courtesy of The Mansell Collection, London.

9.44   For advice on these derivations I am indebted to Prof. G. Devoto, University of Florence, and to Prof. G. B. Pellegrini, University of Padova. See Ernout-Meillet 1939 p. 599 ff. and Benveniste 1945.

Ch. 10 title page: the 22 volumes of Galen's works in the Kühn edition of 1821–1833.

10.1 From the front page of the Venetian edition of Galen published *apud Iuntas,* 1609 (7 vols.).

10.2 From Figuier 1866 opp. p. 378. Dr. J. Walsh, who discusses this painting in detail, suggests that Galen probably worked at a better operating table—and not with a *toga* (Walsh 1926 p. 180).

10.3 From the Museo Nazionale, Naples. With permission from Prof. A. de Franciscis, Soprintendenza alle Antichità, Naples.

10.4 From a color slide kindly provided by Nell C. Juliand for Time-Life Books. Published in Hadas 1965, pp. 50–51 (Great Ages of Man, *Imperial Rome,* photo by Pierre Belzeaux © Time Inc.). With kind permission from Issa Salem El Assouad, Directeur-Délégué des Recherches Archéologiques, Tripoli, R. A. U. The mosaic is at the Musée des Antiquités, Tripoli.

10.5 For details the artist, Mr. Axel Ernst, used documents from the Fossa Sanguinis of Neuss (Wortmann 1971) and the original description of Prudentius (Hymn. X, 1006–1050).

10.8 Ape hand, from Singer and Underwood, *A Short History of Medicine* (1962 p. 63 Fig. 25), courtesy of the Clarendon Press, Oxford. Snake Skeleton, courtesy of V. Aellen, Director, Museum of Natural History, Geneva.

10.9 From Buffon, *Histoire Naturelle,* Paris, Impr. Royale, 1766, Tome XIV, Plate VII.

10.10 From Livon, C., *Manuel de vivisection,* Paris, J.-P. Baillière, 1882. Livon has taken these illustrations from works of Claude Bernard.

10.11 Adapted from Daremberg 1854 I p. 505.

10.12 From *Oeuvres d'Oribase,* Bussemaker and Daremberg 1862 Vol. 4 p. 692.

10.13 For help in preparing this drawing I am indebted to Prof. J.-A. Baumann, Head, Dept. of Anatomy, University of Geneva.

10.14 Courtesy of C. K. Divakaran, Dean, Gujarat Ayurved University, Dhanvantari Mandir, Jamnagar, India.

10.15 Recipe from the 1676 edition of M. Charas, *Pharmacopée Royale Galénique,* Paris (p. 277). Composition and drawing by Miss Judith D. Love of the Rhode Island School of Design.

10.16 From NEED I p. 205.

10.17 Courtesy of Dr. F. E. Ducommun, Nyon, Switzerland.

10.18 Redrawn after Schöner 1964. With permission from F. Steiner Verlag, Wiesbaden, Germany.

10.20 Map based on Hazard 1952 (maps 9, 11).

Page 423: Temple of Poseidon, Cape Sounion, Greece, courtesy Lise Piguet.

COLOR PLATES

3.1 Courtesy of the New York Academy of Medicine.

3.2 Courtesy of the Trustees, British Museum, London. Papyrus of Ani (14th sheet).

3.3 Malachite from Lukuni (Siberia). Courtesy of Prof. M. Vuagnat, Institut des Sciences de la Terre, University of Geneva.

3.4 Chrysocolla from Israel.

3.5 From Desroches-Noblecourt, *Toutankhamon,* Paris, Hachette (1963 p. 6). Courtesy of Prof. S. Curto, Museo Egizio, Turin, Italy.

3.6 Experiment by Dr. D. Kekessy, Institute of Hygiene, University of Geneva.

3.7 The honey from Paestum was generously provided by Prof. Mario Napoli, Soprintendenza alle Antichità, Salerno, Italy. It is now being chemically analyzed. Provisional study shows that the mass probably includes the whole hive, i.e. wax and honey. (The surface melting was caused by floodlights).

3.8 This scheme of the Egyptian vascular system is drawn according to the longest of the three vessel lists (forty-six vessels, Eb 854 to 854-o, GMÄ IV-1/1–3; plus gloss Eb 855-c, ibid., p. 5, which mentions the "receiver vessel"). Breasted gives fifty vessels (Sm 110) rather than forty-six for the following reason: in the Ebers papyrus, after the "ear vessels" are mentioned (Eb 854 f), the text says "two vessels to his right shoulder, two to his left"; Breasted takes these as four additional vessels, but Grapow reads the text as if it meant "two [of the ear vessels mentioned previously] are to the right side, two to the left." None of the forty-seven *metw*, receiver included, is identifiable with any actual blood vessel. One paragraph states that "there are *metw* in [man] to every part of the body" (Eb 854a, GMÄ IV-1/1), but curiously none goes to the kidneys. The kidneys seem to have been entirely neglected by Egyptian medicine; no name for them is known. Detail of heart copied from a hieroglyph painted on a coffin dating 1878–1842 B.C., Boston Museum of Fine Arts, No. 20.1822-27/21.962. For checking the layout of this scheme, especially the *whdw* detail, I am much indebted to Dr. R. O. Steuer.

4.1 My interpretation. References in text.

4.2 See 4.1

4.3 Quotations supporting the ten sketches may be found as follows (see also LTT X, index). (1) Washing or soaking with wine: *Use of Liquids*/LTT VI 127 #4, 129 #5; *On Wounds* #1/A II 794 = LTT VI 401; warm wine: *Mochlicon* #33/A II 674 = LTT IV 375 (on open fractures); vinegar: *On Wounds*/A II 809 #17 = LTT VI 433 #27. (2) No dressing: *On Wounds* #1/A II 794 = LTT VI 401; *Wounds in the Head* #13/A I 457 = LTT III 231; *On Joints* #40/A II 602 = LTT IV 173. (3) Suture: see note 4.136. (4) Dry powders: *On Wounds*/A II 802 #7 = LTT VI 417 #13. (5) Wine on bandage: see note 4.60. (6) Sponge, leaves: *On Wounds*/A II 796 #1 = LTT VI 405 #2. (7) Wool: *On Wounds*/A II 808 #14 = LTT VI 429 #24; *On Fractures* #29/A II 537 = LTT III 517; etc. (8) Plaster directly on wound: *On Wounds*/A II 803 #8 = LTT VI 419 #15. (9) Plaster above linen pad: *On Wounds*/A II 799 #4 = LTT VI 411 #11. (10) Plaster around the wound: *On Wounds* #1/A II 795 = LTT VI 403; A II 798 #3 = LTT VI 409 #10; *On the Physician*/LTT IX 419 #15.

7.1 From Yazdānī, *Adjantâ*, 1954 Plate XXIII. Reproduced with permission of the New York Graphic Society and of UNESCO (Division of Cultural Development, Paris).

7.2 Major workers of *Eciton burchelli* (Westwood) kindly provided by the late Dr. T. C. Schneirla, American Museum of Natural History. Photographed in my laboratory with the assistance of Dr. I. Joris.

9.1 See note 9.77.

9.2 Codex "Urbinate" No. 1367, p. 1, verso. Courtesy of Biblioteca Apostolica Vaticana, Vatican City (see Sabbadini 1900 p. 306).

Index

Diaphragm wounds, as cause of laughter, 198–199

Diet: in Egypt ("mooring stakes"), 95–96, 97–98; of wounded hero (Homer), 142; cheese as "inflammatory," 142, 162; Hippocratic triad (starving, purging, bleeding), 179, 205, 419; starving as a cure, 179; also for wounds, 182, 188 (Hippocr. Coll.); special diet for wounded (Hippocr. Coll.), 189; Chinese dietician, 236–237; prescribed in China, 251, 253; no starving in China, 257; in India, 275, 291, 297; starving for fever (India), 304; compared in Greece, China, India, 310; starving for wounds in Alexandria, 335, 337; in Celsus, 355; unhealthy in Greece, 418; starving as a cure, after Galen, 419

Dilators: See Surgical instruments

Diokles of Karystos: spoon of, 143, 359, 361; on keeping bite wounds open, 184–185

Dioscorides, Pedanius, 113, 154, 338, 352, 353, 390, 413

Disease: causes of, natural and supernatural, in Mesopotamia, 59–60; in Egypt, 125, 129–130; mechanisms of (Hippocr. Coll.), 176–183, 192; in India, mechanisms of, 276, 296, 311; stars as causes of, 285; physical causes of, 296; fever is most important cause of, 303–304; plethora as mechanism of (Erasistratos), 333–337; in Pliny, 347–348. See also Hippocratic medical theories

Dislocation of shoulder: treatment (Hippocr. Coll.), 162–166; in Rome, 341

Dissection. See Anatomy; Decay

Distillation in Mesopotamia, 50–51

Domestication and castration, 24

Doshas, defined, 276, 513–514 n 98. See also Indian medicine

Drain. See Drainage; Surgical instruments

Drainage: suppuration as, 102; with linen or tin drain (Hippocr. Coll.), 157–158, 196; wounds kept open for (Diokles), 184–185; with tube, lost after Hippocrates, 205, 367; acupuncture as, 247–248; different concepts in Greece, India, China, 310; incomplete suture for wound (Celsus), 367. See also Surgical instruments

Drakon (the snake), in Asklepieion, 201–205

Dressings. See Wound dressings

Drill, fire: used as cautery, 96–97; in Egypt, 100; in Greece, 168–169. See also Surgical instruments

Drugs, ancient, difficulty of evaluating, 61–65. See also Antibiotics; Antiseptics; Balsam; Centaury; Dung; Ephedra; Hellebore; Henbane; Honey; Mouse; Myrrh; Oil; Opium; Resin; Tranquilizers; Vinegar; Wine; Wound dressings

Dryness: is natural state (Hippocr. Coll.), 143; but exception thereto, 490 n 75

Dung: as a drug on sores in Mesopotamia, 63; on wounds in Egypt, 108–109; in India, 297; for wounds and ulcers (Pliny), 349; as

a caustic (Celsus), 370; for wound dressings (Galen), 399; on wounds (Talmud), 478 n 138

E

Ears: cautery on, 174, 379; "cauliflower," 174–175; lobes pierced, in Bible, 379, in India, 285–288, in Rome, 379–381; lobes stretched, in Egypt, 516 n 172, in India, 286, 287, 532 n 238, in Africa, 288–292, in Rome, 279, 381; lobes torn in India, 288–292; plastic surgery on lobes, in India, 289–291, in Rome, 379, 381; earrings to protect eyes in Switzerland, 516 n 173. See also Surgery, plastic

Eau Dalibour. See Copper; Zinc

Ebbell, B., 73, 93, 100

Ebers papyrus. See Papyrus, Ebers

Egypt, 69–71; medical history, sources, 71–73; hieroglyphic writing, 75–84; lack of surgeons to treat wounds, 84–86; surgical knives, 86–90; and Smith papyrus, 90–105; use of meat, salt, and opium for wounds, 105–111; use of green pigments, 111–115; use of grease, honey, and lint, 115–120; use of myrrh, 121–124; use of magic in medicine, 125–128; concern with decay and ukhedu, 129–130; embalming, 130–139; heritage of Egyptian medicine, 139–140; links with Greek medicine, 192

Egyptian medicine: in relation to Mesopotamia, 69, 71; to China through embalmers (?), 135; to Greece, 192; to India, 272. See also Papyrus—Ebers, Kahun, Smith

Embalming: archaic hieroglyphic determinative for, 104; by bees, 120–121; Egyptian procedure for, 130–139; resins for, 135–137; spontaneous, in peat bogs, 138; Egyptian word for, 138–139; honey for, 139

Empyema: operation for, in Mesopotamia, 52; in Hippocr. Coll., 52, 156–158; in India, 294–297; in Rome, 372–373. See also Abscess; Clay

Enaima: drugs for fresh wounds (Hippocr. Coll.), 154, 185, 193, 196–197, 205; in Rome, 369–370; effectiveness as antiseptics, 498 n 243. See also Antiseptics

Enema: in Mesopotamia, 48; monthly in Egypt, 129, 522 n 45; for wounds (Hippocr. Coll.), 188, 193, 198; for snakes, 294; in India, 296, 297, 298; for elephants, 303; doctor of, in Alexandria, 317. See also Syringe

Enhemes. See Enaima

Environment, physical: importance in Greek medicine, 195, 242; in Chinese medicine, 242, 243; in Indian medicine, 271, 285, 300. See also Wind

Ephedra: as ma huang in China, 349, 351–352; in Pliny, 349–353; ephedrine, 349, 351

Index

Galen (*Cont.*)
Sushruta, 278, 410–411; on Erasistratos, 327–333; emphasized bleeding and starvation, 337; on "contemplation of wounds" to study anatomy, 355; last flash of Greek medicine, 394; life, 395–398; and Hippocrates, 396; practiced dissection and experiment, 396–397; treatment of wounded gladiators, 398–403; used Chinese silk, 403; treatment of hemorrhage, 403–405; practiced dissection and vivisection, 405–408; recurrent laryngeal nerve, 407–409; never mentioned the "fifth sign" of inflammation, 412–413; and theriac, 415–417; no significant contribution to treatment of wounds, 417–419; translations of, by Nestorians, 421

Galene, 415. *See also* Theriac

Gangrene: defined, 5–6; in Hippocr. Coll., 6; caused by tourniquet, 15; by Clostridia, 16; by tourniquet, 152–153; of limbs, not treated by amputation, 191–192; of jaw, 197; of hand, 199

Gardner, Robert G., 20

Gargas cave, 19–22

Germanicus, 377–378

Ghee: defined, 272; Hindu use as drug, 272, 287, 293, 295, 297, 303

Gladiators: invincible if did not blink, 347; wounded, useful to study anatomy, 354; contest, 382; Galen and, 398–405; liver and blood of, as drugs, 403

Glossocomion, 409

Glossopetrae, 255, 345–346

Gods. *See* Religion

Golden section, geometry of the, 178–179

Granulation tissue, 2–4, 6, 119, 155

Grease: Egyptian use for treating wounds, 102, 115–116, 118, 120; resistant to decay, 120. *See also* Butter; Honey and Grease; Oil

Greek medicine, historical sources, 141. *See also* Hippocrates, Hippocratic Collection; Diokles; Erasistratos; Galen; Homer

Green pigments, Egyptian, for treating wounds, 111–115. *See also* Copper

Gum: Egyptian use for bandaging mummies, 94; defined, 210; for chewing, in antiquity, 210

Gymnastics, in Greek medicine, 179–180

H

Hammurabi, Code of, 43–46, 381. *See also* Law

Hands: prehistoric imprints of, 19–22; mutilation of, 22, 23; "hand-of-a-god" in cuneiform texts, 60; touching wounds with, in Egypt, 99–100, 104–105; touching among chimpanzees, 105–106. *See also* Fingers; Pulse

Harvey, William, 332

Hatshepswt, Queen, 122–123, 209

Headache Mountains, 257, 259, 261, 294

Healing, methods of: three, in Mesopotamian medicine (drug, knife, sorcery), 40; five, in Chinese medicine (psychology, diet, drugs, acupuncture, clinical medicine), 253; three, according to Celsus (diet, drugs, surgery), 253; three, according to Charaka (magic and religion, diet and drugs, control of mind), 275. *See also* Wound healing

Heart: Sumerian pictogram and cuneiform for, 33; as site of intelligence in Mesopotamia, 48; Egyptian hieroglyphs for, 76, Plate 3.8; feces rising to (Egyptian theory), 130; anatomy of (Hippocr. Coll.), 329–332; site of intelligence (Hippocr. Coll.), 329–330; congestive failure of, modern treatment compared to Alexandrian tourniquet, 336–337; poisoned, said not to burn, 377–378; cannot be site of intelligence (Galen), 401; bone in (Aristotle), 513 n 97

Hebrew. *See* Jewish

Hedra, defined, 166, 168

Hellebore: possibly mentioned in Mesopotamian tablet, 63; as arrow poison, 145, 147; as cause of convulsions, 181; medical use of, in Greece, 188–191. *See also* Spasm

Hemorrhage: primitive handling of, 15; from the nose, in Akkadian text, 53–54; few references to, in Egyptian papyri, 96; cautery for hemostasis in Smith papyrus, 96–97; muscle tissue for modern hemostasis, 106; charms for hemostasis, in Egypt (?), 128, in Homer, 142, in India, 298; in Hippocr. Coll., bleeding limb should be raised, 150, 153, cold applied around wound, 150, warmth around head, 150; treatment of, by venesection (Hippocr. Coll.), 152–153; kills, 152, but from wound is good, 197–198 (Hippocr. Coll.); hemostasis after castration in China (1929), 254; bleeding vessels not tied in Greece or India, 276; hemostasis in India, 298, 311; why arteries give blood not air (Erasistratos), 333; stopped with juice of *Ephedra* in Rome, 349; hemostasis (Celsus), 362–365; cautery and cupping for hemostasis in Rome, 364; Galen's treatments of, 400, 403–405. *See also* Bleeding as a "cure"

Hemostasis. *See* Hemorrhage

Henbane. *See* Anesthesia

Herbs: in Mesopotamian pharmacy, 48; "herb" same as "drug," in Akkadian, 48, 49; in Egyptian papyri, 108; herb garden in India, 268, 269, 280; found in Roman hospital, 384–385, 387–388; centaury for wound treatment in Rome, 387–389. *See also* Anesthesia; Drugs; Ephedra; Hellebore; Sélinon; Spices; Thyme

Hercules, 387; knot of, on bandages, 349

Herodotos: on Babylonian medicine, 67; on Egyptian physicians, 71; on Egyptian embalming, 94, 133, 135; on Egyptian

Incas, Peruvian, and trepanation of skull, 25–26. *See also* Indians, American

Incense (frankincense): Egyptian hieroglyphs for, 99, 133; in Egyptian prescriptions, 124, 133; in Greek wound drugs, 154, 176; importance of, as gift to gods, 208; geographic origin of, 211–215; as antiseptic, 219; and the Spice Curtain, 226; in China, 255; in India, 273. *See also* Myrrh; Resins

Incision. *See* Surgical instruments; Wound

India, 261–263; literary works of, 262, 264; and King Ashoka's edicts carved in rock, 264–266. *See also* Indian medicine

Indian (Hindu) medicine, correlations: with China, 257, 288, 300, 302, 310; with Greece, 260, 267, 273, 275, 276, 278, 285, 302, 304, 308, 310–312; with Egypt, 272; with Mesopotamia, 276–277; with Rome, 374–381; with Galen, 410–411; with Jundi Shapur, 420–421; vaidya, iatrós, and yang i compared, 310–312

———— practice: "arrow-doctor," 266–271; experimental surgery, 269–270; treatment of arrow wounds, 271–275; anatomy of "deadly points," 275–278; treatment of snake bites and use of ligatures, 278–285; piercing and stretching earlobes, 285–288; surgery to reconstruct earlobes, 288–292; ideal hospital (Charaka), 292–294; treatment for empyema and anesthesia with wine, 294–297; treatment for broken nose, 297; for wound and ulcer, 297–300; for a thorn in the foot, 300–302; amputation, 302, 311; treatment for fever, 303–304; sutures with ant heads, 304, 306–308; decline after antiquity, 417

————, theory: importance of religion, 273, 275, 283–284, 285, 311; the four pillars (doctors, drugs, nurse, patient), 275; role of magic, 275, 279, 282, 303; theory of the four doshas, 276, 291, 296, 311; admixture of fantasy, 293, 294, 298; fasting, purging, bleeding, 296–297; venesection essential, 297, 300; auscultation, not of lungs, 299. *See also* Ayurveda; Bleeding; Cataract; Diet; Ethics; Hemorrhage; Physician; Purging; Snake; Specialists; Surgeon; Vomiting

Indians, American: use of balsams, 218; sutures with ant heads, 304. *See also* Incas

Indiká, 264

Infection: effect on wound healing, 2–6; and origin of bacteria, 16; oldest, 16–18; in primitive man, 19, 21, 28; in surgery in the 1800s, 28, 420; infected wounds, in Mesopotamia, 52–53, 54, 58–60, 65; favored by foreign bodies, 94; in Egypt, 97–104; in Hippocr. Coll., explanation of "decay" in wounds, 181, 183, suppuration said to prevent inflammation, 184, 497 n 325, used to cleanse bruised wounds, 183–184; in wounded Greek patients, 193, 194, 196, 197, 201; treatment of, in China, 245–247, 254–257; causes and treatment of, in India, 296–300; in Celsus, 362–370. *See also* Abscess; Bacteria; Clostridia; Empyema; Inflammation; Pus; Tetanus

Infirmaries. *See* Hospitals; Wounded

Inflammation: explained, 2–6; acute, defined, 373–374; four cardinal signs of (Celsus), 370, 372–374; Virchow (not Galen) and the fifth cardinal sign, 412–413; *in Mesopotamian texts*, spelling of, 54–58; may also be read as "fever," 56; *in Egyptian texts*, 97–100; hieroglyphic spelling of, 98–99; incantations against (?), 127, 128; *in Hippocr. Coll.*, mechanism of, in wounds, 180–182; said to be prevented by suppuration, 184, 497 n 235; in wounded Greek patients, 193, 199; Greek clay method for diagnosis of, 157, similar Indian method, 273; *in China*, due to excess yang, 248; treatment of, 245–252; and "hot disease," 247; *in India*, treatment for, 300; *in Alexandria*, mechanism of (Erasistratos), 333–335; *in Celsus*, caused by blood clots or lint retained in wounds, 367; of wounds, prevented by hemorrhage, 362; *in Galen*, not necessary for wound healing, 400

Ink: in Hippocr. Coll., black material (ink?) used to detect cracks in skull, 169; Pliny's chemical reaction, 345, Plate 9.1, 493 n 148; similar to shoemaker's blacking, 399, 526 n 77; used on wounds by Galen, 399

Iron: meteoric origin and use of, in Egypt, 86–90, 104; and steel in India, 271; rust on wounds, in Rome, 371, 389; scrap metal as source of drugs, in Roman hospital, 389

Isis, 125, invoked in charm, 127

-itis, as ending, origin of, 158

J

Jade axe, Chinese, found at Troy, 258

Jerome, Saint, 393–394

Jewish: ruler embalmed in honey, 139; King Solomon and incense trade, 211–212; defense of Mecca balsam shrub, 211, 502 n 27; slave had ear perforated, 379; admiration for Galen, 398; medicine at Jundi Shapur, 420; in Talmud, names for "physician," 476 n 44, treatment for wounds, 478 n 138, for snake bite, 488 n 35. *See also* Bible

Jundi Shapur, University of, 420–422

Jung, C. G., and the *I Ching*, 235

K

Kahun Papyrus. *See* Papyrus Kahun

Kanam jaw, 8

Keloid, 6

Knives. *See* Reeds; Surgical instruments, knives

Koehler, W., on grooming among apes, 12

Ktesibios, of Alexandria, 323–326, 332

Index

Mummies: Egyptian, 88, 107; produced in beehives, 120–121; perfume in, 137, 211; natural by tanning in peatbogs, 138; of Han lady in China, 255–257. *See also* Embalming

Mummification. *See* Embalming

Museum, Alexandrian, 314–315, 354; destruction of, 337–338

Muslim: pre-Muslim Arabia, 211–212, 227; admiration for Galen, 398; role in revival of Greek medicine, 420–421; tolerance toward Christians, 420–421, 537 n 100. *See also* Arab

Mustapha Aga, 91

Myrrh: in El Amarna tablets, 120–124; for embalming in Egypt, 122, 135; in Greek énaima, 154; as endearing word, 207; imported to Egypt, 208–209, 215; geographic origin of, 211–215; in Hippocr. Coll., 215; by Persians on wounds, 215; for burns (Celsus), 215; bacteriostatic properties of, 217–218; as wine preservative, 224; and Spice Curtain, 226; Indian, of inferior quality, 377. *See also* Incense; Resins; Trees

N

Nadi-Sveda, Hindu fomentation apparatus, 295–296. *See also* Anesthesia

Natron, 139; for embalming in Egypt, 131–135; as detergent, 133

Neanderthal man, 8–9; alleged amputation in, 9; dental infection in, 19

Needham, Joseph, 240

Needle, surgical. *See* Surgical instruments, needles

Nefertiti, 121–122; in hieroglyphics, 78

Nei Ching. See Huang Ti Nei Ching

Nero, 341, 390, 415

Nerves: of the armpit (Hippocr. Coll.), 165; tendons called *neura* (Hippocr. Coll.), 198; Galen's "nerve of the voice" anticipated by Sushruta, 278, 410–411; as components of tissue (Erasistratos), 333–334, 523 n 68; Galen's "nerve of the voice," 406–409; discovered by Alexandrians, 495 n 206

Nestorians, as transmitters of medical knowledge, 420–422

Nestorios, 420

Nose. *See* Fractures; Surgery, plastic

Novaesium hospital, medical instruments and herbs at, 384–388

Nursing, importance in India, 275, 291, 292–293

O

Oculists, Gallo-Roman, so-called, 364, were not oculists, 529 n 165. *See also* Collyrium

Odyssey. *See* Homer

Oesypum, grease of wool, 490 n 87. *See also* Wool

Oil: in Mesopotamian dressing, 48, 52, 53, 58; for wounds in Bible, 53; antiseptic property of sesame, 53; does not spoil, 120; olive, in Greek salve, 176; on ulcers in China, 238; hot, for hemostasis in India, 311; in wound dressing (Galen), 399

Oleoresins, 210, 218

Onion: in embalming, 135; antibiotic effect of, 135; as "bitter root" for wounds (?) (Homer), 143; in moxa, 249; on wounds in Talmud, 478 n 138; on burns (Ambroise Paré) 486 n 261

Opening of the Mouth, ceremony of, 88–89, 107

Opisthotonos. *See* Tetanus

Opium: used in Egypt (*shepenn*), 108–111; and poppy capsules in Greece, 144–146; not in ancient China, 253; applied externally (Celsus), 370; decoction of, with henbane, 387; in theriac, 415–416

Organ: water-organ invented by Ktesibios, 323, 326; played while gladiators fought, 401

"Orgasm" in wounds (Hippocr. Coll.), 175

Osiris: myth of, 125; decay in corpse of, 127

Osteomyelitis: in fossils, 8, 10, 16–17, 19, 28; in Greek patients, 196, 197

Ostrakon, 161, 195, 316, 317

P

Pain. *See* Anesthesia

Papyrologists, 315–318

Papyrus (as a plant), 84–85; uses of, 140; for chewing, 210

———, Ebers: and Egyptian chronology, 72; translation of, 73; and surgical knives, 86, 89–90; on operating for varicose veins(?), 90, 154; on surgical bleeding, 96; on inducing a wound to suppurate, 101–102; on "diseased" wounds, 104; on opium infusion, 111; on "wadj of boat," 111; on myrrh for wounds, 124; on use of magic in applying remedies, 125–126; on loosening bandage, incantations for, 127; on burns, incantations for, 128; on vascular system, 130, Plate 3.8; concept of "fixation" in, 192. *See also* Egypt; Papyrus—Kahun, Smith

———, Kahun: Sumerian tablets older than, 47; and Egyptian chronology, 72; oldest medical papyrus, 73; veterinary and gynecological content of, 434

———, Smith: and Egyptian chronology, 72; translation of, 73; surgical knives not mentioned in, 86, 253; history of, 90–91; on contending with wounds, 92–99; on wounds "diseased" and not "diseased," 99–104; on touching wounds, 104–105; on treatment of wounds with fresh meat, 105–107; no reference to bleeding in, 106; on treatment of an infected wound, 108–111; on use of green pigment for wounds, 111–115; on use of grease, honey,

Index

Wound dressings
Praxagoras of Cos, 330
Prescriptions: principal form of cuneiform
    medical texts, 36; Akkadian, 37, 38, 52, 59,
    63; Sumerian, 46–51; principal form of
    medical text in Egypt, 76; total of nine
    hundred Egyptian, 76; in Smith papyrus,
    92, 95, 97, 98; in Ebers papyrus, 101–102,
    124; énaima in Hippocr. Coll. (for fresh
    wounds), 154, 185; to induce suppuration,
    184; zinc salve, 176; énaima in Celsus, 369.
    See also Drugs; Herbs, Magic; Wound
    dressings
Prevention, concept in China, 235, 242–243
Priest. See Religion
Probes. See Surgical instruments
Prognoses: Mesopotamian treatise of, 36, 54;
    importance of (Hippocr. Coll.), 170–171,
    193, 199, 200; death as "beautiful," 171;
    criteria for, in Indian medicine, 278, 300
Proud flesh, 4–6, 118
Psychosomatic effects: in Nei Ching, success
    of acupuncture depends on "patient's own
    will," 243; spirit can injure the body,
    243–244; in India, subjugation of the mind
    as a cure, 275
Psychotherapy, 68, 128, 152; in temples of
    Asklepios, 201–205; Socrates on treating
    body and soul, 206; role in Chinese
    medicine, 253; in India, 296, 311. See also
    Magic; Psychosomatic effects; Religion
Ptolemy I, 314, 321
Public physicians. See Physicians, public
Pulse: in Chinese medicine, 238, 245–247
Pump: invented by Ktesibios, 323, 325; heart
    as, 329–333
Purging: in Egypt, 129; in Hippocr. Coll.,
    154, 162, 188; for preventing pus, 161–162,
    174; for teatment of erysipelas, 169; by
    "syrmaism," 174; for "orgasm" in
    wounds, 175; as part of triad (starving,
    purging, bleeding), 179, 205, 419; with
    hellebore, 181, 188–191; for treating
    wounds, 194, 198; in China, 257; of brain,
    in India, 280; by sneezing, 297; for fever,
    304; Galen on, 419. See also Enema
Pus: nature and formation of, 2–6; "good
    and laudable," 4, 102, 183–184; Akkadian
    word for, 59; Akkadian charm against, 67;
    Egyptian hieroglyphs for, 101; Smith and
    Ebers papyri on, 101–104; types of
    (Hippocr. Coll.), 157, 183; prevented by
    purging, 161–162, 174; arises from
    stagnating blood, 180–182; prevented by
    bleeding, starving, purging, 182, 205, 419;
    can be normal event in wound healing,
    183–184; suppuration prevents
    inflammation, 184, 497 n 235; Greek drugs
    to prevent 185; if produced by wound,
    suture must be avoided (Sushruta), 296;
    blood clots become pus (Celsus), 367;
    wounds can heal without suppurating

(Galen), 400. See also Abscess; Empyema;
    Wound healing
Pwnt, land of, 120, 122–123, 209
Pythagoras, 178, 179

R

Reeds, knives made from: in Egypt, 89–90;
    in Rome, 90; in India, 90, 302
Religion: in Mesopotamia, ritual
    prostitution, 54; gods as cause of disease,
    59–61; priests of Sekhmet, 86, 480 n 54;
    Egyptian ceremonies, 88–89, 107; Egyptian
    incantations, 125–128; resin and, 136,
    207–208, 219; in Greek medicine, 201–206,
    311; and perfumes, 207–208; and incense,
    208; and sulphur, 224; priest-doctor in
    China, 239; in India, 273, as medicine of
    "first order," 275, 311, snake worship,
    283–284; and gadgets in Alexandria, 321;
    Pliny the Elder on, 343; as motivation for
    hospitals, 393–394; from anatomy to
    (Galen), 397–398, 409; taurobolium, 403.
    See also Buddha; Christian; Jewish;
    Magic; Mantra; Muslim; Nestorian;
    Zoroaster
Rennet, as styptic in Rome, 349. See also Fig
    tree sap
Repair. See Wound healing
Reserpine. See Tranquilizers
Residues, Greek theory of. See Hippocratic
    medicine
Resins: in prehistory, 14; as adhesives, 14,
    210; in Mesopotamia, 50, 64; in Egypt, 94,
    124; for embalming, 135–137; and religion,
    136, 207–208, 219; in Greece, 154, 215;
    defined, 210; in treatment of wounds,
    215–220; as antiseptic, 217–220; Chinese
    use of, 255; in Roman wound dressings,
    369. See also Antiseptics; Balsam;
    Galbanum; Gum; Incense; Ladanum;
    Mastich; Myrrh; Perfume; Russian;
    Turpentine
Rhazes (Rāzi), 421
Rig Veda, 278
Roger II the Norman, 239
Roman medicine: long practiced without
    physicians, 339; introduction of
    Asklepios, 339; and Greek physicians,
    339–341; folk remedies, 348–349; use of
    Ephedra against bleeding and asthma,
    349–353; Celsus and his surgery, 353–370;
    debt to Indian medicine, 374–381; and
    plastic surgery, 379–381; army hospitals,
    381–390; army physicians, 390–391;
    civilian infirmaries, 390–393. See also
    Celsus; Hospitals; Physicians; Pliny the
    Elder
———, correlations: with Greece, 328–374,
    381–394; with Alexandria, 328, 354, 363;
    with India, 374–381; with Mesopotamia,
    381; with China, 403

Index

Vessels (*Cont.*)

Alexandrian medicine, 330–337; vein-to-artery connections (synanastomoses) (Erasistratos and Galen), 333–335; in Sanskrit, *dhamani*, 536 n 60. *See also* Arteries; Heart; Hemorrhage; Ligatures; Veins; Venules

Veterinary medicine: in Mesopotamia (surgery), 46; in Egypt, mentioned in Kahun papyrus, 72, 73, 434; in China, 236; Chinese veterinarians ranked by number of dead animals, 238; veterinarians cannot both with theory (Celsus), 392

Vinegar: as preservative, 131; used on wounds, (Hippocr. Coll.), 154; noise of boiling vinegar compared with sound of auscultation (Hippocr. Coll.), 169–171; in énaima, 185; as antiseptic, 186–188; as infectious disease of wine, 221–223; problem of wine turning into, for people of antiquity, 221–224;' inspired Pasteur to study human infections, 224; in China, used for pickling, 256; is hemostatic (Celsus), 362; painful when cleaning wounds (Celsus), 367. *See also* Wine

Violence: and human evolution, 6–8; in primitive art, 19–22; nonviolence of Ashoka, Indian king, 264–266; wounds as means of human communication, 417

Virchow, Rudolph, 420; and the fifth cardinal sign of inflammation, 412–413

Vitruvius, 323; and *hospitalia*, not hospitals, 533 n 287

Vivisection: human, in Alexandria, 327, disapproved by Celsus, 354–355; on animals (Galen), 405–409. *See also* Surgery

Vomiting as a cure: induced every month by the Egyptians, 129; induced by "syrmaism" (Hippocr. Coll.), 174, considered part of purging, 179, with hellebore, 188–189; may help against inflammation, 193, as Greek first aid for wounds, 194; in India, induced with drugs called *vamya*, 280; important part of Indian treatment, 297. *See also* Purging

Vraṇa. *See* Ulcer

Vulnerarius, wound-specialist in Rome. *See* Specialists

W

Wadj: meaning "green, fresh," 107; meaning green pigment, 111–113. *See also* Copper

Walsh, J., 401

War. *See* Wounded

Warmth: good for wounds (Hippocr. Coll.), 143, 166, 176, 181. *See also* Cold

Washing. *See* Wound, washing

Water-organ. *See* Organ

Weather. *See* Environment, physical

Weber, Neal A., 306

Weidenreich, Franz, 19

Wells, Calvin, 9, 245

Wheeler, W. M., 304, 306

Whirl of inflammation, in Smith papyrus, 100

Wind, (internal): in Greece, 180, 310; in China, 243, 310; in India, 276, 293, 299, 310, auscultation for, escaping from an ulcer, 299; as a cause of disease, 310

Wine: antiseptic properties of, 48, 186–188; on wounds (Hippocr. Coll.), 150, 154, 161; antiseptic properties due to polyphenols, 187–188; bacterial diseases of, compared with wound infections, 221–224; not the natural end-product of fermentation, 222; sulphur dioxide as preservative of, 222; spices and ancient preservatives of, 222–224; pasteurization of, 224; diseases of, important step in Pasteur's work on human infections, 224; in China, Imperial service of "Wine Men," 236, 238; present in character *i* for "physician," 239; possibly used in China for anesthesia, 251, 254; in India, given for anesthesia, 289, 295; no mention of anesthesia with (Hippocr. Coll.), 295; adulteration of, as current practice (Pliny), 343, 344; may do more harm than good (Pliny), 344; vats can cause asphyxia (Pliny), 345; for cleaning wounds (Celsus), 367; and Galen, 399–400. *See also* Antiseptics; Vinegar; Wound

Wishful thinking: effectiveness of wound-healing drugs, 176, 189; trusting a physician as evidence of (Pliny), 348; theriac as example of, 414

Women: a woman physician in Egypt, 82–84, 480 n 38; social position of, in antiquity, 82–84; in India, lowly condition of, 266; and Indian physician, 280; and Indian treatment of fever, 304–305; discussed by Pliny, 343–344. *See also* Cosmetics; Ethics

Wool: grease of (oesypum), used on fresh wounds (Hippocr. Coll.), 154; greasy, for dressings (Hippocr. Coll.), 165, 166; greasy, for inducing suppuration (Hippocr. Coll.), 184; and honey for sores (Pliny), 348. *See also* Lint; Oesypum

Wound: evolutionary role of, in shaping defense reactions of cells and tissues, 1; biology of, basic notions, 1–6; medical problems created by, 14–19; in primitive art, 19–23; from accidental, to surgery, 24–28; as means of human communication, 417. *See also* Anatomy; Etymology; Writing: Chinese, Coptic, cuneiform, Greek, hieratic, hieroglyphic, Sanskrit, Sumerian

———closure. *See* Adhesive tape; Ants; Surgical instruments, fibulae; Suture

———contraction: explained, 3–4, 6; "Turtle experiment," 155–156; exploited to hold head of humerus in place (Hippocr. Coll.), 164–166

———"diseases" (complications that may disturb wound healing), 3–6; in Smith papyrus, first known reference to

Index